PRINCIPLES OF MODERN
IMMUNOBIOLOGY:
Basic and Clinical

PRINCIPLES OF MODERN
IMMUNOBIOLOGY:
Basic and Clinical

BYUNG H. PARK, M.D.

Associate Professor of Pediatrics
University of California at Los Angeles
Medical School
Harbor General Hospital
Torrance, California

ROBERT A. GOOD, M.D., Ph.D.

President and Director
Sloan-Kettering Institute for Cancer Research
New York, New York

Lea & Febiger · 1974 · Philadelphia

Library of Congress Cataloging in Publication Data

Park, Byung H.
   Principles of Modern Immunobiology: Basic and Clinical

   1. Immunopathology. 2. Immunology. I. Good, Robert A., 1922- joint author.
II. Title. [DNLM: 1. Immunity. 2. Immunologic diseases. QW504 G646i 1974]
RC585.P37   616.07′9   73-13831
ISBN 0-8121-0436-6

Published in Great Britain by Henry Kimpton Publishers, London

PRINTED IN THE UNITED STATES OF AMERICA

Preface

Principles of Modern Immunobiology: Basic and Clinical is intended for practicing physicians and surgeons, as well as for graduate students of biology and medicine. Over the past 25 years immunobiology has made great advances, and it is now clear that immunity to infection, once thought to be the primary function of the immune system, is but a part of a much broader general biologic function that has evolved during the past 400 million years. This function appears to be designed primarily for recognition and elimination of foreign bodies and preservation of the integrity of the individual. Thus immunobiology has now emerged as a multidisciplinary subject encompassing most of the biologic sciences. Further, the recent implications and application of immunobiology in cancer, transplantation, and in many forms of so-called autoimmune diseases have provided additional stimulus for new interest in this science. Practicing physicians and surgeons and students and teachers of all branches of the biologic sciences have become increasingly aware of the importance and necessity of acquainting themselves with the recent advances in the field of immunobiology. We have been motivated to write this book by the evidence at every hand that immunobiology is not only expanding as a discipline but is also penetrating into more and more areas of clinical medicine, as well as general biology.

To a great extent immunology has traditionally been taught as a body of pre-existing facts. Consequently, students are not aware of the way in which current states of the art have been developed out of the past. For this reason we have provided for each subject a short historical introduction to facilitate understanding. The combination of the theoretical and pragmatic is as old as the science of immunobiology, dating in fact from the very beginning of immunobiology. We believe that the most critical test of the validity of the works of basic immunobiology can be made at the bedside by clinicians and that the most crucial questions in immunobiology have often originated from bedside observations and interpretations of natural experiments, i.e., the patient. Thus immunobiology is a branch of basic science that is intimately related to clinical medicine.

In this book we have not tried to offer a detailed account and documentation of the entire field of immunobiology with massive intrusion of footnotes and references. Rather we have chosen to present the subject in a form that we consider to be maximally readable. We have attempted to provide our audience from diverse fields a single text that covers principles of both basic and clinical immunobiology. It is our intent to present a bird's-eye view of the entire field of modern immunobiology.

For these purposes this book is divided into two Parts. Part I, Principles of Basic Immunobiology, is intended to provide orientation to lead our readers directly to the essential points in the shortest space and time. Part II, Principles of Clinical Immunobiology, will provide more practical information for general physicians and surgeons, as well as for house officers finding their way to understanding the clinical problems related to immunobiology without themselves becoming professional immunobiologists.

We realize that the current view and practice in the Minnesota School of Immunology are represented to a certain extent throughout this book. Presentation of a comprehensive and integrated view has been facilitated, we believe, by accepting the coherence of a single basic perspective. The selected references and further readings are provided only as a guide for those who wish to study further and are not necessarily full accounts of the contributions of the many scientists who have developed the discipline of modern immunobiology.

This book would not be possible without the generous guidance of the publisher, especially Mr. Edward H. Wickland, Mr. Thomas Colaiezzi, and Ms. Isabelle Clouser. We appreciate the special help from our secretarial staff—Miss Inez Fyten, Mrs. Ellen Werth, Miss Hae Hiang Song, Mr. Patrick Burns, and Miss Susan Saloka—and from Miss Judy Kempa and Miss Connie Finstad for the illustrations. The staff of the Biomedical Library of the University of Minnesota, especially Mr. Glenn Brudvig, Professor and Head of the Biomedical Library, and Mrs. Shari Hopkins have provided invaluable assistance in preparation of the manuscript.

Our original work that provides much of the basis of our analysis and many of the essential facts in this presentation has been supported by the Minnesota and American Heart Associations, the Minnesota Arthritis Foundation, the John A. Hartford Foundation, the National Foundation March of Dimes, and the National Institute of Health of the United States Public Health Service (AI-00798, AI-08677).

BYUNG H. PARK
ROBERT A. GOOD

Contents

Contents

Appendix

Part I
PRINCIPLES OF BASIC IMMUNOBIOLOGY

1

Contributions of Immunobiology to the Medical Sciences

It is impossible to understand the present without knowing the past.

GOETHE

William Harvey (1578-1657) wrote the distinguished physician Jan Vlakfeld at Haarlem:

> Your much esteemed letter reached me safely, in which you not only exhibit your kind consideration of me, but display a singular zeal on the cultivation of our art. It is even so, Nature is nowhere more accustomed more openly to display her secret mystery than in cases where she shows a trace of her workings apart from the beaten path; nor is there any better way to advance the proper practice of medicine than to give our minds to the discovery of the usual law of Nature, by the careful investigation of cases of rarer forms of disease. For it has been found in almost all things, that what they contained is useful and applicable, is hardly ever perceived unless we are deprived of them.*

This beautiful prose by Harvey summarizes what we want to say here.

Immunobiology began by the interpretation of a natural experiment when Edward Jenner (1749-1823) became aware of the shiny face of the milkmaid at a time when the disfiguring plague, smallpox, was a common medical problem in Europe and England. The legacy, derived from Jenner's contribution in the later part of the eighteenth century, was (1) the first practical use of immunobiology in the protection of man, (2) the first association of hypersensitivity with resistance to infection, (3) the first use of the attenuated virus in immunization, and (4) the first glimpse at the interference phenomenon that is now being translated into molecular terms with our understanding of the interferon and its potential for use in treatment or prevention of virus infection.

Jenner's experiment of Nature is only one of many. Other key experiments of Nature in the development of immunobiology include Louis Pasteur's (1822-1895) neglected cholera culture which led to the attenuated bacterial vaccine. An analysis of serum sickness by von Pirquet

---

*In *Circulation of Blood* (1908), translated by L. Willis: New York, Dutton & Co., pp. 200-201.

(1874-1929) showed for the first time that immunity can sometimes be detrimental to man when his immunologic forces are turned against him. In 1921 in a fascinating analysis of Küstner's own hypersensitivity to boiled fish protein, Prausnitz and Küstner gave us not only the first evidence of passive transfer of hypersensitivity in man but also evidence of active production of desensitization and of fixation of certain kinds of antibodies to the tissue. Philip Levine's concern with Mary Seno (1937), whose sensitization to her husband's Rh+ cells by her fetus produced a fatal disease of the fetus and a severe transfusion reaction in Mary herself, gave us our first understanding of the pathogenesis of erythroblastosis fetalis. Ray Owen's fraternal twin cattle (1947) showed us tolerance or immunodeviation, that negative immunologic adaptation which someday may be put to man's benefit and be as powerful a tool as the positive immunologic adaptation we now use in immunization. These are only a few among the many experiments of Nature that have led the way in developing our understanding of immunobiologic processes.

The decreased worldwide incidence of smallpox can be attributed in large part to the immunization with the vaccinia virus that derived from Jenner's observations. Similarly, the poliomyelitis vaccine, the inactivated attenuated form of wild poliovirus, gave us a widely distributed and effective means of prevention of poliomyelitis. With the extension of our understanding of immune processes it is now altogether possible to prevent most cases of erythroblastosis by a simple, widely distributable means of treatment with antibodies at the time the sensitizing foreign red blood cells are present in the mother's circulation.

With the measles virus we also have the potentiality for mass immunity, although there has to this time been some difficulty in achieving the necessary wide distribution and general acceptance. Also initiated by the practical application of immunobiology has been the decline of diphtheria, pertussis, and tetanus (more apparent in military medicine) as destructive and fatal diseases.

Major contributions of immunobiology of the past include:
1. The prevention of many viral and bacterial diseases.
2. The discovery of the immunologic basis for transfusion.
3. The analysis, definition, and prevention of erythroblastosis fetalis.
4. The beginning of understanding the pathogenesis of serum sickness.
5. The application of serology as a powerful diagnostic tool in analyzing infection.
6. The introduction of skin testing to define both present and past infection.

Now, let us consider the immunobiology of the present. First of all, what is the present? There are many different ways of looking at the present. To some, it started about 30 years ago; to others, especially new students, it began only last year; to still others it will begin in a few months. For this discussion we choose to consider the immunobiology of the present as starting some 30 years ago when one of us began studies of immunobiology. Then we knew something about serology and humoral immunity processes. Now we can define five major classes of immunoglobulins and the subclasses and amino acid sequences of some. Not only did we not know the molecular basis of immunity, but we also lacked knowledge of the cells responsible for the immunologic process. Many of the organs that are now known to be extraordinarily important to immunology were functional enigmas. We can now write a scheme (of course, in the process of constant modification) that reflects the great advances of our knowledge and indicates how the immune system develops and is organized (page 28) (Fig. 3-5). Developing and understanding the relationships indicated in the scheme have derived, in large part, from interpretation of experiments of Nature and critical experimentation and analysis in both ontogenetic and phylogenetic perspective. We now have evidence that the yolk sac cells, which themselves in the yolk sac can only differentiate to fetal erythrocytes, can become pre-thymic cells, which, after proliferating and differentiating in the thymus, become post-thymic (T) cells. Then, upon stimulation with antigens they can give rise to a variety of active substances that act to amplify the influence of the (T) cells, sometimes by a factor of many thousands. We also know that these same yolk sac cells can enter another line of differentiation which, in the bird, we have defined as being of bursal origin. These cells are called post-bursal (B) cells.

The bursa is a strange lymphoepithelial organ seated at the dorsal aspect of the posterior end of the gastrointestinal tract. It differentiates the cells capable of synthesis and secretion of the immunoglobulins. The immunoglobulins in turn utilize another kind of biologic amplification mechanism in getting to the effector processes. How these cells migrate to the various parts of the body where they reside and function at different stages of development is a complex story which will be recounted later (page 25). It is important here to understand that cells of the yolk sac travel to the fetal liver and thence to the bone marrow. Each site gives rise to the precursor stem cells that can ultimately achieve the vital immunologic process. The immunologic function once engaged by antigen utilizes several biologic amplification systems that are capable of engaging, in turn, the effector components among which phagocytosis, inflammation, coagulation, and vascular reactivity seem fundamental. Here again we see the crucial influence of the thymus gland that we did not understand at all when we began the long trek 30 years ago. The congeries of immunoglobulin molecules recruited by special lymphocytes and plasma cells engage the effector mechanisms by an entirely different set of amplification processes than are used by the cells differentiated and educated in the thymus.

In almost every branch of medicine immunobiology has made a major contribution to the substance of the discipline. For example, rheumatology is essentially a clinical application of immunobiology, and though that may not be right, it has become a popular trend at this juncture. Certainly from immunobiologic analysis we are learning much about autoantibodies and about different kinds of immunoglobulins and cryoglobulins that are involved in some way in the pathogenesis of rheumatoid arthritis. We have evidence that antigen–antibody complexes are present in the joints and that the complement system and the other amplification systems are being activated in the rheumatic joint. We can even begin to separate immunologically several forms of rheumatoid diseases in children and to understand in immunobiologic terms the manifestation in the joints and kidneys in lupus erythematosus and other collagen diseases.

Similarly, in endocrinology obvious autoimmune processes seem basic to the expression of, and even to be the cause of certain endocrinologic disorders. On the other side of the coin, highly sensitive radioimmunoassays for both peptide and non-peptide hormones have permitted us to define for the first time the nature of many endocrinopathies and have been responsible, it seems to us, for a veritable revolution in endocrinology. These sensitive new techniques permit us to quantitate precisely trace amounts of hormonal substances that we used to try to assay by crude bioassay techniques.

The dermatologic diseases are no exception. We now have diagnostic autoantibodies for pemphigoid and pemphigus. In erythema nodosum, and erythema multiform bullosum, immunologic processes are now analyzable and represent a definable base of the disorders. The pathogenesis of contact allergy is based on a cell-mediated immune mechanism; the pathogenesis of certain drug and chemically induced hypersensitivities and a number of other skin diseases have been analyzed in immunobiologic terms in recent years. Thus we are beginning to define in immunobiologic terms many of the dermatologic diseases which heretofore have been represented in mere morphologic descriptions.

In cardiology, immunobiology has also played a major role. For example, in rheumatic fever it is clear that immunologic mechanisms play a crucial role. Autoantibodies directed against components of the cardiac tissue cross react in a dramatic way with components of the streptococcus that is known now to be an etiologic agent in this disease. Subacute bacterial endocarditis, the cardiac transplantation, and the analysis of virus-induced cardiac disease all must be understood and achieved in immunobiologic terms. In hematology we can take almost any of the hematologic diseases and dissect them in immunobiologic terms. In renal diseases it certainly is hard for the modern renologist not to consider the immunobiologic processes that contribute to the pathogenesis of kidney injury. The pathogeneses of lupus nephritis, serum sickness, and even of the lung and kidney lesions of the strange Goodpasture syndrome have all been analyzed and defined in immunobiologic terms. The processes involved in hypertensive diseases, as well as in neurologic diseases, can also be looked at in this perspective. As we learn more and more about these diseases in molecular terms, our immunologic approaches will become more and more vital to our understandings.

We are beginning to define allergic processes based on reaginic antibodies and are thus lifting the cloak of black magic from the field of allergy. The discovery of the IgE molecule by the Ishizakas who were aided by studies of an unusual myeloma by Johannson et al., opened a new way of understanding the allergic processes.

All areas of general medicine must be viewed in immunobiologic terms. Not any less prominent is the field of oncology. A deficiency of the immune function is clearly evident in myeloma and Hodgkin's disease. We have evidence from immunologic analysis that chronic lymphatic leukemia can now be defined as a disease of the B-cell system (page 570). Most chronic lymphatic leukemias studied during the last year or so have been shown to be malignant monoclonal deviations of the B-cell line. Tumor specific transplantation antigen and carcinoembryonic antigens must be defined immunologically and studied in experimental animals and in man. Every tumor has at its surface specific antigens that are looked upon by the host as foreigners. They are not like most foreign antigens being eliminated from the body. As a matter of fact, it seems clear that whenever the malignant adaptation is successful some sort of abrogation of immunologic resistance has occurred. This shows up, for example, in neuroblastoma, in carcinoma of the breast, and in carcinoma of the colon. In the latter we are beginning to use carcinoembryonic antigens, as we now call them, to detect persisting tumors. Perhaps such antigens can be used diagnostically early in disease to show the presence of very small tumors and to show whether metastasis has occurred. So it is with most processes related to oncology. An essential relationship between immunity and malignancy seems to exist, and the nature of this relationship will be considered in detail in Chapter 15.

We must also reflect on modern tissue and organ transplantation therapy. At the present time, this still must be a poorly distributed form of medical therapy, but dramatic things are being accomplished. It is almost predictable that surgery will be relegated within the period of our functional medical lifetime to a reconstructive and transplantation surgery. The use of antilymphocyte serum has greatly facilitated successful kidney transplantation. Even in the management of burns in recent years immunobiologic tools have proven useful. For example, a heptavalent vaccine has been developed against the major types of Pseudomonas aeruginosa, a frequent killer of burned patients. Its application provides a new component of the therapeutic armamentarium that can prevent many of the frequently destructive infections that occur in patients with burns.

New immunodeficiency diseases that are being defined regularly in our clinic and in clinics around the world sometimes can be treated effectively. Gamma globulin and plasma infusions by the "buddy system" introduced by Stiehm and Fudenberg represent dramatic immunologic treatment in many cases. In some instances these diseases can be completely corrected by a form of cellular engineering. We have even begun to glimpse the usefulness of a new kind of molecule in immunobiology, the transfer factor of Lawrence. This transfer factor, though poorly understood, seems to have therapeutic usefulness and to be a powerful means of amplifying or recruiting cells to a specific immunologic adaptation. These then are some accomplishments of immunobiology of the present, and they are only a beginning.

As to the future, better and better immunologic tools are being used to define with more and more precision the role of immunologic processes in human disease. A thorough definition of experimental immunologic models is paying off in understanding that surely can be translated into improved diagnosis and therapy. Immunologic intervention and immunodeviation are already being thought of as immunologic engineering that can form the basis of immunotherapy to be used in the clinic in the treatment of many human diseases. An immunologic method for specifically removing substances from the circulation makes possible removing substances like carcinoembryonic antigen, the antigen–antibody complexes, and even toxins, e.g., drugs like digitalis in overdosage or other substances in accidental poisoning. Any molecule to which the specificity of the immune mechanism can be directed can be selectively removed from the body by affinity separation techniques.

We have begun to understand the importance in tissue injury of antigen–antibody complexes. The application of this knowledge has given a new perspective to the understanding of human diseases.

It was postulated by Burnet that forbidden clones are responsible for the autoimmune antibodies. It is becoming clearer that not forbidden clones but "forbidden" antigens, antigens that are out of place or antigens that have been modified in some way, are producing autoimmunity. Further, autoimmune assault is generated most often when for one reason or another the host's immune response is defective. These relationships will be considered in detail in Chapter 15. Surely as understanding of autoimmune diseases increases, they will become vulnerable to effective therapy and prevention.

A powerful tool that promises much for the future is immunogenetics. Recent studies revealed that a particular region of a single somatic chromosome of mice, dogs, monkeys, pigs, and man controls how we differ from one another, whether we respond to antigen, and what kinds of disease we are prone to. This extraordinary chromosomal region so vital to immunity is inherited usually as a single genetic component.

The biologic amplification systems (page 136) have been defined in precise molecular and even genetic terms. The complement system that can amplify immunity on molecular basis at least 300-fold, the kinins, the kallikrein systems, and phagocytosis are parts of the amplification and effector systems. A new third biologic language appears to be the means by which the lymphocyte signals the macrophages to turn on. Already there is evidence that inflammation, vascular reactivity, and exocytosis can be controlled by drugs and by certain immunoglobulin molecules.

The transplantation era is already here because kidneys are being transplanted regularly with real success. Usually a kidney from a matched sibling donor is not rejected. One of our patients is a boy who has now had his mother's kidney in his body for more than 12 years. That kidney is functioning even better in his body than is the kidney that remains in his mother's body. The long-term survival rate for kidney transplants is more than 80 percent when the kidneys come from live donors and more than 70 percent when they come from cadaver donors.

Five years ago we transplanted bone marrow from a sister to her brother who had combined immunodeficiency. This boy still has his sister's marrow. His blood type has switched from A to O, and all of his blood-forming cells can be identified as being of female origin. Bone marrow transplantation in this case cured not only a fatal genetic disease, but a second marrow transplant cured also an acquired, immunologically based pancytopenia. Over and over again throughout the world matched marrow transplants have corrected combined immunodeficiency and aregenerative anemias. Ultimately we will be able to treat with organ and cellular engineering inborn errors of metabolism that lead to early death from cardiac and vascular damage. Without question we will bring new and powerful tools to therapy in all branches of medicine.

Study of the immunodeficiency diseases continues to increase our understanding of basic immunobiology. This is a two-way street. The questions coming from the clinic, critical questions derived from patients with rare and unusual diseases, are taken to the laboratory for definition, and the answers from laboratory analysis will be flowing back to the clinic with increasing frequency. The same thing is happening now in the study of the amplification mechanisms. We are learning more and more about the extraordinary relationships, which we have called collectively the third biologic language. This language operates to control social relationships between cells, is responsible for recognition of foreignness and surface contact with antigenic sites and communication from surface to nucleus by way of signals that rule so many biologic processes. This is going to be as powerful a language as is the DNA-RNA language when we learn to speak and manipulate it.

Specific immunosuppression, immunologic tolerance, and immunodeviation will ultimately bring the transplantation era that will make it possible to transplant all of the tissues that have up to now been impossible. Immunologic intervention is being developed by use of solid immune adsorption column techniques that make it possible to dispose of many unwanted substances.

Immunity is being applied to cancer therapy to eliminate minimal residual tumors. Further, the development of methods of diagnosis and immunization may provide mass immunity against some agents that are causing neoplasia. These methods may also be adapted to eliminate and prevent many of the autoimmune diseases. We are now just beginning to understand the critical relationships. A vaccine derived from herpesvirus of turkeys is already preventing the common malignant disease of the lymphoreticular system in chickens, and current research promises that soon we can have a vaccine against leukemia in cats.

We are beginning to understand the relationship between nutritional deprivation and pestilence on one hand and nutritional hyperadequacy and immunodeviation on the other. Nutrition is being considered as a biologic tool, as well as a chemical tool, for specifically manipulating one or another of the immunologic systems (page 189).

Another concern is the relationship between aging and immunity. Much of the autoimmunity and some of the malignancy that is associated with aging may indeed be attributable to immunodeficiency and thus should be manipulable (page 194). Immunologic tools can contribute to the legacy of health. What do we mean by the legacy of health? We all know people who have never been sick. This legacy of health is what we ideally can give to everyone.

In seeking to achieve these goals we are constantly looking for complete solutions which can be widely distributed rather than partial solutions which are often expensive and difficult to distribute. Nature's experiment will always be there to point the way. Why are clinical experiences and questions such powerful tools in the development of medical science? What scientists do is to play a variation of the parlor game, Twenty Questions, but with the "unknown." Starting with a specific question that is clearly indicated by the experiment of Nature, they analyze the problem by asking questions until highly relevant solutions can be obtained.

In achieving this goal, we must continue to cultivate our art and skill in recognizing and interpreting the experiments of Nature. We should acknowledge our wild and unconventional impulses, but at the same time maintain a highly critical and often combative attitude toward one another. Immunobiology, like all developing sciences, thrives on and needs such interaction.

SELECTED REFERENCES

Burnet, F. M. (1959): *The Clonal Selection Theory of Acquired Immunity*. Nashville, Tennessee, Vanderbilt University Press.

Jenner, E. C. (1796): *An Inquiry into the Causes and Effects of Variolae Vaccine*. London, Low.

Lawrence, H. S. (1955): J. Clin. Invest. *34*:219.

Levine, P., and Stetson, R. E. (1939): JAMA *113*:126.

Owen, R. D. (1945): Science *102*:400.

Prausnitz, C., and Küstner, H. (1921): Z. Bakt. *86*:160.

Stiehm, E. R., Vaerman, J. P., and Fudenberg, H. H. (1966): Blood *28*:918.

von Pirquet, C. F., and Schick, B. (1905): *Die Serum Krankheit*. Leipzig, Wier. Translated by B. Schick (1951): *Serum Sickness*. Batlimore, Williams & Wilkins Company.

FURTHER READINGS

Burnet, F. M., and White, D. O. (1972): *Natural History of Infectious Disease* (4th ed.). New York, Cambridge University Press.

McQuarrie, I. (1944): *Experiments of Nature and Other Essays*. Lawrence, University of Kansas.

Parish, H. J. (1968): *Victory with Vaccines*. London, E. S. Livingstone, Ltd.

2

Immunity, Hypersensitivity, and Immunobiology

The pestilence can never breed the smallpox, nor the smallpox the measles, nor the crystals or chickenpox, any more than a hen can breed a duck, a wolf a sheep, or thistle figs; and consequently one sort can not be a preservative against any other sort.

THOMAS FULLER (1654-1734)

As Fuller said some 250 years ago, the specificity of a contagious disease and the immunity against it was well recognized long before the discovery of the specific causative agents of contagious disease. The Ancients recognized in their wisdom that one seizure with a certain disease affords protection against subsequent attacks of the same kind. Thucydides of Athens observed that those persons who recovered from plague never caught the disease a second time, even though they nursed the sick during the epidemic of plague. The ancient Chinese went a step further; they practiced the inhalation of the powder prepared from the scabs of smallpox lesions to obtain immunity without inducing suffering from the actual disease. These efforts represented the first known examples of artificial active immunization (induction of the immune state).

The term *immunity* in its broadest context means "to be exempt or safe from taxation, military service, obligation, or from epidemic diseases." Since immunity was first recognized as a *resistant state* that followed a certain type of natural infection, immunology (a study of immunity) in its early days of development was primarily concerned with the mechanism(s) of such a resistant state in individuals. The foundations for an understanding of immunity were laid with the invention of the microscope, the recognition of microorganisms, and the advent of Pasteur's germ theory of contagious diseases. The ancient idea of the specificity of a contagious disease and the immunity to it became clearer and could be explained in terms of specific causative microorganisms of each disease. Up to this time, the phenomenon of immunity was looked upon at the level of whole animals: the animal that resisted the challenge of infection was said to have immunity against that particular disease. What constituent of the body is responsible for this immunity? Why and how does this immunity come about? The search for the explanation of such a remarkable phenomenon continued.

A fortunate accident in the laboratory led Pasteur in 1881 to develop the first method of attenuating a virulent strain of bacteria into a harmless strain and to use this attenuated bacteria for the "vaccination" in a manner similar to that used by Jenner in "variolation" for smallpox. The term *vaccination* was coined by Pasteur in honor of Jenner's contribution and has subsequently been used to mean the administration of not only bacteria but also virus and other substances to obtain future immunity against disease. Salmon and Smith in 1886 used dead bacteria for vaccination, and Roux and Yersin in 1888 employed attenuated toxin (toxoid) for successful immunization. Thus, it became clear that not only living microorganisms, but also non-living substances such as dead bacteria and bacterial products could render animals immune.

Two of Pasteur's pupils, Roux and Yersin, in 1888 discovered poisonous properties in the culture media of diphtheria bacilli. Almost at the same time, von Behring and Kitasato showed that cultures of tetanus bacillus were still highly toxic for animals after all the bacilli had been removed by filtration. Two years later in 1890 at Koch's Institute, von Behring and Kitasato showed that the blood serum of animals injected with diphtheria toxin developed the capacity of neutralizing the poison so that an amount ordinarily fatal could then be injected with impunity. Moreover, when removed from the immunized animals and injected into another animal, this serum could protect the recipient against the challenge of toxin (this is the first example of passive immunization). This substance or factor in the serum of immunized animals was called an *antitoxin*. The neutralizing ability of such serum against bacterial toxin represents the first demonstration of the how and the first inquiry into which component of the body is responsible for the immune state. This discovery represents an extraordinary stimulus to humoral pathology. For a few exciting months it seemed as if infectious diseases were all to be conquered through the use of specific antitoxins. Sadly it soon became apparent, however, that the original hopes were overoptimistic, for the antitoxin treatment was found applicable to only a relatively small number of the infectious diseases.

A humoral defense was soon recognized, however, to be directed not only against the toxins of bacteria but also against the germs themselves. Buchner in 1889 demonstrated the innate capacity of blood to kill bacteria and gave an explanation of why the blood was known to resist putrefaction. In 1894 Pfeiffer found that cholera vibrios injected into the peritoneal cavity of a guinea pig that had been immunized against the same organism quickly lost its motility, became granular, and finally went to pieces. In contrast, no dissolution of cholera vibrios was observed in normal controls. The serum of the immunized animals had acquired the capacity to carry out this destruction, and the substance was called *"bacteriolysin."* About the same time, a related phenomenon was discovered by a number of investigators in "agglutination" of bacteria, and the term *agglutinin* was born. Gruber and Durham (1896) found that bacteria isolated from a patient could be identified by their behavior with antiserum of a known preparation. Widal reversed the test procedure; he noted that a patient's serum could be tested with bacteria of a known type and his disease could be identified by the specific agglutination reaction. The well-known Gruber-Widal test for typhoid fever resulted from these investigations. A new method of diagnosis of disease by serologic means was thus opened.

In the following year, Kraus discovered that when he mixed clear filtrates from bacterial cultures with antisera to the same bacteria a cloudiness or precipitate occurred. He named this phenomenon the *precipitin reaction.* Because of its specificity this reaction has proved useful for the identification not only of bacteria, but also of many kinds of protein and particularly of minute amounts of blood. One of the practical applications of the precipitin reaction has been identification of the specific origin of blood stains in forensic medicine.

Bordet and Gengou in 1900-1902 discovered that the serum of animals immunized to red blood cells acquired specific capacity to dissolve other red blood cells of the same type. The factor in the serum of the immunized animals was called "hemolysin." Moreover, they recognized that an additional factor called "alexin" was required for this reaction, and the alexin could be found in non-immunized animals. The factor alexin was later termed "complement." Their recognition of the role of the two components in the hemolytic reaction led to their development of the *complement-fixation reaction.* A modification of this test, devised by Wassermann in 1906, has had immense application, especially in the diagnosis of syphilis.

Many other specific substances of similar nature were found to be present in the serum of immunized animals. These peculiar substances or factors (antitoxins, agglutinins, hemolysins, precipitins) were then collectively called "antibodies." Likewise, the substances (toxin, bacteria) that generate such antibodies in the serum of the immunized animals were called "antigens." The antibodies are formed not only as a result of infection but also as a consequence of the administration of certain poisons of large molecular size, such as toxin from bacilli, higher plants (ricin, abrin), and animals (venoms). A new line of serologic research was initiated, and serology was separated from the question of immunity to infectious disease. It became clear that immunization against microbes and toxins was only a special instance of a general biologic principle and that the same mechanism was operating when innocuous materials, such as cells, proteins derived from a foreign species, or even synthetic chemicals, were injected into animals.

Metchnikoff in 1884 observed that the mobile cells of starfish larva in fluid can engulf solid particles. He later showed that the leukocytes of blood could also engulf and destroy disease-producing bacteria. He named these cells "phagocytes" (eating cells), and the process of engulfment "phagocytosis" and proposed the famous theory of phagocytosis or cellular immunity as a counterpoint to the humoral theory of immunity. Buchner, Pfeiffer, and others showed that fresh whole blood could destroy bacteria to some extent even before immunization (natural immunity) and still better after immunization. Metchnikoff proved this identical fact for phagocytes and phagocytosis. Both the so-called natural (native or original immunity) and the immunity acquired by specific immunization could be explained on either cellular or humoral grounds. This controversy was partially solved in 1895 when Denys and LéClef showed that the serum of an animal immunized against a given disease specifically enhanced the phagocytic activity. Wright and Douglas in 1903 proposed the term *opsonin* for the phagocytosis-enhancing factor in the serum of immunized animals. Immunity then can be classified into two broad categories: natural (innate) immunity and acquired immunity (Table 2-1).

Ehrlich in 1897 and in 1900 put forward a general theory of immunity, the famous "side chain" or receptor theory. The fundamental notion of this theory was that the ability of toxin to combine with antitoxin and the lethal action of toxin represent two separate activities. He assumed that the toxin molecule possessed two distinct reactive sites: the haptophore which combines with antitoxin and the toxophore which expresses the toxicity (page 54). Ehrlich's side chain theory has had a profound influence in stimulating fundamental research in immunology.

Table 2-1. Classes of Immunity

Immunity	Examples
Nonspecific (innate, natural)	Phagocytosis, lysozyme, interferon, c-reactive protein, properdin, complement system, conglutinins, inflammatory response, genetic factors, stress, physical and chemical factors, temperature, hormones
Specific (acquired)	
passive natural	Maternally derived Ig in babies
passive induced	Protection by preformed heterologous or homologous antibodies
active natural	Exposure to infection
active induced	Immunization with toxoid or killed or attenuated organisms
adoptive	Transfer of immunocompetent cells

Some forms of immune reaction, rather than providing a protection or safety to the affected individual, can occasionally produce severe and sometimes fatal results. These are known as *hypersensitivity reactions,* a form of allergy. These reactions are mainly due to tissue damage caused by effects of pharmacologically active substances such as histamine, which are formed under certain conditions of antigen-antibody combination. Portier and Richet in 1902 made the first observation of the fatal hypersensitivity reaction in a dog receiving extract of the Actinia (sea anemone). The development of hypersensitivity to relatively harmless substances was termed by these authors *anaphylaxis,* in contrast to prophylaxis. A local anaphylaxis was produced by Arthus in 1903 (Arthus phenomenon). The term *allergy* was originally coined by von Pirquet in 1906 to describe the altered reactivity of an animal following exposure to a foreign antigen, and included both immunity and hypersensitivity. Over the years, however, the meaning of the term has become restricted to refer only to the hypersensitivity (of adverse type) that may be associated with the development of the immune response to a foreign substance. Various classifications of hypersensitivity reactions have been proposed, and probably the most widely accepted is that of Coombs and Gell (Table 2-2).

Rapid advancement in protein chemistry resulted in a new turning point in understanding the immunologic mechanisms. Tiselius and Kabat opened up new fields of immunochemistry in 1938 when they studied the migration of human serum protein in an electric field. They showed that the serum could be separated into albumin, α-, β-, and γ-globulins and that the antibody activity of immune serum was in fact found only in the γ-globulin fraction. Thus, more precise quantitative studies of antigen-antibody reaction were made possible. The question then is: what organ or what type of cell in the body is responsible for the production of γ-globulin, i.e., antibody? The role of plasma cells and lymphocytes in the production of γ-globulin was shown by Fagraeus in 1948 and by Coons in 1955. The essential role of the thymus gland in an immune response was shown independently by Good and his colleagues in Minnesota and by

Table 2-2. Hypersensitivity

Immediate type, antibody-mediated

    Type I   : Anaphylactic reaction
    Type II   : Cytotoxic or cytolytic reaction
    Type III : Toxic complex syndrome

Delayed type, cell-mediated

    Type IV : Delayed type skin reaction
                  Corneal reaction
                  Homograft rejection

Miller in England in 1960. The essential role of the bursa in chickens in the production of antibodies was first shown by Glick in 1957.

A new theory was needed to accommodate these new discoveries in immunology. Burnet in 1959, reacting to arguments of Jerne, Talmage, and Lederberg in favor of the selectional instead of the instructional theory of antibody synthesis, put forward the *clonal selection theory* to explain not only how an immune response takes place following immunization, but also why there is no immune response to the self-component of the body (page 56).

Immunology in its original meaning was a study of immunity (resistance to infection). From the exponential growth of knowledge concerning the mechanism of immune responses, we can group together those biologic activities responsible for preserving individuality, the mechanisms of specifically adaptive responses, and the analysis and basis of immunologic memory at cellular level. This discourse has far reaching implications in embryology, genetics, cell biology, molecular biology, transplantation, the mechanisms of oncogenic adaptation, in addition to the well-known contribution to analysis of immunity to disease. Thus, immunology has been expanded to a scope far wider than that originally developed—immunobiology.

SELECTED REFERENCES

Arthus, M. (1903): C. R. Soc. Biol (Paris) 55:817.
Bordet, J., and Gengou, O. (1901): Ann. Inst. Pasteur (Paris) 15:289.
Buchner, H. (1889): Centralbl. Bacteriol. 5:817.
Burnet, F. M., and Fenner, F. (1949): *The Production of Antibodies.* Melbourne, Macmillan.
Coombs, R. R. A., and Gell, P. G. H. (eds.) (1963): *Clinical Aspects of Immunology.* Philadelphia, F. A. Davis Company.
Coons, A. H. (1956): Int. Rev. Cytol. 5:1.
Coons, A. H., and Kaplan, M. H. (1950): J. Exp. Med. 91:1.
Denys, J., and LéClef, J. (1895): Cellule 11:177
Durham, H. (1897): J. Path. Bact. 4:13.
Ehrlich, P. (1900): Proc. Roy. Soc. Biol. 66:424.
Fagraeus, A. (1948): Acta Med. Scand. (Suppl. 204) 130:1.
Glick, B., and Chang, T. S. (1956): Poult. Sci. 35:224.
Good, R. A., Dalmasso, A. P., et al. (1962): J. Exp. Med. 116:773.
Gruber, M. (1896): Wien. Klin. Wschr. 9:183.
Gruber, M. (1896): Munchen. Med. Wschr. 43:206.
Gruber, M. (1901): Munchen. Med. Wschr. 48:1827.
Jerne, N. K. (1955): Proc. Nat. Acad. Sci. U.S.A. 41:849.
Kraus, M. (1897): Wien. Klin. Wschr. 10:736.
Lederberg, J. (1959): Science 129:1649.
Metchnikoff, E. (1884): Arch. Pathol. Anat. Physiol. Klin. Med. 96:177.
Miller, J. F. A. P. (1961): Lancet 2:748.
Pasteur, L. (1881): Comptes rendus des travaux du congrès international des directeurs des stations agrononiques, Session de Versailles, pp. 151-152.
Pfeiffer, R. (1894): Z. Hyg. 18:1.
Portier, and Richet, C. (1902): C. R. Soc. Biol. (Paris) 54:170.
Roux, E., and Yersin, A. (1888): Ann. Inst. Pasteur (Paris) 2:629.
Roux, E., and Yersin, A. (1889): Ann. Inst. Pasteur (Paris) 3:273.

Salmon, D. E., and Smith, T. (1884): Proc. Biol. Soc. (Wash.) 3:29.
Talmage, D. W. (1957): Ann. Rev. Med. 8:239.
Tiselius, A., and Kabat, E. A. (1938): Science 87:416.
von Behring, E., and Kitasato, S. (1890): Deutsch. Med. Wschr. 16:1113.
von Pirquet, C. E. (1911): Arch. Intern. Med. 7:259.
Widal, F. (1896): Lancet 2:1371.
Wright, A. E., and Douglas, S. R. (1903): Proc. Roy. Soc. Biol. 72:357.

FURTHER READINGS

Brock, T. (1961): *Milestones in Microbiology*. Englewood Cliffs, New Jersey, Pren-
tice-Hall, Inc.
Burnet, F. M., and White, D. O. (1972): *Natural History of Infectious Diseases*. (4th
ed.). New York, Cambridge University Press.
Clendening, L. (1942): *Source Book of Medical History*. New York, Dover Publica-
tions, Inc.
Long, E. R. (1928): *A History of Pathology*. Dover edition (1965): New York, Dover
Publications, Inc.
Metchnikoff, E. (1905): *Immunity in Infectious Diseases*. New York, Cambridge
University Press.

3
Central Lymphoid Systems

EXPERIMENTS OF NATURE

In 1951 a 54 year old man came to the University of Minnesota Hospital with a history of recurrent pneumonia. The roentgenogram of his chest showed a mass in the mediastinum; his serum protein showed a high albumin-globulin ratio with a strikingly low gamma globulin. The mediastinal mass was later found to be a benign thymoma. The patient suffered at least 17 episodes of life-threatening infections during the next 3 years, and finally died of fulminating hepatitis. This unique experiment of Nature, i.e., the association of thymoma, hypogammaglobulinemia, and impaired immunity in a patient, led to the postulate that the thymus gland may play a role in some way in the development of adaptive immunity. The occurrence of two such rare conditions in a single patient would be more than a chance association. This postulate, derived from clinical observation in a patient, initiated a series of experiments in laboratory animals; the thymus gland was removed from adult and young rabbits, and the antibody responses of these rabbits examined. The results: no demonstrable impairment in antibody response after thymectomy. Why? Does the thymus have nothing to do with adaptive immunity? We could not be sure but thought perhaps our laboratory experiments, rather than our experiment of Nature, were being incorrectly interpreted.

A fortunate laboratory accident provided a new direction in the study of thymectomy and adaptive immunity. In 1954 Glick was studying the effect of bursectomy in early life on the subsequent development and growth of the chicken. He, too, was disappointed to find that the bursectomized chickens grew just like normal chickens. Some of Glick's bursectomized chickens were unintentionally used by Chang for the class demonstration of antibody response in chickens. Nine of the chickens bursectomized as newly hatched birds six months earlier were injected with Salmonella typhimurium-O antigen. Six chickens died immediately after injection. Two survived, but surprisingly, there was no demonstrable antibody response. This unexpected accidental finding led Glick to postulate that the removal of bursa early in life might have rendered the chicken incapable of antibody formation. The succeeding experiments by Glick and Chang showed clearly that this was the case. The reports by

Glick and Chang that the chicken is incapable of making antibody when the bursa is removed immediately after hatching were confirmed and extended by Mueller et al. in Wisconsin. If the bursa is removed later in life, little or no impairment of antibody response is to be found. This discovery of the subsequent impairment of adaptive immunity when the bursa has been removed early in life provided our Minnesota group with a new impetus to re-examine the early failure of demonstrating the effect of thymectomy in rabbits. The thymus was removed from the rabbits in the immediate neonatal period. The depression of antibody response was readily demonstrable in neonatally thymectomized rabbits, and deficient development of antibody formation to certain antigens and of allograft immunity was noted in neonatally thymectomized mice. The same year, Miller in England, while investigating the influence of thymus in virus-induced leukemia in mice, discovered that neonatal thymectomy caused a severe depletion of lymphocytes, a marked deficiency of rejection of foreign skin grafts, and a so-called runting disease. Thus, a new exciting stage was set for the study of thymus and bursa in relation to the development of adaptive immunity.

THE THYMUS

In man, the thymus anlage is generated from the epithelium of the third and fourth pharyngeal pouches at about the sixth week of gestation. Mesodermal elements start to aggregate around the epithelium. By the eight week, the thymic anlage is differentiated into a compact epithelial structure. Although some thought for a time that thymic epithelial cells differentiated to lymphocytes, abundant evidence shows that mesenchymal cells entering the thymus and proliferating in the presence of epithelial cells differentiate into the thymic lymphoid cells (thymocytes). Experiments by Moore et al. in chickens and Davies et al., Stutman and Good, and Moore in mice have proved that mesenchymal cells originating in the yolk sac develop into immunologically competent cells within the thymus. The developmental process reflects an odyssey in which the precursor cells reside first in yolk sac, then in fetal liver, and finally in the marrow of the bone. Post-thymic cells, after developing full immunologic competence, circulate through blood and lymph and tend to reside in specialized regions of bird or mammalian peripheral lymphoid tissues as was shown by Cooper et al. and by Parrott et al. In the postnatal period, the thymus clearly accepts bloodborne cells mainly originating from bone marrow. The thymus, which is probably the main source of lymphoid proliferation in mammalian embryonic life, develops its characteristic lymphoid appearance and the Hassall's corpuscles by the third month of gestation. It becomes a prominent lymphoid organ when the spleen and lymph nodes are still poorly developed and is the first organ in all animal species to become predominantly lymphoid.

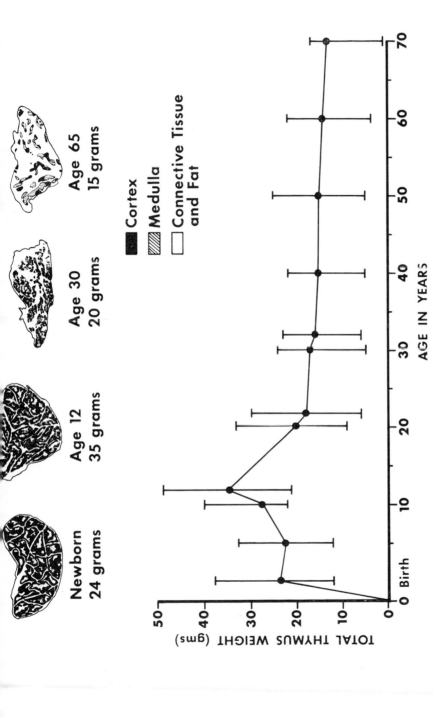

Fig. 3-1. Mean weight of the human thymus at various ages in 462 cases of sudden death from known causes. The vertical bars represent one standard deviation. The weight of the thymus is maximal at puberty and thereafter declines. Progressive changes take place in thymic components with age; there is loss of cortex and increase in fat and interstitial connective tissue (CT). [From the data of Young, M., and Turnbull, H. M. (1931): J. Path. Bact. 34:213; and of Hammar, J. A. (1938): Z. Migr. Anat. Forsch. 44:425.]

In man, the thymus varies greatly in size and weight at different ages (Fig. 3-1). It reaches its maximal relative size just prior to birth. At birth it weighs about 11 gm. Growth of the organ continues throughout childhood, and the maximum size is reached about the twelfth year, when the average weight is approximately 35 gm. A gradual involution beginning shortly after puberty continues until old age, when the thymus is often smaller than in the newborn (natural involution). Involution of the thymus is characterized by a decrease in weight and volume, a decrease in the ratio of cortex to medulla, and microscopic evidence of cell degeneration. Involution of the thymus may also be induced by trauma, stress, illness, X-irradiation, steroid hormones, cytotoxic drugs, lactation, and pregnancy (accidental involution). Thus, whatever its function in the body economy may be, the thymus must be exercising its most important influences early in life. These influences reach a maximum during childhood and decline progressively with age.

The human thymus is located in the anterior mediastinum. It has two lobes (right and left), surrounded by fibrous capsules. In 20 percent of humans aberrant nodules of thymic tissues are found mostly in the neck along the pathway of their normal descent, rarely at the base of the skull or at the root of the bronchus. Each thymic lobe is divided by septa from the capsule into lobules, which appear in section to be totally separate from one another but actually are joined in the center of the lobe. The lobules contain an outer cortex and a central medulla (Fig. 3-2).

The cortex appears dark in a hematoxylin-eosin stained section due to the crowded nuclei of small lymphocytes which show many mitotic figures. These lymphocytes are invested with a fine epithelial lattice which is inconspicuous in the cortex. Phagocytic cells in the cortex contain vacuoles with ingested nuclear debris and PAS positive granules.

The medulla, a pale-staining area, consists mainly of epithelial cells and scattered lymphocytes. The epithelial cells have a prominent cytoplasm which is slightly eosinophilic. In places the epithelial cells are aggregated in whirled patterns to form Hassall's corpuscles (thymic corpuscles), the significance of which remains enigmatic. The epithelial cells are connected by desmosome bridges and are not phagocytic. The epithelial reticulum of the thymus is almost entirely cellular. Unlike the spleen and lymph nodes, there are no extracellular fibers. Mesenchymal reticulum is a relatively minor component of the thymus found only around the blood vessels. Myocytes (myoid cells) and skeletal muscle fibers have been described in the thymus of certain animals, including man.

Thymus lymphocytes do not make antibodies. Plasma cells are present only along blood vessels in connective tissue of the normal thymus. Their number varies greatly from individual to individual and from species to species and can be markedly increased if antigen is directly injected into the thymus. Unlike the lymph node and the spleen, the thymus does not

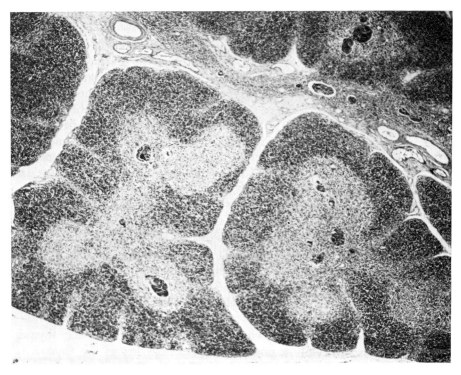

Fig. 3-2. Microscopic picture of normal human thymus. The dark areas represent the cortex and the light areas the medulla.

show such changes as an increased mitotic activity, germinal center formation, or increased plasmacytopoiesis after immunization, e.g., injection of antigens at a peripheral site. The study of the incorporation of tritiated thymidine shows that the thymus is engaged in active lymphopoiesis at a higher rate than are any other lymphoid tissues such as the spleen or the lymph nodes. It is a major organ for production of lymphocytes. Of the lymphocytes in the mouse, Metcalf classified about 1 percent as being large ($> 11\ \mu$), about 10 percent as being medium (7 to 11 μ), and the rest as being small ($< 7\ \mu$). The large lymphocytes transform continuously into medium-sized ones, which in turn transform into smaller lymphocytes. The large and medium lymphocytes probably undergo three to four cycles of cell division a day. The reason for this intense lymphopoiesis is not known. Unlike lymphopoiesis elsewhere, the thymic lymphopoiesis is independent of antigenic stimulation. In the fetus, which is relatively shielded from antigenic stimuli, lymphopoiesis of the thymus is marked but is low or absent in other lymphoid tissues. In germ-free animals thymus lymphopoiesis persists essentially unchanged, but the lymphopoiesis in the lymph nodes and the spleen is much less active than

After neonatal thymectomy, mice appear to survive for a time, but eventually a wasting disease (runting disease) develops. This is probably a manifestation of infection secondary to the immunologic deficiency, for it is not seen as regularly in germ-free mice. The effects of thymectomy in adult animals develop more slowly and are not as pronounced as those produced by neonatal thymectomy. However, if the thymectomy in the adult is followed by sublethal or lethal irradiation coupled with salvage by marrow transplantation, the effects of thymectomy in adult life are like those of neonatal thymectomy. This finding indicates that the adult animals have sufficient stock of thymus dependent post-thymic cells outside the thymus to function normally for a long period in the absence of the thymus. These differences explain why our earlier efforts to demonstrate the effects of thymectomy by extirpation in older animals were not successful. Neonatal thymectomy affects cellular immunity more profoundly than it does humoral immunity. The number of circulating eosinophils may fall after thymectomy and can be restored by thymus graft. Congenital absence of the thymus gland in nude mice and in man (DiGeorge syndrome) results in cellular deficiencies similar to the immunodeficiencies that are observed in thymectomized or thymectomized-irradiated animals.

The thymus is easily grafted in almost any part of the body. The entire adult organ, fragment, or rudimentary fetal thymus can be transplanted to the subcutaneous tissue, under the kidney capsule, in the spleen, or in the anterior chamber of the eye. Any number of thymuses may be grafted into one animal, and all develop normally, indicating apparent lack of feedback mechanism in thymic development. The thymus graft will restore immune function in the animal lacking thymus. If the thymus graft is from a genetically identical strain (isograft) the thymus graft will persist. By contrast, thymus grafts from a genetically different strain of the same species (homograft) will be rejected when the recipient becomes immunologically competent, and consequently the animal will become immunologicaly deficient again at a later time. The graft of the adult thymus can cause graft-versus-host (GVH) disease (page 233) when it is implanted in an immunodeficient recipient. The GVH disease can be minimized by grafting fetal thymus instead of adult thymus or thymus matched according to the major histocompatibility determination.

In recent years, extensive investigations of thymic functions have established that the thymus is essential for the develoment of adaptive immunity. The thymus seems to provide the microenvironment for the differentiation and proliferation of primitive stem cells migrating from the bone marrow, to elaborate a humoral factor that influences immunologic competence of lymphocytes elsewhere, and to foster cell-mediated immunity. The exact mechanisms of this function, however, are not yet fully understood.

Abnormal thymus function is associated with many clinical diseases, including some immunodeficiencies. The pathogenesis of myasthenia gravis and of other autoimmune diseases is known to have some link with thymic malfunction. The role of thymus in the development of lymphoid malignancy has been the subject of intensive investigation. Involution of the thymus with age may be associated with progressive loss of some immunologic functions with age in man and experimental animals. (These topics will be discussed in the appropriate chapters.)

THE BURSA OF FABRICIUS

The bursa of Fabricius, a lymphoepithelial organ so far found only in birds, develops from the dorsal part of the urodeal-proctodeal plate forming the cloaca. By the twelfth day of embryonic life, it contains numerous epithelial buds. By the fifteenth to sixteenth day, lymphocytes appear and large follicles with a dense cortex and lightly stained medulla develop in these buds. Formation of the lymphocytes in the thymus begins 5 to 6 days earlier than it does in the bursa. In adult chickens, the bursa is round or pear-shaped and is located on the posterior wall of the cloaca. Finger-like longitudinal folds (plicae) project from the inner mucous membrane and are thickened by the lymphoid nodules (Fig. 3-4). Lymphoid cells in the bursa have been shown to originate from the yolk sac and later

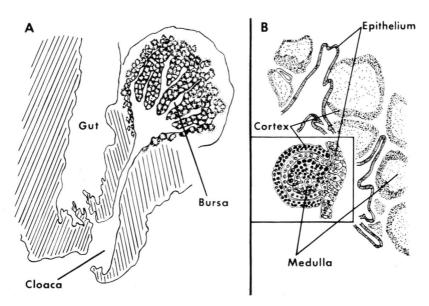

Fig. 3-4. Bursa of Fabricius (embryo). A. The relationship of the bursa to the gut and cloaca in the embryo is shown. The bursa develops in its own cloacal diverticulum. B. The lymphatic follicles are directly subjacent and continuous with the epithelium. [From Jolly, J. (1915): Arch. Anat. Micr. Morph. Exp. 16:363. By permission of Masson et Cie, Paris.]

from blood. The lymphopoiesis in the bursa has, to date, seemed to be independent of antigenic stimulation and as such to be similar to the thymus lymphopoiesis. Recent studies by Van Alten and Meuwissen have shown that certain antigens injected directly into the lumen of the bursa, even during development, can stimulate antibody production in this organ. The bursa appears to provide a special microenvironment for the incoming lymphoid stem cells to differentiate and mature into immunocompetent antibody-producing cells. These lymphocytes then migrate to specified regions of the lymph nodes and the spleen. In mammals these thymus independent areas are found in the far cortical areas and medullary cords of the lymph nodes (Fig. 4-6) and the mantle, germinal follices, and perifollicular regions of the spleen (Fig. 4-7). These are the bursa dependent or the thymus independent areas.

The natural involution of the bursa begins between 7 to 13 weeks after hatching, which is about the time of puberty in this species. The involution can be caused artificially by injecting the young bird with androgenic hormones (hormonal bursectomy). Further, the bursa can be prevented from developing if such hormones are injected into the egg early in embryonic life.

A new interest in the function of the bursa was aroused in 1954 with an accidental discovery by Glick, Chang, and Jaap. The removal of the bursa in a 12 day old chicken was associated with a marked depression of antibody formation. In 1959, Meyer et al. prevented the development of the bursa by injecting 19-nortestosterone into a 5 to 6 day old embryo. Such bursa-less chickens failed to develop capacity to produce and secrete antibodies but showed little or no abnormality of cell-mediated (thymus dependent) immunity.

The inability of bursectomized chickens to produce antibodies can be corrected by the transplantation of syngeneic bursal cells from young chicks. Recent work by Toivanen et al. showed that the restoration of immune function can be achieved only when a functional bursa is used. The involuting or involuted bursa was not effective. After the involution of bursa, the bone marrow cells which previously could not restore long-term immunologic competence became capable of this kind of restoration. These findings indicate that certain stem cells of the B-cell line may be transferred to the bone marrow after the bursa begins to involute. Bursa also is the site for development of lymphomatous cells in a form of virus-induced avian leukosis.

Since the bursa of Fabricius exists only in birds, an extensive search for an equivalent in mammals is still in progress. Archer et al. in 1963 suggested that certain gut-associated lymphatic tissue (GALT) such as that in certain follices of the appendix, Peyer's patches, and sacculus rotundus of rabbits may have a function equivalent to that of the bursa. In mice, the bone marrow may function as a bursa equivalent, but further study of these important relationships is needed.

Recent studies by Cooper and his associates in Birmingham seem to indicate that in birds the switching of immunoglobulin-producing cells from production of IgM to IgG occurs only within the bursa in chickens. How this occurs in mammals is enigmatic, but manipulations with anti-IgM antisera in mice indicate that a developmental step involving IgM production is essential to all antibody-producing cells in both mammals and birds.

COMPONENTS OF THE IMMUNE SYSTEM

At the moment, the central lymphoid tissues consist of the thymus in mammals and the bursa of Fabricius in the chicken. The works of Szenburg and Warner (1962) extended and corrected by Cooper et al. (1965) established the concept of two components of immune response postulated by Good in 1957. The thymectomy in birds depresses cell-mediated immunity, whereas bursectomy abolishes humoral immunity. This dichotomy is more pronounced when sublethal X-irradiation is coupled with thymectomy and/or bursectomy at hatching. Removal of the bursa in ova at 15 to 17 days may produce agammaglobulinemia and inability to produce any antibody. By contrast, complete thymic extirpation in ova or in newly hatched chicks interferes with cellular immunity but not with development of immunoglobulins or ability to produce antibodies. The models of immune deficiency produced by such means are summarized in Table 3-1.

Most immunologists have long been concerned with the problem of accounting for the two kinds of immunity—cellular and humoral. The study of the chicken model provided the basis for a concept of two separate immune systems, i.e., the lymphocytes of bursal origin (B-cells) control the humoral immunity (production of antibody), and the lymphocytes of thymic origin are responsible for the cell-mediated immunity (transplantation immunity, delayed hypersensitivity). The concept of two components was both guided by and reenforced by clinical observa-

Table 3-1.   Models of Immune Deficiency

| Thymus | Bursa | Irradiated Chicken | | Equivalent Human Disease |
		Cellular Immunity	Humoral Immunity	
+	−	+	−	Bruton-type—X-linked infantile agammaglobulinemia
−	+	−	+	DiGeorge syndrome

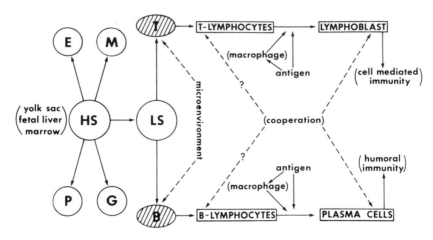

Fig. 3-5. Schematic presentation of the two components of the immune system and of the migration, maturation, and differentiation of stem cells into immunocompetent cells and their interactions.

tions. In the patient with DiGeorge syndrome, where the thymus is congenitally absent or rudimentary, the cell-mediated immunity is selectively depressed. In the patient with Bruton-type agammaglobulinemia, the humoral immunity is selectively impaired, but the cell-mediated immunity remains intact. Thus, the two-component concept of the immune system in chickens provided a new insight for better understanding and classification of the immunodeficiency disease in man.

The relationship of the central lymphoid organs and the migration and differentiation of the stem cells to become immunocompetent lymphocytes are summed up in Figure 3-5.

SELECTED REFERENCES

Archer, O. K., Sutherland, D. E. R., and Good, R. A. (1963): Nature 200:3377.
Cooper, M. D., Peterson, R. D., and Good, R. A. (1965): Nature 205:143.
Davies, A. J. S., et al. (1966): Transplantation 4:438.
Ford, C. E. (1963): Lancet 1:359.
Glick, B., and Chang, T. S. (1956): Poult. Sci. 35:224.
Good, R. A. (1957): In Host Parasite Relationships in Living Cells, Felton, H., et al. (eds.). Springfield, Illinois, Charles C Thomas, pp. 68-161.
Kincade, P. W., and Cooper, M. D. (1973): Science 179:398.
Metcalf, D. (1964): In The Thymus, Defendi, V., and Metcalf, D. (eds.). Philadelphia, The Wistar Institute Press, p. 53.
Meyer, R. K., Rao, M. A., and Aspinall, R. L. (1959): Endocrinology 64:890.
Miller, J. F. A. P. (1961): Lancet 2:248.
Moore, M. A. S., and Owen, J. J. T. (1965): Nature 208:959.
Moore, M. A. S., and Owen, J. J. T. (1966): Develop. Biol. 14:40.
Mueller, A. P., Wolfe, H. R., et al. (1962): J. Immun. 88:354.
Parrott, D. M. V., De Sousa, M. A. B., and East, J. (1966): J. Exp. Med. 123:191.
Sainte-Marie, G., and Leblond, C. P. (1964): J. Hemat. 23:275.
Stutman, O., and Good, R. A. (1971): Transpl. Proc. 3:923.

Szenberg, A., and Warner, N. L. (1962): Nature *194*:146.
Toivanen, A., Toivanen, P., and Good, R. A. (1973): Int. Arch. Allerg. In press.
Van Alten, P. J., and Meuwissen, H. J. (1972): Science *176*:45.
Warner, N. L., Szenberg, A., and Burner, F. M. (1962): Aust. J. Exp. Biol. Med. Sci. *40*:373.

FURTHER READINGS

Defendi, V., and Metcalf, D. (1964): *The Thymus*. Philadelphia, The Wistar Institute Press.
Goldstein, G., and Mackay, I.R. (1969): *The Human Thymus*. St. Louis, Missouri, Warren H Green, Inc.
Good, R. A., and Gabrielsen, A. E. (eds.) (1964): *The Thymus in Immunobiology*. (Conference in Minneapolis). New York, Harper & Row.
Hess, M. W. (1968): *Experimental Thymectomy, Possibilities and Limitations*. New York, Springer-Verlag.
Kobayashi, T., and Ushida, D. (eds.) (1971): *The Thymus: Basic and Clinical Studies*. Tokyo, Keio University Press.
Metcalf, D. (1966): *The Thymus*. New York, Springer-Verlag.
Wolstenholme, G. E. W., and Porter, R. (eds.) (1966): *The Thymus: Experimental and Clinical Studies*. Boston, Little, Brown and Company.

4

Peripheral Lymphoid Tissues

LYMPHOCYTES

The lymphocytes, which were first described by William Hewson of England in his series of papers published by the Royal Society during the 1770's, are the major cellular elements involved in the immune responses. Paul Ehrlich in 1879 introduced a staining technique of blood cells and described the morphology of lymphocytes. He considered the lymphocytes to be nonmotile and incapable of growth or further differentiation and to have no recognizable function. This unfortunate dogma prevailed during the next half century, although many controversial arguments about this point were presented. The first link between the lymphocytes and the immune response was made by Hellman and White in 1930. They observed the so-called reaction center (germinal center) in the lymph nodes of immunized rabbits. McMaster and Hudack in 1935 demonstrated the formation of antibody (agglutinin) in the lymph nodes of immunized animals. Finally in 1945 Harris and his colleagues concluded that the lymphocytes of the lymph nodes are the source of antibody.

In the peripheral blood the lymphocytes, according to a morphologic concept, consist of at least five broad functional subgroups: (1) thymus derived (T) cells, (2) bursa derived (B) cells, (3) precursors of monocytes, (4) primitive stem cells, and (5) partially differentiated stem cells. According to their size, the lymphocytes are classified into small (5 to 8 μ), medium (8 to 12 μ), and large (12 to 15 μ) lymphocytes (Fig. 4-1). The average man produces about 6.5×10^{10} lymphocytes daily. This is more than three times the daily output of thoracic duct lymphocytes. Everett and his colleagues, using radioactive thymidine labeling, calculated that the small lymphocytes of the thymus are formed at a rate of 20×10^6 cells per hour in a 100 gm rat. In mice, the rate of production in the mesenteric and cervical lymph nodes was 0.94×10^6 and 0.63×10^6 cells per hour, respectively. The human body contains 70 gm of lymphocytes in the bone marrow, 3 gm in the circulating blood, 100 gm in the lymph nodes, and 1,300 gm in the remaining tissues. The average weight of a lymphocyte is estimated to be in the order of 64×10^{-12} gm. One antibody-producing lymphocyte can produce *in vitro* about 3×10^{-12} gm of antibodies in 24 hours.

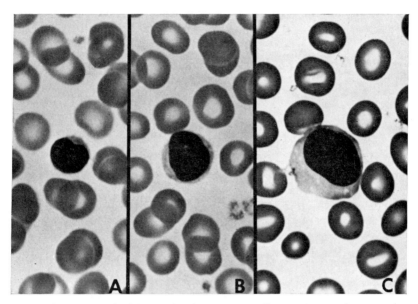

Fig. 4-1. Photomicrograph of human lymphocytes: A. small; B. medium; C. large.

Lymphocytes are motile cells that move at an estimated 4 to 40 μ/min on a glass surface at 37° C. When they move around, lymphocytes tend to assume the so-called hand-mirror form, i.e., the nucleus is in the front with the cytoplasm behind, like a tail. The lymphocytes may display pinocytosis and phagocytosis to a limited degree. They can traverse endothelial cells in the postcapillary venules, and the majority of them function as recirculating cells (Fig. 4-2). In man the life span of short-lived lymphocytes is said to be about 13.5 days, and that of long-lived ones ranges between a few months to many years (up to three years or more). The proportion of long-lived lymphocytes to short-lived lymphocytes varies in different organs as shown in Figure 4-3. Only a small portion of the lymphocytes produced in the thymus are long-lived lymphocytes, but these cells ultimately become the majority of the long-lived lymphocytes in other tissues.

The lymphocytes contain several enzymes (lipolytic, oxidative, proteolytic and nonspecific esterases). They synthesize plasma protein (α-, β-, and γ-globulins), complement components (page 150), and antihemophilic factors. Upon encounter with specific antigen, the T-lymphocytes release lymphokines, e.g., macrophage migration inhibition factor (MIF), and a host of other substances (page 73). The B-lymphocytes transform into plasma cells after encounter with antigens and both synthesize and secrete antibodies. Recently the immunoglobulin receptor molecules have been postulated and demonstrated to be at the cell surface of B-

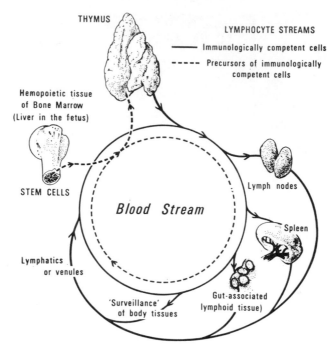

Fig. 4-2. Diagram to show circulation of lymphocytes in the body. Lymphopoietic stem cells arise in the bone marrow and reach the thymus via the blood stream. Within the thymus, stem cells become immunologically competent lymphocytes, emigrate to the blood stream, and circulate between the tissues, lymphatics, and blood stream. The bursa dependent lymphocytes are believed to follow a similar circulation. [From Goldstein, G., and Mackay, I. R. (1969): *The Human Thymus.* St. Louis, Missouri, Warren H. Green, Inc. By permission of William Heineman Medical Books Ltd., London.]

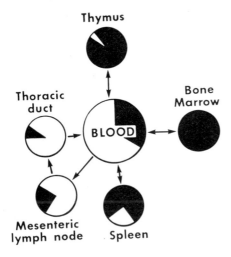

Fig. 4-3. Proportion of lymphocyte population. The white areas in the circles represent the percentages of long-lived small lymphocytes; the black areas represent the percentages of short-lived small lymphocytes. [From Everett, N. B., Caffrey, R. W., and Rieke, W. O. (1964): Ann. N.Y. Acad. Sci. *113*:889.]

Table 4-1. Lymphocytes Bearing Membrane-bound Immunoglobulins

Source	Immunoglobulin-bearing Lymphocytes (Mean and Range)			Total Mean (%)
	IgG (%)	IgM (%)	IgA (%)	
Blood:				
Controls (adults)				
(7 patients) ..	15·6 (14–19)	6·5 (4·4–9·5)	5·4 (3·6–9·4)	27·5
DiGeorge syndrome blood	32·9	26·6	23·7	83·2
Lymph nodes:				
Controls (infants)				
(2 patients) ..	9·9 (5·3–14·4)	5·8 (5·6–6·0)	4·4 (3·6–5·2)	21·1
DiGeorge syndrome	24·3	17·8	10·6	53·0

From Gajl-Peczalska, K. J. et al. (1972) Lancet *1*:1344.

lymphocytes. Taking advantage of these molecules (e.g., γA, γG, γM), one can now identify by immunofluorescence each cell carrying each class and subclass of immunoglobulin on its surface (page 585). The proportion of such cells in the peripheral blood and lymph nodes is shown in the Table 4-1. The surface receptor molecule of T-lymphocytes has not been identified as yet. Therefore, the presence of T-lymphocytes in the blood or in the lymph nodes can be measured only by the phytohemagglutinin (PHA) stimulation test. PHA is known to stimulate T-lymphocytes selectively and to induce blast transformation and mitosis (page 584). The T-lymphocytes are mainly responsible for cell-mediated immunity (page 65), and the B-lymphocytes, for humoral immunity (page 77).

Certain small lymphocytes possessing immunoglobulin receptors at their surfaces are believed to transform into plasma cells after contact with antigen. The most conclusive evidence of this relationship is derived from the recent experiments which showed that plasma cells containing antibody developed from suspensions of small lymphocytes in a cell-tight chamber placed within the homologous host. The plasma cell precursor almost certainly differentiates into a B-lymphocyte plasmablast, then transforms to intermediate transitional cells, and finally to mature plasma cells. The experimental support for this developmental sequence stems largely from the works of Fagraeus, who explanted tissue fragments and cells from rabbit spleens at various intervals during the antibody response to typhoid bacilli. She then studied the morphology and location of the cells in the spleen, and found most of the antibody to be produced by what she called "transitional" cells between plasmablasts and the mature plasma cells. The several stages of plasma cell maturation are illustrated in

Figures 4-4 and 4-5. The characteristic features of the mature plasma cell are (1) eccentric nucleus with coarse chromatin, (2) large cytocentrum centrosome and well-developed Golgi apparatus, (3) large basophilic cytoplasm, and (4) abundant rough endoplasmic reticulum (RER) (Fig. 4-6). These characteristic features may not be readily recognizable in

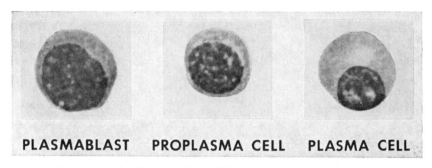

PLASMABLAST   PROPLASMA CELL   PLASMA CELL

Fig. 4-4. Photomicrograph of plasma cells in different stages of maturation.

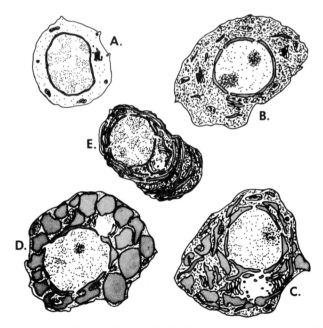

Fig. 4-5. Schematic view of several stages in the life cycle of plasma cells. A. Lymphocytic stage, which may be a plasma cell precursor. B. A "blast" form with polyribosomes, segments of rough endoplasmic reticulum (RER), nucleoli, nuclear pores, and other cellular elements. C and D. Plasma cell of intermediate or transitional character with dilated perinuclear spaces and dilated endoplasmic reticulum (ER) both containing antibody. E. Small plasma cell, Marschalko cell, displaying polarized nucleus and cytoplasm, distribution of heterochromatin in chunks along the inner nuclear membrane, prominent centrosome including Golgi and centrioles, and deeply basophilic or pyroninophilic (=RNA) cytoplasm. This cell is a near terminal form, past the peak of antibody production. The intermediate cells turn out most of the antibody.

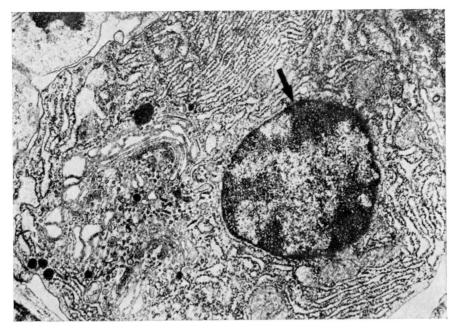

Fig. 4-6. Electronmicrograph of mature plasma cell. Flattened, expanded ergastoplasmic lamellae and contracted nucleus with peripheral dense chromatin clumps (arrow) are shown. (From Humphrey, J. H., and White, R. G. (1970): *Immunology for Students of Medicine.* Oxford, Blackwell Scientific Publications, Ltd.)

the earlier stages of development. The cytoplasm is basophilic (deep blue color) in basic stain and pyroninophilic (red color) with methyl green pyronin (MGP) staining. This characteristic staining is a function of the abundant ribonucleic acid (RNA) in the cytoplasm and can be abolished by pretreatment with ribonuclease. Plasma cells produce antibodies of immunoglobulin nature, and these antibodies are synthesized in the cytoplasm of lymphocytes and plasma cells. Aggregates of such immunoglobulins and antibodies may be concentrated in the Russell's bodies of the plasma cells.

The lymphocytes carry abundant histocompatibility antigens (page 224) at their surfaces. Antiserum prepared against lymphocytes (or thymocytes) is called antilymphocyte serum (ALS). The gammaglobulin from ALS is called antilymphocyte globulin (ALG) and is a potent immunosuppressive agent especially depressing the cell-mediated immunities.

Many lymphocytes are quite sensitive to the destructive effect of X-irradiation, nitrogen mustard, cyclophosphamide, or adrenocortical steroid hormones. Mature plasma cells are less sensitive to irradiation, and the ultimate fate of lymphocytes at the end of the life cycle is not known.

The secretory stages of lymphocytes and plasma cells may be a terminal stage of differentiation. It is clear, however, that T-lymphocytes can divide.

LYMPH NODES

The lymph nodes are found along the path of collecting lymphatics. The lymph flow passes through the lymph nodes to reach the main lymphatic vessels and join with the venous flow. In newborn infants and germ-free animals, the lymph nodes remain small and underdeveloped. When they are exposed to a variety of antigenic stimuli from that sea of microorganisms which makes up their present natural environment, a typical feature of lymph node structure develops.

The functions of lymph nodes appear to be (1) filtration of flowing lymph, (2) phagocytosis of foreign material, e.g., antigens, (3) production of antibodies against the incoming antigens, and (4) support for the proliferation and circulation of T- and B-lymphocytes. In a virus infection, the lymph node may be the site of virus proliferation. The filtered lymph flow in the efferent vessels is enriched by humoral substances (e.g., antibody) and by cellular elements (e.g., lymphocytes). Each node or set of nodes receives lymph flow from a distinctly separate region of the body (e.g., inguinal nodes receive lymph flow from the leg).

The lymph node is encapsulated by dense fibers (Fig. 4-7). Connective tissue branching from the inner surface of the capsule irregularly subdivides the interior. The capsule is pierced at several points by the incoming afferent lymphatic vessels from the outside. The afferent vessel has a valve at the junction of the capsule to prevent reflux. The lymph flow first reaches the subcapsular (marginal) sinus, then the intermediate (radial) sinus between the large nodular mass of lymphocytes, i.e., primary and secondary nodules, and then the medulla where the lymphocytes are grouped in the form of branching cords (medullary cord) converging into the hilus. The lymph flow leaves the node from the hilus via efferent vessels. The primary nodules consist of uniformly small lymphocytes. The primary nodule, once it contains the germinal center, becomes a secondary nodule. These nodules contain a very special form of reticular cells, the denditric reticular cells which are capable of fixing antigens at their surfaces. The subcapsular area that is occupied by the primary and the secondary nodules is the far cortical area. Between this far cortical area and the medullary cord, there is a band with ill-defined margins called the deep cortical region. Since this area is populated mainly by thymus dependent lymphocytes, it is referred to as the thymus dependent area. The far cortical area and the medullary cord are populated mainly by the bursa or bone marrow dependent lymphocytes; hence this is called the T independent area.

Germinal centers are found in lymph nodes, the spleen, the tonsils, and

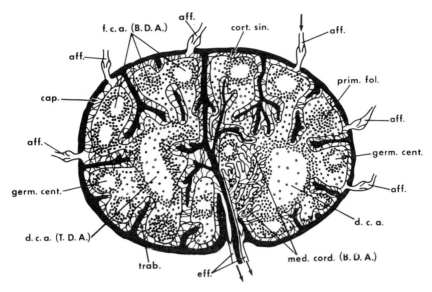

Fig. 4-7. Diagrammatic representation of a typical lymph node of an adult man. The arteries and the veins are not shown here. aff., afferent lymphatic; cap., capsule; cort. sin., cortical sinus; d.c.a., deep cortical area; eff., efferent lymphatic; f.c.a., far cortical area; med. cord., medullary cord; prim. fol., primary follicle; trab., trabecuale; germ. cent., germinal centers within "secondary" lymphoid nodules of the cortex; B.D.A., bursa dependent area; T.D.A., thymus dependent area.

the Peyer's patches, but usually not in the thymus of young mammals. These centers are collections of lymphocytes and related cells which arise from primary nodules. Flemming in 1885 referred to them as germinal centers because of the large number of dividing cells. Hellman in 1921 used the term *reaction center* because he thought that the incoming toxin was destroyed here.

SPLEEN

The spleen reacts with blood-borne antigens from the systemic circulation, in contrast to the lymph nodes which react mainly with the lymph-borne antigens from the local area. In a sense, it is a large settling chamber through which the blood may move slowly. Its functions are to (1) provide the site of differentiation for the lymphocytes and the hematopoietic stem cells, (2) trap the blood-borne foreign and altered endogenous particles (systemic filter) by virtue of its sinuses, ellipsoids, and enormous phagocytic activity of the reticuloendothelial system, (3) provide reservoir space for the circulating blood, and (4) form certain types of antibodies, especially IgM antibodies, after stimulation by antigens in the circulating blood. The spleen may be necessary for life during infancy when the total reserve capacity of the lymphatic tissue is small, and the spleen occupies a relatively large fraction of the abdomen. Sple-

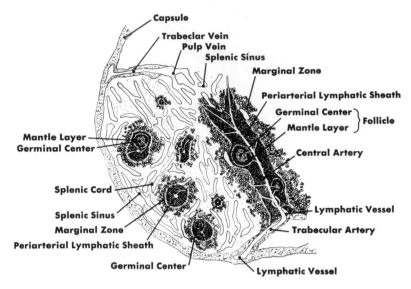

Fig. 4-8. Schematic view of spleen. [From Weiss, L., and Tavassoli, M. (1970): Seminars Hemat. 7:373.]

nectomy is more precarious in infants than in adults. Recently critical studies established that the major function of the spleen is twofold. It produces antibody after intravenous antigenic stimulation and with the phagocytes removes particulate matter that has not been opsonized by specific antibody.

The human spleen, as in most mammals, is surrounded by a capsule of dense, thick connective tissue (Fig. 4-8). From the internal surface of the capsule arise many trabeculae (connective tissue) which subdivide the inner space. The branches of the splenic artery enter the hilus, then follow the trabeculae upward, and branch out. When the branched artery reaches about 200 μ in diameter, the artery leaves the trabeculae and becomes surrounded by a sheath of lymphoid tissue. The artery is then called the *central artery,* and the surrounding lymphoid tissue, which is scattered throughout the spleen, is called the *white pulp.* The central artery branches out further through the lymphatic sheath and reaches the red pulp, where it becomes the penicilliary artery and then the ellipsoid. The red pulp appears like a matrix or background region in which white pulp is embedded. The white pulp usually occupies less than 50 percent of the spleen, but it may expand to 75 percent during an immune response. In severe hemolytic anemia, the red pulp may occupy more than 90 percent of the spleen. After leaving the ellipsoids, the route of arterial blood flow is disputed, i.e., via open circulation or via closed circulation. In any case, the venous blood flow is channeled to the venulae from the sinusoid and the postcapillary venulae, and enters into the veins in the trabeculae.

The white pulp is a cylindric structure with a central artery running through the longitudinal axis. Since it resembles a sheath of the artery, it is termed the *periarterial lymphatic sheath.* The sheath consists of a reticular network packed with lymphocytes and other free cells, e.g., macrophages, plasma cells, granulocytes, and a few red cells. The lymph nodules and germinal centers may appear within the sheath. The shell of small lymphocytes that accumulate around the germinal center is called the mantle (Fig. 4-7). Immediately outside the periarterial lymphatic sheath lies the *marginal zone,* which is characterized by a densely meshed reticulum containing many arterial trunks, a few sinuses, and a variety of free cells. The marginal zone gradually merges with the red pulp.

BONE MARROW

The bone marrow is the principal source of the lymphoid stem cell in postnatal life and is one of the largest organs in man. Its weight is estimated to be between 1500 gm to 4000 gm, comparable to the weight of the liver. It is the only general hemopoietic tissue in the healthy adult. In the human infant, most of the marrow cavity is filled with hemopoietic compartments (red marrow). With age the red marrow recedes to the cavities of the skull and the trunk bones.

The nutrient artery enters the marrow cavity through the cortex, bifurcates to become the central longitudinal artery, and then after division, the arterial capillaries. Venous blood returns from the venous sinus to the central longitudinal artery and then to the nutrient vein. The space occupied by these vessels is termed the *vascular compartment.*

The hemopoietic compartments contain erythrocytes, granulocytes, lymphocytes, megakaryocytes, monocytes, macrophages, plasma cells, mast cells, and their precursor stem cells. Till and McCulloch have established the existence of various kinds of stem cells in the bone marrow. This was done by their study of spleen colonies of mice which were heavily irradiated and injected with normal bone marrow cells. The morphologic identification of stem cells is not regularly possible.

The lymphocytes comprise 10 to 20 percent of the total nucleated cells in bone marrow. In patients with lymphopenic agammaglobulinemia (combined immunodeficiency syndrome or Swiss-type hypogammaglobulinemia) the proportion of lymphocytes is markedly decreased, and plasma cells are absent from the marrow.

Neither human nor mouse marrow properly obtained contains significant numbers of fully competent thymus dependent lymphocytes. Immunoglobulin-producing cells, θ positive incompletely developed T-cells, and T-cells, however, are readily demonstrable in the bone marrow.

Further, the marrow contains many B-lymphocytes and fully differentiated immunoglobulin-producing lymphocytes and plasma cells.

Transplantation of marrow can protect lethally irradiated animals from death and secondary disease. Recently, the transplantation of marrow into infants with combined immunodeficiency disease resulted in a complete reconstitution of immunologic function (page 555). Marrow transplantation also has been shown to have therapeutic value in other diseases such as aplastic anemia, neutropenia, and it could even be of value in leukemia.

The interactions between the thymus, the spleen, the lymph nodes, and the bone marrow in maintaining the integrity of the lymphoid system and immune function are reflected in Figure 4-2.

SELECTED REFERENCES

Fagraeus, A. (1948): Acta Med. Scand. (Suppl. 204) *130*:1.
Flemming, W. (1885): Arch. Mikr. Anat. *24*:50.
Harris, T. N., et al. (1945): J. Exp. Med. *81*:73.
Hellman, T. J., and White, G. (1930): Virchow. Arch. (Path. Anat.) *278*:221.
McMaster, P. D., and Hudack, S. S. (1935): J. Exp. Med. *61*:783.
Till, J. E., and McCulloch, E. A. (1961): Radiat. Res. *14*:213.

FURTHER READINGS

Cottier, H., et al. (1967): *Germinal Centers in Immune Responses*. New York, Springer-Verlag.
Craddock, C. G., Longmire, R., and McMillan, R. (1971): Lymphocytes and the immune responses. New Eng. J. Med. *285*:324.
Elves, M. W. (1967): *The Lymphocytes*. Chicago, Year Book Medical Publishers Inc.
Ling, N. R., (1968): *Lymphocyte Stimulation*. Amsterdam, North-Holland Publishing Co.
Yoffey, J. M., and Courtice, F. C. (1970): *Lymphatics, Lymph and the Lymphomyeloid Complex*. London, New York, Academic Press.

5

The Afferent Limb of Immune Response

ANTIGENS

The word *antigen* was originally defined in terms of its function, i.e., substances which induce the animal to produce antibodies were called collectively antigens. An antibody was defined as a substance in the blood of immunized animals which reacts specifically with the antigen. This definition is a circular but operational one. The inadequacy of these terms became apparent as a result of subsequent studies which showed that a certain substance could induce only cellular immune response without any demonstrable antibody formation. Furthermore, it was also shown in some instances that the antigen could provoke adverse hypersensitivity or specific unresponsiveness in animals (allergy, negative immunologic adaptation, tolerance, or immune paralysis). Therefore, a new term *immunogen* has been proposed for any substance that induces the immune response of any kind. Such an altered state of immunity (allergy in its original sense) may or may not have any beneficial value, even though the word *immunogen* has the connotation for a protective property. The term *antigen* is then reserved for a kind of immunogen that generates the antibody and reacts with the antibodies *in vitro* and *in vivo*.

Landsteiner introduced the term *hapten* to describe substances that react specifically with antibody *in vitro* or *in vivo,* but which themselves are unable to induce antibody formation unless attached to other molecules (usually protein). The hapten is also called an *incomplete antigen* because of its inability to induce an immune response by itself. The protein to which the hapten is attached (conjugated) is called the *carrier protein.* A *haptenic group* is a chemical group of hapten which reacts with the combining site of an antibody. Since the hapten has only one combining site for the antibody (univalent), it is sometimes used for inhibition studies of antigen-antibody reaction (page 108), and such inhibition is called *haptenic inhibition.*

Some important factors that influence the antigenicity (or immunogenicity) of any substance are (1) the rate of administration, (2) the dose of antigen, (3) the method of antigen preparation, (4) the degree of "foreignness" of antigen to the recipient, (5) the sensitivity of the method detecting the immune responses, (6) the age and sex of the recipient, (7) the size of antigens, (8) the metabolism of antigens in the recipient, (9) the presence or absence of adjuvants, and (10) the digestibility and the solubility of antigens.

Most of the proteins, certain carbohydrates, and a few lipids (phospholipid and sphingolipid) are antigenic. Recently, nucleic acid and synthetic polypeptides have also been found to be antigenic. Studies of the latter lower molecular weight substances have provided important information concerning essential components of the structure of antigenic molecules.

PROTEIN

Early investigators found empirically (1) that animals make antibodies readily against the proteins from different species (foreign protein), (2) that animals usually do not make antibody against their own protein or tissues, and (3) that proteins antigenic for one animal may not be antigenic in another animal of the same species. The proteins from remotely related sources such as bacteria, viruses, eggs, milk, and plants usually are better antigens for rabbits, guinea pigs, and mice than are the proteins from phylogenetically closer sources. Exceptions to this rule are so-called autoantigens which may induce antibodies directed against host constituents, e.g., the antithyroid antibody present in Hashimoto's disease, and anti-red cell antibodies in autoimmune hemolytic anemias (page 196).

Most protein molecules, except for a few, are known to be immunogenic. Proteins with molecular weights of 40,000 or more are generally potent immunogens (e.g., albumin, 40,000 to 60,000; γ-globulin, 6×10^6; and virus particles, about 40×10^6). These are known to be the most powerful antigens. When the protein is adsorbed on the floccules of aluminum hydroxide (alum precipitate), the antigen acts more regularly to induce antibody, and the antibody response is usually of greater magnitude than when the antigen is used alone.

An antigen found only in a certain member of a species, but not in the other members, is called an *isoantigen*. The isoantigens are inherited according to Mendelian genetics. The most important of all isoantigens are well-known blood group antigens and histocompatibility antigens (page 239). The isoantigenic differences in the IgG molecule of rabbits are called *allotypes;* in man they are recognized immunochemically as Gm factors on the heavy chain component and InV factors on the light chain component of the molecule. These have also been referred to as the isoantigen G-determinants (page 99).

The exact chemical structure of the antigenic determinant in protein molecules is being defined, for example, Eylar's work on the myelin molecule which is capable of inducing experimental allergic encephalomyelitis (page 449). The primary sequence of amino acid and the secondary and tertiary structures of the peptides are believed to control the antigenicity of the protein molecules.

POLYSACCHARIDES

Many of the polysaccharides in the cell membrane are not by themselves immunogenic, but determine the specificity of protein antigens to which they are attached. A few polysaccharides, however, are known of themselves to be immunogenic. Since the polysaccharides of the cell membrane may contain nitrogen, in considering the antigenicity of carbohydrates one should always be sure that the molecule acts by itself and not as a haptenic component linked to a protein. The polysaccharides of helminths and mollusks are nitrogen free and appear to be antigenic in rabbits and guinea pigs.

The bacterial polysaccharides have been studied most extensively. The polysaccharides of pneumococcus, staphylococcus, Haemophilus influenzae, Salmonella typhosa, meningococcus, and Mycobacterium tuberculosis are known to be antigenic. Avery and Heidelberger in 1923 were first to isolate the antigenic polysaccharide from pneumococcus. Purified polysaccharides are clearly antigenic for humans and mice, but usually not in rabbits and guinea pigs (species specificity of antigens). More than 70 types of pneumococci have been classified according to the antigenic difference of their capsular polysaccharides. In addition to the capsular polysaccharide antigens, pneumococci contain protein antigens that are common to all types. H. influenzae (types A, B, C, D, and E), Neisseria meningitidis (types I, II, and IIIα), and β-hemolytic streptococcus are also classified according to polysaccharide antigens contained in their capsules. Each type of specific polysaccharide has a different chemical structure.

The cell wall of many gram-negative bacteria contains a complex of protein-lipid-carbohydrate (lipoglycoprotein), or of lipid-carbohydrate (lipopolysaccharide). Some of these are toxic to animals, and are called endotoxins. Salmonella bacilli contain a somatic antigen (O-antigen) and a flagella antigen (H-antigen), both of which are lipopolysaccharides. More than 20 different types of pneumococcus have specific O-antigens. The antibodies against the capsular polysaccharides of pneumococci are capable of protecting against pneumococcal infection in man and animals and were used extensively in the treatment of pneumococcal infection in man before antibiotic therapy was available.

Blood group antigens of man, discovered by Landsteiner in 1900, are naturally occurring antigens in the red cells. There are six genotypes (OO, AO, AA, BO, BB, and AB), but only four phenotypes (O, A, AB, and B). Therefore, it is assumed that there are three allelic genes (O, A, B) and that the A and the B genes are dominant over the O genes,

There are at least 12 different blood group systems in man besides the ABO system. Among these the MN system and the Rh system are clinically important. The Rh system, after having been recognized by Levine and Stetson from a fascinating experiment of Nature, was defined by Landsteiner and Weiner in 1940. The transplacental sensitization of the mother by her fetus results in a severe hemolytic disease of the newborn (page 349).

Blood group substances are found in other tissue cells (e.g., sperm, liver, muscle, spleen, kidney, and lung) as well as in secretions (saliva, gastric juice, amniotic fluid, seminal fluid, and cervical mucus). They are present on red blood cells early in their individual differentiation, e.g., the normoblast stage. Individuals who secrete the blood group substances (e.g., into their saliva) are called *secretors,* and the secretion is controlled by a *secretor gene.* Blood group A and B substances are found in the saliva of about 80 percent of individuals whose red blood cells have corresponding blood group antigens. The H substance, a biosynthetic precursor of A and B substances, is found in the secretions of individuals producing both A and B blood group substances, as well as in the secretion of 80 percent of those with blood group O. Persons who do not secrete A, B, or H substances have the Lewis[a] substance, a precursor of H substance, in their secretions.

The blood group substances are composed of glycolipids containing fatty acids, sphingosine, and mucoproteins. The serologic specificity resides in the carbohydrate moieties of glycolipids (Table 5-1).

The simplest polysaccharide antigens are dextran and levan. By virtue of their relatively simple structure, the polysaccharide antigens have been used extensively to define antigenic determinants and antibody combining sites of the antigen molecules. Kabat and his colleagues investigated the capacity of various glucose units (linked $1 \rightarrow 6$) to inhibit the precipitation of dextran by antidextran antibodies (haptenic inhibition). The inhibitory capacity of glucose chains rose to a maximum when the number of glucose residues was increased to 6 or 7 units. From this experiment,

Table 5-1.   Site of Serologic Specificity

Gene	Structure	Specificity
—	β-Gal-($1\rightarrow3$ or 4)-GNAc - - - $\uparrow$ α1,2 Fuc	H
A	α-GalNAc-($1\rightarrow3$)-β-Gal-($1\rightarrow3$ or 4)-GNAc - - - $\uparrow$ α1,2 Fuc	A
B	α-Gal-($1\rightarrow3$)-β-Gal-($1\rightarrow3$ or 4)-GNAc - - - $\uparrow$ α1,2 Fuc	B

the maximum size of the antigenic determinant of dextran was estimated to be 34 $\times$ 12 $\times$ 7 Å.

Heterophil Antigens. The antibody against type XIV pneumococci agglutinates and lyses human red blood cells (Type -A). Since the polysaccharides of pneumococci and human blood group substances are apparently unrelated, the antibody reacting with both is called the *cross-reacting antibody,* and the reacting antigens are called *cross-reacting antigens.* An antibody that cross reacts with different antigens in many phylogenetically distinct species is called a *heterophil antibody.* The antigens capable of these cross reactions are called *heterophil antigens.* In 1911 Forssman injected emulsions of liver, spleen, kidney, adrenals, testes, and brain tissues of guinea pigs into rabbits. To his surprise the rabbits produced an antibody which reacted not only with the tissues of guinea pigs, but also with the red blood cells of sheep. This antibody, called *Forssman antibody,* belongs to one of the many heterophil antibody systems. Another example of a heterophil antibody was found in serum of a patient with *infectious mononucleosis* as describd by Paul and Bunnell. This antibody, which cross reacts with the red blood cells of sheep, is called the *Paul-Bunnell antibody.* All heterophil antibodies thus far identified cross react with red blood cells of one kind or another. Therefore, it is potuslated that the heterophil antigens, whose exact chemical nature is not known, may contain polysaccharides that determine the antigenicity of the molecule.

LIPIDS

Purified lipids do not appear to elicit an immune response unless combined with a foreign protein (*combined immunization*). Antibodies against lecithin, cephalin, and cholesterol have been produced by this means. The foreign protein or serum is said to act as a carrier, but the exact mode of its action is not known. The lipid molecules in this case function as a hapten.

Lipids constitute parts of the endotoxins, blood group substances, and the heterophil antigens. The antigenicity of these substances is controlled by carbohydrate moieties, not by lipids. Heidelberger explained the lack of immunogenicity of lipids by the lack of repeated structure in the lipid molecules. *Cardiolipin* and *cytolipin* are two important lipid haptens. Cardiolipin, the specific hapten of the Wassermann antigen that is used universally in a serologic test for syphilis (STS) was originally discovered in beef heart; hence it was named cardiolipin. It is now found in a wide variety of plants and in animal tissues. It consists of three glycerol molecules esterified with two phosphates and four molecules of unsaturated fatty acid (Fig. 5-1). The cytolipins are made up of sphingosine. One of the cytolipins, cytolipin-H, has a lactose group which determines the specificity of the molecule.

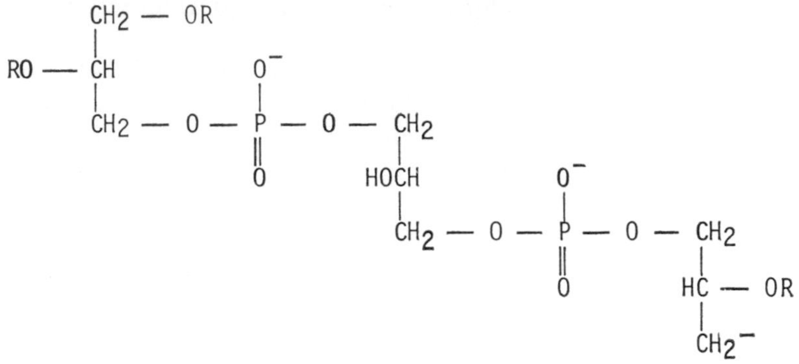

$$
\begin{array}{l}
\text{CH}_2 \text{ --- OR} \\
\quad | \\
\text{RO --- CH} \qquad\qquad \text{O}^- \\
\quad | \qquad\qquad\qquad | \\
\text{CH}_2 \text{ --- 0 --- P --- 0 --- CH}_2 \\
\qquad\qquad\qquad\quad \| \qquad\qquad | \\
\qquad\qquad\qquad\quad \text{0} \qquad\quad \text{HOCH} \qquad\qquad \text{0}^- \\
\qquad\qquad\qquad\qquad\qquad\qquad | \qquad\qquad\quad | \\
\qquad\qquad\qquad\qquad\quad \text{CH}_2 \text{ --- 0 --- P --- 0 --- CH}_2 \\
\qquad\qquad\qquad\qquad\qquad\qquad\qquad \| \qquad\qquad\quad | \\
\qquad\qquad\qquad\qquad\qquad\qquad\qquad \text{0} \qquad\qquad \text{HC --- OR} \\
\qquad\qquad\qquad\qquad\qquad\qquad\qquad\qquad\qquad\qquad | \\
\qquad\qquad\qquad\qquad\qquad\qquad\qquad\qquad\qquad\quad \text{CH}_2{}^-
\end{array}
$$

Fig. 5-1. Cardiolipin.

NUCLEIC ACID

For many years nucleic acids were said to be nonantigenic. However, it was later found that the lysates of T_4 bacteriophages could induce rabbits to form a specific antibody directed against nucleic acid. The extension of this is found in a human disease called *lupus erythematosus* (page 372). Antibodies to single-stranded DNA and double-stranded DNA were found in the sera of patients with this disease. It is now possible to make DNA antigenic by boiling and cooling preparations of DNA rapidly so that the DNA molecule separates into a single strand to which *bovine serum albumin* (BSA) may be attached. Further, an antiribonucleic acid antibody can be readily induced by intravenous administration of ribonucleic acid (RNA).

SYNTHETIC POLYPEPTIDES

A dream of the immunologist is to have antigens whose exact chemical structure of the antigenic determinants is known. Synthetic polypeptides may be just such antigens. Studies of such antigens provide useful information as to the size, the shape, and the amino acid sequence of the antigenic combining site. They may also be useful in defining the exact chemical nature of the inducing components that distinguish the antigen from the haptens. Various methods for the synthesis of homopolymers and copolymers of peptides are available.

Polymers containing single amino acids were generally found to be nonimmunogenic. Copolymers of glutamine-lysine in the ratio of 6:4 were found to be weakly immunogenic. There are many synthetic polypeptides that are known to be immunogenic.

Some important concepts developed from the study of synthetic polypeptides are that (1) the antigenic site of molecules must be accessible to the hypothetic "recognizing machinery" of immunogloblin-producing cells, (2) the D-polypeptides are generally more immunogenic than are

L-polypeptides, and (3) molecules with net charge density between +75 to −75 percent were most immunogenic. One usually cannot prove the non-immunogenicity of a substance but can only infer it because under different conditions a substance may be shown to be either haptenic or immunogenic.

Synthetic polypeptides can be coupled with antigenic hapten such as the DNP (2.4-dinitrophenyl) group. DNP or DNFB (dinitrofluorobenzyl) is used as a skin sensitizing agent for the evaluation of capacity to mount specifically cellular immune responses in man.

CHEMICALLY MODIFIED ANTIGENS

Landsteiner immunized rabbits with azoprotein to which he attached aniline or one of a number of acid derivatives of aniline. The rabbit produced an antibody specific to each of these chemically modified antigens (Table 5-2). This pioneering work opened a new field of immunology and greatly influenced the theory of immune response.

During the last few decades a variety of techniques for attaching low molecular chemicals to proteins and synthetic polypeptides have been developed; for example, (1) iodination, (2) diazotization and the coupling through the aromatic amino group, (3) isocyanate ($R-N=C=O$) or isothiocyanate ($R-N=C=S$) reaction with the free amino group of proteins, (4) the mixed anhydride reaction for coupling the carboxyl group to the amino group, (5) the carbodiamide reaction for coupling

Table 5-2. Chemically Modified Antigens and Their Specificity

Antiserum against Azoprotein coupled with the Hapten	Azoproteins coupled with			
	Aniline	4-Aminobenzoic acid	4-Aminobenzene sulfonic acid	4-Aminobenzene arsonic acid
	NH_2	NH_2 / COOH	NH_2 / SO_3H	NH_2 / AsO_3H_2
Aniline	+ + +	−	−	−
4-Aminobenzoic acid	−	+ + + ±	−	−
4-Aminobenzene sulfonic acid	−	−	+ + + ±	−
4-Aminobenzene arsonic acid	−	−	−	+ + + +

After Landsteiner, K. (1962): *The Specificity of Serological Reactions.* New York, Dover Publications, Inc.

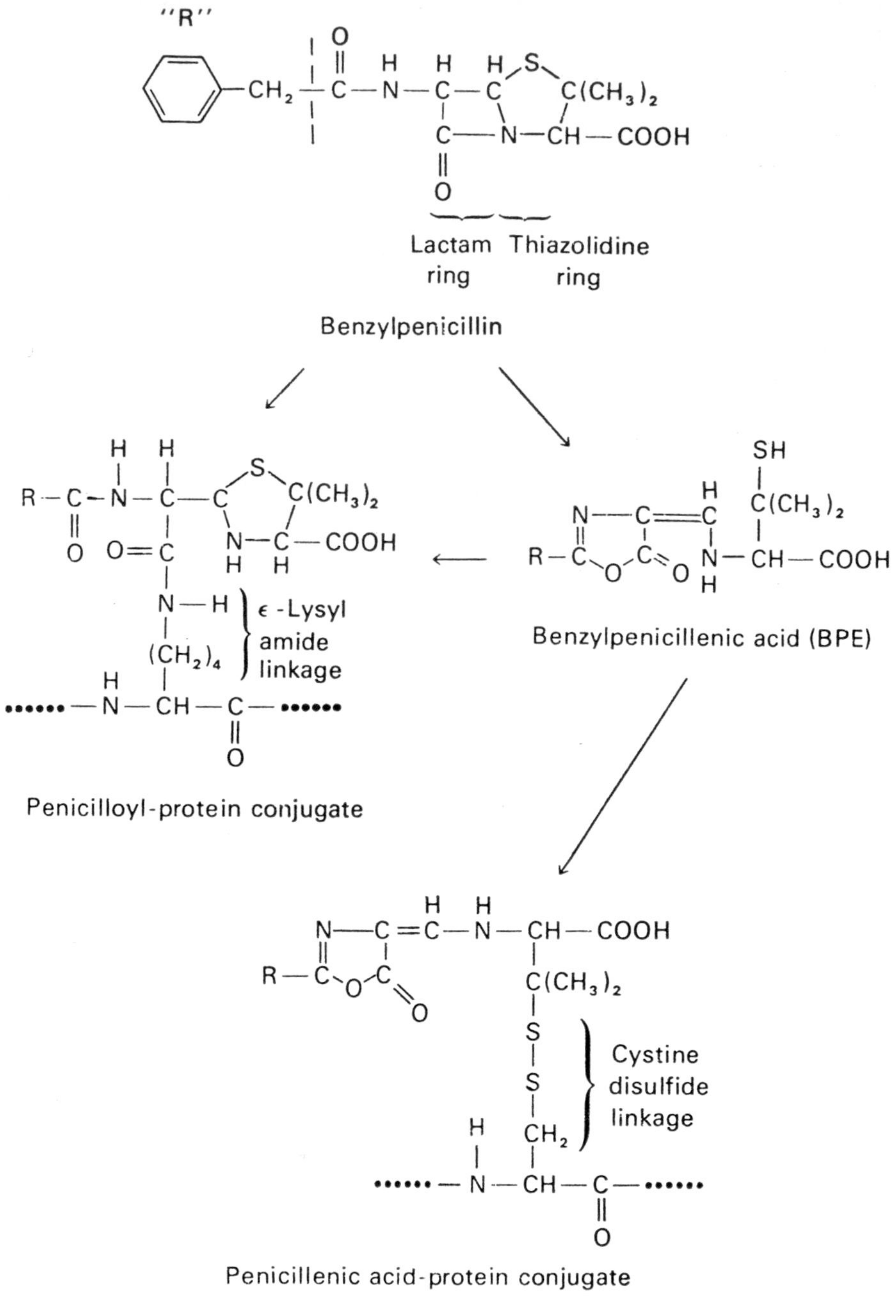

Fig. 5-2. Coupling of penicillin with protein. Penicillin may combine with the amino groups of proteins or with the sulfhydryl groups.

of carboxyl group to the amino group, (6) the coupling of penicillin to the amino group of proteins, (7) the coupling of the dinitrophenyl group to the free amino groups of proteins, (8) the coupling of ribonucleosides to the free amino acid of proteins, and many other methods have been used. The chemical reactions for the coupling of the dinitrophenyl group and penicillin are shown in Figure 5-2.

The low molecular weight compounds attached to the proteins are called *haptens*, and the chemical groups in the protein to which the hapten is attached is called the *haptenic group*. Since the haptenic groups appear to be an important part of the antigenic determinant, they are also sometimes called the *immunodominant groups*.

Aromatic rings, sugars, steroids, peptides, purines, and pyrimidines have been attached to proteins and conjugated to either antigens or antibodies for different purposes. For example, fluorescent compounds (fluorescein and rhodamine) and electron dense materials (ferritin) have been used to trace antigens and antibody molecules in the tissues.

ROUTES, DISTRIBUTION AND FATE OF ANTIGENS

Antigenic or haptenic substances enter the body by a variety of routes. The most common routes by which antigens gain access to the body in natural immunization, e.g., infection and foods, are the respiratory tract and the gastrointestinal tract. The skin and the mucous membrane are important routes for simple chemical haptens. Substances that can pass the placental barrier can also be immunogenic for both mother and fetus (transplacental immunization).

In artificial immunization, the antigens or haptens are introduced either into the blood stream, e.g., injection, transfusion, or transplantation, or locally, e.g., subcutaneous, intradermal injection or contact with the surface of the skin.

One of the central questions of current immunobiology is how the antigens find their way to appropriate cells and how they are recognized, processed, and distributed so that they can effectively engage the cellular systems responsible for the specific components of the immune reaction. These complex biologic processes are gathered under the the term *afferent limb of the immune response*. Unfortunately at this time many uncertainties characterize our knowledge of these relations, and much work is still to be done before we fully understand the afferent limb.

Antigens tagged with either colored materials or radioactive substances have been convenient tracers to determine distribution of antigen in the body. The foreign antigen injected into the blood stream, for example, will follow the general features of blood circulation reaching the liver, spleen, and bone marrow where the veins and arteries are connected by the sinusoids. In the sinusoid the antigens come in contact with the phagocytic cells which may ingest the antigens with varying efficiency. The foreign proteins introduced by the subcutaneous route are carried by the lymph to the lymph nodes and then to the veins. In the lymph nodes, the lymph passes through the sinusoids which are also lined with phagocytic cells. Foreign proteins may diffuse through the basement membranes of the vessels with the diffusion rate being proportional to the radius of the molecule. Particles or large molecules from the capillaries may escape through the gaps between the lining cells into the extravascular spaces.

Substances that persist in the extravascular space for a relatively longer period (e.g., foreign protein, some synthetic polypeptides) have three phases of clearance: an initial equilibrium phase, the phase of slow elimination due to catabolism of the free antigen, and the final phase of more rapid disappearance of antigens due to the enhanced phagocytosis of immune complexes by the phagocytic cells (immune clearance) (Fig. 5-3). In contrast, substances such as flagellar antigens, polypeptides composed of D-amino acids, and those of the high molecular weight or particulate antigens have a generally short half-life in the circulation (1 to 2 percent of injected antigens being found in the blood 12 hours after injection).

Most protein and synthetic polypeptides injected by almost any route are disseminated rapidly throughout the body, broken down, and then excreted rapidly. Frequently one can find less than 1.0 percent of the injected material in the entire lymphoid tissue 48 hours after adminis-

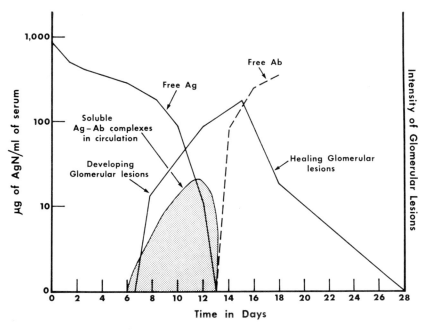

Fig. 5-3. Three phases of antigen (Ag) clearance are shown in the curve of Free Ag. The initial decline represents the equilibrium phase, followed by catabolic phase, and final rapid decline due to immune clearance.

tration. Substances that are not easily ingested by phagocytic cells will persist in the extracellular fluid for some time. Once the foreign substances are ingested, the duration of antigen retention depends on the digestibility of the compound by the phagocytic cells. Substances such as pneumococcal polysaccharides and D-amino acid polypeptides may persist within cells for long periods because they are not readily digested by the phagocytes.

How much of the antigen injected is actually involved in the induction of immune response? Probably only a small amount of injected foreign antigen needs to be active. For example, less than 1.0 percent of hemocyanin (a total amount of 2 gm was given to a rabbit) is said to be involved in the induction of immunity. This fact has made it difficult to assess the functional significance of antigen distribution and metabolism in immune responses. There is always much "noise" in the methods for analyzing these important questions.

Where are the antigens trapped? Some general features of the antigens captured in the mammalian lymphoid system have been derived from the studies of Nossal and Ada. The antigen introduced subcutaneously will reach the draining lymph nodes within a few minutes to a few hours and then be taken up by macrophages in the lymph node medulla. Some permeable antigens may diffuse into the extravascular space of the cortex of the lymph nodes or the white pulp of the spleen. The long-term retention of antigens may occur in the macrophages of the medulla and in the follicles of the lymph nodes, as well as in the marginal zone and the follicles of the spleen. The antigens may be retained in the phagosomes (page 161) of macrophages, and on the surface of the dendritic reticular cells of the follicles in the node. The follicular trapping of the antigens on the surface of the dendritic reticular cells is dependent on the presence of antibody, but the trapping of the antigen by the macrophage is probably independent of the antibody. The site of the antigen retention is not the same site as that of the antibody production. The dendritic reticular cells appear to be a mechanism for surface trapping of antigens and of fundamental importance in the development of immune response. The antigen taken up by the neutrophils appears to play no major role in immune response. Macrophages may play an enhancing role in the immune response by "processing the antigen" in some way (e.g., RNA-complex or super antigen), but the exact mechanism of this influence is not yet understood.

Do the "natural" antibodies play a role in trapping antigens and in the induction of primary immune response? Kim, Bradley and Watson in their studies of "immunologically virgin" newborn piglets showed that the initiation of phagocytosis and the induction of immune response take place in such animals in which antibody is not detectable by the most sensitive techniques available.

When the antigens enter the body, they do not simply behave like a gas entering a box. In fact, there appears to be an elaborate mechanism for the distribution, storage, catabolism, and disposal of antigens, but we are still far from knowing the exact mechanisms involved in the *afferent limb immunity*. It is certain, however, that the mechanism by which the antigens are handled must be influencing the entire immune response, i.e., the phenomena of positive feedback and negative feedback, the activation of lymphocytes, and the origin of diversity of the immune response. Whatever the exact mechanism may be, the antigens, having reached the site where they can contact lymphoid cells, are ready to meet with lymphocytes to induce proliferation, differentiation, and production of antibodies. How they do it is discussed in Chapter 6.

SELECTED REFERENCES

Avery, O. T., and Heidelberger, M. (1923): J. Exp. Med. 38:81.
Eylar, E. H., et al. (1969): Arch. Biochem. 129:468.
Forssman, J. (1911): Biochem. Z. 37:78.
Heidelberger, M. (1956): *Lectures in Immunochemistry*. New York, Academic Press.
Kabat, E. A. (1968): *Structural Concepts in Immunology and Immunochemistry*. New York, Holt, Rinehart and Winston, Inc.
Kim, Y. B., Bradley, S. G., and Watson, D. W. (1966): J. Immun. 97:52.
Landsteiner, K. (1900): Z. Bakt. (Orig.) 2:357.
Landsteiner, K. (1901): Wien. Klin. Wschr. 14:1132.
Landsteiner, K. (1921): Biochem. Z. 119:294.
Landsteiner, K., and Weiner, A. S. (1940): Proc. Soc. Exp. Biol. Med. 43:223.
Levine, P., and Stetson, R. E. (1939): JAMA 113:126.
Nossal, G. J. V., and Ada, G. L. (1971): *Antigens, Lymphoid Cells and the Immune Response*. New York, Academic Press.
Paul, J. R., and Bunnell, W. W. (1932): Amer. J. Med. Sci. 183:90.

FURTHER READINGS

Day, E. D. (1972): *Advanced Immunochemistry*. Baltimore, The Williams & Wilkins Company.
Heidelberger, M. (1939): Bact. Rev. 3:49.
Hogland, R. J. (1967): *Infectious Mononucleosis*. New York, Grune & Stratton.
Jenkin, C. R. (1963): Advances Immun. 3:351.
Landsteiner, K. (1962): *The Specificity of Serological Reactions*. Springfield, Illinois, Charles C Thomas.
Plescia, O. J., and Braun, W. (eds.) (1968): *Nucleic Acids in Immunology*. New York, Springer-Verlag.

6
Theories of Immune Response

Theories are only hypotheses, verified by more or less numerous facts. Those verified by the most, are the best; but even then, they are never final, never to be absolutely believed.

Theory must be continually altered to keep pace with the progress of science and must be constantly resubmitted to verification and criticism as new facts appear.

CLAUDE BERNARD

NUTRITIONAL THEORY

Pasteur in 1880 proposed perhaps the earliest theory of immunity against the microbial diseases. He observed that the culture medium used for the isolation of certain bacteria failed to support the growth of the same bacteria a next time unless a fresh medium was added. Since he did not have a chemically defined medium at that time, he had no way of knowing the exact component(s) of the medium he might have supplemented for the one used. Whatever the exact component(s) might have been, an essential part of the nutritional requirement for the microbes was thought to be exhausted in the medium. He extended this idea to the *in vivo* counterpart, i.e., the phenomenon of immunity. He postulated that an animal becomes immune to the second attack of a microbial disease because the essential substance required for growth of microbes has been exhausted. Therefore, the microbe could no longer grow in the animal. This theory could well explain the phenomenon of specific immunity to a microbial disease in terms of the depletion of the specific nutrient, but could not accommodate newer findings: (1) immunity can be induced by using non-living bacteria; (2) various kinds of antibodies (antitoxins) are found in the sera of immune animals; (3) immunity can be transferred to another animal by giving serum from the immune animals.

SIDE CHAIN THEORY

Ehrlich, in 1900, in his Croonian Lecture, entitled "On the immunity with special reference to cell life," proposed a general theory of immunity in terms of antibody formation, which is known as the *side chain theory*.

CLONAL SELECTION THEORY

In 1957, Talmage and Burnet independently proposed a theory of cell selection. According to this theory, antigens can react with many kinds of cells rather than with globulin, as postulated by Jerne. The antigens react with the appropriate cells and induce the cells to make a specific antibody. These theories of cell selection were further advanced by Burnet (1959). According to this theory, many different kinds of clones of cells, capable of recognizing different antigens, develop spontaneously by the process of random somatic mutation. In this concept a surface receptor for the antigen is essential and Burnet postulated that the receptor is the antibody itself. An antigen will selectively react with the specific clone and induce further differentiation of the cell to produce a specific antibody. During the process of random mutation, a clone of cells, which will react with one's own body antigen, may develop. Such clones are rapidly eliminated by early contact with the self antigens before they can develop further (forbidden clone). This would explain the phenomenon of self tolerance and would predict the induction of tolerance in fetal life, an explanation supported by the studies of Medawar and his co-workers. This theory also explains the pathogenesis of so-called autoimmune disease by postulating the appearance of the forbidden clones which react with components of one's own tissue. This hypothesis, although it avoids the difficulties of instructive hypotheses, still cannot explain the following problems: (1) how the genome of an individual could contain sufficient genetic information to code for the production of all the enormous variety of antibodies which theoretically are possible and (2) how an individual cell expresses only one or two of these immense possibilities. However, the clonal selection theory at the present time is considered to provide the best means of accounting for many of the features of immunologic responses.

THEORIES FOR ORIGIN OF DIVERSITY OF ANTIBODY MOLECULES

As our knowledge of the structure of antibody (the immunoglobins) (page 91) has advanced, many theories have been proposed to account for the genetic basis of the diverse structure of immunoglobulins. The main features of the immunoglobulin structures that we are trying to account for can be summarized as follows: (1) The immunoglobulins are composed of pairs of heavy (H) and light (L) polypeptide chains. The heavy chains vary according to the class of immunoglobulin. (2) Each L (light) and H (heavy) chain has a constant part whose amino acid sequence is similar in all classes, and a variable part whose amino acid sequence differs in different classes of molecules. (3) The antibody specificity is due to the unique sequences of amino acids in the variable part.

The germ line theory postulates that separate genes controlling the synthesis of all possible L and H chains are present in the zygote, and consequently in every diploid cell in the body. Only a single pair of genes, e.g., one for the L, and one for the H chain, may be expressed by any cell at a given time. The problems with the germ line theory are to explain (1) how genes controlling the detailed structures of the variable parts of the L and H chains required to make all possible specific antibodies could be stable during the entire evolution of any species, (2) how the genetic drift could be avoided during the entire course of evolution, and (3) how the ancestors of any species could have all the genes for antibodies which would have no survival advantage for them.

The somatic mutation theories on the other hand, postulated that the zygote contains relatively few genes controlling immunoglobulin synthesis, and the great diversity of immunoglobulin structures is due to the random mutation of lymphocytes during the lifetime of the individual. This hypothesis provides an attractive alternative to the germ line theory, but it is known that the frequency of somatic mutation in a given cell is only about one in a million. The frequency of mutation to account for the diversity of antibodies would be too high to accept easily. Another difficulty of this theory is how one part of each L and H chain (variable part) is subjected selectively to variation. To explain this latter phenomenon, it was proposed that a "scrambler" gene, or generator of diversity (GOD), causes crossing over selectively in that part of the cistron controlling the variable parts of immunoglobulins.

ACTIVATION/INDUCTION THEORY

Various theories of the adaptive immunity so far reviewed have attempted to explain the following major features of immune response:

1. Animals can be induced to make an infinite number of specific antibodies against an infinite number of foreign antigens (either natural or synthetic).
2. The antibody is produced by lymphocytes and plasma cells.
3. Animals do not make antibody, as a rule, against their own body components.
4. The antibody specificity is due to the unique sequence of amino acids in the antibody molecule.
5. Immunologic tolerance (or negative adaptation or unresponsiveness) can be specifically induced by antigens.

The following characteristics of the immune response have not been fully considered in any one of the theories outlined above:

1. The existence of two components of the immune system, i.e., the cell-mediated immunity and humoral immunity.
2. Regulation of cellular immunity mainly by the thymus and of humoral immunity by the bursa, or bursa equivalent.

3. Absence of the antigen from the thymus or the bursa.
4. Independence from known antigenic stimulation of lymphopoiesis in the thymus and in the bursa.
5. Dependence of certain antigens on T-cells and of others on B-cells.
6. Activation of the lymphocyte to proliferate by nonspecific mitogen such as PHA, as well as by specific antigen.
7. Separate sites in the lymph node for the thymus derived (T) lymphocytes and the bursa derived (B) lymphocytes.
8. Cooperation of T-cells and B-cells in some instances of antibody formation.
9. Residence of the receptors for the activating substance in the membrane of responding cells.
10. The "processing" of antigen by macrophage.
11. The phenomenon of the transfer factor.
12. The phenomenon of antigenic competition.
13. Induction of "true" primary immune response in immunologically virgin animals without detectable "natural" antibodies.

The activation theory that we propose will accommodate these additional facts (Fig. 6-2). This theory postulates (1) that the post-thymic

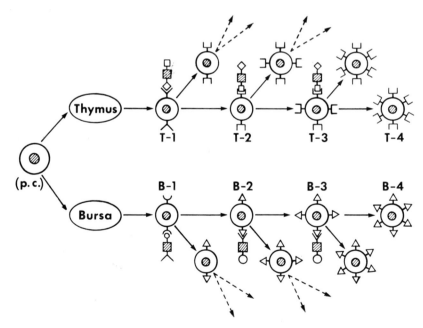

Fig. 6-2. Proposed scheme of the activation induction process. The *activating component* of immunogen reacts with the receptors of T-1 or B-1 cells, i.e., *activation*. The activated T-1 or B-1 cell will transform and divide to give rise to progeny, i.e., B-2 or T-2 cells which will display receptors for the *inducing component* of immunogens. The inducing component of the immunogen will then react with B-2 or T-2 cells to *induce* further differentiation and proliferation.

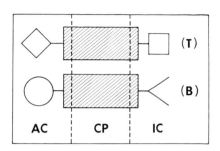

Fig. 6-3. Proposed model of immunogen based on the activation induction theory. AC. Activating component. CP. Carrier portion. IC. Inducing component. (T). Immunogen directed against thymus dependent cells. (B). Immunogen directed against bursa dependent cells.

(T-1) cells and the post-bursal (B-1) cells have a limited multipotentiality and (2) that the immunogen has two components, one for the induction of antibody specificity and one for the activation of either B-1 or T-1 cells (Fig. 6-3).

The functions of the thymus and the bursa are to produce T-1 cells or B-1 cells, which (1) carry cell surface receptors that will react with the activating component of the antigen and (2) have receptors that differ, so that an antigen will react with either T-1 cells or B-1 cels, but not necessarily with both. However, since induction of an immune response by one immunogen often activates both T-cell and B-cell immunities, we must assume that most antigens carry activators for receptors on both T-cells and B-cells.

An antigen carrying an activating component for B-1 or T-1 cells will combine with the group of B-1 or T-1 cells that carry corresponding receptors. This step will activate the B-1 or T-1 cells to transform. The antigen-receptor complex will be invaginated into the cell while the activated cells enter the S-phase of the cell cycle and become hypermutable. The antigen-receptor complex will combine with the RNA of activated cells and influence the synthesis of the new DNA, so that the induction component of the antigen will be copied into the DNA molecules. The progeny of the activated cell will carry a new kind of specific cell receptor that will react with the inducing component, but not with the activating component of the antigen. These newly formed progeny cells are B-2 or T-2 cells. They may carry more than one receptor, i.e., they may carry two or three identical receptors which will react more readily with the inducing component of the antigen. Thus, the limited multipotential T-1 cells or B-1 cells have differentiated, or have been induced to become unipotential cells (B-2 cells or T-2 cells) specific for the inducing component of the antigen, i.e., *induction*. B-2 or T-2 cells then will readily react with the inducing component of the antigen and proliferate to produce progeny that will carry more of the same kind of receptor (B-3 cells or T-3 cells) and become a clone of immunocompetent cells. The receptors of B-2 and B-3 cells are the membrane-bound specific immunoglobulins. Since the B-cell series has a terminal differentiation to secretory cells, contact of the immunoglobulin receptors with antigen induces not only synthesization but also selectively secreting immunoglobulin molecules. Morphologically this event is signaled by the appearance of lymphocytes and plasma cells containing a cellular machinery highly organized for immunoglobulin synthesis and secretion, e.g., the well-developed rough endoplasmic reticulum and Golgi apparatus in cells that at an earlier stage of development showed minimal evidence of such machinery.

The receptors of T-2 and T-3 cells have not been defined chemically. The B-3 cells synthesize immunoglobulins which can be demonstrated at their surface. The B-4 cells are both synthesizing and secreting immunoglobulins, but as specialized cells they no longer have immunoglobulin receptors on their surface. In contrast, the T-3 and T-4 cells do not synthesize or secrete demonstrable amounts of any known immunoglobulin-like molecules. The immunologic functions of T-3 and T-4 cells are executed by secreting such substances as the macrophage migration inhibition factor and lymphokines upon stimulation by the specific antigens. We postulate that the T-2 cells and possibly T-3 cells may synthesize the transfer factor, this factor being nothing but the molecule consisting of the activating component and the inducing component of an immunogen for the T-1 cells. Since the transfer factor is devoid of the major part of the rest of the immunogenic molecule, this deficiency should easily account for its low molecular weight and its resistance to proteolytic enzymes. The activating component of transfer factor will react with and activate the T-1 cells. Since it will carry the same inducing component (determinant group), the T-2, T-3 and T-4 cells will carry the same specificity as the original whole molecule of the immunogen.

The phenomenon of antigenic competition can be explained in this model by postulating that the pool size or the available number of B-1 or T-1 multipotential cells at any given time is rather limited. Since any immunogen carrying activating components for either B-1 or T-1 cells may react with a larger proportion of existing available B-1 or T-1 cells, the second challenge of a different immunogen must be met with a slow or minimal response until the depleted pool of B-1 or T-1 cells is restored. The T-1 or B-1 cells do not carry the receptors for the activating component of self antigen, i.e., self unresponsiveness (or self tolerance). The breakdown of self unresponsiveness is due to the appearance of the hidden part of the immunogen molecule which happens to function as an activating component of the self immunogen to cross react with the receptors of T-1 or B-1 cells of its own. Induction of acquired tolerance is achieved by postulating the abortive activation, i.e., the progeny of T-1 or B-1 cells fail to express the proper receptors on the surface of the membrane on which the inducing components of the antigen can react.

At the same moment, it is postulated that there would be fewer than 100 kinds of B-1 cells which account for the different genetic codes for

the constant part of the different classes of immunoglobulins and different allotypes of immunoglobulin. The codes for the variable parts of immunoglobulin are generated or remodeled at the time of activation of B-1
cells via a mechanism similar to the scrambler gene, or generator of diversity (GOD). The T and B cell cooperation phenomenon is explained by
postulating that the receptor of B-1 cells can be modified by the product
of T-1 or T-2 cells (lymphokine) so that the activating component of
antigen can react better with the modified B-1 receptor than with the
unmodified B-1 receptor. (This could happen in the lymph nodes or in the
spleen, where the T and B cells are close to each other.)

The existence of a forbidden clone, so disappointing as a mechanism
of autoimmunity, can be replaced by the concept of a *forbidden immunogen*. The forbidden immunogen implies that the hidden activating component of immunogenic molecules appears and is available to the pre-
existing receptor of one's own T-1 or B-1 cells. This can be a consequence
of endogenous or exogenous processes, i.e., bacterial antigens cross react
with the host's tissue antigen. The hidden activating component then
happens to react to the T-1 or B-1 cell and initiates the sequence of immune response. However, when that activating component accompanies
an inducing component which cross reacts with the host's tissue component, it may not be expressed operationally as a forbidden immunogen
(abortive activation).

The malignant adaptation can take place by a number of mechanisms:
(1) immunodeviation, i.e., the interplay of the blocking antibody, the
cytotoxic antibody, and the killer cells, and (2) immunologic nonresponsiveness. The immunologic nonresponsiveness can be consequent to perturbation at four levels:

1. Abortive or inappropriate activation.
2. Depletion of corresponding T-1 or B-1 cells.
3. Lack of receptor for the activating component on T-1 or B-1 cells—
   true self tolerance.
4. Lack of activating component on the antigen.

It is postulated that tolerance exists because, among the 100 or so receptors for immunogen, none is present to accommodate the activating
component of the host immunogen. To account for this, one must postulate some mechanism for gene exclusion. One possibility is that while
dividing in the central lymphoid organ, e.g., thymus or bursa, the potential immunoresponsive clones for most host immunogens are eliminated
as proposed by Jerne. Thus autoimmunity would always be consequent
to responses to host immunogens not effectively excluded by this means,
e.g., myelin peptides, thyroglobulin, or immunogens of the host which
cross react with those of non-self origin. A substance may not be immunogenic because of the lack of an activating component, although it has a
good inducing component. This concept can also explain species specific

response, i.e., a substance can be immunogenic to one species of animal, but not the other. Depletion of any subgroups of T-1 or B-1 cells can take place with aging. Breakdown of tolerance can be explained (1) by the appearance of hidden activating or inducing components of immunogens, (2) by the appearance of abnormal T-1 or B-1 cells which carry the receptors for the activating component of self antigen, and (3) by the failure of central lymphoid organs to eliminate cells with forbidden receptors, as in aging.

The antigen can be taken up by the macrophage and made more immunogenic. This is accomplished by modifying (1) the activating component so that it can have an increase in the affinity for the receptor on B-1 or T-1 cells or (2) the inducing component so that it minimizes the frequency of abortive activation. In this way, we can explain why some antigens can be more immunogenic after macrophage processing. Furthermore, certain soluble antigens may be paralytogenic because they have a propensity to react with B-1 or T-1 cells to give rise only to the abortive activation. Therefore, the animal will be temporarily non-responsive (paralysis) until the number of corresponding depleted B-1 and T-1 cells are restored. If the immunogen is long-lasting, the duration of unresponsiveness will be prolonged because the new wave of B-1 or T-1 cells will be consumed continuously until the immunogen is exhausted.

Fishman's super antigen or RNA-antigen complex can be an informational RNA functioning like a transfer factor that was induced by the immunogen. Macrophages may carry receptors like those on B-1 or T-1 cells, and other somatic cells may also carry a few or all of B-1 or T-1 type of receptors. RNA of macrophage, primed by antigen contact, could produce an RNA which transfers to proliferating cells information that contributes to the specificity of the antibody. This RNA could act more readily on the duplicating DNA during cell division.

The concept of abortive activation would simply imply that T-2 or B-2 cells may carry receptors on their surface different from those anticipated because, in responding to the activating component and engulfment of the immunogen, they have produced inappropriate copies that act as inefficient receptors or have no capacity to act as receptors for the second stimulation by the inducing component of the immunogenic molecule. Such T-2 or B-2 cells would thus be unable to react with the original immunogen to achieve antibody synthesis. Considering this in superficial terms, we might say that the animal is not responding to an immunogen or that the substance may not be immunogenic to the animals. However the T-2 or B-2 cells may actually have been activated to become T-3 and B-3 cells and actually be expressing different kinds of surface receptors. But, we may not be able to detect this response, since we are testing for the response to the original immunogen and not testing for the response that has been achieved.

This theory is compatible with the known features of immunity, including the recent information concerning carrier specificity, cooperative interactions between T- and B-cell immunities, and the new information which derives from the two-component concept of the immunity systems. In addition it predicts the following:

1. Some nonimmunogenic molecules may be made immunogenic by coupling them to known activators.
2. Immunogens will be fractionable into activating and inducing components. If the T-cell immunity derives from proliferation of cells that possess the T-activation receptor, T-cell immunity should be achieved by stimulation with the activator alone. Perhaps this is what already has been achieved in the experiments by Benacerraf and Gell.
3. Antigenic competition will tend to sort with respect to activators rather than with respect to inducers.
4. High dose tolerance produced to one antigen from depletion of B-1 or T-1 cells should give unresponsiveness to other competing antigens.
5. Malignant adaptation achieved by the so-called true tolerance mechanism should be reversible by coupling a new activator to the inducer.

The new concepts that are introduced here are (1) that activation of T-cell and B-cells is potentially separable and (2) that activation involves attachment of inducer to the cell surface and potential engulfment of the inducer so that with the B-cell line at least, and possibly with the T-cell, it can achieve reverse transcription and production of new receptors and secretory products for which the cell was not originally programmed genetically.

With this conception the T-1 or B-1 cells possess a limited number of receptors which make it possible for them to be activated to proliferate by the activating component common to many antigens. The process of activation would include engulfment of the whole immunogen, and the inducing component could then act via a reverse transcription process to induce the replicating cell to produce a product. In B-cells this product would be immunoglobulin which would appear at the surface membrane of the cell as a secondary specific receptor for the immunogen. Further encounter with the inducing component of the immunogen could thus induce further proliferation and terminal differentiation to a secretory cell and produce specific antibodies in a great abundance. For T-cells the activating portion of the immunogen could induce production of more cells with the specific activation receptors complementary to the activating molecules. Thus the possibility that T-cell immunity is less specific than B-cell immunity would have to be entertained, and some evidence favoring this view has been presented.

This theory proposes (1) that chemical dissection of immunogens will separate that part of the molecule which can activate lymphoid cells (T-1 or B-1 cells) from the other part of the molecule which can induce B-cells to produce specific antibody and (2) that T-cell immunity may be achieved as well by the activating part as in the complete immunogens. Since reverse transcription is essential to this concept for B-cells at least, the postulate would insist that evidence for reverse transcription be present at least in the activated B-cell population.

SELECTED REFERENCES

Alexander, J. (1932): Protoplasma *14*:296.

Benacerraf, B., and Levine, B. B. (1962): J. Exp. Med. *115*:1023.

Billingham, R. E., Brent, L., and Medawar, P. B. (1956): Phil. Trans. Roy. Soc. (London, Series B) *239*:357.

Breinl, F., and Haurowitz, F. Z., (1930): Z. Physiol. Chem. *192*:45.

Burnet, F. M. (1959): *The Clonal Selection Theory of Acquired Immunity.* Nashville, Tennessee, Vanderbilt University Press.

Burnet, F. M., and Fenner, F. (1941): *The Production of Antibodies.* Melbourne, Macmillan.

Ehrlich, P. (1900): Proc. Roy. Soc. Biol. *66*:424.

Fishman, M. (1961): J. Exp. Med. *114*:837.

Gell, P. G. H., and Silverstein, A. M. (1962): J. Exp. Med. *115*:1037.

Jerne, N. K. (1955): Proc. Nat. Acad. Sci. U.S.A. *41*:849.

Landsteiner, K. (1945): *The Specificity of Serological Reactions.* Cambridge, Massachusetts, Harvard University Press.

Mudd, S. (1932): J. Immun. 23:81.

Pasteur, L. (1880): C. R. Acad. Sci. *91*:673.

Talmage, D. W. (1957): Ann. Rev. Med. 8:239.

FURTHER READINGS

Bretscher, P. A., and Cohn, M. (1968): Nature *220*:444.

Makela, O., and Cross, A. M. (1970): Progr. Allerg. *14*:145.

Pauling, L. (1940): J. Amer. Chem. Soc. *62*:2643.

Smithies, O. (1967): Science *157*:267.

Talmage, D. W. (1959): Science *129*:1643.

7
Cellular Immunity

DELAYED HYPERSENSITIVITY

When immunogen (or hapten) is applied to the skin of sensitive individuals, one of two kinds of skin reactions can be observed: (1) an immediate reaction characterized by the appearance of a wheal and erythema at the site of application, starting within a few minutes, and reaching its maximum intensity in 10 to 20 minutes, or (2) a delayed skin reaction characterized by the appearance of erythema at the site of application, starting in 2 to 4 hours, and reaching its maximum reaction with induration in 48 to 72 hours; hence it is called delayed hypersensitivity.

Perhaps the first description of a delayed hypersensitivity skin reaction under controlled conditions was made by Jenner in 1798. He noted that a papular erythematous lesion of the skin developed at the site of inoculation of vaccinia virus and reached its highest intensity in 24 to 72 hours in persons who had previously been vaccinated. He called this lesion "reaction of immunity" and marveled at the fact that increased inflammation rather than decreased inflammation was associated with the state of immunity. In 1890, Robert Koch described a classical form of hypersensitivity in guinea pigs infected with tubercle bacilli. When live tubercle bacilli were injected into the skin of infected guinea pigs, a dark indurated nodule appeared at the site of the injection after 24 hours and spread to become a sloughing ulcer. In the uninfected control animal, the inoculated site remained quiet and healed with a small nodule. This reaction is known as the Koch phenomenon and can be produced not only by live tubercle bacilli, but also by dead bacilli and by a cell-free extract of the bacilli, e.g., tuberculin. The first clinical use of Koch's phenomenon was reported by Epstein in 1891, who showed that the skin reaction to the old tuberculin could be produced in children and found this test to be useful for the diagnosis of tuberculosis in children. Further extension of Epstein's observation was made by Von Pirquet. Mantoux developed a method of intradermal injection of tuberculin, the Mantoux test, which has been of great value in clinical testing.

The immunologic significance of Koch's phenomenon (i.e., tuberculin-type skin reaction) was not clear at that time. It was not until 1925 that

Zinsser distinguished the tuberculin type of skin reaction from other forms of hypersensitivity skin reactions, such as the Arthus reaction. He pointed out that the reaction to tuberculin could take place without demonstrable circulating antibodies. This reaction he called "delayed hypersensitivity" or "bacterial allergy," since this phenomenon could also be found in a number of other bacterial infections, e.g., Salmonella typhi (typhodin), Pfeifferella mallei (malein), and Brucella abortus or brucellin (abortin).

How does the delayed type of hypersensitivity take place when there is no demonstrable specific antibody? Another 17 years elapsed before a clue to the solution of this puzzling problem was found. In 1942 Landsteiner and Chase succeeded in transferring a delayed hypersensitivity skin reaction to picryl chloride in guinea pigs with leukocytes from the peritoneal exudate of sensitized animals. Chase in 1945 extended this observation to tuberculin skin reactions and transferred the skin sensitivity by the leukocytes of peritoneal exudate of guinea pigs with positive tuberculin reaction. It was later found that not only the leukocytes from the peritoneal exudate, but also leukocytes from the peripheral blood and from the lymph nodes were equally effective in transferring delayed hypersensitivity. Therefore, it could be concluded that the sensitized leukocytes in the peritoneal exudate, peripheral blood, and nodes confer the skin sensitivity to the recipient animals. Alternatively one could also speculate that a trace amount of antibody attached to the cell surface may be responsible for the transfer. Lawrence, who showed in 1955 that an extract of peripheral blood leukocytes from sensitized humans is capable of transferring the tuberculin skin sensitivity to the tuberculin negative recipient called the substance in the leukocytes the "transfer factor." Thus far, the transfer factor as described by Lawrence is limited to human systems and has never been unequivocally demonstrated to operate in any animal model. This difficulty has interfered with the molecular definition of such a potentially important substance.

Since delayed hypersensitivity can only be transferred by leukocytes from sensitized persons, the term *cellular immunity* or *cell-mediated immunity* is now used to describe those types of immunity in which humoral antibodies cannot be demonstrated, but sensitized cells can transfer the sensitivity that is revealed by the delayed skin test reaction. The delayed hypersensitivity skin reaction is only one of many manifestations of cellular immunity. This form of immunity plays a major role in solid tissue allograft rejections, in the development of manifestations in some autoimmune diseases, in bodily defense against certain bacteria, certain viruses, and many fungi, and in the defense against cancer.

INDUCTION OF DELAYED HYPERSENSITIVITY

The introduction of a proper immunogen into an appropriate animal leads to the development of delayed hypersensitivity (induction). After a certain interval, the subsequent challenge with the same immunogen results in the manifestation of delayed-type hypersensitivity (elicitation). The induction phase corresponds to the primary phase of antibody production, and the elicitation phase corresponds to the secondary response. By contrast to the humoral immune response, the manifestation of delayed hypersensitivity cannot at present be measured quantitatively. Despite the difficulty of its quantitation, delayed hypersensitivity and cellular immunity occupy a central area in the rapidly advancing field of modern immunobiology.

What kind of immunogen can induce the delayed-type hypersensitivity? The protein component of various kinds of microorganisms has been found to be related to the development of the delayed allergies. A wide variety of chronic and acute infectious diseases caused by bacteria, viruses, fungi, and protozoa have been shown to be accompanied by the development of delayed hypersensitivity. The elicitation of the delayed hypersensitivity skin reactions with protein extracts of these organisms has been a powerful tool for the diagnosis of diseases produced by them (Table 7-1).

A frequent route for producing delayed hypersensitivity is introduction of immunogens via percutaneous absorption following the application of substances of low molecular weight to the skin, e.g., nickel salts, urushiol from the primrose or poison ivy plant, paraphenylenediamine (hair dye),

Table 7-1. Delayed Hypersensitivity Skin Reactions Used for Diagnostic Purposes in Man

Diseases	Test substance
Tuberculosis	Old tuberculin, purified protein derivative (PPD), filtrate of culture, modified by heat
Leprosy	Lepromin: suspension of leprosy bacteria obtained from infected skin and lymph node
Brucellosis	Brucellin: filtrate of Brucella melitensis or Brucella abortus Brucellergen: nucleoprotein of the bacteria
Glanders	Mallein: a filtrate of culture of glanders bacillus
Tularemia	Protein extract of Pasteurella tularensis
Candidiasis	Candida albicans
Dermatomycosis	Trichophyton
Coccidioidomycosis	Coccidioidin
Histoplasmosis	Histoplasmin
Mumps	Killed virus
Psittacosis	Killed virus
Lymphogranuloma inguinale (venereum)	Extract of yolk sac of infected egg
Cat-scratch fever	Extract of affected lymph node
Hydatid disease	Casoni antigen: hydatid cyst fluid
Leishmaniasis	Extract of the culture

and DNCB (dinitrochlorobenzene), or picryl chloride. It is believed that these substances combine with a body component, presumably proteins in the skin, which can then act as a sensitizing immunogen. Finally, transplantation antigens and tumor specific antigens can also induce delayed hypersensitivity, i.e., cell-mediated immunity, which is generally believed to play a major role in transplantation rejection (page 229) and the prevention or recovery from cancer development (page 201). Other unique features for the induction of delayed hypersensitivity are that (1) it is more easily induced by the use of so-called adjuvants; (2) the protein molecules are mainly effective for such induction, but the polysaccharides seem not to be effective; and (3) the size of the determinant group of the antigen appears to be larger than that involved in humoral immune responses.

What kind of specific tissue response takes place in the lymphoid system after the immunogen is introduced? The lymph nodes draining the site of the sensitized area of the skin enlarge markedly during the ensuing four or five days. On the second day of response, a small number of pyroninophilic "transformed" lymphocytes develop in the deep cortical areas (thymus dependent areas) of the lymph node (page 37, Fig. 4-7). These pyroninophilic lymphocytes reach a maximum number on the fourth day. At their outer limits these expanded deep cortical regions with their organized cortical nodules adjoin the outer regions of the cortex; inwardly they abut on the medulla of the node. By the autoradiographic study of sections of these lymph nodes, it has been shown that the cells in the deep cortical area proliferate actively to give rise to their daughter cells, which are small lymphocytes. The onset of delayed hypersensitivity coincides roughly with the appearance of these labeled (newly formed) small lymphocytes in the circulation at four to five days after exposure to immunogen. When the skin is removed 12 hours after applying the immunogen, the entire cellular changes in the lymph node will continue to develop, followed by a subsequent development of delayed hypersensitivity. This finding indicates that the initial induction process must have been completed within 12 hours of application.

The foregoing changes during the sensitization process in production of delayed hypersensitivity appear to be in sharp contrast to those observed in the humoral immune response (page 77). These differences are illustrated schematically in Figure 7-1.

The differences in the degree and ease of induction of delayed hypersensitivity are determined by (1) genetic factors, (2) age, and (3) sex. Ontogenically, the ability to develop delayed hypersensitivity appears at a well-defined moment in many species quite early in fetal life, and in species like man the capacity of cell-mediated immune response is present by the time of birth and differs only quantitatively from that of adults. Tuberculin sensitivity may be poorly expressed in the neonate, probably

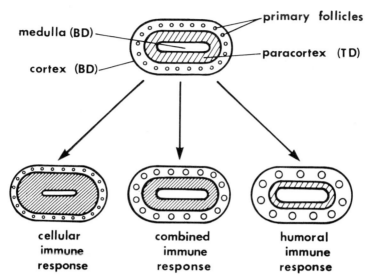

Fig. 7-1. A schematic illustration of cellular, humoral, and combined immune responses. [From Turk, J. L. (1967): *Delayed Hypersensitivity*. New York, John Wiley & Sons, Inc.]

due to a deficient capacity of the skin to sustain the hypersensitivity reaction.

MANIFESTATION OF DELAYED HYPERSENSITIVITY

The characteristic delayed type of skin reaction appears at 5 to 6 hours and reaches a maximum at 18 to 48 hours. In bacterial allergy (e.g., tuberculin reaction) the reaction is characterized by the early appearance of an erythematous papule followed by the development of an indurated lump. In contact allergy, e.g., contact dermatitis, the prominent lesion is a vesicle formation. Histologically the lesions show initial infiltration of polymorphonuclears (at 2 to 3 hours) at the site, followed by the characteristic local perivascular accumulations of mononuclear cells (monocytes, lymphocytes, and macrophages). The distribution of the infiltration is largely determined by the distribution of the eliciting immunogen (Fig. 7-2). More than 80 percent of the mononuclear cells are monocytes which resemble lymphocytes by light microscopy, but have distinctive features of monocytes on electron microscopy. These histologic features are seen in the lesions of contact allergy, graft rejection, and many autoimmune diseases such as thyroiditis and experimental allergic encephalomyelitis, as well as in the classical form of the tuberculin type of skin reaction. Phylogenetically cell-mediated immunity, e.g., allograft rejection, has been demonstrated in representative forms of all vertebrates and may actually exist in some invertebrates, e.g., the earthworm.

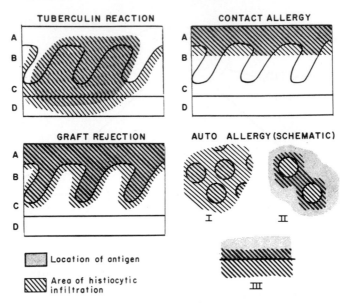

Fig. 7-2. Relationship between tissue location of antigen and areas in which mononuclear cell infiltration and parenchymal damage occur. A. Surface epidermis. B. Follicles and upper dermis. C. Deeper dermis. D. Subcutaneous fat and muscle. I. Islands of antigen-containing parenchyma, e.g., in testis. II. Islands of vascular and connective tissue, e.g., in central nervous system. III. Parallel or interpenetrating arrangement, e.g., in adrenal, peripheral nerve, uvea, meninges. [Fom Waksman, B. H. (1960): In *Cellular Aspects of Immunity* (Ciba Foundation Symposium) Wolstenholme, G. E. W., and O'Connor, M. (eds.). London, Churchill, p. 280.]

The entire reaction of delayed hypersensitivity is believed to be initiated by a small number of sensitized lymphocytes which, upon stimulation by the immunogen, release a variety of humoral factors (the mediators of cellular immunity). The migration inhibition factor (MIF) released from the sensitized lymphocytes causes monocytes to accumulate at the site of the injected immunogen. These monocytes then are transformed into macrophages or so-called "angry macrophage." The angry macrophage then releases lysosomal enzymes that can damage the tissue and provoke an intense inflammatory reaction (Fig. 7-3).

Jones and Mote described a skin reaction similar to the delayed hypersensitivity which occurs during the early stages of humoral immune response to "pure" proteins. This reaction, which is known as the Jones-Mote reaction, has several characteristic features: (1) it is transient; (2) it can be transferred by peripheral blood leukocytes; (3) the induration of skin is minimal; and (4) the accumulation of plasma cells can be observed in the late stage of reaction in contrast to the classical delayed hypersensitivity reaction.

Recent studies by Turk have demonstrated that the Jones-Mote phenomenon is greatly enhanced but that antibody production is almost completely suppressed by a single appropriately timed injection of cyclophosphamide. This result strengthens the linkage of the Jones-Mote phenomenon to the cellular (T-cell) immunities, dissociates it from the humoral immunities, and reveals the potential that humoral immunities have for obscuring the manifestation of cellular immunities.

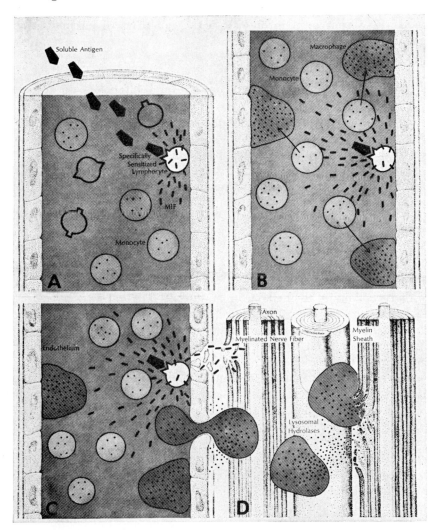

Fig. 7-3. Steps in a delayed hypersensitivity reaction. A. Soluble antigen encounters a sensitized lymphocyte in a venule. The antigen combines with cell-bound antibody, and MIF is released. B. The MIF makes passing monocytes sticky and may also affect the venular endothelium. Monocytes are activated and gradually transformed into macrophages. C. Activated macrophages force their way through the endothelium and vessel wall. D. Release of lysosomal hydrolases, which attack both vessel wall and parenchymal elements. The parenchymal target is represented by the myelin sheath. [From B. H. Waksman (1971): In Immunobiology, Good, R. A. (ed.). New York, Sinaver Assoc.]

A delayed hypersensitivity reaction can be observed in the cornea of a highly sensitized animal. The corneal reaction is characterized by a milky white opacity increasing up to 24 to 48 hours after the application of the immunogen to the cornea and is particularly useful in demonstrating delayed hypersensitivity when the animal has circulating antibodies responding to the immunogen, as well as delayed hypersensitivity. The corneal reaction is absent even in animals with high titers of circulating antibodies.

MEDIATORS OF CELLULAR IMMUNE RESPONSE

The first step in the manifestation of delayed hypersensitivity is the interaction of the sensitized lymphocytes and the appropriate immunogen. It is not known, however, what type of molecule on the surfaces of the sensitized lymphocytes interacts with the antigenic determinant of the delayed type of hypersensitivity. This indeed represents one of the major unsolved problems of modern immunobiology. It may be an unknown kind of immunoglobulin, e.g., Ig-X. Some have proposed that small amounts of IgM at the surface of T-lymphocytes are responsible; others postulated that a small portion of immunoglobulin molecule, e.g., the combining site of light chain or heavy chain determinants, is responsible; still others have contended that buried immunoglobulins are responsible for the specificity of the cellular immunities. To date, however, no direct molecular basis for the cell-mediated immunities has been demonstrated. Since quantitative methods for measurement of cell-mediated immunities have been introduced, questions have been raised concerning the precise specificity of cell-mediated immunity. These reactions may be much less specific than are the antibody responses. Nonetheless, the sensitized lymphocytes undergo a blast transformation as a result of their interaction with the antigenic determinant. The transformation of the sensitized lymphocytes important to expansion of the lymphocyte population itself may not be essential to the triggering of lymphocytes to contribute to subsequent cellular infiltration or to the production of lymphokines that are released by lymphocytes after contact by specific antigens.

The lymphokines thus far described have a wide variety of biologic and chemical properties and have the potential to influence in many different ways the development of inflammation and the bodily defense to it. Recent estimates, for example, have proposed that the biologic influence of a single lymphocyte reacting with antigen can be amplified by a factor of several thousand in influencing the cellular immune mechanism.

Among the many factors produced by the sensitized lymphocytes (Table 7-2), the migration inhibition factor (MIF) is known to exert powerful

Table 7-2. Possible Mediators of Cellular Immunity (Lymphokines)

1. Migration inhibition factor (guinea pig, mouse, rat, human)
2. Macrophage spread inhibitory factor (guinea pig, mouse)
3. Macrophage aggregating factor (guinea pig)
4. Skin reactive factor (guinea pig)
5. Products of antigen recognition (PAR) (mouse, rat)
6. Lymphotoxin (mouse, human, guinea pig)
7. Cloning inhibitory factor (human)
8. Inhibitor of DNA synthesis (human, mouse)
9. Chemotactic factor (guinea pig)
10. Blastogenic factor (guinea pig, mouse, human)
11. Interferon (human)
12. Transfer factor (human)
13. Lymph node permeability factor (rat, guinea pig)
14. Cytophilic antibodies (rat, guinea pig, mouse, human)
15. Direct lymphocyte-target cell cytotoxicity (mouse, human, guinea pig, rat)

effects on the normal monocytes and peritoneal exudate cells. The release of MIF by sensitized lymphocytes is triggered by the same antigens that elicit the delayed hypersensitivity skin reaction. This indicates that the release of MIF by lymphocytes is immunologically specific and correlates well with *in vivo* and *in vitro* effects. The MIF was shown to be a protein molecule (MW: about 50,000 to 70,000), synthesized by the lymphocytes within 6 to 9 hours after the interaction with the immunogen. The effects of MIF on the monocytes *in vitro* appear to be (1) to render the monocytes "sticky" to the vessel wall and inhibit the migration (Figs. 7-3, 7-4), (2) to increase the survival and the differentiation of monocytes in culture and lead to an "activated" state characterized by an increase in size and pinocytic activity and a decrease in the basophils of the cytoplasm

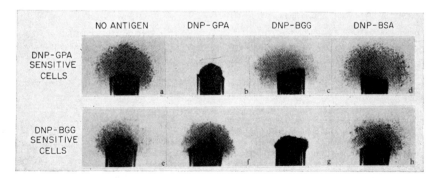

Fig. 7-4. *In vitro* reactions of sensitized cells. Inhibition of migration of sensitized guinea pig peritoneal exudate cells (macrophage) out of capillary tubes in culture in the presence of specific antigen. Cells from animals sensitized with conjugates are affected only by conjugates containing both hapten and carrier protein used initially for sensitization. This "carrier specificity" is characteristic as well for elicitation of skin reactions and other *in vitro* reactions of sensitized cells. Preparations were photographed at 24 hours. [From David, J. R., Lawrence, H. S., and Thomas, L. J. (1964): Immunology 93:279. By permission of The Williams & Wilkins Co., Baltimore.]

(i.e., angry macrophage), and (3) to produce these effects on monocytes without reference to immunologic specificity.

These angry macrophages are believed to be instrumental in the destruction of bacteria, fungi, viruses, and perhaps parenchymal cells that often occurs in cell-mediated immune responses, e.g., graft rejection and autoimmune thyroiditis. It is interesting to note that only a small number of sensitized lymphocytes can trigger the remaining large number of monocytes and mononuclear cells to participate in the cell-mediated immune reaction. *In vivo* cell transfer experiments show, for example, that only a small fraction (2 to 8 percent) of the mononuclear cells accumulated at the site of a cell-mediated immune response are the sensitized lymphocytes, which trigger the entire sequence of the manifestation of the delayed hypersensitivity reaction. The direct injection of MIF into the skin has been shown to elicit a skin reaction similar to that observed in delayed hypersensitivity. Recently it has been shown that certain macrophages have surface receptors to which MIF can attach. These receptors are trypsin and chymotrypsin sensitive but are resistant to the influence of neuraminidase.

FACTORS INFLUENCING CELLULAR IMMUNE RESPONSE

The cellular immune responses are susceptible to all the agents known to affect the immune response in general (Chapter 17). The depletion of the pool of thymus derived (T) lymphocytes in particular, results in the general unresponsiveness in cell-mediated immunity. This general unresponsiveness can be achieved by (1) neonatal thymectomy in many animals, (2) X-irradiation, (3) radiomimetic drugs, (4) antileukocyte serum (ALS), (5) prolonged corticosteroid treatment, and (6) pyridoxine deficiency. The induction phase of cellular immunity can also be blocked by a massive dose of unrelated immunogen administered at the same time. The established cellular immunity can be eliminated or minimized by all the procedures that deplete the T-lymphocytes, e.g., thoracic duct drainage.

A specific tolerance or unresponsiveness to a particular immunogen can be achieved by the exposure to an immunogen in the early stage of the ontogenic development of immunity, e.g., in fetal life, or by a repeated exposure of the immunogen during the postnatal period (Chapter 16). The specific abolition of existing cellular immunity (desensitization) can also be achieved to a certain degree by a repeated exposure to a large dose of the immunogen, but such a desensitization lasts only a few days and often seems to be related to the state of competing humoral immunity.

In contrast to the humoral immune response, the cellular immune response cannot be transferred passively by the serum containing the specific antibody. When proper studies have been carried out, it has been shown to be transferred by the lymphocytes of sensitized donors in man and in all species, and the mechanism of transfer in man appears to be the strange dialyzable "transfer factor." The manifestation of the cellular immunity is hindered by (1) the depletion of the effectors, i.e., monocytes, macrophages, vascular permeability, and coagulation factors and (2) the so-called blocking, enhancing, or deviating antibodies (Chapter 16).

Benacerraf and Gell in 1959 demonstrated the difference in specificity between the antigen-antibody reaction and the delayed hypersensitivity reaction (Table 7-3). In their work they showed that the hapten and a region on the carrier portion of the immunogen are involved in cell-mediated immunities. This phenomenon of carrier specificity may indicate that the area of the immunogen involved in cell-mediated immunity is greater than that involved in antigen-antibody reactions. It was later found, however, that the carrier specificity can also be demonstrated in the early phase of induction of humoral immune responses. If sensitization is accomplished with one protein and its hapten, a secondary response in humoral immunity occurs when a second exposure is presented by the same hapten on another carrier. However, cell-mediated immunity is expressed only to the first hapten carrier combination (Table 7-3 and Fig. 7-4).

Sulzberger, and later Chase, observed that animals fed allergens that are potent developers of delayed hypersensitivity in normal animals may be made specifically unresponsive to subsequent parenteral administration of these antigens. This fascinating phenomenon has never been fully explained but will be considered later with the phenomena of immunologic unresponsiveness, tolerance, and negative adaptation.

IMPAIRED CELLULAR IMMUNITY IN MAN

Capacity to develop and express cellular immunity can be assessed by (1) testing the pre-existing hypersensitivity state and (2) provoking delayed hypersensitivity by an active immunization.

Patients with Bruton-type (X-linked infantile) agammaglobulinemia

Table 7-3. The Difference in Specificity between Humoral and Cellular Immunity

Animal Immunized against a Carrier Hapten Molecule Tested with	Antigen-Antibody Reaction*	Delayed Hypersensitivity†
Carrier-hapten molecule	+	+
Carrier alone	−	+
Hapten alone	+	−

*Hapten specificity in humoral immunity.
†Carrier specificity in cellular immunity.

ordinarily have full vigor of their cell-mediated immunity, even though they can make no circulating antibody. By contrast, patients with DiGeorge syndrome lack cellular immunity and patients with ataxia-telangiectasia, Wiskott-Aldrich syndrome, and the common variable forms of immunodeficiency have varying degrees of deficiency of the cell-mediated immune response. Other patients with apparently normal T-cell systems seem to have deficits of delayed allergic responses and other kinds of cell-mediated immunity because they are defective in the biologic amplification systems, e.g., production of lymphokines or response of effectors that are ordinarily engaged by the T-cell immunity.

Various viral infections (measles, mumps, influenza, and others) are known to be associated with the temporal depression of pre-existing cell-mediated immunity *in vivo* and *in vitro*. Cell-mediated immunity is also depressed in patients with sarcoidosis, Hodgkin's disease, rheumatoid arthritis (sero-positive), Sjögren's syndrome, primary biliary cirrhosis, and secondary syphilis, and in patients receiving various chemotherapeutic agents and X-irradiation. In patients with chronic lymphatic leukemia, both the cellular and humoral immunities are depressed. A selective depression of the cellular immune response is associated with lepromatous leprosy and chronic mucocutaneous candidiasis.

SELECTED REFERENCES

Benacerraf, B., and Gell, P. G. (1959): Immunology 2:53.
Benacerraf, B., and Levine, B. B. (1962): J. Exp. Med. 115:1023.
Chase, M. W. (1945): Proc. Soc. Exp. Biol. Med. 59:134.
Chase, M. W. (1954): Int. Arch. Allerg. 5:163.
Epstein, A. (1891): Prag. Med. Wschr. 16:13.
Jenner, E. (1798): An Inquiry into the Causes and Effects of Variolae Vaccinae. London.
Jones, T. D., and Mote, J. R. (1934): New Eng. J. Med. 210:120.
Koch, R. (1890): Deutsch. Med. Wschr. 16:1029.
Landsteiner, K., and Chase, M. W. (1942): Proc. Soc. Exp. Biol. Med. 49:688.
Lawrence, H. S. (1949): Proc. Soc. Exp. Biol. Med. 71:516.
Lawrence, H. S., (1954): J. Clin. Invest. 33:951.
Mantoux, C. (1919): Presse Med. 18:10.
Sulzberger, M., and Baer, R. L. (1938): J. Invest. Derm. 1:45.
Turk, J. L. (1967): Delayed Hypersensitivity. New York, John Wiley & Sons, Inc.
Zinsser, H. (1925): Proc. Soc. Exp. Biol. Med. 22:35.
Zinsser, H., and Mueller, J. H. (1925): J. Exp. Med. 41: 159.

FURTHER READINGS

Bloom, B. R., and Glade, P. R. (1971): In Vitro Methods in Cell-mediated Immunity. New York, Academic Press.
Lawrence, H. S. (1970): New Eng. J. Med. 283:411.

8
Humoral Immune Response

INDUCTION OF ANTIBODY FORMATION

The exact process of induction of antibody formation is unknown, but we do know that the immunogens in some way induce the lymphoid system to produce antibody. The first step must be the encounter of the immunogen and the responding cells in the lymphoid system. Several possibilities exist for interaction of immunogen with the immunocompetent lymphocytes to induce the production of antibody: i.e., (1) the immunogen may enter the cells and direct the DNA, mRNA, or polyribosome of the cells to produce a specific protein (antibody); (2) the immunogen may simply interact with the cell surface receptor molecule, a homologous antibody, and initiate a "surface to nuclear signal" that tells the cell to divide and undergo a terminal differentiation and then begin to produce and secrete its natural product, antibody; (3) the immunogen is taken up by the lymphoid cells or by other phagocytosing cells, which may modify the immunogen and release the "processed" immunogen, which in turn stimulates the antibody-producing cells by mechanisms as indicated above in (1) or (2); or (4) the immunogen may combine with the pre-existing repressor in the cell and de-repress the capacity to produce specific antibody. Most evidence supports the second possibility.

Immunogens introduced intravenously are quickly localized to the spleen, liver, bone marrow, kidney, and lungs. Within 24 hours the amount of immunogen in the spleen and liver is very small, and by 48 hours more than 80 percent of most immunogens has been excreted via urine. The immunogens introduced into the foot pad or into the subcutaneous tissue are localized mainly in the draining lymph nodes, and only small amounts of immunogens are found in the spleen.

It has been shown in nonimmunized animals that at least a portion of immunogen is taken up by the macrophages in the medullary cords of the lymph nodes, in the red pulp of the spleen, and in the cells lining the sinuses of the cortex of the lymph nodes. By contrast, in previously immunized animals, immunogens are localized mainly at the surface of dendritic macrophages of the cortex of the lymph node. From these observations, it is postulated (1) that the "antigen-processing" by macrophages may be needed for the induction of primary immune response, and (2) that in the previously immunized animal, the immunogens are localized on the surface of the dendritic macrophages so that the "memory cells" can encounter those immunogens easily and be stimulated to proliferate and produce antibody.

What do we mean by "antigen-processing"? We can only speculate from vast data (1) that the macrophages within the lymphoreticular system may differ from other phagocytic cells so that the immunogenic component of the foreign substances is preserved or potentiated during the usual process of degradation by the lysosomal enzymes of the phagocytes, (2) that the immunogen within the macrophages may induce the formation of information RNA which in turn can direct a specific antibody formation by the lymphocytes, or (3) that the RNA of macrophage forms a complex with the immunogen and that this combination acts as a *super immunogen* in some way perhaps by facilitating the entry of immunogen into lymphocytes. It appears that the RNA-immunogen complex formed within macrophages may be necessary to induce a primary immune response, whereas the same immunogen injected for the second time interacts with the pre-existing antibody on the surface of macrophages. Consequently, instead of being taken up into the cells, the immunogen molecules seem to be localized around the surface of the dendritic processes. Attempts to locate the immunogen in the lymphocytes and plasma cells that actually produce antibody have always met with great difficulty, and the results are usually negative or inconclusive. Part of the difficulty is due to the extremely small number (estimated to be 150 cells in 10^8 mouse spleen cells) of lymphocytes that is capable of responding to any given immunogen by antibody production.

What is the nature of the small fraction of lymphocytes that interact with the immunogen? How can such cells arise in the first place? These are the central questions of immunobiology to be answered in the future. It looks, however as though lymphocytes having a specific antibody at their surfaces, especially antibody of the IgM class, may be driven by antigen to a terminal differentiation to antibody-secreting cells.

In any case, the introduction of immunogen is usually followed by a "lag phase" before any antibody can be detected in the circulation. Here again, the definition and the duration of lag phase can vary, depending on the sensitivity of the method used for detecting the antibodies. During the first 24 to 48 hours after the introduction of immunogen, an active synthesis of both mRNA and rRNA is known to take place; this is followed by a morphologic change in the lymphocytes, i.e., transformation, cell division, and differentiation to a veritable factor for synthesis of immunoglobulin. These steps appear to be necessary for the initiation of antibody production at least in volume. These morphologic changes occur prominently in the red pulp or at the edges of the white pulp of the spleen and in the medullary cords or in the mantle zones surrounding germinal centers in the cortical areas of the lymph node.

These newly differentiated antibody-producing cells can be identified by (1) their characteristic pyroninophilic cytoplasm and nucleus containing blocks of chromatin apparently arranged in a wheel-spoke pattern (plasma cell, Fig. 4-4) and (2) the presence of immunoglobulin and antibody molecules in the cytoplasm, which can be shown by immunohistochemical methods (page 129). During the periods of cellular proliferation following encounter with an effective immunogen, the size of the lymphoid organ increases. By the end of the first week, after exposure to immunogen, the organ involved returns to normal size. The typical plasma cells appear to be short-lived, averaging only 2 to 3 days. On the other hand, memory cells appear to be long-lived (890 to 6745 days in man). The memory cell for antibody production seems to resemble a small lymphocyte (Fig. 4-1A). The memory cells are postulated to provide the link between the primary and the subsequent immune response. Makinodan and Albright have shown that the number of progenitors of responding cells to an "antigen" in the spleens of unimmunized mice is approximately 170, but after contact with immunogen by replication this population of responding cells may have expanded 1000-fold by the fourth day. The average generation time of these cells in mice is estimated to be about 8 to 9 hours; thus the progenitor cells probably have divided as many as ten times during this interval.

How long does the immunogen persist in the body? The well-known long-lasting immunity following certain viral infections, e.g., smallpox and yellow fever, is believed to be mainly due to the presence of persisting virus probably as "latent virus" in the host tissues. With nonreplicating immunogens great differences exist in the persistence of the immunogen in the body. In part, these differences are a function of metabolism of the immunogen. Certain bacterial immunogens such as pneumococcal polysaccharides are known to persist in mouse tissue for more than a year, and in man up to 20 years. This persistence may account for the long-lasting immunity of the host to these immunogens. Not all immunogens, however, persist for such long periods, and most humoral immune reactions wane with time, probably as a function of loss of contact with active immunogen.

PRODUCTION OF ANTIBODY

From the moment of birth, no animal in its natural environment can be free of immunologic stimulation. For example, a circulating antibody against sheep red blood cells can be found in mice that have never been purposely immunized against the sheep red blood cells. Therefore, we must assume that some of the naturally occurring immunogen may have induced the production of an antibody that cross reacts with the antigenic component of the sheep red blood cells. Such an antibody is called *natural antibody*, and the immunogen, *natural antigen*.

When the animal is kept in a so-called germ-free environment and fed an "antigen-free" diet, the level of natural antibody is extremely low. Therefore, one can assume that the natural antibodies differ only quantitatively from the conventional antibodies produced by intended immunization. Since natural antibodies can react with a wide variety of bacterial, viral, and red cell antigens, the question arises as to whether any intended administration of a given immunogen can ever induce a "true" primary immune response unless the animals are kept under immunogen-free conditions.

Kim and his co-workers studied the immune response in "immunologically virgin" piglets fed with antigen-free diets. They showed a number of interesting features of immune response in these piglets: (1) the immune response could be induced in the absence of natural antibody, (2) the initial production of antibody is a 19S immunoglobulin which they considered to have an antigenic relationship to IgG molecules, but this identification has been disputed by other investigators who consider this primordial immunoglobulin to be IgM, and (3) the existence of antigenic competition is more readily demonstrable. Prior to antigenic stimulation there were few B-cells and most of the circulating lymphocytes were T-cells. The experimental data on primary immune response of animals in conventional environments may all have to be re-examined and be repeated in the germ-free animals.

When immunogen is introduced to an animal, antibody production by the animal follows a characteristic pattern: (1) the lag period, or the lag phase, (2) the logarithmic phase, (3) plateau, and (4) the phase of decline (Fig. 8-1). During the logarithmic phase, the production of antibody exceeds catabolism, and during the declining phase the catabolism exceeds production. Glenny and Südmersen in 1921 showed that the initial pattern of antibody production after the first immunization is markedly different from that of antibody production after the second immunization. The former is called *primary immune response*, the latter, *secondary* or *anamnestic response*. The primary response is sluggish, weak, short-lived, and composed mainly of 19S IgM immunoglobulin. By contrast, the secondary response is swift, powerful, prolonged, and composed mainly of 7S IgG immunoglobulin (Fig. 8-2). Differences between primary and secondary immune responses are somewhat artificial and based largely on limitations of the methods of quantitating the antibody responses. With sufficiently sensitive methods both IgM and IgG imunoglobulins can be shown to be produced in the primary as well as in the secondary immune response. However, a 19S IgM molecule may be detected much more easily than are 7S IgG molecules in systems like the hemagglutination

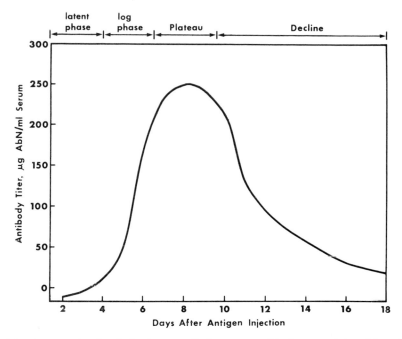

Fig. 8-1. An example of typical primary antibody response. The latent period is followed by a logarithmic rise in antibody titer, a period of plateau, and a decline phase.

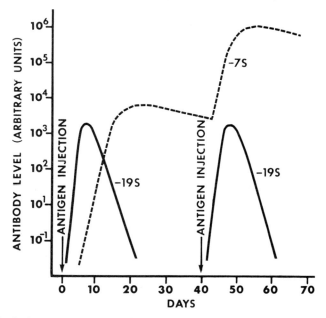

Fig. 8-2. Antibody activity in IgM and IgG immunoglobulins in the primary and secondary immune response. [This idealized diagram is based mainly on data of Uhr, J. W., Finkelstein, M. S., and Baumann, J. B. (1962): I Exp. Med. 115:655. By permission of the Rockefeller University Press.]

assay where molecule for molecule the efficiency of IgM may exceed that of IgG by as much as 750 times.

The duration of the lag phase, or latent period, can vary greatly, depending on the method of antibody detection. For example, in the classical works of Glenny and Südmersen on diphtheria antitoxin, the lag phase was three weeks, but in the recent work on the anti-bacteriophage ϕX 174, the lag phase was 20 hours. More recently, antipneumococcal polysaccharide antibody could be detected in mice within 4 hours and anti-avian erythrocyte antibody in guinea pig lymph nodes within 7.5 minutes following antigenic stimulation. Since animals on which these experiments were performed were not germ-free, one cannot be sure that these recipients are experiencing the "true" primary immune response.

More investigations by extremely sensitive methods are needed to determine whether a "true" primary response requires a longer lag phase. The "true" primary response must involve, according to the theory stated in Chapter 6, a two-step differentiation of potential antibody-producing cells. Thus one would expect differentiation from multipotent B stem cells to unipotent B-2 cells to require time. A primary response should show a longer lag phase than a second encounter with immunogen where the cells have only to be differentiated from B-2 to B-3.

The first antibody to be detected as usually measured is 19S IgM immunoglobulin, and the rate of production follows a logarithmic curve. The length of time for the twofold increase in the antibody concentration is called "doubling time." The 7S IgG, which is said to appear after the IgM globulin production, enters the logarithmic phase. At the end of the logarithmic phase, the 7S IgG production decreases much more slowly than does the 19S IgM. These relationships are schematically shown in Figure 8-2, and the relationship of the actual rate of antibody production and the concentration of circulating antibody is shown in Figure 8-3. Again it must be stressed that the differences, especially on the upswing of these curves, may be largely artificial. Appropriate stimulation of IgG production properly analyzed should give a curve parallel to that of IgM.

Phylogenetically, a humoral immune response can be demonstrated in all species of vertebrates. It is generally lacking in invertebrate species studied to date. Invertebrates need more study in this perspective, but thus far the humoral responses in these species have been less specific and based on molecules quite different from those responsible for humoral immune response in vertebrates. In the wax moth and cockroach, for example, nonspecific agglutinating bactericidal and lytic substances, as well as some substances reacting more specifically with immunogen, have been described. Phylogenetically, the most primitive immunoglobulin molecules defined in the sharks, rays, and primitive fish, like paddlefish (Polyodon) and dogfish, resemble IgM molecules and have high carbohydrate concentration and similar structural characteristics to the IgMs

I*BGG ELIMINATION & ANTIBODY RESPONSE

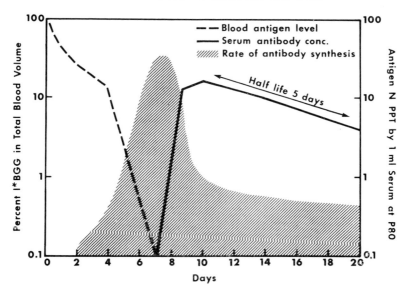

Fig. 8-3. Serum concentration of antigen and estimated rate of antibody synthesis following a primary injection of bovine gamma globulin in rabbits. [From Dixon, F. J. (1954): J. Allerg. 25:487.]

of more recent vertebrates. Much variation occurred in these primitive species in the degree of polymerization of these molecules, but only one basic class of immunoglobulin is present. Beginning with lungfish and extending to the amphibia and reptilia and on into birds and mammals, multiple immunoglobulin classes appeared. The second class of immunoglobulin has many characteristics similar to the IgG molecule of mammals and man. Thus as we progress along the phylogenetic scale, we see increasing differentiation toward the multiple classes of immunoglobulins so extensively elaborated in man and other mammals.

Ontogenetically, the onset of immunoglobulin formation closely follows structural differentiation of lymphoid organs. The onset of synthesis of IgM usually precedes the onset of IgG synthesis. There appears to be a definite progression in time from noncompetence through partial competence to full immunocompetence. For example, the fetal opossum can form antibody against the flagella antigens of Salmonella typhi by the twelfth day after conception which is equivalent to a human fetus at 8 weeks of gestation, or a rat fetus at 11 days of gestation. Antibody against the BGG (bovine gamma globulin) could not be demonstrated at this stage. In lambs, the antibody to bacteriophage ϕX 174 could be detected at 38 to 40 days of gestation, to ferritin at 66 days, to homograft rejection at 80 days, and to crystalline egg albumin at 121 days of gestation. Antibody formation to other antigens did not seem to become possible until well after birth.

Extensive studies by Solomon and his students have revealed that the time of onset of antibody-producing capacity relates directly to the time of development of the peripheral lymphoid tissues. Thus, although rats and mice do not produce significant antibody until after birth, sheep and humans can produce antibody long before birth. The beginning antibody-producing capacity in all four species relates to the time of appearance of lymphoid cells in the peripheral lymphoid tissues.

BIOSYNTHESIS AND SECRETION OF ANTIBODY MOLECULES

The early studies showing that radioactively labeled amino acids are incorporated into antibody proteins indicated a *de novo* synthesis of antibody molecules. The synthesis of antibody molecules is known to follow the general pattern of protein synthesis: (1) transcription of information from DNA into RNA, (2) translation of such information from RNA into polypeptide chains, and (3) assembly and release of the complete γ-globulin molecules as antibody. Recent advances in molecular biology have provided important information concerning the biosynthesis of antibody molecules at subcellular levels.

The immunogen reacts with appropriate lymphocytes and initiates transformation and proliferation of the cells. This is accompanied by an increased synthesis of DNA and RNA in the cells. Further experimental evidences show that immunization causes not only an increased synthesis of the RNA. Therefore, certain antibiotics, e.g., actinomycin D (at transcription) and streptomycin (at translation) can interfere with the antibody production.

In addition to the process of synthesis of the antibody molecule, the antibody-producing cells are extraordinarily equipped after differentiation to act as antibody-secreting cells. At the ultrastructural and biochemical level the organization of the antibody-producing cells is very like that of the secretory cells of the pancreas and salivary glands. For example, in recent years extensive investigations, especially those by Uhr and his colleagues, and by Choi, Knopf, and Lennox with myeloma cells, have defined the process of secretion of antibody in quite precise terms. As the antibody molecules are secreted in great numbers by these highly specialized cells, a regular process of addition of carbohydrate to the molecule and transport of the molecule to the outside of the cell takes place. It is by this process that antibody molecules can be efficiently delivered to the body fluids. Contact of an antibody-producing cell with antigen or immunogen seems to be essential to direct this terminal differentiation of the cell to become a secretory element. The product of this synthesis and secretion is the immunoglobulin molecule. The basic structure of all mammalian molecules is similar. It comprises two light and two heavy polypeptide chains joined by disulfide linkages. Details of the structure of these molecules are considered in Chapter 9.

Where is the antibody molecule synthesized and assembled? The newly synthesized protein was found to be associated with the polyribosomal fraction of cytoplasmic extracts, and the synthesis of the polypeptide chain probably proceeds in an orderly manner from the amino (N) terminal to the carboxyl (C) terminal amino acid. From these findings, a model has been proposed which predicts that each ribosome aligned on a monocistronic strand of RNA will carry a nascent polypeptide chain growing proportionally to the length of RNA assembled in the ribosome (Fig 8-4).

According to the calculations by Williamson and Askonas, the polysomes associated with the heavy chains consist of about 15 ribosomes, which would contain about 1350 nucleotides. This is a sufficient number for coding protein molecules of 450 amino acid residues. On the other hand, the polysomes associated with the light chains consist of 7 ribosomes, which is sufficient for coding protein molecules of 200 amino acid residues.

If the heavy and light chains are synthesized on separate polysomes, how are they assembled to make a complete immunoglobulin molecule? Experimental evidence has shown that these separate chains are assembled in the membrane-bound endoplasmic reticulum (ER) prior to or associated with the process of secretion. It takes approximately 60 seconds to make an H-chain, 30 seconds to make an L-chain, 2 minutes to assemble

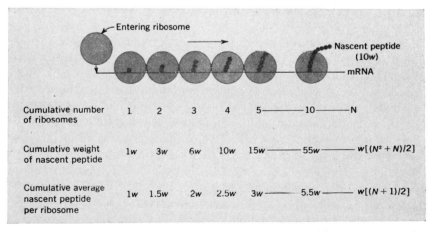

Cumulative number of ribosomes	1	2	3	4	5————	10————	N
Cumulative weight of nascent peptide	1w	3w	6w	10w	15w————	55w————	$w[(N^2 + N)/2]$
Cumulative average nascent peptide per ribosome	1w	1.5w	2w	2.5w	3w————	5.5w————	$w[(N + 1)/2]$

Fig. 8-4. Schematic representation of the increment in nascent peptide with an increasing number of ribosomes in a polyribosomal chain. The ribosomes are spaced evenly along the mRNA strand with the active sites separated by a distance of approximately one ribosome diameter. In moving this distance along the mRNA, each ribosome is assumed to acquire an increment of nascent peptide (w) represented diagrammatically as ●. [From Kuff, E. L., and Roberts, N. E. (1967): J. Molec. Biol., 26:211.]

the L and H chains, and 30 minutes to secrete the whole immunoglobulin molecule.

FACTORS INFLUENCING ANTIBODY RESPONSE

Adjuvants. The immune response to weak immunogens can be increased markedly if the weak immunogens are injected together with one
of a number of nonspecific stimulating agents called adjuvants. Freund
and McDermott in 1942 showed that injection of a suspension of tubercle
bacilli in an oil-detergent mixture (complete Freund's adjuvant) together
with immunogen markedly increased the antibody response. For the adjuvant to be effective, the aqueous solution of immunogen must be
thoroughly emulsified in the adjuvant. Freund's complete adjuvant increases both delayed hypersensitivity and antibody production, whereas
Freund's incomplete adjuvant (an oil–detergent mixture) mainly stimulates the production of antibody. The incomplete adjuvant is not by itself
immunogenic. Other known nonimmunogenic adjuvants are paraffin oil,
peanut oil, lanolin, mineral gels (aluminum hydroxide, calcium phosphate, aluminum phosphate), silica particles, cellulose, acrylamide gel,
and polynucleotides.

The tubercle bacilli in Freund's complete adjuvant are, of course,
strongly immunogenic by themselves, and can be shown to be a good
adjuvant even in the absence of the oil-detergent mixture. The adjuvant
activity of tubercle bacilli appears to be associated with a peptidoglyco-
lipid molecule derived from the wax D-fraction of the bacterial cell wall.
Examples of antigenic adjuvants are gram-negative bacteria such as Bordetella pertussis, endotoxins, acid-fast bacteria, phytohemagglutinin, and
antibody.

If the adjuvant is given before the immunogen, or given into sites different from the immunogen, the immune response is increased in a manner similar to that of simultaneous injection of both adjuvant and immunogen at the same site. However, giving the adjuvant after the immunogens often results in an increased humoral immune response with a decreased or no response of cellular immunity, i.e., *immunodeviation.*

About three weeks after the injection of immunogen in adjuvant (complete or incomplete), a granulomatous lesion develops at the site of injection. There the immunogen can still be identified in the oil-containing
vesicles of the foamy macrophage.

The exact role of adjuvants in immune response is not clear. It is presumed that the effects of adjuvants are due to (1) the delay in absorption
and elimination of immunogen resulting in a prolonged antigenic stimulation, and (2) the ability to stimulate phagocytosis of macrophages and
enhance the "processing of immunogen." These explanations seem to us
inadequate and further definition of adjuvant function is in order.

Immunosuppressive Agents. X-irradiation and radiomimetic cytotoxic

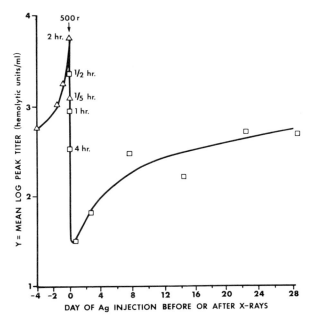

Fig. 8-5. The effect of irradiation on antibody production in a group of rabbits injected with sheep erythrocytes at various times before and after irradiation with 500 R. [From Humphrey, J. H., and White, R. G. (1963): Oxford, Blackwell Scientific Publications.]

drugs (Chapter 17) affect both primary and secondary responses of antibody production; delayed hypersensitivity is somewhat less affected. The time between the immunosuppressive treatment and the administration of immunogen is shown to be an important factor (Fig. 8-5). The greatest depression of immune response is generally found when the immunogens are given 24 to 48 hours after the immunosuppressive treatment; if the immunogens are given 2 to 4 hours before the immunosuppressive treatment, the antibody production may curiously be increased. The mechanism of immunosuppression is mainly based on disruption of DNA molecules of sensitive lymphocytes. The capacity of phagocytosis by macrophages is not necessarily decreased by this treatment. Thymectomy affects the humoral immune response to a somewhat lesser degree than it does the cellular immune response, but in the mouse and to some extent in other mammals certain antigens and the IgG component of antibody response are almost completely dependent on the presence of a thymic influence or an influence of the thymic dependent cell population.

Immune Paralysis. Sulzberger in 1929 and Chase in 1959 showed that guinea pigs can be rendered specifically unresponsive if the immunogens are fed before a parenteral challenge (Sulzberger-Chase phenomenon). Felton in 1949 showed that mice which received larger doses (0.5 to 5.0 mg) of pneumococcal polysaccharides failed to make antibody response

(Felton's paralysis), whereas a smaller dose (0.5 μg) resulted in good antibody response. With protein antigen Smith and Bridges showed that a tolerant state could be produced in young rabbits given a sufficiently large dose of antigen and that the tolerance produced was dose dependent and finite. Mitchison in 1964 showed that both low doses and high doses of certain immunogens can render animals unresponsive to a subsequent immunization. Normally, an animal does not make an immune response to its own tissue component (self tolerance or natural tolerance). This specific unresponsiveness is called *immunologic tolerance, immunologic paralysis,* or *negative immunologic adaptation.* The exact mechanisms are not known, but the phenomenon may be due to the depletion of immunologically competent cells, or to a mechanism of abortive activation (page 61).

The tolerant state to defined antigens has been much studied in recent years, especially by Weigle. His contributions reveal that low dose tolerance seems to involve only the thymus dependent cells and that high dose tolerance involves both thymus dependent and thymus independent cells. The tolerant state can be broken by introduction of immunogen closely related to the tolerance-inducing antigen but containing chemical components closely related to those of the tolerogen.

Antigenic Competition. When two different immunogens, each of which can elicit a primary response on its own, are mixed and administered in the same amounts and by the same route, the response to one of them may be largely or wholly suppressed. This phenomenon was first described by Michaelis in 1902 and is known as *antigenic competition;* the mechanisms have not been fully elucidated. Antigenic competition can be shown when the two antigens are given separately within a short interval. In this case, the antigen given as a secondary stimulus competes more effectively than the primary (first) antigens. It is not clear whether antigenic competition can be abolished by induction of tolerance. As a matter of fact, it has been shown that a form of antigenic competition may even exist in tolerance induction. The extraordinary expression of apparent antigenic competition in a virgin immune response studied by Kim and his co-workers suggests that in a primary response the relatively limited number of cells potentially to be driven by antigen to antibody-producing cells is a limiting factor in production of antibody. This finding could argue for the theory that immunologic commitment of cells by antigen occurs in initiation of an immune response.

Desensitization. It is possible to produce a state of immunologic unresponsiveness in an animal that has been sensitized and is expressing a delayed immune response. This is done by repeating an injection of a small amount of antigen for a prolonged time. This procedure is known as "desensitization." The effect is usually transient. The term *desensitization* is also used to describe a different phenomenon, i.e., the prevention of immediate allergic manifestations, e.g., hay fever, by injecting allergens repeatedly during the season. In this case the mechanism of "desensitization" seems to be due to the production of so-called blocking or competing antibodies. Even in the desensitization in cell-mediated immunity it seems likely that competing antibodies may underlie the loss of ability to express the hypersensitivity by another form of immunodeviation.

Influence of Antibody. The humoral immune response can be suppressed specifically by passive administration of specific antibody. The passively administered antibody appears to regulate the production of antibody via a feedback mechanism in normal immune response. For example, when IgG immunoglobulin of any specificity is given to animals shortly after the immunization, the production of IgG antibody is suppressed, but the production of IgA and IgM antibody may not be affected. However, IgG antibodies may repress not only IgG but also IgM and IgA antibody production and sometimes even cell-mediated immunities (class specific). When a specific antibody is given, under certain conditions the production of the specific antibody is selectively suppressed. On the other hand, Uhr has shown clearly one can quantitatively regulate (suppress or enhance) the production of antibody by removing antibody from circulation.

At present there are six biologic functions of the antibody in regulating the production of antibody: (1) the passively administered antibody can suppress the humoral immune response via a feedback mechanism, the primary response being more easily suppressed than the secondary response; (2) the antibody can modify the immune response by selectively suppressing the synthesis of a class of immunoglobulin; (3) the antibody can compete for the incoming immunogen with the immunogen-binding cells and force the recruitment of cells capable of making high affinity antibody; (4) the antibody can shift the specificity of immune response against one determinant to the other determinant of the same immunogen molecule; (5) the antibody may present an excessive stimulation of sensitive lymphocytes; and (6) the antibody may play some regulatory role in cellular immune response.

The regulation of humoral immune response by passive administration of antibody has been successfully applied recently in the prevention of Rh-sensitization in pregnant women and has resulted in a dramatic reduction of Rh-hemolytic disease in newborns (page 349).

ABNORMAL PRODUCTION OF ANTIBODY

The capacity to produce antibodies may be totally absent, as in patients with a congenital disease called Bruton's agammaglobulinemia, (page 289) and in infants with combined immunodeficiency disease (page 305). Decreased capacity to produce antibody can be developed later in life without any known cause (primary immunodeficiency) or as a consequence of other diseases (secondary immunodeficiency). Patients also may have deficiency in the production of any one kind of immunoglobulin or a combination of two or more kinds of immunoglobulin, as in patients with common variable forms of immunodeficiency diseases (page 310).

On the other hand, an abnormally increased production of immunoglobulin (hypergammaglobulinemia) may be observed in patients with various neoplastic conditions, e.g., multiple myeloma, leukemia, lymphoma, and chronic bacterial and viral infections. These diseases will be discussed in more detail in Part II of this book.

SELECTED REFERENCES

Chase, M. W. (1959): Ann. Rev. Microbiol. *13*:349.
Choi, Y. S., Knopf, P. M., and Lennox, E. S. (1971): Biochemistry *10*:668.
Felton, L. D. (1949): J. Immun. *61*:107.
Freund, J., and McDermott, K. (1942): Proc. Soc. Exp. Biol. Med. *49*:548.
Glenny, A. T., and Südmersen, H. J. (1921): J. Hyg. (Camb.) *20*:176.
Kim, Y. B., Bradley, S. G., and Watson, D. W. (1966): J. Immun. *97*:52.
Kim, Y. B., Bradley, S. G., and Watson, D. W. (1967): J. Immun. *98*:868.
Kim, Y. B., Bradley, S. G., and Watson, D. W. (1967): J. Immun. *99*:320.
Kim, Y. B., Bradley, S. G., and Watson, D. W. (1968): J. Immun. *101*:224.
Makinodan, T., and Albright, J. F. (1967): Progr. Allerg. *10*:1.
Michaelis, L. (1902): Deutsch. Med. Wschr. *28*:733.
Mitchison, N. A. (1964): Proc. Roy. Soc. (Biol.) *161*:275.
Smith, R. T., and Bridges, R. A. (1958): J. Exp. Med. *108*:227.
Solomon, J. B. (1971): *Fetal and Neonatal Immunology*. Amsterdam, North-Holland Publishing Co.
Sulzberger, M. B. (1929): Arch. Derm. Syph. *20*:669.
Uhr, J. (1970): Cell. Immun. *1*:228.
Weigle, W. O. (1967): *Natural and Acquired Immunological Unresponsiveness*. Cleveland, Ohio, The World Publishing Company.
Williamson, A. R., and Askonas, B. A. (1967): J. Molec. Biol. *23*:201.

FURTHER READINGS

Cinader, B. (ed.) (1968): *Regulation of the Antibody Response*. Springfield, Illinois, Charles C Thomas.
Siharff, M. D., and Laskov, R. (1970): Progr. Allerg. *14*:37.
Uhr, J. W., and Möller, G. (1968): Advances Immun. *8*:81.

9
Immunoglobulins

A major advance in immunobiology was the discovery of antibody molecules, the *immunoglobulins*. A turning point of this advancement was made in 1938 when Tiselius and Kabat narrowed the antibody activity of immune serum to the gamma globulin fraction of serum proteins (Fig. 9-1). The gamma globulins were first designated by Tiselius in 1937 as distinct groups of serum proteins, which have an electrophoretic mobility of 10×10^{-5} cm^2, volt^{-1}, sec.$^{-1}$ at pH 8.6. The gamma globulins having an isoelectric point of 7.3 migrate most slowly towards the anode in an electrophoretic field at pH of 8.6 (Fig. 9-1). A further advance was made by Kunkel et al. in 1951 and by Putnam in 1953 when they showed (1) that the myeloma protein in the serum of patients with multiple myeloma belongs to the gamma globulin fraction of serum protein and (2) that the myeloma proteins are heterogeneous in their electrophoretic motility and in their antigenicity. Each individual myeloma protein was shown by Kunkel to be both immunochemically distinct and immunologically related to all other myeloma proteins.

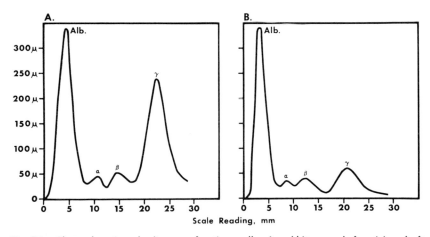

Fig. 9-1. Electrophoresis scale diagram of anti-egg albumin rabbit serum before (a) and after (b) absorption of the antibody. This shows that antibody molecules reside in the gamma globulin fraction of serum. [From Tiselius, A., and Kabat, E. A. (1939): J. Exp. Med. 69:119. By permission of the Rockefeller University Press.]

The next major step in our understanding of antibody molecules was made in 1959 when Porter isolated gamma globulins from the serum of rabbits immunized with egg albumin and digested the globulins with a plant enzyme, papain, in the presence of cysteine, hoping to find a smaller unit of molecule containing antibody activity. The antibody molecules were cleaved in such a way by the enzyme that (1) they were no longer precipitated with the antigen, egg albumin, (2) the digested antibodies had the capacity to inhibit the precipitation of egg albumin by intact antibodies, (3) when the digested antibodies were exposed to cold temperature, a portion of this mixture formed precipitation spontaneously and crystallized, and (4) the soluble portion, not the precipitated portion, retained the inhibitory capacity of precipitation with egg albumin.

Porter was fortunate to use rabbit gamma globulins in his experiment, since it was subsequently found that only rabbit gamma globulins crystallize in this experimental condition. However, under special conditions, similar crystallines can be formed with human gamma globulins, myeloma globulins, and guinea pig globulins. Porter's experiment provided two dramatic bits of information about the antibody molecules: (1) a portion of the antibody molecules can be crystallized, and (2) the antibody molecules can be reduced in size and yet retain some of their biologic activities.

Human gamma globulins can be similarly split into three fragments by papain with minor modification of Porter's procedures. Two of the three fragments are identical and are designated the Fab (antigen binding) fragments. The third fragment can be separated from the other two by

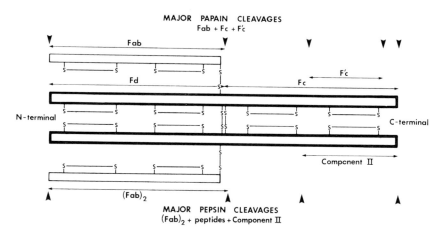

Fig. 9-2. A hypothetical model of an immunoglobulin molecule consisting of two heavy (H) chains and two light (L) chains. Pepsin cleavage results in (Fab)₂ fragments, peptides, and component II (F'c), while papain cleavage results in Fab fragments and Fc fragment. [Modified from Porter's original model in Gellhorn, A., and Hirschberg, E (eds.). (1962): *Basic Problems in Neoplastic Disease*. New York, Columbia University Press, pp. 177-194. Courtesy of Dr. G. W. Litman.]

crystallization, column chromatography, or electrophoresis and is designated the Fc (crystallizable) fragment (Fig. 9-2). Thus each gamma globulin molecule consists of two identical Fab fragments and one Fc fragment. The Fc fragment of IgG, for example, has a molecular weight of 48,000, the Fab fragments have a molecular weight of 52,000, and both fragments have a sedimentation coefficient of approximately 3.5S.

Edelman and Poulik working with myeloma proteins in 1961, showed that gamma globulin molecules can be split into two components by mild reduction with thiols (compounds containing — SH group) in the presence of urea. The two components consist of polypeptides: the heavy (H) chain (MW: 50,000) and the light (L) chain (MW: 20,000). About 75 percent of an IgG molecule is H chain, and the remaining 25 percent is L chain.

Porter found that heavy chain preparations could be precipitated specifically with antiserum against both the Fab fragments and the Fc fragment prepared in goats. On the other hand, the light chain preparations reacted only with antiserum against Fab fragments. These findings imply that the Fab fragments are composed of L chains and portions of H chains (Fd fragment), and the Fc fragment is composed of H chains only. From the data, Porter in 1962 proposed a four chain model of the structure of gamma globulin (Fig. 9-2).

The gamma globulins, however, were shown to be extremely heterogeneous in terms of their molecular size, molecular weight, antigenic determinants, and molecular charges. Consequently, different names were given to each of the subgroups by different investigators. It became increasingly clear that attempts to designate these antibody-containing proteins in terms of their physicochemical properties could never be entirely satisfactory.

The terminology used to describe gamma globulins was complex until an international agreement was reached in 1964 to include all of these subgroups of antibody molecules in a single generic term *immunoglobulin* on the basis of their common properties and to subdivide them into classes and subclasses on the basis of their antigenic differences. Somewhat similar classes and subclasses have been found in several species of mammals studied (mouse, rabbit, and horse). Table 9-1 shows the classes of human immunoglobulins presently recognized. Two symbols (Ig or γ) are used for immunoglobulin and are accompanied by a capital letter indicating the antigenic class, i.e., IgG for one form of 7S gamma globulin, IgM for 19S macrogammaglobulin, IgA, IgD, and IgE. Alternatively these can be written as γG, γM, γA, γD, γE, respectively.

HETEROGENEITY OF IMMUNOGLOBULINS

The serum immunoglobulins comprise an extraordinarily heterogeneous array of molecular types. The initial intimation of this heterogeneity came

Table 9-1. Nomenclature, Molecular Weights, and Serum Concentrations of Known Classes of Human Immunoglobulins

WHO Nomen- clature	IgG, γG	IgA, γA	IgM, γM	IgD, γD	IgE, γE
Molecular weight	140,000	160,000 (×2)	900,000	—	200,000
Serum concentra- tion (mg/100 ml)	800-1600	60-420	50-200	3	—
Old terminology	γ, 7Sγ, γ₂, γss	β₂A, γ, A	β₂M, γ, M 19S γ-macro- globulin		

from the experiment of Heidelberger and Kabat and their associates in the 1930s. They found that the injection of pneumococci into horses resulted in the production of antipneumococcal antibodies of varying molecular sizes and electrophoretic mobilities.

Serum protein molecules can be separated according to the differences in their net charges by electrophoresis in supporting media (filter paper, cellulose acetate membrane, and agar gel) or by ion exchange chromatography in ion exchange resins such as diethylaminoethyl (DEAE) cellulose. Though these methods are highly sensitive for the separation of many proteins, they are to some extent inadequate for separating immunoglobulin molecules in more detail.

By use of ultracentrifugation, the immunoglobulins can be separated according to their sedimentation coefficient into 7S or 19S classes. The 7S fraction has a molecular weight of about 140,000 and corresponds to the slowest migrating gamma globulin in electrophoretic analysis and to the first peak of eluates from DEAE column chromatography with 0.01/M buffer at pH 8. The 19S fraction has a molecular weight of 900,000 and corresponds to the faster portion of gamma globulin in electrophoresis. The immunoglobulins in serum thus constitute a family of protein molecules which are heterogeneous but nonetheless related.

Antigenic analysis of the immunoglobulins has provided another method for differentiating immunoglobulin molecules. Since the immunoglobulins can be used as immunogens, antibody directed against the immunoglobulins of one species can be raised in a different species of animal, and antigenic differences in each immunoglobulin can thus be identified. In 1953, Grabar and Williams developed a technique of *immunoelectrophoresis* (page 95), which combines the electrophoresis of serum

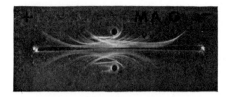

Fig. 9-3. Immunoelectrophoresis of normal (upper) and agammaglobulinemic (lower) serum.

proteins followed by a specific precipitation with an antiserum placed in a well parallel to the electrophoretic axis. By this technique more than 30 different serum proteins, including the different immunoglobulins, can be identified.

That antibody activities may be associated with more than one kind of serum protein was established by the study of another experiment of Nature, i.e., agammaglobulinemia, a genetic disease with lack of antibody response (page 289). In immunoelectrophoresis studies in 1956, Gitlin and his co-workers showed that three groups of proteins were missing from the serum of patients with agammaglobulinemia. A demonstration of typical patterns of immunoelectrophoresis of serum from a patient with agammaglobulinemia is shown in Figure 9-3.

Since the definition of immunoglobulin is based on immunologic properties, i.e., the presence of antibody activity and of common antigenic determinants in the molecules rather than on physicochemical properties of the proteins, the families of immunoglobulins are classified by their antigenic differences. Antiserum specific for one of the immunoglobulin classes is used for the classification.

How are the specific antisera obtained? When rabbits or other animals are immunized with whole molecule, L-chain or H-chain of human IgA, for example, the antiserum produced by these animals usually reacts not only with IgA, but also, to a lesser degree, with IgG and IgM largely because each immunoglobulin contains determinants shared by the other immunoglobulins. The antibodies reacting with IgG and IgM can be precipitated and removed by adding IgG and/or IgM (absorption) so that the remaining supernatant reacts only with IgA (monospecific antiserum). In a similar manner, an antiserum monospecific for IgG and for IgM can be obtained. Each of these specific antisera gives a single precipitin band (page 120) with normal serum, indicating that normal human serum contains IgG, IgA, and IgM, the three major immunoglobulins, whereas these are missing from the serum of patients with agammaglobulinemia. With these specific antisera, most of the pathologic myeloma proteins (page 572) could be classified into one of the three major immunoglobulin classes.

A fourth class of immunoglobulin, IgD, was found in 1965 by Rowe and Fahey in an atypical myeloma protein which did not react with any of the known anti-IgG, anti-IgA, or anti-IgM sera. Although antibody activities had not been detected in this protein, the protein clearly represented a distinct immunoglobulin class, and it was designated IgD.

A fifth class of human immunoglobulin was discovered in 1966 by the Ishizakas and Hornbook as a result of their studies on reaginic antibody (page 106). The antiserum specific for this protein was obtained by immunizing rabbits with a reagin-rich fraction of serum protein from patients with ragweed allergy. The antiserum did not react with any of the known classes of immunoglobulins, i.e., IgA, IgG, IgM, IgD, but gave a precipitin band with a reagin-rich fraction of serum protein. This new class of immunoglobulin was designated IgE. More recently, discovery of patients with IgE myeloma has facilitated further definition of this new class of immunoglobulin in terms of its chemical and immunologic aspects.

HEAVY (H) AND LIGHT (L) CHAINS

Immunoglobulin molecules, being protein molecules of fairly large size, can have many antigenic determinants. Some of these determinants are common to all classes of immunoglobulins, whereas others are specific for each class of immunoglobulins. The antigenic determinants that confer specificity on the different classes are the properties of the heavy chains or, more precisely, of the Fc portions of the heavy chains. Each class of immunoglobulin has an antigenically unique type of heavy chain. These are designated as γ, α, μ, δ, and ϵ chains for IgG, IgA, IgM, IgD, and IgE, respectively.

Where does the common antigenic determinant of immunoglobulin molecules reside? Another experiment of Nature, i.e., the Bence Jones protein in myeloma, led to further understanding of the heterogeneity of immunoglobulin molecules. The common determinants of immunoglobulins are found in Bence Jones proteins, the urinary proteins of myelomatosis, for they give a precipitin reaction with antisera prepared against any class of normal human immunoglobulin. In contrast, the antiserum prepared against Bence Jones urinary protein from one patient precipitates with only some, but not all, individual Bence Jones proteins obtained from other patients with myelomatosis.

Careful examination of the pattern of the precipitation reaction between antisera from normal immunoglobulins and Bence Jones proteins revealed that there are two mutually exclusive antigenic types of Bence Jones proteins. The antigenic type is identical to that of the myeloma proteins in the serum of the same patient. These same antisera against individual Bence Jones proteins precipitate with normal immunoglobulins of all classes and also with light chains from any normal immunoglobulins.

From these observations it can be concluded (1) that the Bence Jones proteins can be divided into two antigenically distinct types, (2) that only one type of Bence Jones protein is present in the urine of an individual patient with myelomatosis, (3) that the Bence Jones proteins are

Table 9-2. Molecular Formulas of Human Immunoglobulins

Immunoglobulins	Molecular Formulas		
IgG	$(\gamma_2\kappa_2)$	or	$(\gamma_2\lambda_2)$
IgA	$\left.\begin{array}{c}(\alpha_2\kappa_2)\\ \text{and}\\ (\alpha_2\kappa_2)_2\end{array}\right\}$	or	$\left\{\begin{array}{c}(\alpha_2\lambda_2)\\ \text{and}\\ (\alpha_2\lambda_2)_2\end{array}\right.$
IgM	$\left.\begin{array}{c}(\mu_2\kappa_2)\\ \text{and}\\ (\mu_2\kappa_2)_5\end{array}\right\}$	or	$\left\{\begin{array}{c}(\mu_2\lambda_2)\\ \text{and}\\ (\mu_2\lambda_2)_5\end{array}\right.$
IgD	$(\delta_2\kappa_2)$	or	$(\delta_2\lambda_2)$
IgE	$(\varepsilon_2\kappa_2)$	or	$(\varepsilon_2\lambda_2)$

antigenically identical with the light chains of normal immunoglobulins, (4) that normal immunoglobulins carry light chains of the two distinct antigenic types, and (5) that the common antigenic determinant of immunoglobulins of all classes resides in the light chains.

Further studies with type-specific antisera revealed that the two different light chain determinants are carried on separate immunoglobulin molecules. These two types of immunoglobulins are designated *type K* and *type L,* and are present in all classes of immunoglobulins. For all immunoglobulins, the proportion of type K is 60 percent, and of type L, 30 percent; the remainder has neither specificity. The light chain specific for K type immunoglobulin is called κ-chain, and for L type, λ-chain. Thus, the molecular formulas for each class of immunoglobulin can be written in terms of antigenic difference. These formulas are shown in Table 9-2. Apparently both κ and λ chains are not found on the same immunoglobulin molecules, and a single cell produces only one type of light chain.

SUBCLASSES OF IMMUNOGLOBULINS

Studies on myeloma proteins revealed a further degree of heterogeneity in immunoglobulin heavy chains. Using rabbit and monkey antisera to individual myeloma proteins, Grey and Kunkel in 1964 found three antigenic subclasses of IgG molecules. In the same year Terry and Fahey used monkey antisera to normal human IgG to distinguish three subclasses of IgG molecules. Comparison of the findings of these two groups of investigators revealed that two of the three subclasses corresponded, but the third subclass of the one group was different from that of the other group. Therefore, it was apparent that there are four subclasses of IgG molecules and these were designated G_1, G_2, G_3, and G_4. The frequency of the four subclasses in the IgG-myeloma corresponds approximately to the relative proportions of these subclasses in normal serum. Among Caucasians, the proportion of G_1 is 50 percent; of G_2, 24 percent; of G_3, 8 percent; and of G_4, 8 percent. Subclasses of IgA reported in 1966 by Kunkel and Prendergast and by Vaerman and Heremans were designated as Le and He. Further subclassification may be forthcoming with regard to IgA. Evidence for subclasses of IgM has been presented, but is not convincing. To date subclasses of IgD and IgE have not been reported.

ALLOTYPES OF IMMUNOGLOBULINS

The antigenic specificities of different classes of immunoglobulins are represented in all normal individuals of a given species and are called *isotypic specificities*. Two other kinds of antigenic specificities, *allotypic* and *idiotypic* are known to exist and also are under genetic control. The existence of these individual differences in human immunoglobulins was first noticed by Grubb and Laurell in 1956. They found that certain *anti-gamma globulin reactions* (page 392) mediated by human rheumatoid factor in the serum of certain patients could distinguish the antigenic differences between IgG molecules of one group of individuals from those of another. Dray and Young in 1958 and Oudin in 1960, while working with rabbit IgG, reported the antigenic differences in IgG of groups of rabbits. The term *allotypic specificities* was used by Oudin to describe the antigenic differences of IgG molecules in different groups of individuals within the same species. The term *idiotypic specificities* pertains to the antigenic specificities peculiar to a *single* kind of antibody produced by a single individual of the species.

It became clear that animal and sometimes human subjects injected with IgG from another individual of the same species may produce iso-antibodies reacting with the donor's IgG. The situation is similar to that of blood group isoantibody, i.e., individuals can produce antibodies against the immunoglobulins of others, depending on whether they have inherited the same or a different gene controlling the antigenic variants of immunoglobulin.

Two allotype systems are known in man: the *Gm system* and the *InV system*. For obvious reasons the allotypes of human immunoglobulins cannot be studied by deliberate immunization of one person with immunoglobulins or myeloma protein from another person. Such isoimmunization, however, does occur as a result of transfusion of blood or plasma and as a result of the transplacental passage of maternal IgG to the fetus. The fetus may produce anti-allotype antibodies when the mother and the fetus have different allotypes of IgG molecules.

How is the allotypic specificity determined? First, indicator particles coated with an IgG of known allotype are prepared. Red blood cells (Rh positive) are most frequently used as indicator particles coated with an appropriate nonagglutinating immunoglobulin. These red cells are then agglutinable by anti-allotype antibody to the appropriate immunoglobulin coating the surface of the red blood cells. In the test the ability to block the agglutination by an unknown allotype immunoglobulin is determined. The agglutination can be blocked by adding an excess of immunoglobulin of the same allotype with which the red cells are coated, but it will not be blocked if an immunoglobulin of a different allotype is added.

The Gm allotypes are antigenic specificities associated with the Fc portion of heavy (H) chain of human IgG molecules and have not been found in other classes of immunoglobulins. More than 20 distinct Gm allotypes are now recognized and are designated Gm (1), Gm (2), etc., roughly in the chronologic order of their discovery. Particular Gm allotypes are confined to a particular subclass of IgG, e.g., Gm (1), Gm (2), Gm (3), and Gm (4) have been found only on IgG_1 molecules, whereas Gm (5), Gm (6), Gm (10), Gm (11), Gm (13), and Gm (14) have been found only on IgG_3 molecules.

The antigenic specificities of the InV allotype are found only in the type K, L chains. Three InV allotypes—InV(1), InV(2), and InV(3)— are known. These allotypes are controlled by alleles at a single genetic locus. The antigenic determinants of InV(2) and InV(3) have been found to be correlated with whether leucine or valine is present at position 191 in the constant part of type K, L chain. No special amino acid substitution has yet been found to correspond with the InV(1) allotype.

COMBINING SITE OF ANTIBODY

The extent of physicochemical and immunologic heterogeneity among immunoglobulin molecules is indeed striking. Our next questions are: What part of the immunoglobulin molecule recognizes the specific antigenic determinant? What is the mechanism of such specific recognition?

Most natural immunogens, even when chemically pure, have complex molecular structures, express different kinds of antigenic determinants on the various parts of the molecules, and elicit antibodies against each of several determinants simultaneously. Furthermore, the exact chemical structure of these various antigenic determinants is mostly unknown. For this reason the precise information concerning the combining site of antibody molecules has been obtained by use of immunogens to which a chemically defined hapten has been attached artificially (page 47). It is then possible to study the interaction of the hapten with the specific antibody without interference of antibodies directed against the unknown parts of immunogen molecules.

By use of chemically defined antigenic determinants, several interesting findings have been revealed: (1) an antibody against a defined hapten group can be produced within many different classes, subclasses, or allotypes of immunoglobulins of an individual; (2) the combining site of antibody molecules resides in the variable parts of Fab fragment; (3) the specificity of combining sites is due to the difference in primary sequence of amino acids in the variable part of the immunoglobulin molecule; and (4) the size of antigenic determinants can be estimated to be in the order of 3 to 6 glucose residues for dextran, or 8 to 12 amino acid residues for silk fibroin. Therefore, assuming the size of the combining site of antibody to be similar to that of the antigenic determinant, we can conclude that only 10 to 20 variations among the 1320 amino acids of the whole molecule account for immunologic specificities. The observed variations of amino acid sequences of the Fab portion of the light chain and the heavy chain are sufficient to account for the infinite variety of antibody specificity.

BIOLOGIC ACTIVITIES OF IMMUNOGLOBULINS

Traditionaly, antibodies have been described in terms of their visible reactions with antigen, e.g., precipitins, lysins, antitoxins, and agglutinins (page 12). For a long time it was assumed that these various effects of antibodies were caused by one kind of antibody molecule acting under different conditions. This assumption is no longer valid, since it is now clear that different classes, subclasses, and allotypes of immunoglobulin molecules may react with the same antigenic determinant to produce different biologic actions. In other words, precipitin reaction to one antigen can be found in IgA, IgG, or IgM immunoglobulins. However, the biologic activities and functions of different classes of immunoglobulin differ greatly by virtue of their unique molecular structure and chemical and immunologic properties (Table 9-3).

Table 9-3.   Biologic Activities of Human Immunoglobulins

	IgG	IgA	IgM	IgD	IgE
Stable at 56-60%	Yes	Yes	Yes	Yes	No
Transplacental passage	Yes	No	No	No	No
Valence for antigen binding	2	2	10	—	—
Efficiency in serologic tests	Precipitation Complement fixation Toxin neutralization	Variable	Agglutination Hemagglutination Virus neutralization	—	—
Present in milk	+	+	Trace	—	—
Selective secretion by seromucous gland	—	+	—	—	—

IgG. IgG immunoglobulins constitute the major portion (85 percent) of total immunoglobulin in man. IgG is comprised of a continuous range of molecules differing in their isoelectric point (extends α_2-γ_2-globulin region), in their sedimentation coefficient (6.56 $\pm$ 0.385), and in their molecular weight (145,000 $\pm$ 5,000). Normal IgG contains 2.6 percent carbohydrates by weight, associated with heavy chain, an amount significantly less than that found in other immunoglobulins.

Most antibodies to gram-positive pyogenic bacteria, certain viruses, and antitoxins in human adult serum are found among the IgG immunoglobulins. The Fc portion of IgG molecules is known to exert certain biologic functions such as transplacental passage, fixation of complement, fixation to receptors on skin, B-cells, and macrophages and opsonic activity. The IgG molecule is transported across the human placenta; almost all other maternal proteins are excluded from the fetal circulation. From reciprocal studies of agammaglobulinemic mothers with normal offspring and of agammaglobulinemic offspring of normal mothers, it was clear as early as 1955 that of the immunoglobulins, only maternal IgG was passively transported to the fetus. In 1964 Gitlin and his co-workers showed that the Fc fragment, but not the Fab fragment, will cross the human placenta. Brambell in 1966 showed that the transplacental passage is due not to simple filtration, but to an active transport process across the trophoblastic cells of the placenta; the selectivity is mediated only by certain "transmission sites" on the Fc portion of the IgG heavy chain. In healthy adults, the total free IgG is about 80 gm and is distributed equally between the blood and the interstitial tissue. A quarter of the IgG passes across the capillary wall each day, and the same amount returns to the blood via the thoracic duct.

IgG appears to be unique among the immunoglobulins in that the rate of catabolism, the fraction of total intravascular IgG catabolized daily, increases with its concentration in the blood. This phenomenon is peculiar to IgG and is not observed with IgA, IgM, or with other plasma proteins, such as albumin, whose catabolic rates are essentially independent of their concentrations in the plasma (Table 9-4). Consequently, the half-

Table 9-4. Metabolic Characteristics of Human Immunoglobulin

	IgG	IgA	IgM	IgD	IgE
Half-life (days)	25-35	6-8	9-11	2-3	2.1
Production (mg/kg/day)	28-36	8-10	5-8	0.4	—
Carbohydrate (5)	2.5	10	10	—	10.7
Intravascular distribution (5)	40	40	80	75	Mostly extra-vascular

life of the IgG may be much shorter than usual if the IgG levels are markedly raised, e.g., in patients with IgG myeloma, chronic liver disease, or chronic infection (malaria or leishmaniasis). For example, a person with three times the usual serum IgG level will have to produce IgG at about six times the usual rate to maintain the higher level. This phenomenon gives us a possible explanation of why patients with IgG myelomas are prone to suffer from specific antibody deficiency syndromes, i.e., the building blocks for all immunoglobulin synthesis have been directed to production of a single immunoglobulin or myeloma protein. The control of the catabolic rate appears to depend upon the Fc piece of IgG H chain, as also does the active transport across the placenta.

The IgG molecules are suited to their function of combining with a wide variety of antigens of all shapes and sizes. The combining sites are at the N-terminal of the two "arms" (the Fab fragment), with a "knob" at the middle corresponding to the Fc piece. The two arms appear to operate flexibly as though they were hinged together, so that the combining sites can be at a variable distance apart up to the whole length of the arms (Fig. 9-4). This property remains after the Fc piece has been removed, e.g., by enzyme digestion.

At birth the predominant immunoglobulin in the circulation is the maternal IgG, which is selectively transferred across the placenta. The low level of immunoglobulin synthesis by the fetus is attributable largely to the lack of antigenic stimulation in the intrauterine environment rather than to the absence of capacity for an immune response. The levels of IgG fall during the first few months of life as the maternal protein is catabolized and then rise due to increased synthesis by the infant until they reach adult levels by the fifth year.

IgA. IgA comprises about 10 percent of total immunoglobulins in human serum, contains about 10 percent by weight of carbohydrate associated with the heavy chain, and is found in relatively large quantities in parotid saliva, 28 mg; colostrum 151 mg; and in tears, 7 mg per 100 ml.

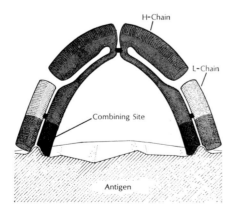

Fig. 9-4. Schematic illustration of IgG molecule showing the two "arms" of N-terminal, with a "knob" at the middle corresponding to the Fc piece. [From Nisonoff. A. (1969): New insights into immunoglobulins. Hosp. Prac. 4:9.]

In contrast, only a trace amount of IgG is found in these fluids. A relatively smaller amount of IgA is present in bile, secretions of intestinal glands, and prostatic fluid.

The IgA molecules of external secretion are principally 11S, whereas those of serum are mainly 7S with only 5 to 10 percent being 11S. The IgA molecules in secretions contain an additional structural unit called the *transport (T) piece* or *secretory (S) piece* that has a molecular weight similar to that of the L chain but is antigenically distinct. More recently, an additional polypeptide chain, the J chain, has been reported to be part of the structure of rabbit and human secretory IgA. Additional studies have revealed that the J chain is not restricted to secretory IgA but exists on other polymeric immunoglobulins such as serum IgA and IgM.

The secretory IgA molecules consist of four H chains, four L chains, and one transport (T) piece. It is believed that the transport (T) piece is added to the IgA molecule during the process of transport through the epithelium of glands or the intestinal surface and that in some way it participates in the active transport of IgA molecules (Fig. 9-5). Thus IgA has a remarkable property of being preferentially secreted into the colostrum, saliva, intestinal juice, and respiratory secretions. The secretory piece of IgA can easily be identified only in the epithelial cells of these secretory glands. The IgA that is transported into the external secretions is largely synthesized locally by plasma cells in the tissue, but a

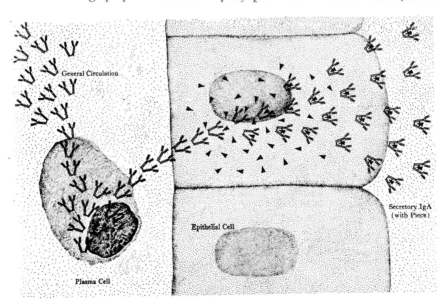

Fig. 9-5. A proposed mechanism for the synthesis and secretion of IgA molecule. IgA molecules are synthesized in the plasma cells and then move in two directions, i.e., into the general circulation and into the epithelial cells where the secretory piece is added before the secretion. [From Tomasi, T. B. (1967): Hosp. Prac. 7:26.]

small amount may derive via the blood stream from elsewhere in the body. Strong evidence for the local synthesis of IgA is that IgA iso-antibodies against red blood cells may be readily detectable in colostrum but not in the plasma.

Since IgA is selectively concentrated in certain secretions, it has been postulated that IgA antibodies may play a protective role at mucous surfaces. IgA molecules appear to be adapted for this purpose, since the secreted form of IgA molecules has a somewhat increased resistance to digestion by proteolytic enzymes and to reducing agents. Antibody activities against Brucella suis, diphtheria bacilli, antitoxin, isohemagglutinin insulin, and ragweed have been demonstrated in IgA.

Selective deficiency of IgA has been shown to be associated with an increased episode of respiratory infections and in increased incidence of autoimmune diseases. Therefore, the role of IgA in the surface of mucous membrane may be both to provide protection against local infections and to prevent the development of the autoimmune process by interfering with absorption of antigens from the surfaces.

IgM. One of the characteristic properties of IgM is its high molecular weight (about 900,000). It constitutes 5 to 10 percent of the total immunoglobulins in the blood. The study of Waldenström-type macroglobulinemia, a pathologically produced IgM molecule, has provided major information about the IgM molecules. Both normal and pathologic IgM show a heterogeneity in ultracentrifuge, i.e., 19S, 29S, and 38S. 19S fractions occupy the major portion of IgM, whereas 29S and 38S fractions are thought to be greater polymeric forms. Further, the 19S IgM molecules are comprised of five identical subunits joined together by disulfide linkages (Fig. 9-6). From this finding one might expect that the 19S IgM molecule would comprise ten identical combining sites. Experimental evidence suggests that some IgM molecules indeed have ten combining sites but others may have only five valences.

These structural characteristics of IgM molecules appear to be well suited for their unique biologic functions, i.e., the protective activity against microbes and other large-sized immunogens that have repeating antigenic determinants on their surface. Some examples of immunogens with such antigenic determinants on the surface are the capsules of pneumococci, the cell wall of gram-negative bacilli, bacterial flagella, and surfaces of viruses. When an IgM molecule combines with these antigens, it activates complement so effectively that a single molecule can lyse the cell. In contrast, the IgG molecules can achieve the same function only when two or more molecules become attached close together on the cell surface. Consequently IgM molecules may become 20 times more active in agglutinating salmonella bacteria, more than 100 times more potent in killing them, and almost 1000 times more effective in opsonizing the bacteria than are IgG molecules.

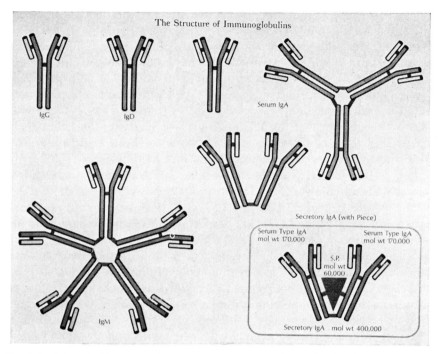

The Structure of Immunoglobulins

IgG

IgD

Serum IgA

Secretory IgA (with Piece)

Serum Type IgA
mol wt 170,000

Serum Type IgA
mol wt 170,000

S.P.
mol wt
60,000

Secretory IgA mol wt 400,000

IgM

Fig. 9-6. Schematic illustration of comparative structure of the immunoglobulins. IgA molecules can form dimer, trimer, or secretory forms. IgM forms a pentamer. [From Tomasi, T. B. (1967): Hosp. Prac. 7:26.]

IgM antibody seems to be produced early in humoral immune response and to appear in the blood stream rapidly and transiently when the immunogen is soluble. Phylogenetically and ontogenetically the IgM is clearly a more primitive immunoglobulin than is IgG. Among the most primitive representatives of vertebrate evolution the antibody molecules appear to be similar to IgM, but a variety of forms including monomers, dimers, tetramers, pentamers, and hexamers may be found in the blood of these primitive species. IgM is almost absent in the blood of the fetus and rises quickly after antigenic stimulation which is usually first encountered in large amounts after birth. For this reason the measurement of the IgM level in the cord blood may have diagnostic value for the detection of intrauterine infection.

IgM in normal individuals is distributed predominantly within the blood stream, presumably because of its large size. It has a half-life of 5 to 6 days, considerably shorter than the 18 to 23 days usually observed for IgG. It does not cross the placenta and is present only in trace amounts in milk or other secretions. In patients with Waldenström's macroglobulinemia, an increased production of IgM molecules takes place in the lymphocytes or plasma cells throughout the body, and these molecules sometimes exhibit auto-antibody activities, e.g., antibodies directed against the I-antigen of red cells.

IgD. IgD was discovered from the study of a rare form of myeloma. A small amount is present in normal human plasma. The half-life is about 3 days. Recently, antibody activity against penicillin, insulin, milk proteins, diphtheria toxoid, and nuclear and thyroid antigens has been demonstrated in IgD molecules.

IgE. The discovery of the IgE molecule was made by the Ishizakas in 1966 during their study of reaginic antibodies. These heat labile skin-sensitizing antibodies are responsible for the anaphylactic type of immediate hypersensitivity in several species, such as man, monkey, dog, rat, rabbit, and guinea pig. The Ishizakas showed (1) that antisera specific for the H chains of human IgG, IgA, IgM, or IgD did not block the reaginic activity, and (2) that a specific antiserum prepared for the reaginic antibodies does not react with any of the other four known classes of immunoglobulins. These evidences indicate that reaginic antibodies reside in a unique class of immunoglobulin. The amount of purified reaginic antibodies was not sufficient for further characterization of this new class of immunoglobulin until a myeloma patient was discovered in 1967 who produced large quantities of IgE myeloma protein. IgE myeloma protein contains approximately 10 percent carbohydrate and has a molecular weight of about 190,000.

IgE antibody activities are inactivated completely in one hour at 56° C. They are susceptible to mercaptoethanol treatment and attach firmly to certain tissues and especially to most cells. Trace amounts of IgE are present in the serum. The antibodies of this class do not precipitate with any antigens nor fix complement. Elevated serum levels of IgE can be found in certain patients with pollen allergies and especially in patients with helminth infections. The function of IgE in bodily defense has not yet been elucidated.

SELECTED REFERENCES

Brambell, F. W. R. (1966): Lancet 2:1087.
Dray, S., and Young, G. O. (1958): J. Immun. 81:142.
Edelman, G. M., and Poulik, M. D. (1961): J. Exp. Med. 113:861.
Gitlin, D., Hitzig, W. H., and Janeway, C. A. (1956): J. Clin. Invest. 35:1199.
Gitlin, D., et al. (1964): J. Clin. Invest. 43:1938.
Grabar, P., and Williams, C. A. (1953): Biochem. Biophys. Acta 10:193.
Grey, H. M., and Kunkel, H. G. (1964): J. Exp. Med. 120:253.
Grubb, R., and Laurell, A. B. (1956): Acta Path. Microbiol. Scand. 39:390.
Heidelberger, M. (1956): Lectures in Immunochemistry. New York, Academic Press.
Ishizaka, K., Ishizaka, T., and Hornbook, M. M. (1966): J. Immun. 97:840.
Kabat, E. A., and Mayer, M. M. (1961): Experimental Immunochemistry. Springfield, Illinois, Charles C Thomas.
Kunkel, H. G., and Prendergast, R. A. (1966): Proc. Soc. Exp. Biol. Med. 122:910.
Kunkel, H. G., Slater, R. J., and Good, R. A. (1951): Proc. Soc. Exp. Biol. Med. 76:190.

Oudin, J. (1960): J. Exp. Med. *112*:107.

Porter, R. R. (1959): Biochem. J. 73:119.

Porter, R. R. (1962): In *Basic Problems in Neoplastic Disease*, Gellhorn, A., and Hirschberg, E. (eds.). New York, Columbia University Press, p. 177.

Putnam, F. W., and Udin, B. (1953): J. Biol. Chem. *202*:727.

Rowe, D. S., and Fahey, J. L. (1965): J. Exp. Med. *121*:171.

Terry, W. D., and Fahey, J. L. (1964): Science *146*:400.

Tiselius, A. (1937): Biochem. J. *31*:1464.

Tiselius, A., and Kabat, E. A. (1938): Science 87:416.

Vaerman, J. P., and Heremans, J. F. (1966): Science *153*:647.

FURTHER READINGS

Bermier, G. M. (1970): Progr. Allerg. *14*:1.

Cold Spring Harbor Symposia on Quantitative Biology (1967): *Antibodies*. Cold Spring Harbor, New York, vol. 32.

Grubb, R. (1970): *The Genetic Markers of Human Immunoglobulins*. New York, Springer-Verlag.

Janeway, C. A., et al. (1967): *The Gamma-globulins*. Boston, Little, Brown and Company.

Kabat, E. A. (1968): *Structural Concepts in Immunology and Immunochemistry*. New York, Holt, Rinehart and Winston, Inc.

Merler, E. (ed.) (1970): *Immunoglobulins, Biological Aspects and Clinical Uses*. Washington, D. C., National Academy of Sciences.

10
Antigen-Antibody Reactions

Serology, the study of the interaction of antigen and antibody, has provided not only the means of studying the mechanisms of immunity but also valuable methods for diagnosis of many infectious diseases, for identification and classification of microorganisms, and for the precise measurement of many trace substances such as hormones and enzymes in the biologic fluids. All these useful applications are based on the extraordinary discriminating power and the specificity of the reaction between antigen and antibody. Thus, with known antigens, we can detect the unknown antibodies by virtue of their specificity.

As we have learned more about the molecular biology of antibodies, many traditional concepts in serology have been modified and replaced by new ones. In the early days of the development of serology, it was assumed that a separate antibody exists for each antigen-antibody reaction, i.e., antitoxins, precipitins, agglutinins, anaphylaxins, hemolysins, bacteriolysins, opsonins. This concept was replaced by Zinsser's *unitarian theory of antibodies,* which proposed that the "same antibody" could perform all these different functions under different conditions. This general concept is still valid in the light of present knowledge, for it can be shown that antibody of a single subclass of immunoglobulin can function as opsonin, agglutinin, precipitin, etc., when it interacts with the antigen under appropriate conditions. On the other hand, a single antigen can induce antibody molecules that belong to several classes and subclasses of immunoglobulins and perform the same kind of reaction, e.g., precipitation and agglutination.

The advancement of immunochemistry has brought further understanding of the nature of antigen-antibody interaction. It is now clear that the initial encounter between antigen and antibody, i.e., *the primary reaction,* does not have effects visible by ordinary means. Under appropriate conditions, however, the primary reactions are often followed by visible manifestations such as precipitation and agglutination. These visible manifestations *in vitro* are called *secondary reactions.* Some of these secondary reactions may take place *in vivo* and initiate further chain reactions which lead to such manifestations as anaphylactic shock and serum sickness. These *in vivo* manifestations are called *tertiary reactions* (Table 10-1).

Table 10-1. Examples of Secondary and Tertiary Manifestations of Antigen-Antibody Interaction

---

Secondary Manifestations (*in vitro*)
  Precipitation
    In solution
    In gel
  Agglutination
    Active, direct agglutination
    Passive agglutination of red blood cells or other particles coated with antigen
    Reverse passive agglutination
    Antiglobulin test (Coombs')
  Complement fixation
  Lysis of red blood cells or bacteria
  Opsonization
  Immune adherence
  Anaphylaxis *in vitro* (e.g., Schultz-Dale test)
  Histamine release from leukocytes
  Virus neutralization (e.g., Jerne plaque technique)
Tertiary Manifestations (*in vivo*)
  Anaphylaxis *in vivo*
  Prausnitz-Küstner (P-K) reaction
  Passive cutaneous anaphylaxis (PCA)
  Toxin neutralization
  Arthus reaction
  Clearance of antigen from circulation
  Clinical allergy
  Immunity against infectious disease

In this chapter, we will survey some basic concepts of the primary and the secondary reactions and their applications. Many aspects of tertiary reactions will be explored in Chapter 11 and in the clinical immunobiology section of this book.

PRIMARY REACTIONS OF ANTIGENS AND ANTIBODIES

The primary interaction between antigen and antibody is the first step in a series of biochemical processes which may or may not result in an overt secondary or tertiary reaction. The primary reaction is invisible, takes a few milliseconds to complete, occurs even at low temperature, and obeys general rules of physical chemistry and thermodynamics. Therefore, the physicochemical aspects of the interaction between antigen and antibody molecules cannot by itself be regarded as a unique phenomenon. What makes the antigen-antibody interaction unique is its specific nature by virtue of the special conformational structure of the antibody molecules (Fig. 10-1).

As early as in 1902, Arrhenius and Madson in Copenhagen suggested that the laws of physical chemistry should also be applicable to the reaction between the antigen and the antibody. Present concepts of antigen-antibody reactions have developed from the work of Landsteiner. The

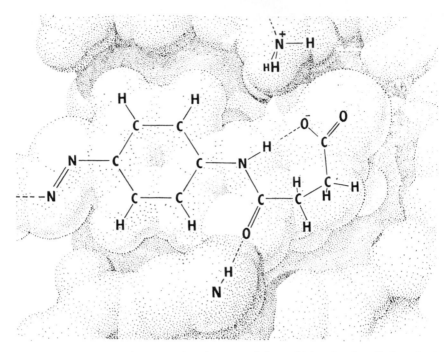

Fig. 10-1. Hypothetical illustration of conformation of the combining site of antibody molecule. The haptenic group of antigen is surrounded by combining site of antibody molecule. [From Pauling, L. (1947-48): Endeavour 7:43.]

antibodies are globulin molecules modified in such a way that the combining sites of the antibody molecule react with the determinant groups of the antigen molecule. The reaction is considered as a reversible phenomenon:

$$Ag + Ab \underset{K_2}{\overset{K_1}{\rightleftharpoons}} Ag \cdot Ab$$

where Ag represents one of the multiple antigenic determinants of an antigen molecule; Ab, the combining site of the antibody molecule; and Ag · Ab represents the complex of antigen-antibody. Further, the concentrations of total combining sites of the antibody molecule and the corresponding antigenic determinants are governed by the law of mass reaction:

$$\frac{(Ag)\ (Ab)}{(Ag \cdot Ab)} = K$$

The determination of the value of K (equilibrium constant) for any particular antigen-antibody reaction is valuable for deriving thermodynamic data which indicate the nature of the bond between the combining site

Table 10-2. Biologic Bonds and Their Strengths

Type of Bond	Strength (K cal.)
Van der Waals'	0.5
Ionic	5
Hydrogen	2-5
Reinforced ionic	10
Covalent	40-140

of the antibody and the determinant groups of the antigen molecule. The K value can be used to calculate the change in free energy that accompanies the reaction between antigen and antibody.

By what force do the antigen and antibody combine? Studies of antigen-antibody reactions during the past 20 years indicate that general physico-chemical forces of intermolecular attraction are involved (Table 10-2). It is postulated that several of the weaker intermolecular forces such as Van der Waals' force, ionic bonds, and hydrogen bonding are most likely the basis of the antigen-antibody binding rather than covalent bonding. This postulate can explain the specificity of the antigen-antibody reaction on the basis of complementarity (fit) between the combining site and the determinant group. It should, however, be recognized that the complementarity need not necessarily be exact. An illustration of this complementarity is shown in Figure 10-1. Thus, the extraordinary specificity of the antigen-antibody interaction derives not from the specific physico-chemical forces involved, but rather from the unique complementarity in the spatial configurations of the combining site of the antibody molecule and that of the determinant groups of antigen.

DETECTION AND USE OF PRIMARY Ag-Ab REACTION

Both physical and chemical methods have been employed for detecting primary Ag-Ab reaction (Table 10-3). The required conditions for detecting a primary reaction are (1) that free and bound antigen can be distinguished precisely, and (2) that the antigen can be distinguished from antibody in the reaction mixture.

For the separation of free antigen from bound antigen, a number of methods are available: differential centrifugation, electrophoresis, precipitation, filtration, and dialysis. For the distinction between antigen and antibody, purified polysaccharide antigen has been used because it is devoid of nitrogen. Recently, antigens with built-in markers have been used. These markers can be in the form of characteristic color, fluoresence, or heavy metals. Since built-in markers are somewhat rare, artificial markers have been developed to label either antigen or antibody, or both. The most commonly used artificial markers are radioactive isotopes (^{131}I, ^{35}S) which can be coupled with the antigen or antibody molecules or with

Table 10-3.   Methods of Measuring Primary Interaction of Antigen-Antibody

---

Quantitative Methods
  Separation of bound antigen from free antigen
    By precipitating antigen-antibody complex with 50% ammonium sulfate or anti-immunoglobulin
    According to the difference in molecular size of free antigen and antigen-antibody complex by equilibrium dialysis, ultracentrifugation, or gel filtration
    By adsorbing antigen to inert surfaces of chromatographic paper, silica, talcum powder, fullers' earth, or dextran-coated charcoal
    Adsorption of specific antibody to polymeric surfaces of polypropylene, polystyrene, or Sephadex
    According to differential electrophoretic mobility of bound and free antigen by disk polyacrylamide gel electrophoresis or by paper (or acetate) electrophoresis
  Measurement of fluorescence of antigen or antigen-antibody complex
    Fluorescence quenching
    Fluorescence enhancement
    Fluorescence polarization
  Isotope-labeled eluates
Qualitative Methods
  Tracing of labeled antigen to antigen-antibody precipitates
    Indirect radioimmunoelectrophoresis
    Radioimmunodiffusion
    Direct radioimmunodiffusion and radioimmunoelectrophoresis
    Immunofluorescence
  Differential electrophoresis of bound and free antigen
    Radio gel electrophoresis
    Free boundary electrophoresis

---

the synthetic hapten. Such labeling permits the ready estimation of free and bound antigen with a higher degree of sensitivity.

Another widely used method of labeling antibody molecules is to couple the antibody molecule with fluorescent dyes. The fluorescent dye attached to the antibody or antigen molecule can be located directly in the tissue section by use of a fluorescent microscope. A third type of substance used for labeling antigens and antibodies is ferritin, a protein from horse spleen, which contains sufficient iron to render it electron-dense in electronmicroscopy.

The separation of primary, secondary, and tertiary manifestations of antigen-antibody interaction has important practical implications, for it was shown by Minden and his co-workers that the results of secondary and tertiary tests are frequently negative despite the presence of antibody detected by primary tests (Table 10-4). Thus the secondary and tertiary tests can be far less informative in telling whether antibodies are present than are tests of the primary antigen-antibody interaction. Further, the results of secondary and tertiary tests did not correlate with the primary tests. This indicates that the *quality* and the *quantity* of antibody are among the important factors to be considered in secondary and tertiary tests. Furthermore, each class of immunoglobulin has a markedly different

Table 10-4. Comparison of Primary Tests with Secondary and Tertiary Tests for Antigen-Antibody Interaction

	Number Positive/Number Studied
Primary Binding Tests	
Ammonium sulfate test	15/15
Radioimmunoelectrophoresis	15/15
Secondary Manifestations	
P-80	3/14
Gel diffusion	1/15
Hemagglutination	10/15
Tertiary Manifestations	
Passive cutaneous anaphylaxis (PCA)	0/14
Prausnitz-Küstner (P-K)	4/12
Clinical symptom after drinking milk	0/15

From Minden, P., Reid, R. T., and Farr, R. S. (1966): J. Immun. 96:180. By permission of The Williams & Wilkins Co., Baltimore.

Table 10-5. Serologic Heterogeneity of the Immunoglobulins

Serologic Reactions	IgG	IgM	IgA
Precipitation	Strong	Weak	Variable
Agglutination	Weak	Strong	Positive
Hemagglutination	Weak	Strong	Positive
Classical complement fixation	Strong	Weak	No activity
Hemolysis and bacteriolysis	Weak	Strong	No activity
Virus neutralization	Positive	Positive	Positive
Toxin neutralization	Positive	Positive	Unknown

efficiency in serologic reactions (Table 10-5). For this reason the primary test should be carried out with tests evaluating secondary or tertiary reactions to demonstrate the presence or absence of antibody.

MEASUREMENT OF ANTIBODY AND ANTIGEN

Many different methods for measuring antibody or antigen have been devised based on either primary, secondary, or tertiary manifestations of antigen-antibody interaction. The choice of any one method depends on many factors such as the nature of the antigen, quality and quantity of the antibody, the degree of precision, and the information required. Some of the methods commonly employed are listed in Table 10-6.

Concentration of antibody is expressed either in terms of absolute weight units, e.g., of antibody nitrogen per ml of sample, in terms of titer, or in terms of units. The titration procedure is to measure the concentration of antibody in serum by adding a constant amount of antigen

Table 10-6. Sensitivity of Various Methods of Detecting Antibodies

Methods	μg of Antibody Nitrogen/ml
Precipitation in gel	3-5
Flocculation test (syphilis)	0.02-0.5
Bacterial agglutination	0.01
Complement fixation	0.01
Toxin neutralization (diphtheria)	0.01
Prausnitz-Küstner in man	0.01
Passive cutaneous anaphylaxis	0.003
Hemolysis	0.001-0.003
Hemagglutinin	0.003-0.006
Radioimmunoassay	0.0001
Mixed hemadsorption	0.0001-0.00001
Phage neutralization	0.001-0.00001
Bactericidal viable count	0.00001

to a row of tubes containing serially diluted antiserum, e.g., 1/10, 1/20, 1/40, 1/80 . . . , and to look for visible effects, e.g., agglutination or precipitation. Titer is expressed as the dilution of the last tube that shows the visible effects of antigen-antibody interaction. Thus, if the dilution of the last tube that agglutinates a pneumococcal suspension is 1/640 the antibody titer of the serum is 640. Further, if the last tube showing agglutination of pneumococcus contains 1 ml volume, the titer of serum is 640 units per ml of serum. The disadvantage of using titration methods is that they do not measure amount of antibody in terms of absolute weight units.

Precipitation

Precipitation means a *throwing down,* and has been used in this sense in chemistry to indicate a solid sediment formed in a liquid reaction mixture. In serology it is used to describe antigen-antibody aggregates that ultimately settle under the force of gravity. The words *flocculation* and *precipitation* are often used indiscriminately in the literature. *Precipitation* is a general term that describes a certain type of visible reaction which follows the union of antigen and antibody, whereas flocculation tells us something about the appearance of such a precipitate, i.e., a loose aggregate (flake) that is easily disturbed by shaking.

The distinction between *agglutination* and *precipitation* is quite easy to draw when frank agglutination of cells is compared with precipitation of soluble antigens. However, it would be difficult to draw a line when we consider an infinite gradation of size of particle from cells, down through virus to macromolecules.

Because it is necessary only to mix two reagents together in order to produce reactions, precipitation and agglutination were the first serologic reactions to be described. Both of them, however, must be clearly distinguished from nonimmunologic, i.e., nonspecific, aggregation due solely to physicochemical processes. The serologic reaction is, of course, initiated by the immunologically specific union between the combining sites of antibody and the determinant groups of corresponding antigen.

The precipitation reaction may be used qualitatively or quantitatively. The great sensitivity of the precipitation reaction, together with its specificity, renders this test of value in detecting and identifying various protein or polysaccharide antigens. Thus precipitation tests are of practical importance in detecting the adulteration of foodstuffs or in differentiating human and animal blood and seminal stains in forensic medicine. These tests are eminently suitable for the detection of even minute amounts of impurities in biologic preparations. Potent antisera can detect as little as 1 μg of protein antigen by the precipitation test.

Dean and Webb in 1926 described a method that allows comparisons of potency of different batches of antiserum. Constant amounts of antiserum are added to tubes containing varying dilutions of antigen, and the tube showing the most rapid precipitation under standard conditions is regarded as containing the optimal proportions of reactants. This method of titration provides a *constant antibody optimal ratio* (Table 10-7). In the *Ramon titration* a constant amount of antigen is added to the tubes containing serial dilution of antisera. This type of titration gives a *constant antigen optimal ratio* and is widely used in estimating the antitoxin contents of horse antisera. Because of the different conditions in the two types of titration, the value obtained for ratios also differs, sometimes up to 30 percent or more. These differences are probably due to the fact that at the higher dilutions of antigen, the concentrations of serum above that required for optimal precipitation often fail to enchance the precipitation and may even slow it down.

Table 10-7. An Example of Constant Antibody Precipitation Reaction

Antigen Dilution	Appearence of Mixture After 1 hour at 37° C	Time of First Flocculation	
1/10	Clear	Prozone	⎫ Antigen
1/20	Clear	Prozone	⎬ Excess
1/40	Opalescent	30 minutes	⎭
1/80	Turbid with floccules	5 minutes =	optimal tube
1/160	Turbid	10 minutes	⎫
1/320	Opalescent	20 minutes	⎬ Antibody
1/640	Opalescent	30 minutes	⎬ Excess
1/1280	Clear	Postzone	⎬
1/2560	Clear	Postzone	⎭

The antibody is rabbit antiserum prepared horse globulin, at a final dilution of 1/10. The antigen is horse globulin diluted initially 1/5 and then by doubling dilutions.
The optimal tube in this experiment is that containing 1/10 antibody and 1/80 antigen; hence the ratio of antigen:antibody is 1:8.

In the precipitation reaction the *zone of equivalence* is the region where the relative proportions of antigen and antibody are such that no antigen, and little or no antibody, can be detected in solution (Fig. 10-2). Normally the zone of equivalence coincides with the region of optimal proportions. On either side of equivalent zone lie the regions of antigen and antibody excess (Fig. 10-2). The precipitation is incomplete in these regions.

Antisera can be divided into two broad categories: *Rabbit (R) type* and *Horse (H) type*. The R-type antisera are characterized by a tendency to form relatively insoluble complexes in both regions, especially in the region of antibody excess. The H-type antisera, on the other hand, tend to have narrow zones of precipitation and to form soluble complexes in the region of antibody, as well as of antigen, excess. The R-type antisera tend to form precipitation at uniform rates through the whole region of antibody excess. Consequently no single optimal proportion ratio can be determined when a constant amount of antigen is titrated. By contrast, the H-type antisera exhibit well-defined ratios with both constant antigen and constant antibody titration methods.

Since horse antisera to polysaccharide antigens are of high molecular

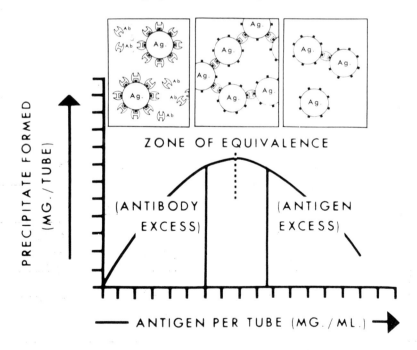

Fig. 10-2. A schematic illustration of a typical precipitation curve. The lattice of antigen-antibody complex is formed optimally at the equivalence zone. The excess of either antibody or antigen results in a less amount of precipitation. [From Gordon, B. L., and Ford, D. K. (1971): *Essentials of Immunology.* Philadelphia, F. A. Davis Company.]

weight (IgM) and do not behave like H-type antisera in the precipitation reaction, the relative proportions of IgG and IgM antibodies in the antisera may be the major factor that determines whether an antiserum belongs to the R or the H type. The capacity to produce precipitation antibody, precipitin, varies greatly in different animal species. For example, it is difficult to obtain precipitin or agglutinin from guinea pigs, although they produce neutralizing antibody quite well.

Several theories have been advanced to explain the mechanism of the precipitation reaction. Marrack in 1934 proposed the *lattice theory*. The lattice theory states that the precipitation is caused by the formation of a network of antigen and antibody molecules held together by specific interaction of their combining sites. This is based on the following postulates: (1) The antigenic determinants are multivalent and hydrophilic. This, combined with a negative charge on the antigen molecule as a whole, produces a water-stable colloid, in which the antigen molecules repel each other while attracting water molecules. (2) The antibody molecule is at least divalent (IgM may have as many as 10 combining sites with five valences), is hydrophilic with negative charge, and forms a stable

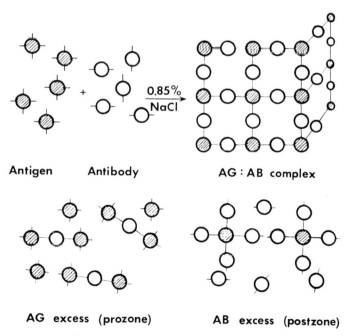

Fig. 10-3. A schematic illustration of the lattice theory of Marrack. The antibody has at least two combining sites. At the right proportion of antigen and antibody in the mixture, they will form an antigen–antibody complex, which is thought to be a form of lattice. The prozone phenomenon is due to antigen excess, and the postzone phenomenon to antibody excess. [From Gray, D. F. (1970): *Immunology*. New York, American Elsevier Publishing Company, Inc. By permission of Edward Arnold (Publishers) Ltd., London.]

colloid. (3) When the antigen and antibody are mixed together in the presence of a suitable electrolyte, the determinants on each surrender their water affinities to become hydrophobic and are drawn together by their corresponding determinants. This is the first stage of the precipitation reaction and it is completed within milliseconds. (4) The negatively charged antigen-antibody complex (primary union) is neutralized by the electrolyte, and a continuous three-dimensional lattice is slowly formed resulting in a visible precipitate of floccules. This is the second stage of the reaction and ordinarily takes several hours to complete (Fig. 10-3).

The lattice theory has stood the test of time and is still adequate to explain many features of serologic reaction. For example, the *zone phenomena* in the precipitation reaction can be explained by the development of lattices in the tubes in the equivalence zone or regions of optimal proportion. Here the proportions favor sequential union between antigen and antibody. In the presence of excess of either antigen or antibody, the reactant in the minority is quickly coated with unattached molecules of the other. This produces a large number of tiny aggregates having occupied combining sites but no capacity to attract each other (Fig. 10-3). The prozone in the area of antibody excess may create a problem in the diagnosis of human and bovine brucellosis by agglutination methods unless serum dilutions are extended beyond the prozone area.

Practical Application of Precipitin Reaction

Ring Test. The simplest form of the precipitin reaction is the ring test extensively used in Lancefield's streptococcal grouping technique. An extract of streptococcal group-specific polysaccharide "C" substance is layered on to groups A, B, C, or G streptococcal antisera prepared in rabbits. By this interfacial technique the reaction is visible as the formation of a white disc or plane at the junction of the two perfectly clear fluids. Under the conditions of the ring test the reaction takes place over a wide range of concentrations as the antigen and antibody diffuse into one another until the optimal ratio is reached. Each precipitin test should be accompanied by control tubes containing immune serum and saline, nonimmune serum, and antigen. No precipitation should be seen in the control tubes. In forensic medicine unknown proteins are identified by using appropriate antisera. This method is suitable for identifying blood and tissues in murder cases or in automobile accidents and horse, kangaroo, or other illegal meat in processed foods intended for human diet. A special adaptation of this method is the capillary tube precipitation technique where the precipitate formed as two solutions diffused together falls to the bottom of the tube and can be roughly quantitated.

Constant Antibody Optimal Ratio Titration. Dean and Webb introduced an arbitrary unit of antibody in a horse globulin-antiglobulin titration. The Dean and Webb unit is that amount of antibody flocculating optimally with 0.00001 ml of the antigen. For example, if 1/16 dilution of an antigen flocculates optimally with 1/2 dilution of antibody, 1 ml of antigen would flocculate with 8 ml of antibody; hence 0.00001 ml of antigen (arbitrary standard) would flocculate with 0.00008 ml of antibody. Therefore, the antiserum under test contains 1/0.00008 = 12,500 units of antibody per ml. This approach represents an early effort at quantitation which is seldom used any more, but the principles involved are commonly employed in quantitations expressed in arbitrary units.

Ramon Flocculation Test. A constant antigen optimal ratio test developed by Ramon is suitable for following the development of antibody response against diphtheria toxin in horses. Fresh toxin is first standardized against an international standard antitoxin and then titrated against the unknown test horse serum. The potency of the unknown serum can be assessed against the standard antitoxin and expressed as "international units."

Agar Gel Diffusion Methods (Immunodiffusion). Greater precision and ability to recognize the multiplicity of components in the mixture of antigen and antibody can be achieved by allowing the reactants to diffuse simultaneously in agar gel. Oudin and Held in 1946 showed that antigen diffusing through a semisolid agar column containing antibody produces a concentration gradient of antigen to form a specific precipitate when optimal proportions are reached with respect to the antibody present. As the antigen migrates down the column, the zone of maximal precipitation may also move down as the initially formed precipitate dissociates in the presence of excess antibody. The rate of movement depends on temperature, the concentration of antigen and antibody, molecular size, and shape. The density of the precipitate depends on the concentration of precipitable antibody (precipitin). A variation of this procedure is to allow both antigen and antibody to diffuse toward each other from the opposite side of the agar column. This procedure is the *Oakley-Fulthorpe* test (*double diffusion in one dimension*).

Mancini et al. in 1965 developed a method for a quantitative radial immunodiffusion. Melted 3 percent agar gel buffered at pH 8.6 is mixed with an appropriate amount of specific antiserum and poured to make a layer 1 mm thick. After the agar is solidified, wells of 1 mm diameter are punched out in the agar plate. An accurately measured volume of antigen is introduced into each of the wells by means of a micropipette. After incubation in a humidified environment, ring-shaped bands of precipitate (halos) are formed concentrically around the wells (*single diffusion in two dimensions*). The diameter of the halo is measured after migration has stopped and is compared with that of the standard reference plate. The diameter of the halo ring has a linear relationship with the amount of the antigen in the well at a given concentration of the antiserum in the agar plate.

5

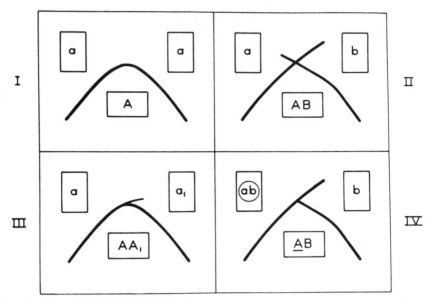

Fig. 10-4. Basic comparative precipitation patterns in Ouchterlony plate technique. I: line of identity, II: line of non-identity, III: line of partial identity, and IV: line of one-sided inhibition, which may indicate the presence of multispecific antigen particles in one of the wells. [From Ouchterlony, O. (1967): In *Handbook of Experimental Immunology*, Weir, M. D. (ed.). Philadelphia, F. A. Davis Co., p. 678.]

This method has been adapted for the quantitative estimation of different classes of immunoglobulins in serum and other body fluids, employing antisera specific for the heavy chains of immunoglobulin classes. It is the most useful method for the estimation of low levels of immunoglobulins in patients with hypogammaglobulinemia.

Ouchterlony, in 1948, devised a precipitin method based on double diffusion in two dimensions in agar plates. This method allows a simultaneous, direct comparison of several antigens or antibodies (Fig. 10-4). When comparing antigen, a reference serum is placed in a well punched in the agar. The homologous antigen and unknown sample are placed in equidistant wells. As the reagents diffuse toward each other, precipitation occurs along the line of optimal proportions. Antigens can thus be compared with respect to their immunologic relationships and be defined as having immunologic identity, non-identity, or partial identity with one another (Fig. 10-4).

The relative distance of the line between antigen and antibody wells depends on the relative concentration of the interacting molecules. When antigen or antibody is in great excess, the line will not form in the agar between the two wells. Instead a precipitate will form in the well containing the lesser component.

Gel precipitation techniques have many advantages over the fluid precipitation. They are useful in analyzing complex mixtures of antigens or antibodies. They permit a simultaneous study of the immunologic components of immune sera and their electrophoretic mobility. They may be used as a rapid diagnostic tool in virus diseases, e.g., small pox or rinderpest, and in many fungal or bacterial tests as well.

Elek in 1948 further adapted gel diffusion as an *in vitro* test for the detection of diphtheria toxin. A strip of filter paper soaked in 1000 units of diphtheria antitoxin is laid on the surface of a serum agar plate. Test organisms, together with control strains, are inoculated as single lines at right angles to the antitoxin strip. When toxin is formed by the growing organism, it diffuses out to meet the diffusing antitoxins, producing a fine, tangential line of white precipitate at the junction (Fig. 10-5). In this way even the rate of production of toxin can be quantitated immunologically.

Immunoelectrophoresis. By combining electrophoresis with double diffusion, Grabar and Williams in 1953 developed a method of separating the antigenic components of complex mixtures, such as human serum. After electrophoresis in agar, ditches are cut in the agar parallel to the direction of migrating serum protein, and antiserum is placed into the ditch. Antibodies diffuse laterally from the ditch, and after three days or so, a series of individual lines of precipitate corresponding to the final

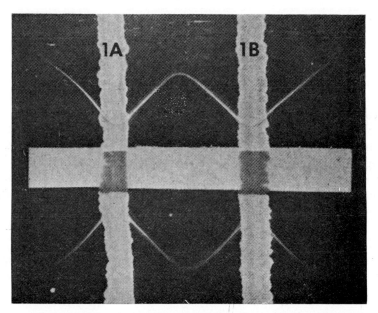

Fig. 10-5. Elek's method for demonstrating toxigenicity of an unknown strain of Corynebacterium diphtheriae. IA, culture streak of known toxin-producing strain; 1B, culture streak of unknown strain. In this instance, both are found to be identical strains. [Modified from Elek, S. D. (1948): Brit. Med. J. 1:493.]

positions of the electrophoretically separated proteins are formed. By this technique human serum can be resolved into more than thirty antigenically distinct proteins. With appropriate controls, the line corresponding with each component can be identified. Micronization of these methods by Scheidegger and Zahnd provided a most useful clinical adaptation of this technique. Methods based on similar principles but using other semisolid phase materials such as cellulose acetate have been employed as additional adaptations of this technique, especially in clinical medicine.

Radioimmunoelectrophoresis. This is a sensitive, quantitative method for the detection of antibodies to antigens such as peptide hormones. The antigen must be available in purified form which can be labeled at high specific activity with an isotope such as ^{131}I. Such antigen is mixed with the developing antiserum and added to the ditch. The antigen diffuses into the gel together with the developing antiserum. Part of this radioactive antigen becomes trapped by specific antibody and is localized in the immunoglobulin precipitate line. The localization of radioactive antigen can be made by autoradiography. Thus, this method permits identification of the immunoglobulin class in which the specific antibodies are present.

Quantitative Precipitation. Heidelberger and Kendall analyzed precipitate formed in the region of optimal proportions of antigen-antibody mixture and quantitated the precipitation in terms of total nitrogen content. If an antigen such as pneumococcal polysaccharide is used, the nitrogen value of the precipitate will correspond with the antibody nitrogen value, since the antigen is nitrogen free. Knowing the amount of antigen nitrogen in the precipitate permits quantitation of the antibody nitrogen by difference. This method can only be applied when the homogeneous antigen is used, since no test tube can be selected as the optimal tube when heterogeneous antigens and antibodies are present.

Quellung Reaction. In 1902 Neufeld described the apparent swelling (German word *Quellung*) of the capsule when bacteria were mixed with appropriate antiserum. The reaction may be due to the binding of antibody molecules to the periphery of the bacterial capsule to form fine precipitate. Thus the bacterial cell wall appears to be swollen without actual swelling of the cell wall.

The capsular swelling test has been extremely useful in the antigenic classification of encapsulated bacteria: Diplococcus pneumoniae, Neisseria meningitidis, and Hemophilus influenzae. Because of the rapidity of the Quellung reaction, the identification of presumed pneumococci in a sputum specimen may take no more than 20 to 30 minutes.

Agglutination

In agglutination, particulate antigens are brought together by antibody. The particles are in general large enough to be seen under the microscope. More usually, in quantitative titrations the flocculation of the suspension is observed with the naked eye. Bacteria, yeasts, red blood cells, or antigen-coated polystyrene latex particles are frequently employed in agglutination tests.

The agglutination test is much more sensitive (10 to 400 times) than the precipitation test in detecting antibodies. Agglutination, like precipitation, is a secondary manifestation that follows primary interaction of antigen and antibody. The two parts of the reaction can be shown to occur optimally under markedly different physicochemical conditions.

The early description of red cell agglutination was made by a German medical student, Creite, in 1869 and by Landois in 1875. The early description of bacterial agglutination was made by Charrin and Roger in 1889 and by Gruber and Durham in 1896. The initial demonstration of immune hemagglutination was made by Ehrlich and Morgenroth in 1900 in goats. In 1901 Landsteiner described human red cell isoantibodies and opened the way to successful blood transfusion, to a better understanding of erythroblastosis, to the discovery of immune tolerance in chimeric twin calves, and to the study of blood group genetics in many other animals.

The same principles are involved in agglutination and precipitation. Under appropriate conditions, agglutination occurs in the test tube containing optimal proportions of the anitgen-antibody mixture. The particulate antigen can be visualized as an inert carrier particle of large size to which multiple antigenic determinants are attached. Therefore we must accept that some form of lattice is formed during agglutination. The prozone and postzone phenomena in the agglutination reaction can also be explained by antigen or antibody excess. The principles are similar to those involved in the precipitation reaction. However, in the agglutination reaction *blocking* (incomplete or so-called monovalent) *antibodies* may prevent agglutination. It has been shown that blocking antibody combines with antigen and inhibits the agglutinating activity of complete antibody added later. The phenomenon associated with so-called incomplete antibody or blocking antibody in agglutinin reactions must now be explained in terms of distribution of antigens on the surface of the particles and quantitative factors related to the nature of the antibody-antigen union, since it is now known that all antibody molecules are at least divalent. Since the blocking antibodies are globulins, particles that are coated with blocking antibody can be made to agglutinate by adding antiglobulin sera (*direct Coombs' test*).

Three hypotheses have been proposed to explain the aspects of agglutination that are not accounted for by a simple lattice theory: (1) the repulsive force between cells, due to the fact that they all carry the same charge, has to be overcome; (2) removal or blockage of the hydrophilic groups on a cell results in their agglutination; and (3) antibodies may be attached to the surfaces of cells but prevented from agglutinating cells because of steric hindrance of antibody molecules resulting from attachment to the cell surface. Pollack et al. have proposed a comprehensive theory to account for all aspects of red cell agglutination. They start with the long-held thesis that the interplay of two sets of forces, *cohesive force* and *electrostatic repulsion,* determines whether charged particles such as red cells or bacteria remain separated or agglutinated in suspension. For example, red cells are negatively charged probably due to the carboxyl groups of sialic acid residues at the surface. In the presence of electrolytes a red cell is surrounded by a diffuse layer of cations forming *zeta potential (Z)* which is defined as

$$Z = \frac{-4.137 \times 10^{-2}}{\sqrt{(D\mu)}} - \frac{3.09 \times 10^{-1}}{D} \text{ volts,}$$

where sodium chloride is the electrolyte, D is the dielectric constant, and μ is the ionic strength. Adsorption of IgG and IgM antibodies to red cells can reduce the surface charge by up to 30 percent.

Bacteria are antigenic mosaics carrying multiple distinct antigens on the surface. These are grouped, for convenience, as flagellar (H), somatic (O, C, M, or T), virulent (Vi), capsular, and exotoxic antigens. An antiserum prepared against typhoid bacilli, for example, contains antibodies directed against Vi, O, and H antigen. Each of these antibodies can be selectively absorbed from the antiserum to become monospecific to H, O, or Vi antigen.

If such monospecific sera are individually mixed with living typhoid bacilli under a cover glass and observed with a microscope, we find that (1) H antibody binds with flagellar antigen, arrests motility, and forms loose agglutinates of bacteria; (2) O antibody binds with the somatic cell wall, resulting in tight clusters, but sometimes leaving the motility intact; (3) Vi antibody fails to arrest motility and to induce agglutination. The complexity of the antigenic structure of bacteria and fungi is only recently being clarified, since scores of antigenic determinants in and on such organisms have been identified by long-term immunization of test animals or continuing infections of man.

Practical Application of Agglutination Test

The Slide Agglutination Test. This simple, qualitative test is widely used for blood grouping, for rapid identification of bacterial species, and in flocculation tests for syphilis.

In blood grouping, the slide agglutination test is most commonly used before the transfusion for cross-matching of donor red cells with the intended recipient's serum. A drop of an approximately 4 percent red blood cell suspension is placed within each area of two circles on a glass slide. A

Table 10-8.   Pattern of Agglutination Observed in the Typing of Human Blood (ABO System)

Blood Group	Genotype	Distribution (%)	Group A Serum	Group B Serum	Red Cell Antigen	Isohemagglutinin in Serum
O	O	45	—	—	none	anti-A anti-B
A	AA or AO	40	—	+	A	anti-B
B	BB or BO	10	+	—	B	anti-A
AB	AB	3	+	+	A and B	none

+: agglutination;   —: nonagglutination

drop of blood group A serum containing agglutinins for blood group B red cells is added to one circle, and a drop of blood group B serum to the other. The glass slide is rocked gently to enhance the mixing of the drop and is observed over 5 minutes for the agglutination of red blood cells. The pattern of agglutination observed in various blood groups is shown in Table 10-8.

In grouping of bacteria, for example, salmonella, a loopful of bacteria taken from young culture is emulsified to give an opalescent suspension in each of several drops of saline on a paraffin-divided slide. To each drop is added a loopful of different group specific anti-O antiserum. One drop without antiserum serves as a control. Gentle rocking of the slide causes visible agglutination within one minute in the drop that contains antiserum specific for the given organism. The control drop and those containing nonspecific antisera remain uniformly opalescent.

The Tube Agglutination Test. This is a standard quantitative test for detailed titration of antibody, especially in patients with enteric infection. Known antigen suspensions are prepared from young, fully virulent cultures in appropriate manner for the preservation of antigen; for example, O suspensions are boiled, H suspensions are formalized, and alcohol extract of Vi antigen is prepared that can be adsorbed on to carrier red cells. The preparations containing the antigen are standardized according to opacity to give a standard concentration and are checked by standard antibody for agglutination.

In the tube agglutination test, a fixed volume of standardized antigen is added to an equal volume of serial dilutions of the patient's serum in normal saline. The result is expressed as *titer,* which is the highest dilution of serum causing visible agglutination at 52°C, for example 1/640, or as its reciprocal, 640.

Serologic diagnosis by agglutination is widely used in enteric infections, brucellosis, leptospirosis, and typhus. The disadvantage of this test is that serologic diagnosis may not be made with certainty until towards the end of the second week of illness, when a rising titer can be demonstrated in paired sera. The advantages of serologic diagnosis are that (1) the diseases can be detected retrospectively when isolation of the causative organism may be difficult or has been missed, and (2) it confirms the bacteriologic diagnosis. Only titers much above the normal range or rising titers in paired sera have diagnostic significance.

Passive Agglutination Test. The limitation of the agglutination test is that it can only be applied if the particles having the homologous antigen at their surfaces are available. For this reason, many antigens have been artificially attached to particulate materials, often by nonimmunologic means. Cells and organic or inorganic particles on which antigen may be attached can be agglutinated (*passive agglutination*). It should also be possible to adsorb antibodies, instead of antigen, to the inert particle and effect agglutination by adding antigen (*reversed passive agglutination*).

Collodion particles have not achieved wide popularity for passive agglutination tests because of the technical difficulty associated with the instability of suspensions and the nonspecific results. The *latex test* devised by Singer and Plotz in 1956 is now in popular use. Latex polystyrene particles coated with a variety of antigens or antibodies are available commercially. Single latex particles of 0.8 to 1.1 μ diameter can adsorb 75,000 molecules of globulin. The mechanism of adsorption is not known. The *bentonite test* employs sodium bentonite particles. Bismuth tannate and barium sulfate particles have also recently been used for agglutination tests.

In recent years, red blood cells have been widely used as carrier particles (*passive hemagglutination test*). Various polysaccharides can be attached directly to the surface of red blood cells. When red blood cells, for example sheep red cells, are treated with tannic acid that acts as a mordant, they will also take up at their surface many protein antigens (Boyden procedure). Polysaccharides derived from the tubercle bacillus can be directly attached to red blood cells and antibodies easily titrated in humans and animals (Koegh procedure). Hormones, viruses, and various tissue antigen can be attached to red cells treated with tannic acid and used to detect minute amounts of antibody with great sensitivity.

Antiglobulin Test (Coombs' Test). The use of the agglutination test has been greatly extended by employment of antisera to human γ-globulin. In 1944 it was found that the Rh negative mothers of erythroblastotic newborns often possess antibodies that do not agglutinate the red cells of newborns under ordinary conditions, but these antibodies can be revealed by a blocking action of agglutination by other agglutinating antibody. When the serum of such Rh negative mothers is mixed with the appropriate red blood cells, no visible reaction is seen. Further, if known agglutinating serum is subsequently added to the mixture, still no agglutination takes place (*blocking*). This is due to the attachment of the *nonagglutinating, incomplete,* or *blocking antibody* to the combining sites of the red cells. However, it was later found that many samples of incomplete or blocking antibody would bring about agglutination in serum or albumin solution rather than in saline. Further, pretreatment of red cells with trypsin, or receptor-destroying enzyme will render them susceptible to agglutination by so-called incomplete antibody.

Red cells carrying such antibodies can be agglutinated by adding antisera directed against human globulin (*Coombs' test*). In the *direct Coombs' test,* red cells that have been coated with antibody (globulin) *in vivo* are agglutinated by antiglobulin antibody; in the *indirect Coombs' test* antibody is adsorbed to the red cells *in vitro* and then the reaction is completed by the addition of antiglobulin antisera. The direct Coombs' test is widely used in the diagnosis of hemolytic disease of the newborn which is caused by maternal antibodies to Rh and other antigens. For unknown reasons, this test is usually negative in hemolytic anemia of the newborn due to ABO incompatibility between the mother and the newborn.

A number of indirect antiglobulin tests have been devised, and these are used not only for the detection of antibodies such as those on the surface of red cells but also for the study of the antigenic structure of imunoglobulins. Many ingenious *sandwich* and *globulin consumption* tests based on the potentialities of the red cell, antigen, antibody, and human gamma globulin interaction have been devised to increase the sensitivity of the test. Some of these are very sensitive immunologic methods. Among the most sensitive of these methodologies are the mixed hemagglutination or mixed hemadsorption techniques described by Fagraeus and her colleagues. The phenomenon is not strictly an agglutination test but rather an adsorption of red cells to the antigen adherent to the glass surface, the red cells being linked by an antiglobulin to the tissue cells, which are coated with an antibody to a surface antigen.

Complement Fixation Test (CFT)

Complement could be described as a function rather than a substance because complement activity is the end result of a chain reaction involving at least eleven separate proteins in normal serum. None of these proteins is an immunoglobulin, and their concentration in blood is not increased by immunization. Complement participates in many antigen-antibody reactions and can cause lysis of cells if the antigen-antibody reaction has taken place on the surface of the cell membrane. This lytic action on the antibody-sensitized cells is utilized in the complement fixation test (CFT).

The complement fixation test is one of the more sensitive serologic reactions. It can detect as little as 0.04 μg of antibody nitrogen or 0.1 μg of pneumococcal polysaccharide antigen. It is the most complex serologic test involving five reagents; antigen, test serum, complement, sheep red cells, and anti-sheep red cell antibodies (hemolysin). The mechanisms of this test are that (1) complement is fixed to antibody-antigen complex; therefore, disappearance of free complement from the mixture indicates the presence of an antigen-antibody interaction; (2) the amount of free complement can be assessed by adding subsequently an indicator system of antibody-sensitized red cells, which will undergo lysis under the influence of free complement; (3) the absence of hemolysis indicates that the complement has been already fixed (or consumed) by antigen-antibody complexes (Table 10-9).

Each of the three reagents used in this system (sheep red cells, hemolytic antibody against sheep red blood cells, and complement) must be separately standardized. Sheep red cells are used as a 3 percent suspension by volume of washed packed cells. The inactivated hemolytic antibody is titrated to determine the minimal hemolytic dilution (MHD). One MHD of hemolytic antibody is defined as the highest dilution of inactivated rabbit antiserum causing complete lysis within 30 minutes at 37° C of one unit volume (e.g., 0.1 ml) of washed 3 percent sheep red cells in the presence of an excess (e.g., 3 MHD) of complement. Alternatively, an end point of 50 percent lysis can be established. One MHD of complement is defined as the highest dilution of guinea pig serum that lyses one unit volume (e.g., 0.1 ml) of washed sheep red cells in the presence of

Table 10-9.　Mechanism and Interpretation of Complement Fixation Test (CFT)

Stage 1	Stage 2	Stage 3		
Test System	Complement Added	Indicator System	Result	Interpretation
Antigen + Positive serum*	Fixed to test system	Sheep red cells + Anti-sheep red cell antibody*	Hemolysis (−)	CFT (+) Antibody present
Antigen + Negative serum*	Remain free, and available for indicator system	Sheep red cell + Anti-sheep red cell antibody*	Hemolysis (+)	CFT (−) Antibody not present

*Serum is heated to inactivate pre-existing complement.

an excess (e.g., 5 MHD) of hemolytic antibody under the same conditions.

A classic example of the complement fixation test is the Wassermann reaction used in the diagnosis of syphilis. Serial dilutions of the patient's serum are mixed with Wassermann antigen or cardiolipin in the presence of complement at 37° C for one hour. Then the indicator system consisting of red cells coated with antibody (sensitized red cells) is added and the mixture is incubated at 37° C for 30 minutes. Appropriate controls are run at the same time. The presence of antisyphilis antibody in the patient's serum is indicated by the absence of hemolysis in the indicator system (Stage 3, see Table 10-9). False positive Wassermann reactions may occur in many diseases, e.g., leprosy, tuberculosis, nonvenereal spirochetal infections, malaria, measles, trypanosomiasis, infectious mononucleosis, mesenchymal disease, and systemic lupus erythematosus.

Immunofluorescence Technique

Coons and his colleagues studied antigenic macromolecules in tissue section by using specific antibody globulin which had been labeled with fluorescent dyes such as anthracene and fluorescein. These dyes were readily linked with antibody globulin. The tissue section had to be prepared in such a way (for example, frozen section) as to avoid damage to the reactivity of the antigen under study with the antibody molecules.

A direct immunofluorescence method employs a single treatment of tissue section with fluorescein-labeled antibody followed by a wash in physiologic buffer saline to get rid of the excess uncombined antibody. The slide is then examined under the fluorescent microscope. The most widely used dyes which fluoresce at the wavelength of 550 to 640 mμ are fluorescein isothiocyanate, lissamine-rhodamine, orange-red, and lemon-yellow. Either antigen or antibodies may be made fluorescent. This method has been used in (1) tracing the distribution of antigens, e.g., viruses, fungi, and bacteria, in the body, (2) tracing the distribution of antibodies in tissues and circulation, (3) locating determinant groups on the surfaces of antigens, (4) locating cytophilic antibodies that tend to stick to cell surfaces, (5) studying valency of antibodies, (6) detecting the presence of antinuclear antibodies in collagen diseases, (7) tracing autoantibody in autoimmune diseases, and (8) locating antigen-antibody-complement complex depositions in tissues. With recent innovations that include intensive incident light sources and even larger beam activation, quantitation of immunologic reactions at cell surfaces by quantitative immunofluorescent methodologies has been possible.

Other variations of this technique are (1) the indirect or double layer technique in which unlabeled specific antibody is combined with the antigen in tissue and then the labeled antibody against that γ-globulin is combined with the unlabeled antibody, (2) the sandwich technique to locate antibody in the tissue by first combining antigen with the antibody in the tissue and then combining the labeled antibody directed against the antigen with the remaining free determinant groups on the antigen, and (3) the indirect method for detection of antigen by having complement attached to antigen-antibody complex and subsequently attaching a labeled antibody directed against one or another of the complement components.

Antibody linked to an electron-dense marker, ferritin, can be used for the localization of antigen (*immunoferritin technique*). This method has been useful in identifying and localizing antigens at the ultrastructural level.

The complexities of the possible uses to which these methodologies can be put is illustrated by the hybrid antibody techniques. Using methods of dismantling and reassembling immunoglobulin molecules, it has been possible to create hybrid molecules that have specificities directed toward antigenic determinants and, for example, marker ferritin molecules. In this way antigen determinants can be localized precisely and specifically within the body, on cell surfaces, or within cells.

Toxin Neutralization Test

The neutralizing capacity of antibodies provides major protective mechanism in several diseases such as diphtheria, tetanus, botulism, and gas gangrene.

Antitoxins are expressed in arbitrary units determined by animal protection experiments. The potency of toxin is expressed as MLD (minimum lethal dose), or the amount of toxin, which injected subcutaneously, will kill a guinea pig weighing 250 gm in 4 to 5 days. The L+ unit of toxin is defined as the amount of toxin which, when mixed with one unit of standard antitoxin and injected subcutaneously, will kill a 250 gm guinea pig in 4 to 5 days. In practice, the assay of antitoxin may be carried out using groups of animals. Death of 50 percent of the animals is taken as a more or less precise end point, i.e. LD_{50}. *In vivo* assay of antitoxin often may fail to agree with *in vitro* titration partly due to the difference in avidity of the antibody molecules.

Virus Neutralization Test

The infective properties of virus can be accurately detected even at a very high dilution of the virus. This allows us to measure the lowest concentration of antibody necessary to neutralize the infective action of these agents. Neutralization of bacteriophage by antibody has been the basis for one of the most sensitive of all techniques for the detection of antibody. The antibody blocks the infectivity of the phage by attaching to the tail of the phage.

Phage particles can be enumerated by counting the number of plaques in an agar layer heavily seeded with bacteria sensitive to phage. TCD_{50} (median tissue culture dose) represents the dose of virus which gives rise to cytopathic change in 50 percent of culture cells, for death of animals (LD_{50}), and for infectivity (ID_{50}). Neutralizing antibody vs viruses can be quantified in terms of capacity to interfere with any of these quantifiable biologic processes.

Passive Cutaneous Anaphylaxis

Ovary introduced passive cutaneous anaphylaxis in 1952. In this procedure, antibody is injected intradermally into the back of a guinea pig. Approximately three hours later the animal is given an intravenous injection of corresponding antigen mixed with a dye, e.g., Evans blue. The vascular reaction at the site of the antibody injection induces extravasation of the dye, resulting in blue discoloration of the injected site of the skin.

Detection of Antibody Produced by Single Cells

Two techniques have been developed and applied successfully to detect antibody produced by single cells. In the *microdroplet method,* single cells which have been isolated from the lymph node or spleen in tiny droplets of nutrient medium by means of a micromanipulator are placed below a layer of paraffin oil and incubated. Antibody production by single cells can be assessed by adding appropriate antigen, e.g., bacteriophage, and checking later for interference with infectivity, agglutination, or fluorescent reaction.

In the *Jerne plaque technique* lymph node cells from animals immunized with sheep red cells are prepared in fully dispersed cell suspension and then incubated for one hour in an agar containing sheep red cells. At the end of incubation, complement is added to the agar plate. Those cells producing antibody against sheep red cells are surrounded by a clear area in the agar produced by the hemolysis. The cells producing the antibody resulting in cell lyses are called *plaque-forming cells* (PFC). The original technique (direct method) detects 19S antibody-producing cells, whereas the modified technique (indirect method) based on adding later IgM anti-immunoglobulin antiserum detects the production of 7S antibodies. By conjugating sheep red cells with various kinds of antigen, this technique can be used to detect antibodies directed against other antigens.

Measurement of Hormones

The hormone is coated with red cells treated with tannic acid. The red cells can be agglutinated by specific antihormone serum. The free hormone in test samples can be measured by virtue of its ability to complete binding of the hormone for the specific antibody and thereby prevent the specific agglutination of hormone-coated red cells (*hemagglutination inhibition test*). This technique, once quite popular, has largely given way to radioimmunoassay techniques for detection and quantitation of hormone.

Other assay methods use radioactively labeled hormones (*radioimmunoassay of hormones*). The principle is that radioactively labeled hormones are added to antihormone antibody. The hormone bound to antibody is separated from the unbound hormone by 50 percent saturated ammonium sulfate (Farr's technique) or by the double antibody technique which adds an excess of precipitating antibody directed against the γ-globulin containing antihormone antibody. In the radioimmunoassay for insulin, for example, labeled and unlabeled insulin compete for anti-insulin antibody. The ratio of bound and free insulin varies inversely with the amount of unlabeled insulin in the test sample. After equilibration the bound and free labeled insulin are separated by paper electrophoresis. The radioactivity in the two separate zones on the paper is counted, and the ratio of bound and free labeled insulin can be calculated. The amount of unlabeled insulin in the test sample is calculated from a standard curve. Many hormones, drugs, and biologicals have been assayed and detected in blood, urine, and in tissue section by this method (Table 10-10). This method and its modifications may be made extremely sensitive, capable of detecting hormones and other substances in small amounts.

Table 10-10. Examples of Detection and Assay of Hormones by Immunologic Techniques

Hormones	*Detection and Measurement*	
Insulin	Chromatoelectrophoresis	2.5 ηg
	Hemagglutination inhibition	10-100 mμg
	Fluorescent antibody technique	β-cells of pancreatic islets
Glucagon	Chromatoelectrophoresis	3 ηg
	Fluorescent antibody technique	β-cells of pancreatic islets
Growth hormone	Hemagglutination inhibition	1-10 mμg
	Precipitin method	1-5 ηg
	Fluorescent antibody technique	Acidophil cells of anterior pituitary
Thyrotropin	Hemagglutination inhibition	1-10 mμg
Corticotropin	Fluorescent antibody technique	Basophil (R-type) cells of anterior and posterior pituitary
Chorionic gonadotropin (in urine)	Hemagglutination inhibition	< 10 mμg
(in serum)	Complement fixation	10 mμg

Equilibrium Dialysis

Marrack and Smith in 1932 used equilibrium dialysis to study the interaction of antigen and antibody. Cellophane dialysis bags containing known amounts of antibody are dialyzed for 18 to 24 hours in a series of buffered solutions containing different concentrations of a hapten small enough to pass freely across the semipermeable cellophane membrane. The concentration of hapten is measured by its color, its fluorescence, or by labeling the hapten with radioactive isotope. When the hapten molecules are bound to the antibody inside the bags, the concentration of hapten is greater inside the bag than outside. The difference would be a function of the total hapten binding capacity of antibody and the average intrinsic association constant of the antibody-hapten interaction.

This technique provides a means of elucidating the nature of antibody and antigen binding sites and the kinetics of the antigen-antibody interaction. However, it cannot at present be used for antigens of large size due to the lack of suitable membranes. If the hapten has propensity to bind serum protein other than immunoglobulins, the antibody must be purified before use.

CROSS REACTION

An antibody produced in response to stimulation of one immunogen may react with some apparently unrelated immunogens. This is called

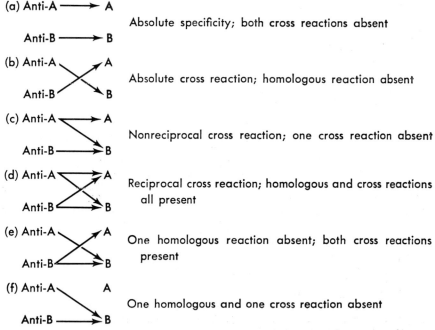

Fig. 10-6. Various types of cross reactions.

cross reaction, the opposite aspect of specificity. Heterophil antibody is a well-known example of cross reaction. Here antibodies induced by viruses or other microorganisms can cause the production of antibodies that recognize and react with sheep red blood cells.

How does cross reaction arise? Several possibilities are that (1) different immunogen may have common antigenic determinants, (2) some immunogen-like cells carry many different antigenic determinants, e.g., group or species specific determinants, (3) heterogeneous antibodies are produced after single immunogen stimulation, or (4) antibody directed against A antigen may react with B antigen due to the conformational similarity of determinant groups of A and B antigen.

Reaction between unrelated antibody and antigen (cross reaction) is generally weaker than the reaction between related antibody and antigen (homologous reaction). However, cross reaction can in some instances be as strong as or stronger than reactions with the homologous determinants. Various types of cross reactions (reciprocal and/or nonreciprocal) are shown in Figure 10-6.

SELECTED REFERENCES

Arrhenius, S., and Madson, T. (1902): In *Contributions from the University Laboratory for Medical Bacteriology to Celebrate the Inauguration of the State Serum Institute,* Solomonsen, C. J. (ed.). Copenhagen, Olsen, Ch. 3.

Charrin, A., and Roger, G. H. (1889): Soc. Biol. 9:667.

Coombs, R. R. A., Howard, A. N., and Wild, F. (1952): Brit. J. Exp. Path. 33:390.

Coons, A. H., Creech, H. J., and Jones, R. N. (1941): Proc. Soc. Exp. Biol. Med. 47:200.

Dean, H. R., and Webb, R. A. (1926): J. Path. Bact. 29:473.

Elek, S. D. (1948): Brit. Med. J. 1:493.

Fagraeus, A. (1972): In *Membranes and Viruses in Immunopathology,* Day, S. B., and Good, R. A. (eds.). New York, Academic Press, p. 535.

Grabar, P., and Williams, C. A. (1953): Biochem. Biophys. Acta 10:193.

Greite, A. (1869): Z. Rat. Med. 36:90.

Gruber, M. (1896): Munchen. Ored. Wschr. 43:206.

Heidelberger, M., and Kendall, F. E. (1929): J. Exp. Med. 50:809.

Heidelberger, M., and Kendall, F. E. (1933): J. Exp. Med. 58:137.

Heidelberger, M., and Kendall, F. E. (1935): J. Exp. Med. 61:563.

Heidelberger, M., and Kendall, F. E. (1936): J. Exp. Med. 64:161.

Heidelberger, M., and Kendall, F. E. (1937): J. Exp. Med. 66:437.

Landois, L. (1895): *Die Transfusion des Blutes.* Leipzig, Vogel.

Landsteiner, K. (1935): *Specificity of Serologic Reactions.* Springfield, Illinois, Charles C Thomas (1936), and New York, Dover Publications, Inc. (1962).

Mancini, G., Carbonara, A. O., and Heremans, J. F. (1965): Immunochemistry 2:235.

Marrack, J. R. (1934): Spec. Rep. Ser. Mid. Res. Conn., No. 194.

Minden, P., Reid, R. T., and Farr, R. S. (1966): J. Immun. 96:180.

Neufeld, F. (1902): Z. Hyg. 15:54.

Ouchterlony, O. (1948): Acta Path. Microbiol. Scand. 25:186.

Oudin, J. (1946): C. R. Acad. Sci. (Paris) 222:115.

Ovary, Z. (1952): Int. Arch. Allerg. 3:293.

Pollack, W., et al. (1965): Transfusion 5:158.

Scheidegger, J. J., and Zahnd, J. (1957): Helvet. Med. Acta 24:499.

Singer, J. M., and Plotz, C. M. (1956): Amer. J. Med. 21:888.

Zinsser, H. (1921): J. Immun. 6:289.

FURTHER READINGS

Chase, M. W., and Williams, C. A. (eds.) (1967): *Methods in Immunology and Immunochemistry*. New York, Academic Press.

Coombs, R. R. A., and Franks, D. (1969): Progr. Allerg. *13*:174.

Crowle, A. J. (1961): *Immunodiffusion*. New York, Academic Press.

Kabat, E. A., and Mayer, M. M. (1961): *Experimental Immunochemistry*. Springfield, Ill., Charles C Thomas.

Weir, D. M. (ed.) (1967): *Handbook of Experimental Immunology*. Philadelphia, F. A. Davis.

11

Complement System and Biologic Amplification Mechanisms

Pfeiffer in 1894 demonstrated that the immune serum of guinea pigs acquires the capacity to dissolve cholera bacteria (Pfeiffer's phenomenon). Bordet in 1895 repeated the experiment and found that Pfeiffer's phenomenon, i.e., immune lysis of bacteria, requires two components of serum: a heat-stable component (56°C for 30 minutes) that is present only in immune serum and a heat-labile component present in both immune and nonimmune sera. Bordet in 1898 described the same phenomenon in the serum of animals immunized with red blood cells of different species and called the heat-labile factor *alexin*. The term *alexin* was later replaced by the new term *complement* proposed in 1899 by Erhlich and Morgenroth, who concluded from their experiments that serum contains two substances: the *interbody* with two haptophore groups and analogous to the immune body, and an *addiment*, which they named *complement*. The first complement fixation test was later developed by Bordet and his associate Gengou. The best known form of the complement fixation test is the Wassermann test for the diagnosis of syphilis.

It was later found that a brief incubation of fresh normal serum with preformed antigen-antibody complex depleted the complement activity of the serum. The works of Pillemer and his colleagues in early 1950s showed that human and guinea pig sera contain at least four distinct components required for the hemolytic activity of complement, two heat-labile and two heat-stable components:

1. C'_1—heat-labile, found in the euglobulin fraction of serum.
2. C'_2—heat-labile, found in α- and γ-globulin fraction of serum.
3. C'_3—heat-stable, inactivated by zymosan.
4. C'_4—heat-stable, inactivated by ammonia or hydrazine.

Sera from different species contain different proportions of complement components, but each component can be exchanged from one species to another, even though different components may be less efficient in interactions across the species barriers. For example, C'_3 is the limiting factor in human and guinea pig sera, whereas C'_2 is limiting in mouse serum. It

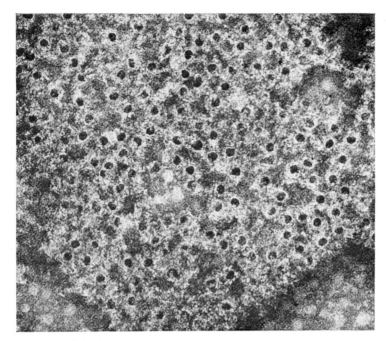

Fig. 11-1. Electronmicrograph of holes on the red cell membrane caused by the action of anti-red cell antibody and complement. The red cells were treated with an autoantibody against red cell membrane from a patient with autoimmune hemolytic anemia and human complement. The dark circles correspond to the holes (pits) in the red cell membrane.

has since been found that C_1 consists of three components linked together and stabilized by divalent cations and that what was originally called C_3 can be separated into six components. Mayer and his colleagues proposed a theory to explain the order and mechanism of interaction of these components. It was assumed that the lysis of the red cell, for example, could be the consequence of inducing a single site of irreversible damage ("hit") at the cell membrane. Consequently, osmotic imbalance due to the free movement of electrolytes leads to the ultimate lysis of cells. Morphologic support for this hypothesis has been revealed by electron-microscopic analysis (Fig. 11-1).

NOMENCLATURE OF COMPLEMENT COMPONENTS

The term *complement* now pertains collectively to 11 proteins or 9 distinct components that constitute a significant proportion of the total serum proteins. Approximately 10 percent of human serum globulin belongs to the complement components. The activation of complement activity is initiated mainly by the antigen-antibody complex, and the components act in specific sequence—a cascade. The biologically active by-products resulting from the activation of some of the components act as mediators of the inflammatory process, alter the vascular permeability, cause chemo-taxis of leukocytes, effect contraction of smooth muscles, and release his-tamine from mast cells. The entire cascade resulting in activation of the final components C8 and C9 leads to lysis of sensitized red blood cells.

In 1968, an international agreement was reached for the definition and designation of each component of complement. The components are des-ignated numerically and represented by symbols: C1, C2, C3, C4, C5, C6, C7, C8, and C9. The three subcomponents of C1 are C1q, C1r, and C1s. The complement dependent cytolysis starts with the interaction of eryth-rocyte (E) and antibody (A) leading the formation of their complex (EA). The interaction of EA with C1 is represented as EAC1, the inter-action of EAC1 with C4 as EAC14, etc. These notations may be abbrevi-ated by indicating only the first and the last reacting components. For ex-

Table 11-1. Physicochemical Characteristics of Proteins of the Complement System

Name	Molecular Weight (1×10^5) (Daltons)	Electrophoretic Mobility	Approximate Serum Concentration ($\mu g/ml$)	Major Fragments
Classic components:				
C1q	400	γ_2	190	
C1r	168	β	?	
C1s	79	α_2	120	
C4(E)	240	β_1	430	C4a, C4b
C2	117	β_2	30	C2a, C2b, C-kinin
C3(F)	185	β_1	1300	C3a, C3b, C3c(β1a), C3d(α2D)
C5(F)	185	β_1	75	C5a, C5b
C6	125	β_2	60	
C7	?	β_2	?	
C8	150	γ_1	trace	
C9	79	α	trace	
Alternate pathway factors				
Properdin	223	β (in agar) γ_2 (in agrose)	trace	
Factor B (C3PA, GBG, $\beta_2$glycoprotein II)	105	β_2	225	a-fragment (GGG) b-fragment (GAG)
Control proteins:				
C1INH(EI)	90	α_2	180	
C3bINA(KAF)	100	β_2	25	
C6INA	?	β_1	?	
Anaphylatoxin INA	310	α	?	

ample, EAC1423 may be written as EAC1-3. Complement components that are enzymatically active may be expressed by placing a bar above the appropriate numeral. Thus $C\bar{1}$ denotes activated C1 and $C\overline{42}$ the C3 convertase. Fragments derived from cleavage of components during reaction are designated with small letters. For example, C3a and C3b are fragments of C3 produced by the action of $C\overline{42}$. Hemolytically inactive forms of components are denoted with the suffix i (e.g., C4i, C3i). Almost all of the complement components have been isolated, purified, and identified immunochemically and chemically. Much of the credit for these achievements must be given to Nelson and Mayer for guinea pig complement and Müller-Eberhard for human complement.

Some of the physicochemical characteristics of the 11 components of complement are shown in Table 11-1. They differ widely in molecular size and electrophoretic mobility. All components of human complement have been purified so that it is possible to perform chemical and immunologic analysis for their detection. Unlike the immunoglobulins, these complement components appear to be antigenically distinct from one another and do not share antigenically identifiable peptide chains. The concentrations of various components of complement in the serum do not appear to be related to their functions in immune hemolysis.

REACTION SEQUENCE OF COMPLEMENT AND GENERATION OF EFFECTOR MOLECULES

Most of the information about the complement system derives from studies of lysis of cells such as the sheep red cells. The cells (E) are treated (sensitized) with appropriate antibody (A) to form an antigen-antibody complex (EA). The interaction of EA with the complement components leads to the generation of a series of intermediates and by-products (Table 11-2).

The first component (C1) comprises three subunits, C1q, C1r, and C1s. The C1q subunit binds to the Fc portion of immunoglobulin of the EA. Under the electron microscope this fascinating molecule looks like a six-fingered hand and appears to be made up of at least 16 separate peptide chains capable of uniting more or less specifically with the Fc component of IgM and IgG. Porter has recently discovered that C1q has many characteristics of collagen, including repeating of the structural composition of the amino acids and a high hydroxyproline composition. In humans, IgG1, IgG2, IgG3, and IgM molecules are capable of initiating reaction with this first complement component. The activated C1, either as bound EAC1 or free in the fluid phase as $C\bar{1}$, or its subunit $C\bar{1}s$, has esterase activity.

Following treatment with C1 esterase, C4 achieves a transient state of activation. In the activated form ($C\bar{4}$), the molecule is able to react with

Table 11-2. Classical Reaction Sequences of Complement Components and Generation of Biologically Active Substances

Reaction Sequences	Biologically Active Substances
(1) EA + C1q,r,s, → EAC1q,r,s, (EAC$\overline{1}$)	
(2) EAC$\overline{1}$ + C4 → EAC$\overline{1}$,4 ↘ C4i	Virus neutralization
(3) EAC$\overline{1}$,4 + C2 → EAC$\overline{1}$,$\overline{42}$ ↘ C2i, C-kinins	C-kinins
(4) EAC$\overline{1}$,$\overline{42}$ + C3 → EAC$\overline{1}$,$\overline{423}$ ↘ C3a	{ Immune adherence / Enhanced phagocytosis } Anaphylatoxin
(5) EAC$\overline{1}$,$\overline{423}$ + C5,C6 → EAC$\overline{1}$,$\overline{423}$,5,6 ↘ C5a	{ Anaphylatoxin / Chemotaxis }
(6) EAC$\overline{1}$,$\overline{423}$,5,6, + C7 → EA1-7 ↘ C$\overline{567}$	Susceptible to lymphocytotoxicity { React with bystander cells / Chemotaxis }
(7) EAC1-7 + C8 → EAC1-8	
(8) EAC1-8 + C9 → EAC1-9	Lysis of bacteria and red cells

a suitable receptor and become bound; if it fails to collide with a receptor within a short period of time, it undergoes inactivation and accumulates as C4i in the fluid phase. C4 may bind either directly to red cell membrane or cell-bound antibody; in both locations it is cytolytically active. During activation C4 is also cleaved by C$\overline{1}$, resulting in C4a and C4b. EAC14 has capacity to neutralize certain virus.

The reaction of C$\overline{1}$ with C4 uncovers the capacity of C$\overline{1}$ to cleave to its other natural substrate, C2. The major fragment of C2 is taken up by the cell to form EAC142. The unaltered form of C2 can also bind directly with EAC14 to form EAC142, and this binding is reversible. The EAC142 complex is extremely labile and reverts to EA14 with a half-life of approximately 10 minutes at 37°C. The decay of EAC142 is accompanied by release of an inactive C2 derivative C2a. The C$\overline{42}$ enzyme (C3 convertase) present on EAC142 cleaves the C3 into two fragments. The major fragment, C3i, either binds to the cell to form EAC1423 or remains in the fluid phase as C3i. A smaller fragment (C3a) is released in the fluid phase and mediates the anaphylatoxin activity. One active site of C$\overline{42}$ is capable of catalyzing the binding of several hundred molecules of C3—a biologic amplification mechanism. It has been postulated that C3 passes through a transient period of activation just as does C4.

The C$\overline{423}$ enzyme of EAC1423 cleaves C5. The major fragment of C5, together with C6, forms an unstable intermediate EAC142356. The minor fragment, C5a, has the activity of an anaphylatoxin and is a powerful chemotactic agent. The C7 interacts with EAC1-6 to achieve a stable EAC1-7. The C567 fragment liberated may react with "bystander" cells and seems to have chemotactic activity. The EAC1-7 cell is then suscept-ible to lymphocytotoxicity.

Following the attachment of C8 to EAC1-7, lysis of cell ensues and proceeds at a slow rate even in the absence of C9. Addition of C9, how-ever, enhances the speed of lytic reaction. It is postulated that C8 is the component which actually causes the damage on the cell membrane and that C9 functions as an enhancing or activating factor. However, electron microscopic studies have revealed that the characteristic "holes" (Fig. 11-1) on the membrane appear earlier in the complement sequence at C5 but that the functional holes do not appear after the action of C8 and C9. In addition to C9, the lysis of the EAC1-8 can be enhanced by phenanthro-lene. Both C9 and phenanthrolene activity can be inhibited by EDTA (ethylenediaminetetraacetate). As with cell lysis the entire complement cas-cade seems to be required for most efficient antibody-mediated bacteri-cidal action of serum.

ALTERNATE PATHWAY OF COMPLEMENT ACTIVATION

Recent studies have disclosed that the terminal components, C3-9, can be activated directly without preceding activation of C142. The first evi-dence for the existence of alternate pathways was shown by Pillemer and his colleagues in 1954 when they described what they called the *properdin system*. Properdin (factor p) is a serum protein that reacts with zymosan at 17°C in the presence of magnesium ions and certain additional non-dialyzable factors to form a complex (PZ), which upon exposure at 37°C electively inactivates C3-9. The additional factors required to form PZ were factor A, a hydrazine sensitive factor, factor B, a heat-labile factor, and an euglobulin fraction of serum. Since the three factors resemble C4, C2, and C1, respectively, it was once postulated that the properdin sys-tem may represent one form of classical reaction sequence initiated by the interaction of natural, low avidity antibody and zymosan at 17°C. However, Gewurz et al. in 1968 showed the initiation of alternate path-ways by bacterial lipopolysaccharide (LPS) which interacts with serum to utilize and destroy components C3-C9 without utilizing significant amounts of C1, C4, and C2. It was later established that the alternate pathway could be engaged, even though the C142 pathway was com-pletely inoperative.

Additional evidence for the alternate pathway is that the anticomple-mentary activity of cobra venom which inactivates C3 selectively oper-ates through this alternate mechanism. This reaction required a cofactor called C3 proactivator (C3PA) by Müller-Eberhard, and has been shown to be immunochemically identical to the properdin factor B, which has a molecular weight of 223×10^3 daltons. Factor B was shown to be absent from the serum of a patient with an abnormal activation of complement.

Factor A appears to be a hydrazine sensitive euglobulin of approximately 180×10^3 molecular weight. Factor $\overline{A}$ has a molecular weight of 30 to 40×10^6 and is also probably the same as the one Müller-Eberhard et al. called C3PA convertase. Factor E has a molecular weight of 160×10^3 and is required for the activation of C3 by cobra venom. A tentative scheme for the overall view of the alternate pathway of complement activation is shown in Figure 11-2.

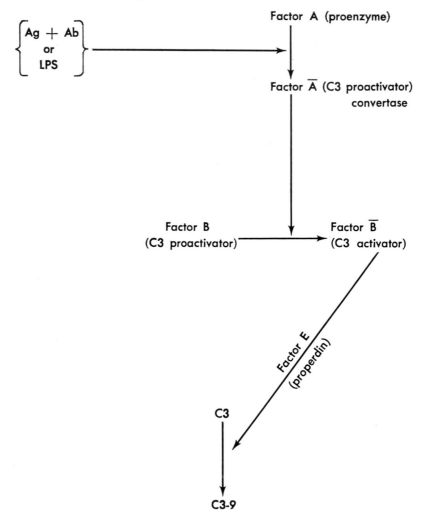

Fig. 11-2. Postulated scheme of alternate pathway for complement activities.

REGULATORY MECHANISMS OF COMPLEMENT ACTIVATION

Complement activation can be inhibited *in vitro* by chelating Ca^{++} or Mg^{++} by citrate or EDTA, and by heat inactivation of heat-labile components. C4 and C3 are destroyed by ammonia or hydrazine. Alkylphosphates combine with the active sites of esterases and block the esterase enzyme activities of C1 and C2 They have no effect on the native form of C1 or C2 unless the latter has already been converted to active forms.

Naturally occurring inhibitors of complement can be found in normal human and guinea pig serum (Table 11-1). The heat-labile α_2-neuraminoglycoprotein (C1INH) inhibits C1 and S1s activity as well as plasma kallikrein. The serum of patients with hereditary angioneurotic edema lacks this inhibitor. Consequently, these patients have recurrent attacks of acute noninflammatory edema in localized areas. If the edema occurs in the larynx, it may lead to death from airway obstruction. Absence of inhibition of C1 esterase activity leads to lowering of serum concentrations of C4 and C2 and thus to secondary deficiencies of these components in serum. This is important clinically, since C1 esterase inhibitor deficiency leads not only to hereditary angioneurotic edema but also to increased susceptibility to kidney disease and lupus erythematosus. The C1INH also inhibits the capacity of $C\overline{1}r$ to activate C1s or to cleave to a synthetic substrate.

The C3b inactivator (C3bINA) destroys the hemolytic, immune-adherence, and phagocytosis-enhancing properties of C3b fragment by cleaving C3b into C3c and C3e. An inactivator of C6 on EAC1-6 complex has been described. Finally an enzyme called *anaphylatoxin inactivator* cleaves the C-terminal arginine from the C3a and C5a anaphylatoxic fragments to render them inactive.

The C4 inactivator can be produced from guinea pig euglobulin and is active only against C4 and not against C2. A hemolytically inactive form of guinea pig C8 can block the ability of EAC1-7 to accept a hemolytically active form of C8. The inactive form of C8 is produced from the hemolytically active form at low ionic strength and pH 7.5. The C3 inhibitor can be obtained by incubating human serum with zymosan and dissociating the inhibitor from the zymosan complex. This inhibitor blocks hemolytic activity and specifically blocks the steps after the formation of EAC142 but does not interfere with immune adherence. Plasmin or fibrinolysin is a proteolytic enzyme derived from its precursor by activation. It destroys hemolytic activity of complement by exhausting the C1s precursor of the C1 esterase. In addition, it activates C1s to $C\overline{1}s$ in the absence of C1q and C1r and also destroys the functional activity of the C1 inactivator. Trypsin is another enzyme that inactivates C1s. Both trypsin and plasmin can cleave C3 and C5 and thus release biologically active fragments.

The serum of cattle and certain ruminants contains a naturally occurring substance which aggregates an immune complex fixed with complement. This substance called *conglutinin* by Bordet and Streng in 1909 is not found in most other species of mammals. Conglutinin has been purified and identified as a specific serum protein with molecular weight of 75,000 and a sedimentation coefficient 7.8S. It is antigenically unrelated to any known class of immunoglobulins.

Substances analogous to conglutinin have been produced by injection of "alexinated" material (fixed with complement) from one animal into another of the same species. These substances called *immunoconglutinins* by Streng in 1930 may be isoantibodies or autoantibodies directed against a hidden determinant group of one of the complement molecules. The hidden determinant groups appear as a consequence of the activation of the native form of complement components. Immunoconglutinins have been shown to have specificity for C3 or C4, and it is possible to find the specificity for other components. Under appropriate conditions the immunoconglutinins may inhibit immune adherence or enhance complement fixation. Immunoconglutinins, which may appear during the course of infectious, collagen, or autoimmune diseases and during immunization, have been identified as being IgM and IgG molecules.

The cascade of complement activation is also modulated by the instability of certain complement enzymes under natural conditions. For example, the C2 portion of $C\overline{42}$ enzyme and the C5 fragment from EAC14235 have extremely short half-lives under natural conditions. This rapid degradation can thus influence the entire sequence of complement activation.

BIOLOGIC ACTIVITY OF COMPLEMENT

Cytolysis. The classic activity of complement is immune cytolysis. This requires antimembrane antibody and all nine components of complement. Recently complement has been found to cause cytolysis independent of antibody participation. This is called nonimmune cytolysis and begins with attachment of C567 to the cell surface to form EAC567. $C\overline{423}$ can effect the formation of EAC567 either in the fluid phase or from the surface of an adjacent $EAC\overline{423}$ cell. Apparently the half-life of the activated forms of C567 is long enough to permit the C567 to combine with the distant cells. When C8 and C9 are added to EA567, cell lysis takes place.

When complement interacts with monocytes or lymphocytes, it may induce lysis of red blood cells. When chicken red cells (E), IgM antibody (A), and isolated complement components are used, EAC142, EAC1-3, EAC1-7 are obtained, and when such cells are incubated with either purified monocytes or purified lymphocytes, lysis can occur. Both EAC1-3 and EAC1-7 can be lysed in the presence of isolated monocytes, but only EAC1-7 could be lysed in the presence of isolated lymphocytes.

Anaphylatoxins. Histamine-releasing substances produced in serum by an antigen-antibody complex may produce symptoms similar to those of systemic anaphylaxis. These substances are biologically active, low molecular weight fragments of the complement components, C3 and C5. Anaphylatoxins are also referred to as C3a and C5a. They cause contraction of smooth muscles or they can change capillary permeability. Both of these manifestations may be inhibited by certain anihistamines, but they are chemically and biologically distinct from each other.

C3 is cleaved by $C\overline{42}$ into the biologically active fragment C3a and a larger fragment C3b. C3a has molecular weight of 7200, contains a greater number of basic than acidic amino acid residues, and migrates toward the cathode on electrophoresis at pH 9. The release of C3a from C3 is enhanced at a pH lower than 5. Biologically active C3a fragment may also be produced by treating C3 with trypsin, C3 inactivator complex, or plasmin. Although the biologic activity of these substances is similar, the chemical compositions may not be identical with that produced by $C\overline{42}$.

C5 is cleaved by $C\overline{423}$ of $EAC1\overline{423}$ and releases biologically active C5a. Treatment of C5 with trypsin produces a similar fragment. The molecular weight of C5a is estimated to be approximately 15,000. An inhibitor of both C3a and C5a activity can be found in whole human serum and has been shown to be a thermolabile 10S pseudoglobulin with electrophoretic mobility of an α-globulin. This protein can inactivate a large molar excess of both C3a and C5a and may play an important regulatory function *in vivo*.

Chemotactic Factors. Antigen–antibody complexes *in vivo* or those suspended in fresh serum *in vitro* are powerfully chemotactic for neutrophils. This influence is evident from studies of the Arthus reaction (page 182). They can be demonstrated *in vitro* and thus quantified by means of a simple device consisting of a chamber divided into two sections by a fine membrane which has pores large enough to allow neutrophils to migrate through, but small enough to prevent random passage of neutrophils (Boyden chamber). Neutrophils in a suitable medium are placed in one half and the test substance for chemotactic activity in the other half of the chamber, and incubated at 37° C for appropriate time. The chemotactic activity of the test substance can be measured in terms of the numbers of neutrophils that migrate through to the other side of the membrane. This method, at best semiquantitative with the classical Boyden chamber, has been rendered quantitative by using a double membrane technique in the lower chamber. By this method, it has been shown that C3a, C5a, and C567 are chemotactic. Further, the treatment of C3a with trypsin abolishes its capacity to contract smooth muscles but leaves intact its chemotactic activity. The mechanism which renders C567 chemotactic has not been fully investigated. Studies of chemotactic activity of C567 complex in C5-deficient mice and C6-deficient rabbits have not revealed the exact role of C5 and C6 in the generation of chemotactic C567 complex. It has recently been shown that lipopolysaccharide (LPS) and inulin can interact with serum to activate the alternate pathway. Both can accelerate clotting of blood from normal rabbits, but not from C6-deficient rabbits. This evidence has been used to implicate the C6 component in intravascular coagulation.

Thus, the by-products of the fluid phase of the complement-component interaction possess permeability-enhancing, chemotactic, and clot-promoting activities, as well as a potential for extending the cytotoxic events to unsensitized bystander cells. The alternate pathway also participates in those events leading to cell lysis, bactericidal function, and clot promotion.

Immune Adherence. In 1953 Nelson described a phenomenon in which particles coated with antigen–antibody complexes in the presence of complement *in vitro* stick tightly to platelets of many species or to red blood cells, but not to platelets, of primates. This reaction, called immune adherence, was considered important in the defense against pathogenic bacteria or virus, since such particles adsorbed to the surface of red cells may be rapidly ingested by phagocytes. Only C1, C4, C2, and C3 are necessary for immune adherence, and the reaction is directly dependent upon the number of bound C3 molecules on the cell surface. Since immune adherence is little affected when serum is grossly deficient in C2, it is apparent that both C3 and C4 can promote immune adherence of human red cells.

Neutralization of herpes simplex virus is achieved by specific antiserum in the presence of C1 and C4. *Histamine release* has been reported to be achieved by complement without the involvement of anaphylatoxins. Recently, *kinin-like activity* was generated from C2 and C4 by treatment with C1 esterase by trypsin.

Interrelationship of Other Systems. The activation of the complement sequence is intimately interrelated with coagulation and the fibrinolytic and kinin-generating systems of the blood. A schematic representation of these interrelations is depicted in Figure 11-3. Activated Hageman factor initiates the clotting sequence, and at the same time interacts with one or more cofactors, Hageman cofactors or plasminogen, to produce plasmin. Plasmin has broad proteolytic activity, including capacity to digest fibrin and fibrinogen, to cleave C3 to yield anaphylatoxin, to activate C1 to $\overline{C1}$, and finally to cleave activated Hageman factor to yield the prealbumin fragments most active in the conversion of prekallikrein to kallikrein. Kallikrein in turn cleaves kininogen to yield bradykinin, a vasoactive and chemotactic substance. Consequent to the kinin-generating system a frag-

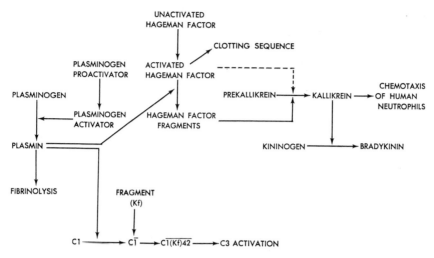

Fig. 11-3.   Interrelations between the coagulation, kinin-generating, fibrinolytic, and complement systems.

ment called Kf is generated, which alters the function of $\overline{C1}$ to make it capable of reacting more efficiently with C4 and C2.

COMPLEMENT AND PATHOGENESIS OF IMMUNOLOGIC INJURY

From the preceding discussion it is clear that the multiple biologic activities of the complement system observed *in vitro* can play a major role as a biologic amplification system in the bodily defense. Similarly the interaction may play crucial roles in the pathogenesis of immunologic injury *in vivo*. Anaphylatoxins cause smooth muscle contraction, peripheral vasodilation, increased vascular permeability, and edema. Chemotactic factors cause the migration of neutrophils into the area of complement activation. As these cells break down or liberate their content, tissue damage may occur. Immune adherence causes the localization of leukocytes to membrane surfaces, especially at sites of deposition of immune complexes. These cells can then damage important membranes, as in the Arthus reaction. Activation of complement is followed by an influx of leukocytes and subsequent destruction of tissue via the inflammatory process *in vivo*.

Arthus Reaction. A form of vasculitis manifested as circumscribed hemorrhagic necrosis occurs following the local injection of appropriate antigen into an animal with circulating antibody or vice versa. This lesion, called the Arthus reaction, is due to the local deposition of antigen, antibody, and complement and does not develop in animals depleted of complement or depleted of polymorphonuclear leukocytes.

Serum Sickness. A generalized disease known as serum sickness is caused by complement-fixing immune complexes in the wall of the vascular system. The immune complexes are deposited beneath and between the endothelial cells along the basement membrane or internal elastic lamina followed by activation of complement, infiltration of leukocytes, disruption of the basement membrane, and medial necrosis. Rabbits depleted of C3 do not develop arteritis, even though the immune complex may deposit on the vessel wall. They can, however, develop evidence of damage to the filtration membrane in the kidney vessels and of damage to membranes in blood vessels, e.g., the Arthus reaction or experimental Masugi nephritis.

Nephrotoxic Nephritis. A self-perpetuating nephritis is caused by the injection of serum containing antibasement membrane antibody. The injected antibody rapidly fixes to the glomerular basement membrane and causes immediate structural and functional injury. This initial stage is followed by the response of the host to the foreign immunoglobulins attached to the basement membrane. The central role of complement in nephrotoxic nephritis can be clearly demonstrated by the fact that tissue damage during the initial phase of this disease can be prevented by the pretreatment of injected antibody with papain or pepsin, which prevents the fixation of complement to the antibody, or by depleting complement in the animals. The complement is consumed during the second-stage of this disease.

It is entirely possible that some components of renal injury may be independent of complement, since the duck anti-rat kidney antibody, an antibody incapable of efficiently fixing mammalian complement *in vitro*, can induce proteinuria immediately after injection. Similarly, serum complement may participate in vascular damage in immune complex diseases but is not essential to major aspects of renal injury in experimental serum sickness.

Participation of complement in the pathogenesis of human diseases is evidenced by (1) alterations of serum complement activity during the disease process, (2) demonstration of complement fixation in the diseased tissue, and (3) increased catabolism of certain components of complement. Since little is known about the rate of synthesis and catabolism of the complement components, except for C3 and C4, a reduction of whole serum complement or of a component cannot be said to be indicative of active participation of complement in a given disease, nor do normal levels of complement or complement components rule out the involvement of complement in the pathogenesis of a given disease.

Complement Component Profiles in Diseases. In systemic lupus erythematosus with nephritis, antigen-antibody complexes are known to be available in the circulation and deposits of antigen immunoglobulin and complement occur in the glomerular blood vessels. The complement profile in the circulation reveals all of the components to be low in the blood. Detailed analysis establishes that both primary and alternate pathways of the complement system are being activated. With effective treatment that alleviates renal manifestations the total complement and all of the individual complement components return to normal more or less in parallel. The complement-component profile usually seen in lupus is illustrated in Table 11-3. A different profile is encountered in the hypocomplementemic membranoproliferative glomerulonephritis of children. In this disease C1, C4, and C2 are all present in normal concentration, but total complement, C3, and C5 are very much depressed. The complement system in this disease shows evidence of activation at the third component and beyond as would occur when the system is activated by the alternate pathway. In acute poststreptococcal hemorrhagic nephritis the very earliest evaluation of the complement profile sometimes reveals evidence of activation via the primary pathway. More often, however, even early in the course of the disease, C1, C4, and C2 are spared while total complement, C3, and later components are depressed. These findings indicate that different mechanisms of activation of the complement system may operate in each of these three human diseases associated with glomerular damage by immunologic mechanisms. Characteristic complement profiles are seen also in human diseases based on genetic deficiencies of complement components. Such profiles have been crucial in defining the relation-

Table 11-3. The Profile of the Change in Serum Complement Components in Various Diseases

Diseases	CH50	C1	C1q	C4	C2	C3	C5	C9
Systemic lupus erythematosus	D	D	D	D	D	D		D
Hypocomplementemic glomerulonephritis	D	N		N	N	D	D	
Poststreptococcal nephritis	D	N		N	N	D	D	
Mixed cryoglobulinemia	D		D	D	D	N		
Autoimmune hemolytic anemia		D		D		D		
Lymphosarcoma		D		D	D	N		
Graft rejection					D			
Rheumatoid arthritis*		D		D	D			

* In synovial fluid.
D = decreased.
N = normal.

ship of complement component deficiencies Clq, Clr, Cls, Cl esterase inhibitor, C3, C3 inactivator, and C7 deficiencies with human diseases like vasculitis, nephritis, lupus erythematosus, and increased susceptibility to infection.

Complement also plays a major role in the pathogenesis of *autoimmune hemolytic anemia, paroxysmal nocturnal hemoglobinuria,* and *hereditary angioneurotic edema.*

SYNTHESIS AND DEVELOPMENT OF COMPLEMENT SYSTEM

Where is the complement synthesized, and how? Since the discovery of complement, most of the early studies were focused on blood leukocytes, the reticuloendothelial system, and liver as potential sites for synthesis of complement. Recent advances in tissue culture techniques and the use of radioactive isotopes have made it possible to study this question more directly and precisely. Three critical criteria have been applied to the interpretation of the results obtained from the *in vitro* experiments: (1) demonstration of net increase in specific protein or activity in question, (2) demonstration of incorporation of radioactive precursor into the structure of the protein or component, and (3) demonstration that the cells putatively synthesizing the component cannot carry out this activity when influenced by antimetabolites that prevent DNA, RNA, or protein synthesis.

Using these criteria wherever possible, the best evidence indicates that (1) Clq is synthesized in macrophages and lymphoid tissue; (2) Clr and Cls are synthesized in separate cells but in many tissues of the body, including epithelial cells of gut, spleen, liver, lungs, and perhaps kidney; (3) C4 is synthesized in liver, lymphoid tissue, epithelial tissues, and fibroblast; (4) C2 is synthesized in liver, spleen, and bone marrow; (5) C3 is produced in bone marrow, liver, lymphoid organs, macrophages, fibroblast, and human lymphoid cell lines; (6) liver is known to produce C6, C8, and C9; and (7) C8 is produced in the lungs, spleen, and kidneys of pigs.

The genetic controls over the synthesis of the complement components are extremely complex. At least nine alleles are known for the genetic control of human C3 synthesis. Taking advantage of this polymorphism of C3, it was shown that the C3 type in the recipient of a liver transplant changed to the C3 type of the donor six days after transplantation.

When does the capacity to make complement develop? All complement components may not develop simultaneously, or the presence of minute quantities may be masked by the faster development of inhibitors. However, total hemolytic activity of complement can be detected in fetal lambs, fetal pigs, and fetal calves almost as early as blood samples can be obtained; e.g., in fetal lambs total complement is already detectable as early as the twenty-third day of a 180 day gestation period, between the thirteenth and eighteenth day of chick embryonation, and the fortieth day of the 115 to 120 day gestation in pigs.

Human cord serum contains less complement than does maternal serum. Both C3 and C4 can be detected in the human fetus as early as the ninth week of gestation. Individual C3, C4, and C5 components and total hemolytic activity are lower in full term and premature infants as compared to the maternal levels and reach the adult levels by three to six months of age. Most of the increase of complement and complement components occurs in the first few days after birth, perhaps as a function of colonization by microorganisms.

Phylogenetically, no hemolytic activity of complement has been demonstrated in the hemolymph of the horseshoe crab, spunculid worm, and starfish thus far studied by classic methods. However, the hemolymph of the horseshoe crab and of the spunculid worm does support cobra-venom-induced lysis of red cell, which may indicate the presence of an alternate pathway and of terminal components of complement.

Among the vertebrates, sea lampreys appear to be lacking the classic complement pathway. However, representative elasmobranches, chondrosteans, holosteans, and teleosts all have complement systems that have striking similarities to the mammalian system, as do amphibians, reptilians, and birds. The classical complement system seems to have developed in parallel with the development of humoral immunity.

Interesting recent evidence presented by Day et al. suggests that elements of the so-called alternate pathway may be extremely primitive and present in some of the simplest phylogenetic deviations among the invertebrates. It is tempting to conclude that the alternate pathway, at least in some of its constituents, is much more primitive than is either the classical pathway or humoral immunity. We thus are inclined at the moment to think of the alternate pathway as the true primary pathway and the classical pathway as one of perhaps several alternate pathways in this fundamental system for destruction of abnormal, damaged, or foreign cells.

DEFICIENCY OF COMPLEMENT FUNCTION

C1q is somewhat diminished in patients with the Bruton type of agammaglobulinemia and is greatly diminished in patients with the Swiss type of combined immune deficiency. C1q is nearly normal in the Nezelof type of immune deficiency disease (thymic dysplasia with normal levels of IgG immunoglobulins) and in the DiGeorge form of thymic aplasia. These findings suggest that a link exists between synthesis of C1q and interactions with or synthesis of immunoglobulin molecules.

In patients with hereditary angioneurotic edema, the functional or absolute deficiency of C1 inhibitor can be demonstrated. Consequently C4 and, to a lesser extent, C2 substrates for the esterase are reduced in the serum of these patients. The catabolic rate of C4 is markedly increased.

C2 deficiency has been detected in humans and shown to be inherited as an autosomal recessive.

Patients with C2 deficiency have been found to exhibit a high frequency of susceptibility to infection, renal glomerular disease, lupus erythematosus, vascular disease, dermatomyositis, rheumatoid manifestations, and nonthrombopenic purpura. Patients with inherited deficiencies of C1r and C1s have been studied and likewise found to exhibit frequent infections, vascular disease, renal disease, and a lupus-like syndrome. Patients with C3 deficiencies based on several different hereditary mechanisms have highly lethal susceptibility to infections, especially pulmonary infections. Patients with C5 abnormality and deficient C5 function have classical Leiner's disease of the skin and enteric infection with gramnegative organisms. A patient lacking only C6 was clinically well, but a patient lacking only C7 had arthritis. Similarly, mice lacking C5, rabbits lacking C6, and guinea pigs lacking C4 show far greater susceptibility to infections than do normal animals. In both man and lower animals deficiency of even a single complement component is associated with diseases of potentially high lethality as would be expected of perturbations in a biologic amplification system so well maintained as a system of interacting proteins through the long eons of history.

SELECTED REFERENCES

Austen, K. F., et al. (1968): Bull. WHO 39:935.
Bordet, J. (1898): Ann. Inst. Pasteur (Paris) 12:688.
Bordet, J., and Gengou, D. (1901): Ann. Inst. Pasteur (Paris) 15:289.
Bordet, J., and Streng, O. (1909): Zbl. Bakt. 49:260.
Day, N. K. B., et al. (1970): J. Exp. Med. 132:194.
Ehrlich, P., and Morgenroth, J. (1899): Berl. Klin. Wschr. 36:481.
Frank, M. M., et al. (1971): J. Exp. Med. 134:176.
Gewurz, H., Shin, H. S., and Mergenhagen, S. E. (1965): J. Exp. Med. 128:1049.
Mayer, M. M. (1961): In *Experimental Immunochemistry* (2nd ed.), Kabat, M., and Mayer, M. M. (eds.). Springfield, Illinois, Charles C Thomas.
Mayer, M. M., Miller, J. A., and Shin, H. S. (1970): J. Immun. 105:327.
Müller-Eberhard, H. J. (1968): Advances Immun. 8:1.
Müller-Eberhard, H. J. (1969): Ann. Rev. Biochem. 38:389.
Nelson, R. A. Jr. (1953): Science 118:733.
Nelson, R. A. Jr. et al. (1966): Immunochemistry 3:111.
Pfeiffer, R. (1895): Z. Hyg. Infektr. 19:75.
Pillemer, L., et al. (1954): Science 120:279.
Streng, O. (1930): Acta Path. Microbiol. Scand. (Suppl. 3) 20:411.

FURTHER READINGS

Kabat, E. A., and Mayer, M. M. (1961): *Experimental Immunochemistry.* Springfield, Illinois, Charles C Thomas.
Lachmann, P. J. (1966): Advances Immun. 6:479.
Nelson, D. S. (1963): Advances Immun. 3:131.
Ruddy, S., Gigli, I., and Austen, K. F. (1972): New Eng. J. Med. 287:489.
Schultz, D. R. (1971): *The Complement System,* New York, S. Karger.
Schur, P. H., and Austen, K. F. (1968): Ann. Rev. Med. 19:1.
Wolstenholme, G. E. W., and Knight, J. (eds.) (1965): *Complement.* Boston, Little, Brown and Company.

12

Phagocytosis System
and Nonspecific Mechanisms
of Host Resistance

The role of phagocytes in the host's defense against an invading organism was proposed by Metchnikoff in 1883. His theory of phagocytosis is also called the cellular theory of immunity or the theory of natural immunity in contrast to the theory of humoral immunity or acquired immunity. This theory was vigorously opposed by many proponents of the humoral theory of immunity who believed that humoral antibodies, not the phagocytes, confer immunity. For example, Nuttall in 1888 discovered the bactericidal activity of defibrinated blood and suggested that the role of the "phagocytic white cells" must be merely to remove the bacteria that had been killed by a heat-stable substance in the blood of normal animals. This view was further supported by Pfeiffer's observation of cholera vibrio in 1884 and by von Behring's discovery of antitoxin in 1890.

A heated controversy between the humoralists and the cellularists continued until Wright and Douglas in 1903 showed that a serum substance, which they called opsonin, enhanced the engulfment of bacteria by phagocytes. It is now firmly established that phagocytosis is the final mechanism by which foreign bodies, including pathogenic organisms, are eliminated from the circulation and that the phagocytes are intimately involved in the induction of the immune response, as well as in the expression of both immunologic defense and immunologic injury.

The essential role of phagocytes in the defense against bacterial infection was further established by Holmes et al. in 1966 in their study of an experiment of Nature, infants with chronic (fatal) granulomatous disease. They showed clearly that these patients succumb to bacterial infection in spite of their normal cellular and humoral immunity because the phagocytes of these patients fail to kill certain ingested bacteria.

THE PHAGOCYTOSIS SYSTEM

Phagocytic ability of varying degrees can be demonstrated easily in different types of cells in tissue culture. The *in vivo* phagocytic capacity of most cells, however, may be quite limited. Metchnikoff recognized two

Table   12-1.   Phagocytic Cells of the Body

Microphages
  Neutrophils
  Eosinophils
Macrophages
  Histiocytes: connective tissues
  Monocytes: blood
  Microglia: central nervous system
  Sinus lining cells: spleen, liver, bone marrow
  Reticulum cells: lymphoreticular tissue, spleen, lymph nodes, bone marrow, thymus

---

major groups of phagocytes, the *microphages* and the *macrophages* (Table 12-1).

The ability to engulf and digest particles is an essential nutritional mechanism in the free-living, as well as in the parasitic, protozoa. The amoeba apparently achieves two advantages by engulfing and digesting microorganisms, i.e., it uses these organisms as a source of food and it protects itself from a fatal infection. Metchnikoff first pointed out that specialized groups of cells called *phagocytes* (eating cells) within the mesenchyma would be of great importance in providing a defense mechanism. He traced the essential continuity of the phagocytes during the evolutionary stages from protozoa, through the primitive metazoa and sponges, to the mesenchymal phagocytic cell systems of higher animals. In the protospongia two types of cells could be distinguished, an outer layer of flagellated cells providing locomotion and an inner core of amoeba-like cells serving for digestion of food and for the defense of the body. The next step in the progress of differentiation is seen in the sponges with a canalicular system lined by entodermal phagocytes in addition to the phagocytes in the mesoderm. With the development of an entodermal layer which could secrete enzymes into the digestive canal, phagocytosis in these cells is no longer necessary. However, the phagocytes of the mesoderm are retained in all higher forms of animals and appear to maintain their primitive ingestive function. These phagocytes act as scavengers for the short-lived cells which are taken up after they die or at the end of their life span (effete cells) and are digested; thus their chemical components are reutilized in the body's economy. The phagocytes also act in the host as a defense against infections. In primitive invertebrate systems with no recognizable humoral immunity, phagocytic cells are very vigorous amoebocytes and can clearly recognize foreign substances.

The term *reticuloendothelial system* (RES) was introduced by Aschoff in 1924 to designate all the actively phagocytic cells, as demonstrated by the capacity to take up significant quantities of vital dyes such as lithium carmine when these are injected into the blood stream in low concentration. The concept of the reticuloendothelial system is primarily a physiologic or functional one, and the cells belonging to this system were originally defined on the basis of their ability to take up vital dyes or carbon particles.

Aschoff recognized three groups of cells with the ability to store vital dyes or particulate materials. The first consists of the endothelial cells of blood and lymph vessels and the fibroblast of connective tissue, but these cells showed only faint vital staining and, therefore, were excluded from the RES. The second is the group of stellate cells in the pulp strands of the spleen or the medullary cords of lymph nodes (reticulum cells or stellate macrophages). The third comprises the lining cells of lymph sinuses and the sinusoids of the liver and bone marrow and similar cells in the adrenal and pituitary glands. The term *reticuloendothelial system* was derived from the fact that one main group, the stellate macrophages of the spleen and the lymph nodes, was thought to form a network, or reticulum, and the other cells to line dilated blood or lymph sinuses. The histiocytes of tissues and the monocytes of blood, a system of wandering phagocytic cells, make up a fourth component of the RES. The system is one of phagocytic cells, but, rather arbitrarily, only the macrophages are included. The microphages, Metchnikoff's term for polymorphonuclear leukocytes, and the megakaryocytes are excluded despite the vigorous phagocytic potential of the latter.

The phagocytic cells that are scattered throughout the connective tissue of various organs are generally called *histiocytes*. For many years the relationship between blood monocytes and tissue histiocytes (or macrophages) was a matter of controversy, but it is now established that monocytes are generated continuously from bone marrow and migrate into the tissues to become histiocytes. Local multiplication of histiocytes is thought to occur at the site of inflammation. This multiplication, however, may be attributable to incompletely differentiated precursors which look much like lymphocytes (M-cells). The lung is particularly well supplied with histiocytes, which are present in the alveolar walls. It has now become clear that the histiocytes and macrophages in special compartments may be separable from one another. For example, the alveolar macrophages and peritoneal macrophages have markedly different metabolic activity. Oxygen consumption is threefold higher in the alveolar macrophages than in the peritoneal macrophages.

BLOCKADE AND STIMULATION OF RETICULOENDOTHELIAL SYSTEM

The cells of the reticuloendothelial system are largely responsible for removal of many foreign materials from the blood stream. They remove, for example, partially denatured proteins by virtue of their extremely fine discriminatory power for detecting minor alterations in serum proteins.

The overall function of the reticuloendothelial system can be therefore measured by injecting intravenously a solution of partially denatured serum albumin, trace-labeled with radioactive iodine, and following its clearance from the blood stream. The rapid removal of the altered albumin in a normal animal is shown in Figure 12-1.

By overloading the cells of RES with relatively large amounts of a colloidal suspension, such as carbon particles in the form of india ink, it is possible to depress temporarily their phagocytic function towards other materials. This is shown by curve B of Figure 12-1 and is called *blockade* of the reticuloendothelial system. It is now clear that the so-called reticuloendothelial blockade comprises two components. One of these is de-

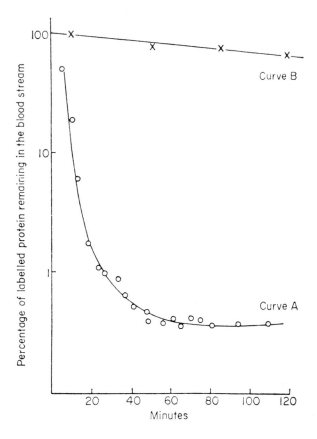

Fig. 12-1. The clearance of heat-aggregated protein from the blood stream. The effect of blockade of the reticuloendothelial system. Human serum albumin, denatured by heating and labeled with radioactive iodine, was injected intravenously into normal rats (o) and rats which had received 50 mg india ink 6 hours previously (x). The india ink temporarily blocks uptake by the reticuloendothelial system. [From Freeman, T., Gordon, A. H., and Humphrey, J.H. (1958): Brit. J. Exp. Path. *39:463.*]

pletion of nonspecific or specific opsonins, and the other is an actual cellular saturation or exhaustion. However, such depression lasts only for a few hours, or a day or two, because the cells have great capacity for proliferation and recovery. It has been postulated that persistent bacteremia in certain infections may be due to overloading of the reticuloendothelial system, but there is no real evidence that this could occur in the ordinary course of disease. However, the impairment of phagocytic function can occur in hemorrhagic shock, and it is quite possible that the clearance mechanism may be diminished and accelerate death.

By accurately measuring the rate of clearance of radio-labeled proteins from the blood stream it has been possible to discover conditions in which the phagocytic activity of the RES is markedly stimulated. Most experimental work has been done in rats and mice, and it is not certain how far the results of these works can be generalized to other species. Stimulation is evident after administration of estrogens, of certain lipids such as glycerol trioleate, and of just the right doses of cortisone.

A finding of considerable interest is that injection of living BCG (bacillus Calmette-Guérin) resulted in a prolonged and considerable increase in the phagocytic capacity of the reticuloendothelial system, which becomes evident about one week after the BCG injection and lasts for three weeks or more. It is possible that this stimulation is a consequence of the development of delayed hypersensitivity. Mackaness and his associates recently reported that phagocytic cells stimulated apparently by factors released from sensitized lymphocytes after contact with antigen can be as much as 10 times more effective in phagocytosis and killing of bacteria, even though the latter have no relationship to the bacteria initiating or provoking the hypersensitivity reaction (angry macrophage).

ELIMINATION OF BACTERIA FROM BLOOD

The body possesses remarkably efficient mechanisms for eliminating bacteria from the blood stream. With most bacterial species, large numbers of living organisms can be swiftly cleared from the circulation.

When large numbers of living bacteria are injected into the veins of an experimental animal, the count of organisms, as revealed by repeated quantitative blood cultures, in general follows the type of curve shown in Figure 12-2. In the first place, the clearance is extremely rapid and the count of bacteria falls from a billion to less than a hundred per ml of blood within 10 minutes. This rapid initial fall in the number of bacteria can be observed with most organisms and is not dependent on pre-existing immunity against the test organism.

Subsequent to this initial phase, the remaining course varies with the virulence of the test organism. As a rule, although a few bacteria may persist for some time, all disappear completely within an hour or so. Exceptions to this general rule are found in the encapsulated virulent strains

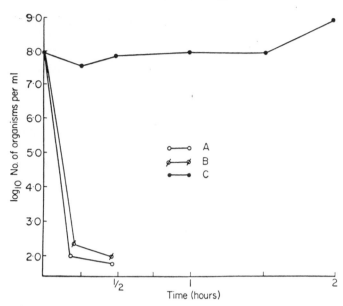

Fig. 12-2. Clearance of organisms from the blood stream of the rabbit. A. Course of bacteremia after injection of avirulent, unencapsulated Streptococcus pneumoniae into a normal previously uninjected animal. B. Course of bacteremia after injection of an 8-hour culture of fully
virulent, encapsulated organisms into a previously immunized animal. C. Course of bacteremia
after injection of an 8-hour culture of fully virulent, encapsulated organisms into a normal previously uninjected animal. Death occurred at 48 hours. [From Humphrey, J. H., and White, R. G.
(1970): *Immunology for Students of Medicine*. Philadelphia, F. A. Davis Company.]

of pneumococcus, Klebsiella, and Bacillus anthracis. An example is shown
in Figure 12-2. With an average 24 hour culture of a virulent type, the
bulk of the organisms will have lost their capsules, and consequently the
initial drop of bacterial counts may assume the usual rapid fall. A few
encapsulated forms will persist, and their multiplication produces an increase of bacteria in the blood that may lead to the death of the animal.
With a young culture of 8 hours or less, the virulent organism will possess capsules and also be in an actively dividing growth phase. In this
case no measurable initial clearance may occur, and the count of organisms in the blood will rise from the moment of injection until the time of
death.

For encapsulated bacteria like the virulent pneumococci, an immune
serum containing specific antibody directed against the carbohydrate of
the capsule can be shown to have a dramatic enhancing effect on the
phagocytic function and clearance of the bacteria from the blood stream.
Experiments with a perfused isolated liver show that encapsulated pneumococci suspended in normal serum can be passed repeatedly through
the liver without removal of bacteria, but such organisms are promptly
removed from the perfusate when they are suspended in immune serum.

Studies with repeated large doses of living bacteria given intravenously suggest that the phagocytic capacity of the RES is rarely, if ever, exceeded *in vivo*. This finding indicates that in bacteremia due to an organism other than the encapsulated species, the continued presence of the organism in the circulation of a normal host is due to the continuous supply of bacteria from an extravascular focus. The simplest example is bacterial endocarditis in which the bacteria-laden vegetations on the heart valves continuously supply bacteria to the circulation.

MECHANISM OF PHAGOCYTOSIS

The neutrophils and monocytes are easily obtained from the peripheral blood or from the peritoneal exudates and have been extensively used for studies of phagocytosis. In a healthy man approximately 20 to 30 $\times$ 10^9 neutrophils are in the circulation at any given time. The half-life of neutrophils in the circulation has been estimated to be about 6 hours, and the neutrophils never return to the circulation again after leaving the intravascular space. An equal number of neutrophils are supposed to be located in a marginal pool along the blood vessel surfaces. For every circulating neutrophil, 50 to 100 mature neutrophils are reserved in bone marrow. The whole life span of neutrophils is estimated to be no more than a few days and the daily degradation is close to 50 to 100 ml of packed neutrophils.

The function of these phagocytes involves a sequence of steps: (1) sticking of phagocytes to capillary endothelium in the inflamed area, (2) locomotion, (3) emigration through the vessel wall into tissues, (4) attraction to the microbes, or chemotaxis, (5) engulfment or ingestion of bacteria, (6) increased metabolism and degranulation, and (7) final digestion or egestion of the foreign material.

A most important initial component of inflammation is the sticking of phagocytes to the vascular endothelium after injury. However, this stickiness of the endothelium is still a poorly understood process. Neutrophils show a striking tendency under certain conditions to stick to foreign surfaces such as glass, or to stick to one another to form clumps. Divalent cations and plasma proteins are required for the sticking; fibrinogen in particular seems to play a role.

One of the most striking properties of phagocytes is their ability to crawl about on the blood vessel walls, in tissues, or on foreign surfaces such as glass. These cells do not usually move for long distances in a straight line, but rather tend to change direction every 20 microns or so by sending out a new pseudopod in random fashion. Under ideal conditions they can travel 35 to 40 microns per minute. The locomotion of the mononuclear phagocytes is similar to that of amoebae. In the movement of neutrophils, however, no cytoplasmic streaming is discernible, and the granules of neutrophils generally maintain their position unchanged during locomotion.

Observation of neutrophil emigration in living tissue under the light microscope shows gradual passage of the cell through a major pathway from lumen to tissue, with cells passing between the junctions of endothelial cells of the capillary or venule during inflammation. Recent electron microscopic studies of the mechanism of emigration have shown that the neutrophils may occassionally be engulfed by the endothelial cells and thus be transported to the outside of the capillary.

Chemotaxis—directed locomotion toward or away from substances or particles in the environment—has been studied for more than 70 years. Direct observation of neutrophil movement by camera lucida has shown clearly that within a certain range of an attractive object, such as a clump of bacteria, the random pattern of movement is changed to a straight line movement toward the intended object of phagocytosis. Chemical attraction of neutrophils to bacteria such as Staphylococcus aureus apparently can operate in the absence of serum, complement, or glucose in the medium.

Recent studies by Boyden showed that complement components participate in chemotaxis induced by antigen-antibody complex. More specifically, it is now known that low molecular weight fragments of the fifth and third complement components (C5a and C3a) represent the most powerful stimuli to chemotaxis. Some evidence that the very large molecular complex, C567, acts as a chemotactic stimulus has also been presented.

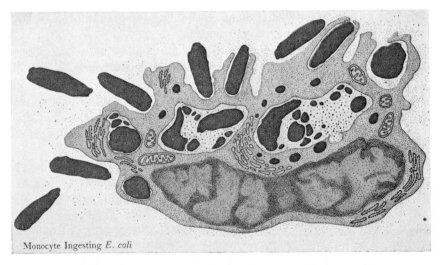

Monocyte Ingesting *E. coli*

Fig. 12-3. A schematic illustration of processes of phagocytosis. [From Douglas, S. D., and Fudenberg, H. H. (1969): Hosp. Prac. 4:29.]

Studies of phagocytosis by electron microscopy have established that the particles do not simply pass through the cell membrane. The objects are taken up by both invagination and flagella-like outfolding of the cell membrane surrounding the particle to be engulfed. The ingested material is thus surrounded closely by a layer of inside-out cell membrane called phagosome. These features of the phagocytic process are shown in Figure 12-3.

The next step in phagocytosis is the fusion of lysosomal granules to the phagosome to form a phagolysosome. During this process the digestive enzymes in the lysosomal granules (Table 12-2) are ingested into the phagolysosome, and the final digestion of ingested material ensues.

Changes in the metabolism of leukocytes occur during phagocytosis. The consumption of O_2 and glucose, the activity of the hexose monophosphate shunt, and production of H_2O_2 are markedly increased as particulate is ingested (Table 12-3). Recently Park et al. showed that the level

Table 12-2. Hydrolytic Enzymes in Lysosomes

Acid phosphatase	Phospholipase
Acid ribonuclease	Acid lipase
Acid deoxyribonuclease	Phagocytin and related bactericidal
Aryl sulfates A and B	proteins
Cathepsins, B, C, D, E	Endogenous pyrogen
Collagenase	Plasminogen activator
Phosphoprotein phosphatase	Hemolysin(s)
Phosphatidic acid phosphatase	Mucopolysaccharides and glycoproteins
Organophosphate-resistant esterases	Beta galactosidase
Beta glucuronidase	Alpha mannosidase
Alpha-L-fucosidase	Beta-N-acetylglucosaminidase
Alpha-1, 4-glucosidase	Cytochrome C reductase
Alpha-N-acetylglucosaminidase	Lysozyme phagocytin
Alpha-N-acetylgalactosaminidase	Basic proteins: (a) Mast cell-active;
Hyaluronidase	(b) Permeability-inducing, independent of mast cells

Table 12-3. Metabolic Changes in Neutrophils during Phagocytosis

1. O_2 consumption increases two- to threefold, and the increase is almost entirely insensitive to cyanide.

2. The glucose consumption and lactate production increase by about 25 percent, especially during the period of actual uptake of particles.

3. The amount of glucose metabolism via hexose monophosphate shunt increases from about 1 percent in cells to 10 percent in phagocytosing cells.

4. H_2O_2 is produced in the respiratory burst.

5. The incorporation of glucose, acetate, phosphate, and lysolecithin into lipid is stimulated suggesting the membrane turnover during ingestion.

of cyclic adenosine monophosphate is also increased within the first 5 minutes of phagocytosis in human neutrophils. The mechanism by which most bacteria are killed following ingestion by phagocytes, especially by the neutrophils, involves an apparent halogen action of the organism which requires H_2O_2 and an enzyme, myeloperoxidase. H_2O_2 production is markedly increased during the response of the phagocytic cell to engulfment of particulate material. Genetically determined deficiency of the capacity to produce H_2O_2, such as occurs in children with chronic granulomatous disease or inability to produce myeloperoxidase, leads to deficiency in resistance to certain microorganisms (page 324).

Ingestion of certain bacteria by phagocytes requires a preparation of bacteria by *opsonins*. The term *opsonin* denotes a serum substance that would enhance phagocytosis. It consists of heat-stable and heat-labile substances. The most important heat-stable opsonins are specific antibodies directed against the surface antigens of bacteria and are referred to as *immune opsonins,* or *bacteriotropins*. This type of antibody combines with the surface antigen of the cell and prepares (opsonizes) it for ingestion by phagocytes.

Recently Quie and his associates have shown that the opsonic properties of antibodies are closely associated with integrity of the Fc portion of the IgG molecule. Further, Johnston et al. demonstrated that pneumococcus opsonized with IgG antibody is not phagocytized unless a small volume of fresh normal serum is added, or purified C1, C4, C2, and C3 are added sequentially.

IMPAIRMENT OF PHAGOCYTOSIS

Phagocytic activity of the reticuloendothelial system is diminished in various morbid conditions such as hemorrhagic shock, severe trauma from burns, diabetic ketoacidosis, and pyrexia. Phagocytic function of neutrophils is reported to be depressed by such therapeutics as colchicine, salicylate, steroids, antibiotics (chloromycetin, tetracycline), and antitumor drugs (6-mercaptopurine, methotrexate).

A deficiency in leukocytic myeloperoxidase has been found to be associated with impairment of candicidal capacity of phagocytes in certain patients with systemic candidiasis. The phagocytes (neutrophils and monocytes) of patients with chronic granulomatous disease characteristically fail to kill ingested bacteria of certain kinds, notably those which produce catalase. An abnormal metabolic response by leukocytes of these patients, especially the deficiency in production of H_2O_2 during phagocytosis, has been implicated as the cause for the killing defect. In patients with the so-called *lazy leukocytes syndrome*, a deficiency in the migration of phagocytes has been associated with an increased incidence of infection.

A deficiency in opsonic activity in the serum is associated with an increased susceptibility to infection, especially pneumococcal infection, in splenectomized infants and animals and in patients with sickle cell disease. The opsonic activity of serum is deficient in patients with agammaglobulinemia and in newborn infants. Recently, Miller and his associates described an infant with increased susceptibility to infection associated with C5 deficiency.

NONSPECIFIC MECHANISMS OF HOST RESISTANCE

In the nonimmunized host, it is sometimes difficult to distinguish between truly nonspecific phenomena involved in resistance to infection and those phenomena mediated by naturally occurring antibody. Nevertheless, nonspecific, sometimes naturally occurring defense mechanisms do operate and play a major role in the host's resistance to infection. First, together with the important but little understood role of the mucous membrane and the skin, the phagocytosis system forms the main protective mechanism of the body. The efficiency of the phagocytic system can be much enhanced by the humoral and cellular immune responses of the host.

A few naturally occurring antimicrobial substances are known, however, and they contribute substantially to host resistance. The contributions of these substances in the host's defense may explain the different susceptibilities of different host-species to the same infection. *B-lysins,* heat-stable substances, are bactericidal for gram-positive bacteria. They are found in the sera of most animals and increase during infection. *Lysozyme,* an enzyme, is found in many body fluids. It lyses gram-positive organisms and enhances the bactericidal action of antibody and complement for gram-negative bacteria. *Interferon,* an inhibitor of viruses indistinguishable from virus-induced interferon, appears quickly in the circulation of mice and rabbits after an injection of bacterial endotoxin. Interferon may be produced by lymphoid cells and other cells after a variety of stimulations. It appears very promptly after these stimuli and thus could contribute substantially to the defense against the virus infection. *Complement* plays an essential role in the elimination of bacteria by phagocytes and in the direct lysis of bacteria by antibodies. Other antibacterial substances in tissues, notably basic polypeptides, have also been identified.

SELECTED REFERENCES

Aschoff, L. (1925): *Handbuch der Krankh der Blutes und der Blutbild, Organe.* Berlin, Springer, 2:473.
Boyden, S. (1962): J. Exp. Med. 115:453.
Holmes, B., et al. (1966): Lancet 1:1225.
Johnston, R. B., et al. (1969): J. Exp. Med. 129:1275.
Mackaness, G. B. (1969): J. Exp. Med. 129:973.
Metchnikoff, E. (1883): Biol. Central Bl. 3:560.

Miller, M. E., Oski, F. A., and Harris, M. B. (1971): Lancet *1*:665.
Miller, M. E., et al. (1968): Lancet *2*:60.
Nuttall, G. H. F. (1888): Z. Hyg. *4*:353.
Park, B. H., et al. (1971): Nature (New Biol.) *229*:27.
Quie, P. G., Messner, R. P., and Williams, R. C. (1968): J. Exp. Med. *128*:553.
Wright, A. E., and Douglas, S. R. (1903): Proc. Roy. Soc. London *72*:357.
Wright, A. E., and Douglas, S. R. (1904): Proc. Roy. Soc. London *73*:128.

FURTHER READINGS

Braunsteiner, H. (ed.) (1962): *The Physiology and Pathology of Leukocytes*. New York, Grune & Stratton, Inc.
Hirsch, J. G. (1965): Ann. Rev. Microbiol. *19*:339.
Karnovsky, M. L. (1968): Seminars Hemat. *5*:156.
Nelson, D. S. (ed.) (1969): *Macrophages and Immunity*. New York, North Holland-American Elsevier Publishing Company.
Williams, R. C., and Fudenberg, H. H. (eds.) (1972): *Phagocytic Mechanisms in Health and Disease*. New York, Intercontinental Medical Book Corporation.
Zucker-Franklyn, D. (1968): Seminars Hemat. *5*:109.

13

Inflammation and Mechanisms of Immunologic Injury

The inflammatory process is thought to be fundamental to the survival of the organism, for without it there could be no protection against noxious external stimuli nor repair of damaged tissue. For example, when a small number of pneumococci are inoculated under the skin of a normal rabbit, a minimal local lesion is produced, but the infection is contained, and the animal survives. By contrast, when the same treatment is given to the rabbit which is rendered unable to mount normal inflammatory response, the infection rapidly spreads, leading to septicemia and sometimes death.

On the other hand, inflammation, like other vital processes, may become aberrant and may be considerably more harmful to the host than the original noxious stimulus that provoked the inflammatory reaction. The inflammatory process is often the final mechanism by which many immunologic reactions are expressed. Horse serum, for example, is an innocuous agent when injected into the skin of a rabbit for the first time, as only minimal inflammation is produced. After a repeated injection, however, horse serum can produce a violent inflammatory reaction that is often destructive to the host. The inflammatory reaction itself is to some extent stereotyped, and it cannot distinguish between instances in which the process is protective and instances in which the process is harmful.

THEORIES OF INFLAMMATION

Although the description of inflammatory reactions involving the skin and the external organs can be found in the recorded history of all ancient peoples, it was Celsus of Rome at the beginning of the Christian era who described the famous *four cardinal signs* of inflammation, i.e., *redness, swelling, heat* and *pain*. Galen of Greece in the second century A.D. added the fifth cardinal sign of inflammation, the *loss of function*. Galen propounded the concept that inflammatory disease is the result of a cause acting locally, and this produces disturbance of function. In other words, corruption produced an abscess which caused interference with function.

It was not until the nineteenth century that the more precise mechanism of the signs and symptoms of inflammation was elucidated. The medieval concept of inflammation was that of a humoral theory, i.e., the inflammation is initiated by an accumulation of heat originating from the heart and followed by an influx of blood, mucus, and bile.

This humoral theory of inflammation was gradually replaced by the vascular theory. John Hunter showed that the redness of inflammation is due to increased blood flow through dilated vessels, and recognized that inflammation is associated with exudation of plasma and the suppuration due to extravasation of small globules.

The discovery of the cell by Schleiden (1838) and Schwann (1839) set the stage for the development of the present cellular-humoral concept of inflammation. Virchow in 1858 showed that inflammation is preceded by cell and tissue injury and that the vascular changes occur subsequent to such cell injury. Cohnheim, Virchow's pupil, made the classical description of the vascular changes in inflammation and described the emigration of leukocytes after observing the circulatory changes in the terminal bed of a frog's tongue and mesentery and in the rabbit's ear. These changes include hyperemia followed by slowing of blood flow. With more severe injury blood stops flowing. These circulatory changes are followed by the margination and sticking of leukocytes and then migration through the vascular wall.

Metchnikoff (1893) emphasized phagocytosis and elimination of the inflammatory agent by phagocytic cells as essential features of inflammation. In his study of the comparative pathology of inflammation he showed that the lowest animals, e.g., sponges, reacted to injury only with phagocytosis by mesenchymal cells. A vascular reaction with emigration of leukocytes was observed in animals with a vascular system consisting of arteries, veins, and capillaries. Thus the participation of the blood and the vascular system in the inflammatory response occurs only relatively late in the phylogenetic scale. Although in higher animals phagocytosis without vascular reaction is not looked upon as inflammatory, the removal of the inflammogenic agent by phagocytic cells is one of the principal functions of inflammation.

With the development of the theory of humoral immunity, various views on inflammation have gradually been synthesized into a general concept. According to Rössle (1934), the vascular system facilitates a rapid accumulation of phagocytes and humoral antibodies in the higher animals. Thus a principal aim of the inflammatory reaction might be *parenteral digestion* of foreign substances. Further, since inflammatory reactions can be triggered by the antigen-antibody reaction, Rössle coined the term *allergic inflammation*.

The physical chemistry of inflammation was studied by Schade (1923) who stressed the initial alteration of cells and tissue in the inflamed area, particularly the accumulation of hydrogen ions and an increase in osmotic pressure. Lewis (1927) showed evidence that the vascular changes of inflammation are mediated by histamine or other similar *H-substances*. Menkin (1940) isolated thermolabile and thermostable substances from inflammatory exudates which increased vascular permeability and promoted emigration of leukocytes. These studies set a new stage for the studies of the mediators of inflammation. The ultrastructure of the vascular alteration has been studied recently by Florey (1961) and others to extend the earlier observations of vascular changes and emigration of leukocytes. (Fig. 13-1).

Despite all the advancements made during the past 80 years or more, we are still far from being able to give a complete account of the entire inflammatory process. Recently Thomas has called attention to the difficulty of reconstructing a whole which really represents a set of interacting processes, each of which may be of value to the bodily defense, but in the aggregate may represent a catastrophe to the tissues and host. It has been believed that inflammation really exists as an entity among biologic mechanisms and that it represents an orderly sequence of timed and coordinated events, staged to occur in such a way that the host is protected

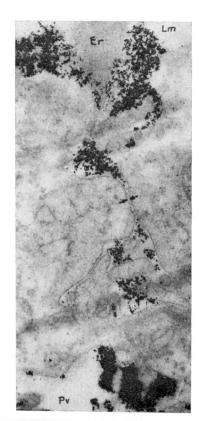

Fig. 13-1. Details of a junctional area between two endothelial cells. Continuity between the lumen (Lm) and the perivascular space (Pv) is easily seen. Thorotrast particles are seen throughout this space. Er: erythrocytes ($\times$ 20,000). [From Peterson, R. D., and Good, R. A. (1962): Lab. Invest. 11:507.]

against a foreign adversary and enabled to minimize damage to his own tissue, kill off the adversary, and finally tidy up the place and make whatever repairs are necessary. However, if one looks closely, there really is no such orderly mechanism. Instead, there are quite a few independent and separate mechanisms which are each sensibly designed for defense of one organism against incursion by another; each of these probably has other uses as well, some of them perhaps unrelated to defense, but there can be no doubt as to their usefulness when tissues are invaded.

When these various components of inflammation do take place all at once, it is often no longer easy to see it as defense; it is more like disease. It is this kind of catastrophe that was originally called inflammation. The host is caught up in mistaken, inappropriate, and unquestionably self-destructive mechanisms by the very multiplicity of available defenses which do not seem to have been designed to operate in net coordination with each other. The end result is often not defense, but an agitated, uncoordinated tactic of war that leads to the destruction of host tissue.

INFLAMMATORY PROCESS

Inflammation, a basic pathophysiologic response of living tissue to injury, is present in some form in all multicellular animals. It comprises a complex series of interacting and to some extent interdependent reactions in the terminal vascular bed that serve to bring phagocytes into the area to defend against the invading microorganisms and set the stage for repair of the injury through proliferation of connective tissue cells and collagen production.

Local inflammatory reaction is characterized by a set series of interrelated events that proceed in a regular sequence independent of the initiating stimulus or the tissue involved. The response can be divided into four stages: (1) increased vascular permeability, (2) emigration of neutrophils, (3) emigration of mononuclear cells, and (4) cellular proliferation and repair. Usually the first recognizable event in an inflammatory reaction is the development of an apparent stickiness of the capillary and venule walls. About the same time or shortly thereafter, increased vascular permeability can be recognized.

Increased Vascular Permeability

This first phase of the inflammatory response follows initial evidence of stagnation of circulation and starts shortly after the stimulation (infection, deposition of antigen-antibody complex, and activation of complement or other physical and chemical irritation). It is readily recognized by the leakage of colloidal dyes through the walls of terminal venules near the capillary-venule junction. Electron microscopic studies have demonstrated that the leakage of colloidal material occurs between the endothelial cells of venules. These endothelial cells are joined by a substance which is altered during the inflammation to permit the free passage of high molecular weight material. The exact chemical basis of this essential feature of inflammation remains enigmatic.

Within 15 to 30 minutes, white blood cells apparently under the influence of chemotactic stimuli accumulate in the area and start to emigrate from the vessels by the same route between endothelial cells used by the exudative fluid. These cells widen the spaces between the endothelial cells to allow the passive escape of a small number of red blood cells. The initial increase in vascular permeability is due to the influence of histamine or a histamine-like substance released locally by mast cells. It may last only a few minutes. However, under most circumstances, these substances are produced continuously for many hours after the initiating event and result in continued exudation of plasma and white blood cells.

Histamine, serotonin, and kinins have been shown to directly mediate the increased vascular permeability. All three substances have a positive charge and may act by combining with acidic mucopolysaccharides or glycoproteins in the blood vessel wall. It is interesting to note that serotonin, active in rodents, does not have this effect in humans or other mammals.

Histamine, which is mostly concentrated in the basophilic granules of tissue mast cells and circulating basophils, forms a complex with heparin. Histamine can be released from these granules by several mechanisms: (1) mechanical disruption, (2) interaction of an antigen with cytophilic antibody on the surface of mast cells, and (3) the generation of anaphylatoxin via activation of the complement system either by classical pathways requiring complement fixing antibody or by alternate pathways (Chapter 11).

Platelets are a rich source of histamine and participate in the inflammatory process by releasing histamine to the local area. In addition to the factors mentioned, sensitized lymphocytes react with specific antigen to produce a platelet-histamine-releasing factor, which is neither antibody nor complement.

Kinins, which are small polypeptides rich in arginine, are released from a plasma alpha-globulin, kininogen, by certain proteolytic enzymes, e.g., kallikrein. Neutrophils contain an enzyme capable of producing kinins from kininogen and may play an important role in sustaining the increased vascular permeability.

The interrelationship of these various factors leading to the generation of histamine and kinins is depicted in Figure 13-2.

Emigration of Neutrophils

Neutrophils begin to emigrate from the affected vessels 15 to 30 minutes after the irritation, and the maximum emigration is usually reached

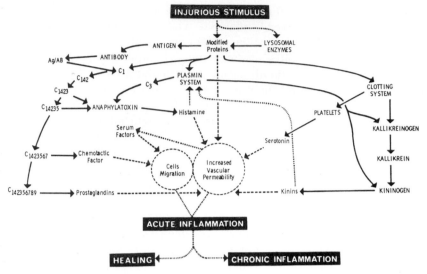

Fig. 13-2. Schematic representation of the interrelationship of various factors leading to inflammatory processes. [From Forscher, B., and Houck, J. C. (eds.) (1971): *Immunopathology of Inflammation.* Amsterdam, Excerpta Medica.]

within 4 to 8 hours. The emigration of neutrophils is dependent upon the presence of specific chemotactic factors which attract neutrophils to the site of the inflammation. First the neutrophils stick to the blood vessel wall and then emigrate out through the junction between endothelial cells; finally they penetrate the basement membrane and enter the interstitial spaces.

These neutrophils actively ingest and digest the foreign substances, furnishing an important first line of host defense against invading organisms or other foreign material. In addition, these neutrophils release substances that maintain the inflammatory response by increasing vascular permeability and by attracting more neutrophils. They facilitate further exudation of both neutrophils and mononuclear cells and set the stage for the predomination of mononuclear cells in the tissues.

Complement components C3a, C5a and possibly $C\overline{567}$ are known chemotactic factors, but the heat-labile neutrophil chemotactic factors in the serum from freshly clotted blood are different from the chemotactically active components derived from complement. Neutrophil granules contain chemotactically active polypeptides, and these factors may play a role in sustaining the emigration of leukocytes. Chemotactic factors can be found in some bacterial products which are active in the absence of serum, plasma, or antigen-antibody interaction.

The intensity and duration of the neutrophil emigration is proportional to the amount of chemotactic factor present in the inflamed area. In

allergic inflammation produced by antigen-antibody-complement interaction, the emigration of neutrophils may last for 24 to 48 hours. However, in inflammation induced by bacteria, the emigration may continue
until all the invading substances have been eliminated. When the amount
of foreign material is such that it attracts a large number of neutrophils and
also stimulates accumulation of fibroblasts and proliferation and synthesis
of collagen, the end result is the formation of a walled-off abscess that may
require drainage before healing can occur.

Emigration of Mononuclear Cells

Usually the third stage of the inflammatory response is the emigration
of mononuclear cells which starts about 4 hours after the initial stimulus
and reaches a peak after 16 to 24 hours. The early appearing mononuclear cells resemble lymphocytes but have a rapid turnover rate and characteristic electron microscopic features of monocytes originating from
bone marrow. The monocytes, which resemble macrophages, appear as a
development of these lymphocyte-like cells at a slightly later stage of
inflammation.

The emigration of circulating mononuclear cells requires the synthesis
of new messenger-RNA and protein within the cells. This process is triggered by some unknown substance liberated from the inflamed site. Such
primed mononuclear cells are then attracted by the chemotactic substances released from the inflammatory lesion by neutrophils. Other
chemotactic stimuli for such mononuclear cells originate from thymus derived lymphocytes that have interacted with antigen. In this instance, the
mononuclear cell infiltration is prolonged and more intense, as in the delayed hypersensitivity reaction. Still other chemotactic substances mentioned above derive from the complement components and these influence
the mononuclears, as well as polymorphonuclears. Finally, connective
tissue components other than those listed also contribute substances chemotactic to mononuclears that have not been defined and the origin of
which remains obscure.

Cellular Proliferation and Repair

Resolution and repair are the final stages of the inflammatory process.
Proliferation of fibroblasts in the area of the lesion starts within 18 hours
and reaches the peak by 48 to 72 hours. Regeneration of parenchymal
cells of the organ involved may take place. During this period the fibroblasts produce acidic mucopolysaccharides and collagen fibers. It has
been postulated that the acidic mucopolysaccharides may combine with
the chemical mediators of inflammation and thereby neutralize the effects
of these substances. The end stage of inflammation may be (1) complete
repair and restoration of function with or without scar formation, (2)
formation of an abscess, or (3) formation of granuloma.

Of particular interest is the formation of granuloma. When the inflammation is induced by microorganisms that survive inside the phagocytes or by foreign substances that are not digested by the phagocytes, granuloma form. In these instances, mononuclear cells surround the lesion, become activated, and develop into so-called epithelioid cells. The latter fuse or proliferate without completing division to become multinucleated giant cells. In addition, fibrous tissue may develop from fibroblasts in the area. In this manner, microorganisms, such as tubercle bacilli, may be walled off and contained for many years. Such bacilli may survive for many years inside the granuloma. In almost all instances granuloma formation due to infection is associated with cell-mediated immunity.

The kinetics of cellular migration during the inflammatory process can be studied by the *Rebuck skin window* technique. A small superficial abrasion is made on the skin, and a sterile coverslip is taped over the area. The coverslip is changed every 2 hours for 24 hours. Emigrated cells are attached to the coverslip, and the morphology of such cells can be identified by proper staining. This technique is widely used as a clinical research tool and for the assessment of the capacity to develop the cellular component of the inflammatory response. Recently quantitative cellular techniques have been used to study this process in man.

SYSTEMIC MANIFESTATIONS OF INFLAMMATION

When the local inflammation is not contained successfully, systemic manifestations of inflammation may take place, namely, fever and leukocytosis. It was thought that fever is a natural adaptation of the host that has beneficial effects in containing certain microbes. It is questionable, however, whether the host cells would function better at temperatures higher than normal in defense against the microorganisms. Fever therapy was used in the treatment of syphilis before the era of chemotherapy, but its effectiveness has not been established.

How is the systemic fever produced in infection or in inflammatory or allergic reactions? A useful model for the study of this question has been the experimental fever produced in animals by injection of endotoxin from gram-negative bacteria. Endotoxin produces fever by stimulating certain cells to release a protein, *endogenous pyrogen,* into the circulation. This protein acts on the central nervous system, especially on the thermoregulatory center, to produce fever. Neutrophils and monocytes produce endogenous pyrogen *in vitro* under a wide variety of stimuli, such as exposure to bacterial endotoxin, phagocytosis of bacteria, or even exposure to inert particles like polystyrene latex particles, antigen-antibody complexes, and a change in the ionic strength and oxygen tension of the medium in which the neutrophils are incubated.

Preformed endogenous pyrogen can be found in the neutrophils and macrophages that have emigrated into the inflamed lesion. Cells other than circulating neutrophils and macrophages may also be able to produce such pyrogen, since fever can be observed in animals and humans that are completely lacking circulating neutrophils and monocytes. This indicates that the production of pyrogen may be a universal property of the reticuloendothelial system and perhaps of many other cells.

Leukocytosis, an increase in the number of white blood cells in the circulation, is another systemic manifestation of inflammation. As a rule, pyogenic bacterial infections produce leukocytosis with an increase in the number of circulating neutrophils. Viral infections are not usually associated with leukocytosis and sometimes may even induce a mild *leukopenia,* a decrease in the number of leukocytes in the circulation.

Leukocytosis can be induced experimentally for diagnostic purposes in man by intravenous injection of endotoxin or cortisone. The peak response of leukocytosis occurs between 4 to 6 hours after the onset of inflammation.

Another systemic manifestation of inflammation is the production of acute phase reactants, or acute phase proteins, mainly by the liver. Blood concentrations of fibrinogen, alpha-2-glycoproteins, C-reactive proteins, coagulation factors, mucoproteins, and complement components are increased. Increased fibrinogen concentration is reflected in the elevation of the erythrocyte sedimentation rate (ESR). *C-reactive protein* was originally discovered because it formed a precipitin reaction with pneumococcal capsular polysaccharide. In general, the C-reactive protein appears in plasma within a few hours after the onset of tissue damage as in infection and disappears shortly after the infection has been contained or the process initiating tissue damage has abated.

The serum concentration of albumin is decreased and that of the alpha-2-globulin and gamma globulin may be increased during chronic inflammation. Microcytic hypochromic anemia is another manifestation of chronic inflammation. This is due to the defect in the ability to utilize iron for hemoglobulin synthesis during active infection or chronic stimulus to inflammation.

MECHANISMS OF IMMUNOLOGIC INJURY

Just as the phagocytosis and inflammatory processes can do more harm than good to the host in certain situations, the immune reactions can often be detrimental to the host rather than providing beneficial defense mechanisms. Von Pirquet was the first to develop the concept of allergy, an altered reactivity, which includes not only immunity, but also hypersensitivity (overreaction) as well as hyposensitivity. Thus immunologic reactions that produce tissue injury in certain conditions are called *hypersensitivity reactions.*

During the past 80 years, our understanding of the phenomenon of the hypersensitivity reaction has progressed steadily. The initial fundamental observations were reexamined (researched) in detail, and new observations have been added continuously, resulting in a more precise formulation of definitions and development of useful immunologic methods for the understanding of the mechanisms of immunologic injury. Analysis of the mechanisms underlying the hypersensitivity reactions indicates a clear distinction between the two principal mechanisms of immunologic injury, i.e., *directed form* and *indirect form*. Directed immunologic inju-

Table 13-1.　Mechanisms of Immunologic Injury

1. *Humoral (precipitinogenic)*	
Directed	Masugi nephritis
	Goodpasture's disease
	Steblay nephritis
	Kay nephritis
	Drug-induced hemolysis (some)
	Hemolysis in Rh disease
Indirect	Immune complex diseases
	Serum sickness
	Lupus nephritis
	Arthus reaction (inflammatory)
	Drug-induced thrombocytopenia
	Drug-induced hemolytic anemia
	Most chronic nephritis
2. *Humoral (reaginic)*	
Indirect (always)	Passive cutaneous anaphylaxis (PCA)
	Urticaria
	Asthma
	Hay fever
	Prausnitz-Küstner reaction (P-K)
	Schultz-Dale reaction
3. *Cellular*	
Directed	Killer action of sensitized lymphocyte against target allogeneic cells (Brunner type)
	Contact allergy
Indirect	Koch's phenomenon
	Cavitation of tuberculosis
	Granulomatous reaction in bacterial infection
4. *Intravascular Coagulation*	
Local	Hemorrhagic necrosis of Arthus reaction
	Local Shwartzman reaction
General	Generalized Shwartzman reaction
	Bilateral cortical necrosis of man
	Hemolytic uremic syndrome
5. *Endogenous Toxin*	Myasthenia gravis
	—the release of toxic substance secondary to indirect cellular or humoral assault.

ries result from the action of the specific antibodies or sensitized cells directed against target cells or tissue constituents; in indirect injuries, innocent bystander cells or tissues are injured because the antigen-antibody reaction happened to take place nearby. Depending on the kind of antibody involved, the humoral type can be subdivided into precipitinogenic (immune complex diseases), cytotropic (reaginic anaphylactic reaction) and cytolytic (immune hemolytic anemia) types. A classification of the many means by which injury to the host may occur as a consequence of immune reaction is presented in Table 13-1.

Anaphylactic (Reaginic) Hypersensitivity

Anaphylactic hypersensitivity depends on the presence of homocytotropic antibodies which are distinguished from other types of antibodies by certain characteristics: (1) they are active only within the same or a closely related mammalian species; (2) they attach to the cell surface of certain cells, primarily mast cells; (3) when the antigen reacts specifically with the antibody on the cell surface, biologically active substances released from the cells cause visible signs and symptoms of hypersensitivity. For this reason, the anaphylactic hypersensitivity reaction is classified as a humoral hypersensitivity of the cytotropic type.

Anaphylactic reactions are, like other hypersensitivity reactions, characterized by a specific initial event, the reaction between antigens and *homocytotropic antibodies* that tend to attach to the cells of the same species. The homocytotropic antibodies belong to different immunoglobulin classes in the different animal species and are still under intensive investigation. Their existence in man was convincingly demonstrated by Prausnitz and Küstner in 1921 in their passive transfer experiment; but during the next four decades attempts to define the so-called reaginic (cytotropic) antibodies were unsuccessful until Ishizaka and co-workers in 1966 showed that the reaginic antibodies of man probably belong to a new class of immunoglobulins, IgE.

This initial observation was confirmed when Johansson and Bennich in 1967 identified a new class of human myeloma protein, which is a counterpart of the IgE. By the development of antisera to the IgE myeloma protein, the IgE in normal sera can be measured quantitatively. It was further shown that IgE possesses several reaginic properties.

IgE and probably other homocytotropic antibodies attach to the surface of cell membrane by means of the Fc part of the molecule. Complement does not participate in this binding. After passive transfer of homocytotropic antibody there is a latent period of 8 to 18 hours before the antigen can elicit an anaphylactic reaction. The period is probably needed for the attachment of the antibodies to the cell membrane. These reactions are most likely independent of the classic complement cascade. Recent evidence, however, suggests that the alternate pathway of complement can be activated by aggregated IgE. It is likely that participation of the complement system from C3 and beyond is involved in reaginic-type hypersensitivity reactions. The observable symptoms are due to release of mediator substances from the recipient cells, e.g., histamine, bradykinin, slow reacting substances of anaphylaxis (SRS-A), acetylcholine, serotonin, and prostaglandins. It is not known why the homocytotropic antibodies are not always fixed uniformly in all tissues, but their dispersal probably depends on the distribution of cells with appropriate receptor for the Fc part of the IgE or other homocytotropic antibodies, e.g., mast cells.

When the antigens (allergens) interact with the antibodies on the cell surface in the skin, a local release of mediator substances, especially histamine from reacting mast cells, will induce a local increase of vascular permeability and dilatation of capillaries. Consequently a localized edema develops which is a common familiar feature of *urticaria*. When these mediators are released locally in the lung parenchyma, bronchial asthma develops which is characterized by (1) edema of the mucous membrane, (2) contraction of bronchial smooth muscle, and (3) increased mucous secretion of bronchial glands. These signs may all be induced by histamine, bradykinin, or SRS-A.

If the specific antigen is suddenly brought into the circulation of an organism with cytotropic hypersensitivity, the antigen-antibody reaction takes place in the same way, but the release of large amounts of mediator substances into the circulation leads to one form of anaphylactic shock. Another form of anaphylactic shock is produced by circulating IgG antibody–antigen complexes which, although not attaching so firmly to the cells by the receptor mechanism, can activate release of histamine and generalized anaphylaxis through the complement activation at the cell surface.

Cutaneous anaphylaxis is also observed experimentally when the local skin site is sensitized by an intracutaneous injection of antibody, and a mixture of antigen and dye is injected intravenously 3 to 6 hours later. Or, both antigen and antibody may be injected into the same skin site to produce cutaneous anaphylaxis. Regardless of the method used, the reaction is called *passive cutaneous anaphylaxis (PCA)* if antibody is injected before antigen has been introduced. When antigen is injected first, the reaction is called *reversed PCA*. Nonspecific irritation may occur after injection of antiserum but generally does not last more than an hour. Thus if antigen is injected intravenously 3 to 6 hours after the intradermal injection of antiserum, irritation of the skin by either antiserum or antigen is unlikely to interfere with the reaction. For this reason, as well as because of its high sensitivity in detecting antibody, this sequence of injections is used in most studies involving PCA. Guinea pigs have been used extensively for the study of PCA, but recently mice and rats have been shown to elicit PCA reactions in which the maximal reaction is not reached until 30 minutes after injection of the antigen.

Prausnitz-Küstner (P-K) reactions in human beings probably correspond to PCA reactions in experimental animals. If serum samples of atopic patients are injected intracutaneously into a normal individual, and the skin site is challenged 24 to 48 hours later by allergen to which the donor is sensitive, the sites show wheal and erythema reactions, which are maximal 15 to 20 minutes after the injection of allergen. The allergic reaction to human reaginic serum and allergen can be observed in the monkey by the same procedure used to demonstrate PCA reactions in the guinea pig.

The *Schultz-Dale reaction* demonstrates that isolated uterine or intestinal strips from sensitized animals will react with contraction upon contact with antigen. Passive sensitization of an isolated guinea pig ileum can be accomplished *in vitro* by incubation of the proper antibody with the ileum. It is of interest, as Halpern et al. (1960) first showed, that normal gamma globulin competing for receptor sites on the intestinal strip can interfere with antibody sensitization of the strip for contraction induced by specific antigen. A protective influence of normal gamma globulin through competition against influence of aggregated gamma globulin is perhaps most clearly illustrated in the well-established increased susceptibility of agammaglobulinemic children to the anaphylactoid reactions produced by intravenous injections of gamma globulin aggregates (Barandun et al., 1962).

Chemical Mediators of Anaphylaxis

The chemical mediators of anaphylaxis form a system which may be regarded as a preformed biologic arrangement that is ready for release when an antigen reacts with homocytotropic antibody on the cell surface. The clinically observable signs of anaphylaxis are due to the accumulated pharmacodynamic effects of these mediators. Among the important mediators are (1) histamine, (2) plasma kinins, (3) slow reacting substance of anaphylaxis (SRS-A), (4) acetylcholine, (5) serotonin, 6) prostaglandins, and (7) *permeability factor dilute (PF/dil)* and *complement-derived anaphylatoxins*.

Histamine [4-(2-aminoethyl)imidazole] (*Fig. 13-3*). Biosynthesis of histamine, a continuous process, involves the action, with the aid of a coenzyme, of the enzyme histidine decarboxylase on the amino acid L-histidine. Histamine is stored in the mast cells which presumably contain the major part of the body histamine. The bronchial tree contains a large number of mast cells, the lung being the tissue with the highest concentration of histamine in the human body. In human blood, histamine is distributed as follows: basophils, 51 percent; eosinophils, 29 percent; neutrophils, 14 percent; and other white cells and platelets, 6 percent.

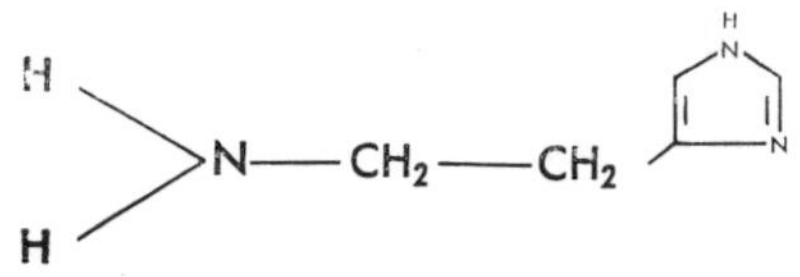

Fig. 13-3. Chemical structure of histamine [4-(2-aminoethyl) imidazole].

The exact mechanism of the release of histamine has not yet been completely elucidated. When antigen combines with homocytotropic antibody on the surface of the mast cell membrane, histamine is released from the mast cell granules into the surrounding tissues by a mechanism involving decrease of cellular levels of cyclic adenosine monophosphate (AMP). Recent evidence suggests that increases of cyclic guanosine monophosphate (GMP) inverse to the decrease of cyclic AMP may be involved in the release of histamine from mast cells. Release of histamine from mast cells upon challenge with antigen occurs not only in tissues spontaneously sensitized in nature but also in passively sensitized tissues of guinea pigs, rabbits, and men. The degree of mast cell degranulation and release of histamine depends on the dose of antigen.

The degranulation of mast cells, however, may be generated by several mechanisms other than interaction of cytotropic antibody and antigen at the cell surface. Infection is one of the well-known causes of mast cell degranulation. In patients dying of asthma, a marked depletion of mast cell granules in the lung tissue is a characteristic feature.

Histamines, of course, play other roles in physiology, e.g., participating in growth and repair of tissues and stimulating phagocytosis and alterations of ground substance. In addition to the well-known role in the inflammatory process, histamine has been implicated as a regulator of circulating homeostasis by maintaining balance with catecholamines.

Constitutional peculiarities seem to exist between allergic and nonallergic individuals. Although the wheal and flare reactions in skin after intradermal injection of histamine are similar, the tissue response to histamine in allergic individuals seems to be characterized by a rather more extensive degree of infiltration of neutrophils and eosinophils than normal. Further, allergic individuals may have greater reactivity of the bronchi and blood vessels to pharmacologically active substances than do normal persons.

The main pharmacologic actions of this powerful amine are:
1. Contraction of smooth muscles.
2. Increase in permeability of capillary vessels.
3. Increase in secretion of mucous glands.
4. Dilatation of the small capillaries and contraction of small arterioles in some tissues.

5. Induction of itching and nausea and an increase in intestinal motility.

The histamine release mechanism can be abolished *in vitro* by incubation at 45°C for a few minutes, be reversibly inhibited at low temperatures, or be influenced by pH and the concentration of divalent cations, Mg^{++} and Ca^{++}. The process requires oxygen and is impeded by several metabolic depressors, especially sulfhydryl inhibitors. It is a swift, energy-consuming, almost explosive process. About 20 seconds after contact with antigen, the antibody effects of histamine can be recorded in tissues. Recently, Lichtenstein and Orange and Austen have shown that both catecholamines and methyl xanthines inhibit histamine release by leukocytes *in vitro*. This finding indicates that decreased levels of cyclic 3',5'-AMP may relate to the release of histamine, whereas increased levels are associated with inhibition of degranulation of mast cells and histamine release.

Histamine is rapidly broken down by oxidation through the action of the enzyme histaminase and by methylation. The metabolites are rapidly cleared from the circulation and are excreted mainly through the kidney.

Many synthetic compounds have been found to antagonize the action of histamine. Most of these antihistamines have a core of substituted ethylamine ($-CH_2CH_2N=$) similar to that in histamine. They probably act by competing for the histamine receptor sites on the effector cells.

Plasma Kinins. It has been known since 1937 by the work of Werle et al. that kallikrein reacts with plasma to form a substance which causes smooth muscle contraction. In 1949 Rocha e Silva showed that trypsin or snake venom added to plasma generates a substance which causes contraction of smooth muscle and dilates the blood vessels. They called this substance *bradykinin*. Antihistamine had no effect on it, and it took about seven times longer for the contraction of smooth muscle to reach a peak than it did with histamine; hence the name, bradykinin (slow to move).

At present three kinins have been isolated, synthesized, and their amino acid sequence established:
1. Bradykinin, a nonapeptide:
   H-Arg-Pro-Pro-Gly-Phe-Ser-Pro-Phe-Arg-OH.
2. Kallidin II, a decapeptide:
   H-Lys-Arg-Pro-Pro-Gly-Phe-Ser-Pro-Phe-Arg-OH.
3. Methyl-lysyl-bradykinin, a hendecapeptide:
   H-Met-Lys-Arg-Pro-Pro-Gly-Phe-Ser-Pro-Phe-Arg-OH.

The biologic activities of these three kinins are similar; the differences are merely quantitative. Bradykinin, the best known and probably the most important of the plasma kinins, causes (1) dilatation of blood vessels, (2) increase in vascular permeability, (3) constriction of bronchial smooth muscle, (4) increased secretion of mucous glands, (5) itching, (6) hyperemia, and (7) pain of skin. Blood plasma and most tissues, including neutrophils, contain kininases, a group of enzymes with uniform specificity and optimum pH. These kininases, and possibly chymotrypsin, decompose plasma kinins rapidly, and the half-life of bradykinin is less than 30 seconds *in vivo*. Numerous studies have established the pathogenetic role of the kinins in experimental animals such as guinea pigs, rabbits, dogs, and rats. But their exact role in pathogenesis of anaphylaxis in man has not been fully explained.

Slow Reacting Substance of Anaphylaxis (SRS-A). Other biologically active, closely related compounds that cause muscle contraction were observed in lung tissue by Kellaway and Trethewie (1940). Since the action of these compounds was slower than that of histamine, they were named accordingly, slow reacting substances of anaphylaxis (SRS-A). SRS-A is liberated from sensitized lung tissue of guinea pigs and man and produces contraction of bronchial muscles. SRS-A generates a marked and prolonged contraction of human bronchioles, but this effect is weak or lacking in bronchioles of cats, dogs, rabbits, and guinea pigs at comparable doses. Higher concentrations are needed to elicit contraction of bronchioles in these experimental animals.

Whereas the pharmacologic effect of histamine on human bronchial muscle is most prominent during the first 3 minutes, SRS-A dominates the constriction after 8 minutes, and is much more prolonged (for many hours) than that of histamine. This may account for some allergic reactions that are resistant to antihistamines. SRS-A is highly soluble in water and has a tendency to combine with lipids. It is unaffected by alterations of pH and can be decomposed by boiling, oxidation, and by action of certain bacteria. SRS-A is readily adsorbed to the surface of glassware and other instruments, a major reason for the difficulties encountered in quantifying its influence in *in vitro* experiments.

SRS-A is not a preformed substance but is produced in the tissues, especially in the lung and blood vessels when a reaction between antigen and cytotropic antibody takes place. It was shown *in vitro* that the production of SRS-A increases within the first 5 minutes after challenge with antigen and continues for hours in the presence of excess antigen. Similarly SRS-A is formed in human asthmatic lung tissue after antigenic challenge and released in sufficient amounts to account for the pathogenetic mechanism of bronchial asthma. So far, three types of slow reacting substances have been studied, but they are not well defined and may belong to a group of related substances. SRS-A appears to be an unsaturated fatty acid, but the precise chemical structure is not known, and its quantitation depends solely on the bioassay method, i.e., its unique pharmacologic activity on the contraction of isolated smooth muscle preparations.

It was believed that the production and subsequent release of SRS-A in the lung tissue and perhaps other tissues is initiated solely by the reaction between homocytotropic antibody and antigen. Recent studies by Austen et al., however, indicate that alternate mechanisms for the release of

SRS-A exist in the rat, i.e., by a reaction between the antigen and IgG, which is apparently not a homocytotropic antibody in the rat. It is known that important differences exist in the immunoglobulin class of homocytotropic antibodies among the different species, but it has not been definitely established whether the human SRS-A system is exclusively activated by the reaction of antigen and homocytotropic antibody, IgE, or by reactions with other immunoglobulins as well. Some evidence, for example, of reaginic IgGs has been presented.

Acetylcholine, Catecholamines, and Adrenergic Receptors. Acetylcholine, which is released in the parasympathetic synapses of respiratory glands and smooth muscles, induces the constriction of the bronchus and the secretion of the mucous glands. No evidence has yet been found to indicate that the release of acetylcholine is initiated by the interaction of homocytotropic antibody and antigen. Further, release of acetylcholine induced by vagus stimulation in asthma attacks can produce bronchial constriction similar to that induced by SRS-A, histamine, or bradykinin. A difference, of course, is that this reaction can be inhibited by atropine.

Catecholamine is a generic term referring to compounds that contain a dihydroxybenzene nucleus (catechol) and have sympathomimetic activity. The two main naturally occurring compounds are epinephrine (Adrenalin) and norepinephrine (noradrenalin). Catecholamines either increase or inhibit the contraction of smooth muscles of the bronchus, depending on the type of receptor on the target cells that are activated.

There are two types of adrenergic receptors, alpha and beta. Catecholamines produce excitation on alpha receptors and inhibition on beta receptors. The adrenergic system of bronchial muscle and bronchial glands is dominated by the beta receptors which, by stimulation, result in the relaxation of smooth muscle and possibly in the inhibition of the glandular secretions. The processes resulting in the relaxation of smooth muscle through the action of beta-adrenergic receptors involve sequential activation of several enzyme systems. By the activation of cyclic 3′,5′-AMP, a second enzyme is activated which in turn activates a third enzyme, which then initiates the breakdown of glycogen to glucose-1-phosphate. The complexities of these interactions are under intensive study and as yet are not completely understood.

Serotonin (5-hydroxytryptamine, 5-HT). The initial assumption that serotonin may play some role in bronchial asthma stems from the clinical observation of patients with the carcinoid syndrome. Asthmatic symptoms were frequently seen in these patients. Although serotonin is found in the mast cells of rats and is released by reaction of antigen and cytotropic antibody in this species, it is not found in human mast cells. Therefore, serotonin may not be of much importance as a mediator of anaphylactic reaction in man.

Prostaglandins. Several compounds in the respiratory apparatus could, by faulty metabolism, disturb the tonus and secretions of the bronchus. The prostaglandins are aliphatic unsaturated fatty acids found in many tissues, including the lungs. Prostaglandins E_1 and E_2 (PGE_1 and PGE_2) relax isolated human bronchial muscle *in vitro*. PGE_{2a}, however, appears to constrict the bronchial muscles. The role of prostaglandins in the pathogenesis of bronchial asthma in man is yet to be established.

Permeability Factor Dilute (PF/dil) and Anaphylatoxin. When plasma is diluted with saline, a permeability factor dilute (PF/dil) is activated which increases the vascular permeability. It has been postulated that PF/dil may be formed in the tissues when the precursor substance in the plasma globulin fraction is diluted by edema fluid created by histamine effects. The exact role of PF/dil in the induction of anaphylactic reaction has not been established.

Anaphylatoxins derived from C3a and C5a (see Chapter 11) induce contraction of the smooth muscle, although they react with different receptors. There are distinct species-related characteristics with regard to the ability to generate smooth muscle contraction and mast cell degranulation. Anaphylatoxin in guinea pig lungs induces asthmatic symptoms *in vivo* which may be prevented by prior use of antihistamines.

It is possible that antibodies other than IgE may initiate similar anaphylactic reactions such as asthma by the activation of the complement system. Indeed, evidence implicating a special subclass of IgG as a reaginic antibody has been presented.

Arthus Reaction

In 1903 Arthus treated rabbits with daily injections of horse serum and demonstrated that if the injection was repeated at intervals of 8 days in a limited area of the skin, a localized, intense, hemorrhagic reaction developed. After appropriate sensitization, this reaction began immediately and infarction, necrosis, and destruction of the skin area ensued. It was later found that such a reaction is dependent on the presence of precipitating antibody in the circulation. This type of reaction involving circulating antibody, of which the Arthus reaction is an extreme manifestation, can elicit tissue damage in several other ways, depending upon the localization and concentration of the antibodies and antigens as complexes in the tissues. Infiltration by polymorphonuclear leukocytes in the blood vessels is essential for the tissue destruction.

Serum sickness is another example of immunologic injury due to circulating antigen-antibody complex. When horse serum is injected into an organism of a different species (in man usually in order to obtain a protective passive immunity), a characteristic clinical syndrome may develop after 8 to 15 days. The most common clinical features are swelling at the site of injection, enlargement of regional lymph nodes, urticarial rashes often starting at the injection site and later involving the whole skin, and less frequently, fever and exanthema with a different morphology. Arthritis, renal disease with or without proteinuria or hematuria, and reduction of the neutrophil count are seen in some patients. The syndrome is usually rather mild, and the symptoms disappear within 3 to 5 days. In some instances, however, a more serious course may occur that includes fatal glomerulonephritis, severe gastrointestinal symptoms, cardiac involvement, and central and peripheral nervous system involvement, and severe arthritis.

Largely due to the works of Ishizaka et al., Germuth, and Dixon and co-workers, the pathogenesis of serum sickness is well understood on the basis of the effect of circulating antigen-antibody complexes. It may be assumed that precipitating antibody in the blood and the homologous antigen, in principle, interact according to the same rules as in other liquid media *in vitro*. In the excess of antigen or antibody, soluble antigen-antibody complexes are initially formed. Subsequently, with the optimal ratio of antigen-antibody concentrations, insoluble precipitates will form. The soluble complexes of antigen-antibody lodge in various tissues and organs, especially in the glomeruli of the kidney. Activation of complement components and other effector mechanisms is initiated by these immune complexes that set the stage for the development of the inflammatory reaction resulting in the damage of the tissue which itself acts as an innocent bystander. Immunologic injury such as that induced by circulating immune complexes formed in serum sickness is seen also in lupus erythematosus and poststreptococcal acute glomerulonephritis.

Masugi Nephritis

In 1933, Masugi immunized rabbits with rat kidney tissue. He then injected the antiserum into rats and produced a nephrotoxic nephritis, a classic model of directed immunologic injury. The pathogenesis of Masugi nephritis is due to the interaction of the antibody with the antigen in the glomerular basement membranes (GBM). The rabbit immunoglobulin and complement have been shown to be deposited in linear fusion along the luminal side of host glomerular basement membrane. The pathogenesis of this injury has been clarified on the basis of animal experiments which have shown that (1) the capacity of heterogenous anti-kidney antibodies (so-called nephrotoxic serum) to induce glomerulonephritis depends mainly on the anti-GBM antibody, (2) anti-GBM antibody can be passively transferred, and (3) as a rule circulating anti-GBM antibody titer is very low in the nephritic animal.

A similar nephrotoxic nephritis can be produced in rabbits by injecting anti-rabbit GBM antibody raised from ducks. Since the gamma globulins of ducks fix complement poorly, only minimal glomerular damage occurs. However, when the rabbit produces antibodies against the duck gamma globulin, a violent glomerulonephritis may develop by the mechanisms similar to those of immune complex nephritis. Here, however, the immunologic assault is directed against antigen foreign to the host, which for immunologic reasons is distributed at the basement membrane. Thus, directed immunologic assault in immunologic injury can be focused against either host or foreign antigens. It is equally clear that induced immune assault can also be directed against either host or foreign antigens. Another variation of nephrotoxic nephritis can be induced in sheep by injecting isolated GBM from human or monkey kidneys. Nephrotoxic nephritis due to a direct immunologic attack on the sheep's own GBM is produced when the host's antibodies directed against human or monkey GBM cross react with its own GBM. This model is known as the Steblay model of autoimmune glomerulonephritis.

The human counterpart of Masugi nephritis is observed in Goodpasture's syndrome.

Hemolytic Diseases

The process of cytolysis by immunologic injury has been studied *in vitro* by employing red cell lysis to activate the complement system. Ample evidence supports the view that the same mechanisms are operating during *in vivo* lysis of red cells in many clinical hypersensitivity disorders and may be a major cause of granulocytopenia, agranulocytosis, or thrombocytopenia. Here again the destruction of the hematologic elements may be consequent to either directed immune assault as in erythroblastosis fetalis or induced antigen-antibody complex type of immune assault as in certain drug-induced thrombocytopenias and hemolytic anemias. In man, blood group incompatibility reactions and autoimmune acquired hemolytic disease are the well-known examples of cell damage due to the directed immunologic injury by the cytolytic antibodies. Drug-induced hemolytic anemia may be due to either directed or indirect immune assault. Detailed descriptions of these clinical conditions are described in Part II of this book.

Shwartzman Reaction

In 1928 Shwartzman induced a local skin reactivity in rabbits by first injecting endotoxin intradermally and later intravenously. This phenomenon is called the Shwartzman reaction. The characteristic lesion of the Shwartzman reaction is hemorrhagic necrosis of the skin due to inflammation and intravascular coagulation at the local site. A generalized form of the Shwartzman reaction, first described by Sanarelli in 1924, is produced by two spaced injections of endotoxin and is based on generalized intravascular coagulation. Among laboratory animals, the rabbit is uniquely susceptible to both local and generalized forms of the Shwartzman reaction. The local Shwartzman reaction is elicited in the rabbit by intradermal injection of a small dose of endotoxin and challenged 24 hours later with intravenous injection of the same preparation. Petechial hemorrhage appears at the site of primary inoculation within a few hours of challenge, rapidly coalesces, and progresses to complete necrosis within another 24 hours (Fig. 13-4A) The interval between so-called preparative and provocative doses is fairly critical, with the outside limits being 6 to 48 hours. The generalized Shwartzman reaction is elicited by injection of both doses intravenously and is characterized by bilateral, hemorrhagic, cortical necrosis of kidneys. Hemorrhagic necrosis often occurs in skin,

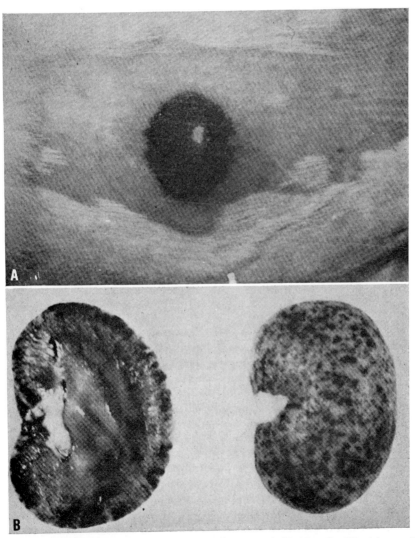

Fig. 13-4. A. Typical local Shwartzman reaction in prepared skin site of rabbit 4 hours after challenging injection of endotoxin. B. Generalized Shwartzman reaction in rabbit kidneys, showing the characteristic bilateral cortical necrosis.

bowel, lung, liver, adrenal, and other organs (Fig. 13-4B). Histologically, in the local Shwartzman reaction cellular thrombi with enmeshed leukocytes and platelets are seen in the small vessels of the dermis, whereas in the generalized Shwartzman reaction thrombi consisting almost entirely of fibrin occlude the glomerular capillaries.

Although many experiments have been done since the local Shwartzman reaction was first described in 1928, it is only recently that its mechanism has been elucidated. It has now been established that nearly all of the remarkable biologic properties of endotoxin can be attributed to the capacity of these lipopolysaccharide molecules to activate the complement system via the alternate pathway (see Chapter 11). At the same time the endotoxin molecule has capacity to attach to platelets and endothelium; the complement activation by the endotoxin can damage these cells and produce intravascular coagulation. The complement-induced injury to endothelium and platelets produces all the essential ingredients of the local Shwartzman reaction and explains the basic events of the generalized Shwartzman reaction. Endothelial damage, platelet activation, the presence of polymorphonuclears, intravascular coagulation, and complement activation all are required to produce this form of tissue injury. It is now clear that endotoxin may not be necessary and that local and generalized Shwartzman reactions can be produced by a variety of events if they occur in appropriate conjunction. For example, local infection by viruses or bacteria or immune complex injury can prepare for the local Shwartzman reaction, whereas antibody-antigen reaction in the circulation can both prepare for and provoke the generalized Shwartzman reaction. The mechanism of hemorrhagic necrosis of the Arthus reaction is very similar to that of the local Shwartzman reaction. Thus, although the Shwartzman reactions are induced by endotoxins under very precise experimental conditions, the analysis of this *quasi*-immunologic reaction reveals mechanisms that play roles of greatest importance in certain forms of immunologically induced tissue injury.

Activation of the effector systems by endotoxin also produces inflammation, fever, and tissue necrosis similar to that found in more conventional immunologic injury. The local Shwartzman reaction is inhibited by alpha blockade but not by beta blockade. The generalized Shwartzman reaction is inhibited by alpha blockade, as well as by making the test animal tolerant to epinephrine.

The clinical counterpart of the generalized Shwartzman reaction is seen during septicemia with certain gram-negative bacteria, e.g., meningococcemia and in the hemolytic uremic syndrome.

Cell-mediated Immunologic Injuries

Just as humoral immunity can often cause a variety of tissue injury, cell-mediated immunity induces tissue injuries via the mechanism of delayed hypersensitivity (Chapter 7). Koch reported in 1891 the first observation of hypersensitivity reaction to tubercle bacteria in a guinea pig. Zinsser in 1923 drew a sharp distinction between an *immediate type* and a *delayed type* of hypersensitivity.

The fundamental biologic importance of the delayed hypersensitivity reaction has been partially elucidated only recently, and the terms *cell-mediated* or *cellular hypersensitivity* have been used in place of delayed hypersensitivity and bacterial allergy.

Besides the importance of cellular hypersensitivity as a major factor determining the course of many infectious diseases, this form of hypersensitivity reaction is known to be fundamentally involved in several other conditions, such as contact dermatitis, solid tissue and organ graft rejections, autoimmune diseases of experimental animals and man, and immunologic attack on tumors. The mechanisms of immunologic injuries in various disease conditions are explored more fully in the second part of this book.

SELECTED REFERENCES

Austen, K. F., and Becker, E. L. (eds.) (1968): *Biochemistry of the Acute Allergic Reactions*. Oxford, Blackwell Scientific Publications.

Barandun, S., et al. (1962): Vox Sang. 7:157.

Brocklehurst, W. E., Humphrey, J. H., and Perry, W. L. M. (1955): J. Physiol. (London) 129:205.

Cohnheim, J. (1867): Arch. Path. Anat. 40:1.

Dixon, F. J., et al. (1958): Arch. Path. (Chicago) 65:18.

Florey, H. W., and Grant, L. H. (1961): J. Path. Bact. 82:13.

Germuth, F. G. (1953): J. Exp. Med. 97:257.

Halpern, et al. (1960): Allerg. Asthma (Leipzig) 6:304.

Ishizaka, K., Ishizaka, T., and Hornbrook, M. M. (1966): J. Immun. 97:840.

Johansson, S. G. D., and Bennich, H. (1967): Immunology 13:381.

Kellaway, C. H., and Trethewie, E. R. (1940): Quart. J. Exp. Physiol. 30:121.

Koch, R. (1891): Deutsch. Med. Wschr. 17:101.

Lewis, T. (1927): *The Blood Vessels of the Human Skin and Their Response*. London, Shaw.

Lichtenstein, L. M. (1969): In *Cellular and Humoral Mechanisms in Anaphylaxis and Allergy*. Movat, H. Z. (ed.). Basel, S. Karger, p. 176.

Masugi, M. (1933): Beitr. Path. Anat. 91:82.

Menkin, V. (1940): *Dynamics of Inflammation*. New York, The Macmillan Company.

Metchnikoff, E. (1968): *Lectures on the Comparative Pathology of Inflammation*. (First published in 1893). New York, Dover Publications, Inc.

Orange, R. P., and Austen, K. F. (1969): Advances Immun. 10:106.

Prausnitz, C., and Küstner, H. (1921): Z. Bakt. 86:160.

Rocha e Silva, M. (1955): In Ciba Foundation Symposium on *Histamine*. London, Churchill, p. 178.

Rössle, R. (1934): Verh. Deutsch. Ges. Path. 27:152.

Sanarelli, G. (1924): Ann. Inst. Pasteur 38:11.

Schade, H. (1923): Verh. Deutsch. Ges. Path. 19:69.

Shwartzman, G. (1928): Proc. Soc. Exp. Biol. Med. 25:48.

Thomas, L. (1971): In *Immunopathology of Inflammation*, Forscher, B. K., and Houck, J. C. (eds.). Amsterdam, Excerpta Medica, p. 1.

Von Pirquet, C. (1906): Munchen. Med. Wschr. 54:1457.

Werle, E., Gotze, W., and Keppler, A. (1937): Biochim. Z. 289:217.

Zinsser, H. (1923): J. Exp. Med. 34:495.

FURTHER READINGS

Aas, K. (1972): *The Biochemical and Immunological Basis of Bronchial Asthma.* Springfield, Illinois, Charles C Thomas.

Cohnheim, J. (1889): *Lectures on General Pathology.* London, New Sydenham Society.

Forscher, B. K., and Houck, J. C. (eds.) (1971): *Immunopathology of Inflammation.* Amsterdam, Excerpta Medica.

Good, R. A., et al. (1969): Fed. Proc. 28:191.

Keller, R. (1966): *Tissue Mast Cells in Immune Reactions.* New York, American Elsevier Publishing Company.

Major, R. H. (1957): *A History of Medicine.* Springfield, Illinois, Charles C Thomas.

Zweifach, B. W., Grant, L., and McCluskey, R. T. (eds.) (1965): *The Inflammatory Process.* New York, Academic Press.

14
The Influence of Nutritional Deficiency and Aging

The nutritional state and the age of individuals are two important factors in the full expression of immune function and bodily defense. The rise and fall of immune function must obey the principle of the natural life cycle of an individual, i.e., maturation and senescence, and is profoundly influenced by the nutritional state of the individual. Therefore, it is important that one should always consider the contribution of nutrition and age to the expression of immunologic capacity.

Historically, the importance of immunity in protecting against infectious diseases was recognized about the same time as was the importance of essential nutrients for health and the existence of nutritional deficiency diseases. The early literature during the first half of the twentieth century is replete with conflicting reports on the effects of nutritional deficiencies on antibody response, both in experimental animals and in man. The apparent association of famine with pestilence led to the assumption that malnutrition may reduce immunity and predispose to infectious diseases. With the advances in our knowledge of the immune system and the development of methodology for precise quantification of both nutritional components and immune functions, it has become possible to initiate more meaningful investigations concerning the influence of nutrition and aging on the immune function.

NUTRITIONAL DEFICIENCY AND SUSCEPTIBILITY TO INFECTION

Nutritional deficiency results in (1) prolonged convalescence, (2) poor wound healing, (3) impaired tissue healing, and (4) increased susceptibility to infection and lowered resistance to disease. Cannon (1945) showed that severe chronic restriction of the intake of protein in animals, with an otherwise adequate diet, resulted in a reduced capacity to produce several kinds of antibodies. Wissler in 1947 showed reduced resistance to infections to be due to the decreased ability of malnourished animals to manufacture antibodies. When depleted animals are passively immunized, they may survive infections as well as do normally nourished controls.

Actual morphologic changes in the tissues of starving individuals may partially explain their increased susceptibility to infection. Superficial necrosis of the mucous membrane of the respiratory tract, the gastrointestinal tract, and the skin frequently is seen. This break in the continuity of normally protective surfaces makes a ready portal for those organisms that are always present. The combination of a weakened tissue barrier, a decreased capacity of the malnourished bone marrow to form leukocytes of both the granulocytic and lymphocytic series (Asirvadham, 1948), and a decreased immune response to invading pathogens may account for the increased severity of infection in the malnourished organism. The susceptibility to and mortality from typhoid fever have been reported to be increased by dietary deficiency of either vitamin A or vitamin D, by administering a diet with low mineral content, or by eliminating animal protein from the diet (Robertson and Tisdall, 1939).

A commonly reported clinical observation is a greatly increased frequency of terminal infections in patients who die with a marked degree of hypoproteinemia. This may be due in part to the mechanical accumulation of pulmonary secretions. Vitamin A deficiency has been reported to decrease resistance to colds. Multiple infections of the skin were common in prisoners of war and in inhabitants of concentration camps. A significantly increased evidence of rheumatic heart disease was associated with poor nutrition. Hypoproteinemic patients receiving a regular hospital diet have a lesser capacity to produce antibody than do those patients being given protein supplements. It is well known that the infection of and mortality from tuberculosis are far greater in populations with an inadequate state of nutrition (Faber, 1938).

The concept that malnutrition could make man more susceptible to infectious disease and also alter the course and outcome of the resulting illness has long been extant in the history of medicine and public health. Circumstantial evidence is plentiful, principally based on clinical experience. Well-controlled observations have been few, and the analysis of influences under field and clinical conditions is so difficult that clear proof to support the concept has been slow to accumulate. It has been much easier to demonstrate that infection is often directly responsible for lowering the state of nutrition. The fact that infectious diseases were widespread in the same regions of the world as those in which malnutrition also prevailed led gradually to a realization that the phenomena might be interrelated.

INFANT FEEDING AND RESISTANCE TO INFECTION

Breast feeding reduces both morbidity and mortality rates, especially the latter. Infants fed with human milk, as compared with those fed cow's milk, demonstrate higher resistance not only to intestinal disorders but also to respiratory diseases. Breast feeding was generally favored in the pre-antibiotic era for the prevention of infectious disease and as the best therapeutic diet—at that time—for infants and young children with chronic often severe acute pyogenic, especially staphylococcal, infections. Similar observations were made in chronic intestinal disorders or severe malnutrition combined with chronic infection.

In general, this effect of human milk in a variety of infections was ascribed not so much to the presence of specific antibodies as to the action of nonspecific factors of unknown origin. In breast-fed infants polio virus might be attacked in the intestinal tract by specific anti-polio antibodies present in human colostrum and milk. Transfer of antibodies from ingested human milk through the intestine into the blood is a negligible factor in resistance to disease, if it occurs at all. However, the possibility remains that dietetic immunization using the local antibody system of the mammary gland may be of great importance in providing resistance to enteric infections under conditions of extensive exposure.

In more recent years improved general hygiene and the use of antimicrobial agents have obscured the superiority of human milk over cow's milk in regard to the rate of morbidity and mortality. However, statistical studies from countries, such as the United Kingdom and Sweden, which are by no means underdeveloped, indicate that these differences may still be demonstrated, even under good hygienic conditions.

Unlike the mixed intestinal flora of infants on cow's milk formula, the intestinal flora of healthy breast-fed infants is characterized by the prevalence of a particular species of lactobacillus, namely, Lactobacillus bifidus. The acid fecal reaction of breast-fed infants, together with the antibacterial fermentation products, i.e., lactate, acetate, and formate, may help to suppress pathogenic or otherwise harmful intestinal bacterial flora, such as coliform and other proteolytic putrefying microorganisms.

The growth of Lactobacillus bifidus in normal breast-fed infants is stimulated by the high ratio of lactose to protein and the presence of a specific bifidus growth factor in human milk. Chemically, the *bifidus factor* belongs to the group of nitrogen-containing carbohydrates. In human milk, the presence of a great variety of such neutral or acidic oligosaccharides and polysaccharides has been demonstrated. Cow's milk contains only 1/40th to 1/50th of the amount of such nitrogen-containing carbohydrates found in human milk.

HUMORAL IMMUNITY IN MALNUTRITION

High mortality rates among children under 5 years of age in developing countries have been regularly associated with the interaction between infections and malnutrition. Further, an increased susceptibility to certain microorganisms such as Pseudomonas aeruginosa and the serious prognosis of measles are believed to be mainly due to the consequences of malnutrition.

Since the classic study of Cannon (1942) which showed the depression of serum gamma globulin levels and depressed antibody response in severe malnutrition, several general concepts have developed: (1) that malnutrition depresses both host resistance and immune responses, (2) that malnutrition of any severity was noted to have synergistic effects with infections by most classes of bacteria, particularly the pyogenic bacteria, and (3) that these synergistic effects are due to the deficient production of humoral antibodies.

Aref and his co-workers in Egypt recently found that serum concentrations of IgG, IgM, and IgA were all below normal in babies with clinical kwashiorkor that developed under the age of 7 months. IgM concentration continued to be very low in kwashiorkor victims as old as 2 years, and it remained low 6 months after adequate nutritional treatment of the disease. IgA concentration, on the other hand, rose to thrice normal in children with kwashiorkor who were 1 to 2 years old. The concentration of IgG was like that of IgA, but with only moderate elevation. IgM levels tended to remain low for long periods following nutritional reconstitution. These results indicate that severe early protein-calorie malnutrition in infancy may suppress IgM synthesis for prolonged periods. The production of IgM represents, both phylogenetically and ontogenetically, the most primitive and basic humoral antibody response. In addition to depression of immunoglobulin development by severe malnutrition early in life, profound deficits of specific antibody synthesis and long lasting influence of severe chronic nutritional deprivation on specific immune responses were observed. Further investigation will clarify the effect of malnutrition on the production of IgM and other immunoglobulins directed toward specific antigenic stimuli.

The low IgA levels in early life followed after 1 to 2 years by elevations three times normal that were observed in the Egyptian study deserve further attention. IgA is synthesized by plasma cells in mucous epithelial surfaces of the respiratory tract and intestine and in nearly all secretory glands. Thus IgA provides the first line of host defense against certain invading microorganisms as well as against any undesired antigenic molecules. Infants in underdeveloped areas of the world invariably would have high frequency of gastrointestinal infection during the first year of life. Recently it has been found that antigenic stimulation via the gut leads not only to production of IgA in bowel secretions but also to the selective production of antibodies of IgA type in the circulation. This mechanism might explain the shift from low IgA levels in younger infants to thrice normal levels in the older infants. Further, IgA might combine with antigens and make them a less effective antigenic stimulator to the IgM- or IgG-producing cells and result in the prolonged depression of IgM synthesis found in those malnourished infants.

CELLULAR IMMUNITY IN MALNUTRITION

The enhancing effects of chronic malnutrition on immunity to Mycobacterium tuberculosis, Pasteurella pestis, several virus diseases, and protozoal infections have also been reported. Moreschi (1909) and Rous (1914) reported the decreased incidence of spontaneous and metastatic tumors in malnourished animals. Little was known then, however, about the influence of malnutrition on cell-mediated immunity.

Recent advances of our understanding of the two components of the immune system and clinical observations on the susceptibility to infection in patients with various forms of immune deficiency disease have stimulated a more precise study of the influence of malnutrition on the function of the immune system. Examination of the types of organisms that were regularly isolated from children congenitally lacking either the humoral (B-cell) or cellular (T-cells) immunity has revealed a striking parallel with many of the groups of organisms involved in synergistic or antagonistic interactions of host resistance and malnutrition previously found in both experimental animals and man. For example, children with congenital agammaglobulinemias (selective B-cell deficiency) suffered chronic infection with the encapsulated high grade pyogenic bacterial pathogens (pneumococcus, Hemophilus influenza, streptococcus, or Pseudomonas aeruginosa) but were rarely troubled by fungal or viral infection or infection with facultative intracellular bacterial pathogens. On the other hand, patients lacking cell-mediated immunity (selective T-cell deficiency) were frequently the victims of progressive viral or fungal infection, tuberculosis, salmonellosis, or atypical acid-fast infection and showed marked increases in the incidence of solid tissue malignant neoplasms. These observations suggest that in some malnourished states the host resistance might be affected in a similar manner to that characterizing patients with B-cell deficiency, but that host resistance mediated by the T-cells might be intact or even enhanced in some forms of malnutrition.

More recently, Jose et al. (1970) reported that malnourished Australian aboriginal children had depressed antibody responses but increased *in vitro* transformation of lymphocytes by the influenza antigen when compared with normally nourished controls. This observation has now been extensively investigated under highly controlled laboratory conditions by Cooper et al. (1970) and Jose and Good (1973).

Protein-deficient mice showed increased responses to phytohemagglutinin (PHA) stimulation and rejected allografts of skin more rapidly than normal, indicating normal T-cell immunity, and such mice showed striking depression of splenic plaque-forming cells and antibody synthesis to sheep red cells. Furthermore, the protein-deficient mice or rats showed markedly reduced serum cytotoxic antibodies and inhibitors (blocking antibody) of the killer effects of T-cells in immunized animals, increased resistance to infection with pseudorabies virus, and enhanced phagocytosis of Listeria monocytogenes by peritoneal macrophages.

In detailed studies using allogeneic and syngeneic tumor immunity systems to quantify precisely cellular and humoral immunities in rats and mice, Jose and Good found that moderate chronic deprivation of protein, protein-calorie, or of specific essential amino acids produces selective deficiency of antibody production while leaving intact or even enhancing cellular immunity. These influences are exerted most strikingly when primary immune responses are assessed, but clear influences on secondary and tertiary antibody responses could also be demonstrated.

With more severe chronic restrictions of protein, protein-calorie, or essential amino acids both cellular and humoral immunity were depressed. Recently Smythe et al. have associated the clinical susceptibility of South African children with severe kwashiorkor to measles with deficits in cellular immunity. Unfortunately, as with other field studies of these complex relationships, it is difficult to separate the consequences from the provoking conditions and further studies are necessary. It seems likely to us, however, that the acute components of the nutritional deprivation in clinical kwashiorkor accounts for the deficiencies of T-cell immunities seen in this condition. By contrast to the situation in kwashiorkor in some areas of world, chronic protein-calorie malnutrition, e.g., in marasmic states, may be associated with preserved cellular immunity and striking deficiencies of antibody production just as it is in experimental animals.

AGING AND IMMUNE FUNCTION

As in other biologic systems, immune function also undergoes profound changes during the life cycle of an individual organism. To understand how the aging process affects the immune system, a comprehensive quantitative study is needed not only of individuals after adulthood, but also of individuals from birth to death, since aging of the immune system may begin surprisingly early in the maturation of the individual.

Although the earliest time for the individual to initiate humoral immune response varies with the test antigen and animal species, there is in general a rapid increase in the ability to synthesize antibody during neonatal and juvenile life (Sterzl and Silverstein, 1967). During these periods the immunocompetent cell population grows much faster than the individual or the organs in which these cells reside. Thus, during the first month of life in mice, the doubling time of body weight and spleen mass is about 14 days, whereas the doubling time of the ability to synthesize antibody is about 4 days. Consequently, the body and splenic weight increase only fourfold during the first 30 days of life, whereas the immunologic capacity of mice, as measured by ability to synthesize antibody, increases more than a hundredfold.

In addition to the meager antibody response of neonates, the antibody molecules produced are primarily limited to the 19S IgM class. In contrast, adults synthesize a wide spectrum of 7S immunoglobulin (IgA, IgG) as well as the 19S IgM. Experimental work in mice indicates that the inadequacy of antibody synthesis in neonates may be the result of a deficiency in the immunocompetent cell population and of environmental factor(s) that have not yet been defined. Bosma et al. (1967) reported a twelvefold increase in the ability to synthesize antibody in mice between 1 and 3 months of age; only about 25 percent of this growth can be accounted for by an increase in the number of immunocompetent cells or potentially immunocompetent cells. This would suggest that much of the difference between one month and three month old mice in ability to synthesize antibody is due to a difference in the differentiation process of antigen-triggered immunocompetent units.

The first indication that the immune system may undergo deterioration as early as adolescence stems from clinical studies on the age-related changes in the natural antibody titers in man. Thomsen and Kettel (1929) reported that isohemagglutinin titers (anti-A and anti-B antibodies) among Europeans rose rapidly to a peak level at about 10 years of age and then declined gradually with advancing age. The titer was found to be 25 percent of the peak level in individuals in their late sixties. Since the occurrence of natural antibodies is due to the stimulation of natural antigens in the environment, the decline of natural antibody titer would mean that changes in the immune system of individuals may be primarily responsible for the age-related changes in these titers. Such assumptions have been supported by animal experiments in which the results were surprisingly similar to those found in man. It was further found that the immune function of mice, as judged by the ability to make humoral immune response, increased rapidly to a peak level during the first few months of life and then began to decline gradually (Fig. 14-1). Further, with advancing age the capacity to synthesize 7S antibody is more se-

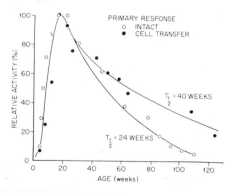

Fig. 14-1. Relative primary antibody-forming activity of BC3F₁ mice and their spleens as a function of age (mean life span, 120 weeks). [From Makinodan, T., and Peterson, W. J. (1966): Develop. Biol. 14:96.]

verely affected than is the capacity to synthesize 19S antibody. In this respect aged mice are similar to neonates.

In man a marked waning of delayed hypersensitivity was noted in
elderly people as evidenced by a decreased number of positive PPD
(purified protein derivative tuberculin) reactions, decreased response
to 2,4-dinitrochlorobenzene (DNCB) sensitization, and decreased lymphocytic response to PHA stimulation. Thus the available clinical and
laboratory evidence clearly indicates that the cell-mediated immune system is weak in the immediate newborn period, reaches a peak level in
puberty, and thereafter declines. Similarly, total serum levels of immunoglobulin tend to rise slightly with age, the rise being accompanied by a
waning of antibody response to new antigens, an overall decrease of immunoglobulin level, and an increase of autoantibodies and paraprotein
or M component (page 573) of gamma globulin. These paraproteins,
formerly thought to occur only in multiple myeloma and Waldenström's
macroglobulinemia, appear to be quite common in elderly people as are
positive assays for the rheumatoid factor.

What is the meaning of constant involution of the immune system with
age? Not only in man, but in all experimental animals having a thymus,
involution of the thymus organ and thymus dependent lymphoid system
begins about the time of sexual maturation. Therefore, it is tempting to
speculate that the involution of thymus function may initiate the process
of aging, and this may serve the evolutionary necessity for eliminating
aged individuals to provide a survival advantage for the species. A programmed involution of the immune system (a biologic clock) in aged individuals is accompanied by an increase in cancer and autoimmune diseases and by a decrease in host resistance to invading organisms. The
concept of *immunologic surveillance* (Thomas, 1959) which may apply
to this question, will be discussed in Chapter 15.

AGING, AUTOIMMUNITY, AND VIRUS INFECTION

From the brief survey in preceding sections, it can be concluded that a
general decline of immune function takes place after puberty as the individual ages. The question then is whether the two are related. Walford
(1962) has emphasized the role of *autoimmune phenomena* in the aging
process and has proposed that the aging process may be one expression
of autoimmunity. He assumed that increasing diversification of immunogenicity of the dividing cell population of the body provokes an immune
response to one's own tissues—*autoimmunization*.

Autoimmunization or *autosensitization* is a pathologic process by which
an antigenic component of one's own tissue cells initiates its own immune
response (Chapter 15). The result may be the production of antibody, or
cell-mediated hypersensitivity which, as in allergic responses to foreign
antigens, can result in tissue damage and disease—*auto-allergic diseases*

or *autoimmune diseases.* For example, Hashimoto's disease, thyrotoxicosis, systemic lupus erythematosus, and many other diseases are now believed to be autoimmune in nature.

How does autoimmunization take place? The immune process was originally conceived as a defense mechanism because of its importance in defending the body against infection. It was later found that immune reactions can be evoked by antigenic components of microorganisms that are not toxins and by many essentially bland components of animals. In other words, the immune system of the body cannot distinguish a harmful from a bland antigen. However, the body does appear to possess a built-in mechanism to prevent immune response directed against its own tissues, the concept of *horror autotoxicus* proposed by Ehrlich. It might have been predicted that under special circumstances this mechanism which maintains *immunologic tolerance* to the individual's own tissue would fail. It was later found that such failure does occur, resulting in the production of autoimmune diseases.

Breakdown of immunologic tolerance then might be due to (1) pathologic changes of the immune system resulting in recognition of its own tissue as foreign or (2) acquisition of new immunogenicity by somatic cells, which will be recognized as foreign. Such changes are believed to take place according to a programmed schedule of genetic expression. However, recent advances in molecular virology, and particularly in elucidation of the pathogenesis of many slow virus diseases, provide a body of new evidence that viruses are extremely powerful candidates for the induction of many biologic processes previously believed to be of genetic or adaptive origin.

Recent examples include the role of rubella virus in causing developmental defects and the multiple autoimmune lesions caused by the virus of Aleutian mink disease. Many unexplained diseases which had earlier been considered to be of genetic origin are now regarded as viral because epidemiologic and virologic studies have established beyond doubt their infectious nature. The pathogeneses of kuru and scrapie (Chapter 33) are excellent examples of this new trend. Mice infected with lymphocytic choriomeningitis (LCM) show clear evidence of assaults by antigen, antibody, and complement, and deposition of amyloid-like material, arteritis, and chronic tissue damage with clinical appearance of accelerated senescence. LCM virus is known to mature by inducing new antigens at the cell surface where it reproduces by budding. Viral infections may thus produce lesions by virtue of biochemical changes in cells which lead to autoimmune responses, autoimmune injury, and perhaps even to immunologic injury and premature aging.

In studies of the intimate relation between waning of cellular and humoral immunity, autoimmune phenomena, and aging one sees dramatic differences between genetically disparate strains of mice. Certain mice, e.g., NZB and AJ, can be considered to be susceptible to autoimmunity; other mice like CBA are highly resistant to development of autoimmunity with aging. When one studies the autoimmune susceptible strains of mice like NZB, AJ, and C57KS, one notes that early involution of immunity functions, particularly T-cell functions, occurs in a striking reciprocal relationship to the development of autoimmune manifestations. The declining immunologic vigor certainly can be assumed to open a door to permit entrance into the body of exogenous microorganisms and antigens of great variety. Further, endogenous organisms, e.g., latent or slow viruses, may be permitted to extend within the body and express a pathogenetic potential. With aging, immunodeficiency may contribute to the development of both autoimmunity and monoclonal expansion of lymphoid and other cell populations and may expose the host to stimulation with immunogens similar to host antigens but capable of abrogating tolerance. Similar phenomena are implicit in the Steblay model of autoimmunity and in Weigle's studies of the pathogenesis of autoimmunity and the breaking of tolerance using defined antigens.

The facts are clear; immunodeficiency, apparently genetically modulated, is a frequent concomitant of aging. Thus immunodeficiency may contribute to susceptibility to autoimmunity, development of malignancy, and even the generalized aging process itself. Much work remains, however, before the precise nature of these relationships and clinically applicable adjustments to them can be forthcoming.

SELECTED REFERENCES

Aref, G. H., et al. (1970): J. Trop. Med. Hyg. 73:186.
Asirvadham, M. (1948): J. Infect. Dis. 83:87.
Bosma, M. J., Makinodan, T., and Walburg, H. E. (1967): J. Immun. 99:420.
Cannon, P. R. (1942): J. Immun. 44:107.
Cannon, P. R. (1945): Advances Protein Chem. 2:135.
Cooper, W. C., Mariani, T., and Good, R. A. (1970): Fed. Proc. 29:364.
Faber, K. (1938): Acta Tuberc. Scand. 12:287.
Jose, D. G., and Good, R. A. (1973): J. Exp. Med. 137:1.
Jose, D. G., Welch, J. S., and Doherty, R. L. (1970): Aust. Paediat. J. 6:192.
Moreschi, C. (1909): Z. Immunitaetsforsch. 2:651.
Robertson, E. C., and Tisdall, F. F. (1939): Canad. Med. Ass. J. 40:282.
Rous, P. (1914): J. Exp. Med. 20:433.
Smythe, P. M. et al. (1971): Lancet 2:939.
Sterzl, J., and Silverstein, A. M. (1967): Advances Immun. 6:337.
Thomas, L. (1959): Discussion in Cellular and Humoral Aspect of the Hypersensitive States, Lawrence, H. S. (ed.). New York, Hocber-Harper.
Thomsen, O., and Kettel, K. (1929): Z. Immunitaetsforsch. 63:67.
Walford, R. L. (1962): J. Geront. 17:281.
Wissler, R. W. (1947): J. Infect. Dis. 80:250.

FURTHER READINGS

Cannon, P. R. (1948): Some Pathological Consequences of Protein and Aminoacid Deficiencies. Springfield, Illinois, Charles C Thomas.
Comfort, A. (1964): Aging: The Biology of Senescence. New York, Holt, Rinehart and Winston.

Pollack, H., and Halpern, S. L. (1952): *Therapeutic Nutrition.* Washington, D.C.
National Academy of Science, National Research Council Publication 234.

Scrimshaw, N. S., Taylor, C. E., and Gordon, J. E. (1968): *Interaction of Nutrition and Infection.* Geneva, WHO Monograph Series 57.

Sigel, M. M., and Good, R. A. (eds.). (1972): *Tolerance, Autoimmunity and Aging.* Springfield, Illinois, Charles C Thomas.

Walford, R. L. (1969): *The Immunologic Theory of Aging.* Baltimore, Williams & Wilkins Company.

Wolstenholme, G. E. W., and O'Connor, M. (eds.). (1967): *Nutrition and Infection.* Boston, Little, Brown and Company.

15

Immunologic Surveillance, Autoimmune Diseases, and Cancer

Immunity can be conceived as an Olympian deity within us transforming chaos into cosmos. Ehrlich in 1901 deemed immunologic inertness to body components a necessary and sufficient condition of life. He showed that goats would produce antibodies against the red cells of other goats, but not against their own, and regarded this as illustrating a fundamental law of nature, i.e., horror autotoxicus. He did not, however, regard this law as inviolable and considered the possibility that some diseases might be due to breakdowns of this law of nature.

One of the greatest developments in medicine during recent years has been the growing recognition of the importance of processes in which the immune mechanisms of the body are turned against the body's own components. Burnet and Fenner (1949), in differentiating between self and not-self body components established in embryonic life, postulated the elimination of anti-self cells from the body and rationalized that auto-immune diseases may develop when this elimination process is ineffective and "forbidden clones" of immunocytes emerge. Jerne in 1956 postulated that each possible antibody is normally represented in at least one cell which could produce it. But some individuals produce antibodies to their own antigens when their physiologic mechanisms break down. The hypothesis for this view is that the primary feature is not an anomaly of extrinsic antigens but a derangement of immunocompetent cells and of the homeostatic mechanism that should prevent the emergence and pathogenetic activity of these immunocytes. The self constituents of the body, not recognized as such, would function as antigens and induce a damaging autoimmune response that sometimes leads to overt disease.

Thomas (1959) suggested that transplantation immunity as defined in the extraordinary analysis of Medawar (1959) must constitute a major part of adoptive immunity and that adoptive immunity as a whole could be viewed as Nature's means of dealing with malignant cells with foreign antigens at their surfaces arising within the body. In contrast to the conventional notion that the chief function of the immune system is to combat infection by invading microorganisms, this hypothesis proclaims that another important, possibly the primary, function of immune mechanisms is to eliminate aberrant host cells, chiefly those that can be the basis of cancer. Burnet (1970) adapted this hypothesis into his theory of clonal selection, coined the term *immunologic surveillance*, and extended it further into the form that if it were not for the double and perhaps correlated "invention" by nature of labile genes controlling histocompatible antigens and of a genetic mechanism for producing a diverse antibody pattern, the vertebrate species would have perished because of its propensity to develop malignant disease. To this view only when a tumor could circumvent this barrier does it become cancer. Thus, the constantly changing concept of adoptive immunity at the cellular level was invoked to explain many aspects of autoimmune diseases and the mechanism of malignant adaptation.

IMMUNOLOGIC SURVEILLANCE

The concept of immunologic surveillance, which had roots in the thought of Ehrlich, stems from the postulate made by Lewis Thomas that a major function of adaptive immunity in mammals is to recognize and eliminate foreign materials arising in the body by somatic mutation or some equivalent process. It is a broad concept and constitutes a part of the still broader concept of internal biologic homeostasis within the mammalian body economy. While presenting his self-regulation concept, Thomas did state, however, that a corollary of his general hypothesis would be that patients suffering from immunodeficiency diseases based on genetic aberration should be expected to have far too much cancer. This prediction has, of course, been amply fulfilled, even though it has not yet been fulfilled in a manner that substantiates the basic theory on which the corollary was fashioned.

If the surveillance process is important, its efficiency will be dependent on the constant presence in the body of a wide range of immunocytes which appear "uncommitted" because they carry receptors that may never meet corresponding antigenic determinants. Surveillance, if it exists, would be a negative factor in the natural history of human cancer. Since the exact mechanism by which cancer develops is not known, the surveillance theory can only predict that in certain clinical and experimental

Table 15-1. Leukemias in Infantile, X-linked Immunodeficiency

Acute lymphocytic leukemia
Malignant lymphoma
Chronic monomyelogenous leukemia
Thymoma with leukemia
Lymphatic leukemia

Table 15-2. Malignancies in Patients with Primary Immunodeficiency

Primary Disease	Cases of Malignancies	% Cancer
Bruton-type agamma-globulinemia	6, all but one leukemia	5-10
Ataxia-telangiectasia	42, many forms of cancer, mostly lymphoreticular	10-15
Wiskott-Aldrich syndrome	16, mostly but not exclusively lymphoreticular malignancies	> 10
Common variable immunodeficiency	> 30, many forms of cancer	5-10
Severe dual system immunodeficiency	3	1-10

conditions where immunologic function is depressed, the incidence of cancer will be more frequent than it would otherwise be. Indeed, a few examples of such conditions are readily available to support the existence of an immunologic surveillance mechanism.

1. Patients with congenital primary immunodeficiency diseases have an unduly high incidence of cancer. (Good, 1972; Tables 15-1, 15-2)
2. In the general population, the incidence of malignant diseases is high in infancy, declines during youth, and rises again logarithmically with age, when the immune function is becoming much less effective.
3. Prolonged administration of immunosuppressive agents, X-irradiation, and immunosuppressive drugs in man and experimental animals results in a high incidence of cancer.
4. Cancer, as well as allogeneic cells, tissues, and organs, can be transplanted to immunosuppressed animals and man across allogeneic barriers.
5. Withdrawal of such immunosuppressive drugs may lead to a complete regression of such transplanted tumors established after immunosuppression, even though the cancer has become widespread throughout the body.
6. Spontaneous cures of clinical cancer, as well as of microscopic cancer, do occur. Cancers in man and animals regularly provoke demonstrable immune reaction.
7. Removal of the thymus gland in certain species of animals, notably in mice, renders the animal more susceptible to induction or transplantation of certain cancers. This same maneuver, however, inhibits development of other cancers, e.g., leukemia that begins in the thymus and mammary adenocarcinoma that seems to require a vigorous thymus dependent lymphoid system for its own development.

8. If properly immunized, an animal may be rendered resistant to the development of cancer.

9. Regressor tumors in experimental systems can be shown to be correlated with effective cellular immunity to the malignancy as in the Moloney sarcoma system and Shope papilloma system.

10. Evidence of multiple adaptive interfaces between immunity and malignancy can be demonstrated, e.g., blocking antibodies, antigenic modulation, sneak-through mechanisms, and inhibition of immunocyte display by tumors.

11. Tumors developing *in vivo* regularly can be shown to have antigens foreign to the host and the host to develop immune responses to the tumor.

12. Dramatic regressions of malignant and widely metastasized tumors of animals and man have been induced to occur by manipulations, e.g., transfer factor treatment, treatment with BCG and other immunologic stimuli, and nonspecific immunization especially capable of provoking cell-mediated immune response.

Thus, Thomas's intriguing suggestion that adaptive immune responsiveness evolved in part at least as a general protective surveillance mechanism in vertebrates to eliminate spontaneously arising neoplasms has generated a great deal of new information concerning the relationship between immunity and malignancy. The primordial lymphocytes develop the capacity to recognize and to react destructively against anomalous "not-self" surface characteristics on altered somatic cells. The operation of such a programmed "policing" system is postulated to be based on a phylogenetic development of an extensive genetic polymorphism of antigenicity, principally the histocompatibility antigens of cell surface molecules, and the diversity of "receptors" on the immunocytes. This combination makes it possible for individuals to distinguish subtle differences between "self" and "non-self" that permit the normal and eliminate abnormal foreign materials.

Some information has appeared which challenges the concept of immunosurveillance as a general concept. In both man and experimental animals with the most generalized and most profound immunodeficiencies cancer has not appeared all over the body. Indeed, cancer and inducible cancers to a variety of agents may be less frequent than normal in such instances. This finding suggests that a subtle balance between immunity and malignancy does exist, but that perhaps immunosurveillance as originally conceived is not absolutely correct. Indeed, patients who have immunodeficiency, although developing far too much cancer, do not develop all kinds of cancers. For example, immunodeficient children develop many different cancers but not an increased incidence of neuroblastoma or Wilms' tumor which are the most frequent tumors of childhood. Instead they tend to suffer from lymphoreticular malignancies and certain epithelial malignancies as in the stomach and colon. The reason for such selective incidence is enigmatic at present.

IMMUNOLOGIC UNRESPONSIVENESS TO SELF ANTIGEN

The capacity of an animal to make an immune response to an antigen might be nullified if the antigen came into contact with the immunologic apparatus while the latter is still immature. This is the idea put forward by Burnet and Fenner to explain why animals, under normal conditions, do not appear to make an immune response against their own tissue components. This idea stems from Ehrlich's earlier observations that antibody is not, as a rule, produced against self components and that the body can identify the self from non-self. Ehrlich's term *horror autotoxicus* derives from his theory of immunity (Chapter 7) in which he postulated that the antibodies represent cell receptors for nutritive or toxic substances manufactured in excess and shed into the circulation, since the body would not make substances, i.e., horror autotoxicus.

Burnet and Fenner in 1949 advanced Ehrlich's idea and proposed the *self marker hypothesis* to explain the remarkable capacity of the immune system for distinguishing between self and not-self; that is, all antigens in the body have a characteristic structure, or *self-marker*. When cells of the immune apparatus come into contact with the body's own antigens during embryogenesis, they are rendered incapable of making an immune response by the so-called self-recognizing units, i.e., natural immunologic tolerance. The *clonal selection theory* subsequently proposed by Burnet postulates that natural immunologic tolerance is due to the failure of the development of effective clones of immunocytes which would react with self antigen and is essentially limited to all the potential antigenic determinants present in the environments in which primary differentiation of stem cells to immunocytes takes place. This theory predicts that tolerance or immunologic unresponsiveness to any foreign antigen will be produced experimentally if the antigen is presented to animals during fetal life. Subsequent experiments showed that this may sometimes be the case (Chapter 16).

Observations by Cinader et al. and the extensive studies by Smith and Bridges showed tolerance to protein antigens to be inducible in immediate postnatal life. The latter investigators found, however, that the development of tolerance was dependent on the dose of antigen and of finite duration that was to some extent dependent on the amount of antigen originally introduced. Earlier studies by Dixon and Maurer and later studies by Mariani et al. showed tolerance to be inducible even during adult life if a sufficient dose of antigen was used or if the immunologic disparity between host and antigen was not too great.

The question, then, is how the mechanisms of surveillance and tolerance could be developed in the immune system. The concept of random mutation by somatic cells has been suggested as the mechanism. Dividing somatic cells are believed to be more susceptible to random mutation. Taking advantage of the observed fact that lymphocytes in the thymus proliferate continuously and only a small fraction spawned in the thymus leaves this organ, it is postulated that the thymus gland may be the site of clonal selection, at least for cell-mediated immunity. By random mutation immunocytes of all kinds may develop continuously. Those clones that will react with self component, *forbidden clones,* are eliminated to bring about natural tolerance, and those clones that survive will function as immunologic surveillance mechanisms.

In general, the receptor site on the surfaces of immunocytes generated by random mutation will unite with varying degrees of avidity with a limited range of antigenic determinants. When such a union takes place, the response of the immunocytes, whether destruction, minor damage, or proliferation, will depend on a variety of factors, such as genetic content, physiologic state of the cell, the mode of antigen presentation, and the local microenvironment. It is also possible that the responding cells may bypass all the intermediate steps and be driven to end stage differentiation. All of these factors may be operative and constitute a *selective pressure.* "Absolute tolerance," therefore, is the exception rather than the rule. In embryonic life, selective pressure may favor the development of self-tolerance or natural tolerance. In postnatal life, the selective pressure may be operative pathologically against the rule of self-tolerance and surveillance mechanisms and may lead to the development of autoimmune diseases and cancer. Further, it may be possible to induce tolerance postnatally to antigens other than self antigens, *acquired tolerance.* The continued presence of antigen may be a necessary condition for selective pressure to achieve prolonged tolerance.

The concepts that immune adaptations in both positive and negative directions involve somatic mutation coupled with selection, however, are incongruous with developing evidence which suggests that specificity of immunity may be a function of point mutations in the germ line coupled with instructional influences capable of inducing the genetic controls, e.g., by reverse transcription (Chapter 7).

PATHOGENESIS OF AUTOIMMUNE DISEASES

The possibility that the autoimmune process might be involved in many diseases has stimulated much of the new line of thinking on the pathogenesis of many diseases. During the decades which followed Ehrlich's observations, autohemagglutinins were occasionally described in association with hemolytic anemia. But the concept of the autoimmune process was largely forgotten until 1938 when Dameshek and Schwartz rediscovered hemolytic anemia associated with an autoantibody, hemolysin. Boorman et al. in 1946 demonstrated by the Coombs' test that the red cells in autoimmune hemolytic anemia are coated with globulin molecules. In the ensuing years major advances have been made in our understanding of autoimmune processes as a cause of many diseases such as rheumatoid arthritis, systemic lupus erythematosus, and Hashimoto's thyroiditis.

How does autoimmunization take place? There are four possibilities by which an individual could develop an autoimmune (auto-allergic) response: (1) hidden or sequestered antigen in the body may induce the immune response by interacting pathologically with the immune system, (2) the self antigen may become immunogenic by alteration of antigenic molecules, (3) foreign antigen may induce an immune response that cross reacts with normal self antigen, and (4) breakdown of self tolerance may occur by mutational changes in immunocompetent cells.

The *sequestered antigen theory* postulates that the antigens of the body which do not normally circulate in the blood become accessible to the immune system under pathologic conditions. Examples of antigens considered to be noncirculating are eye lens proteins, milk casein, thyroglobulin, and antigens of the reproductive system, e.g., sperm. Since the definition of noncirculating antigen is relative to the sensitivity of the detecting method, the observer may easily be lead to a fallacy. It is difficult to decide exactly what criteria should be used to define these hidden determinants.

Altered antigen or *neo-antigen* may arise from chemical, physical, or biologic processes. We know that haptenic chemicals can couple with body proteins and render them immunogenic, e.g., contact dermatitis and penicillin allergy. Physical means of inducing auto-allergy are implicated in photosensitivity and cold allergy. For example, Tan and Kunkel have shown that exposing certain nucleoproteins in the skin to ultraviolet light can produce antigens to which the host reacts as if to foreign substances. Finally, the somatic cell may undergo mutation to acquire new self antigens which would no longer be recognized as self by the body's own immune system and thus would stimulate an immune response.

The *cross-reacting antigen theory* postulates the existence of exogenous antigens that are cross reactive with self antigens. Because of the enormous variety of antigenic challenge that an individual may encounter, the possibility exists that any one of these antigens can induce a cross-reacting immune response. The well-known example of this is the cross reaction between streptococcal M-protein and human heart muscle and its implication in the pathogenesis of rheumatic heart disease. Weigle has extensively studied this means of breaking the tolerant state and has created beautiful experimental models of autoimmunity such as thyroiditis. The Steblay model is another example of this mechanism. Glomerular membranes from man or monkey upon injection into sheep can induce production of antibodies that cross react with the sheep's own glomerular antigens and act as nephrotoxic antibodies producing glomerular disease.

Finally, the *forbidden clone theory* postulates that by random mutation the precursor cells of potentially harmful clones of immunocytes may arise. These forbidden clones develop to mount an effective immune response to self antigen, i.e., breakdown of self tolerance.

Recently Fudenberg (1966) and Williams et al. (1968) suggested that most autoimmune diseases may in fact be due to the action of "slow" viruses topistic to one or another organ tissue. Such viruses are assumed to be able to act pathogenetically only when there is a genetic predisposition to minor immunologic deficiency or when the virus infects *in utero* and induces both an immunodeficient and a tolerant state. Circulating antibody is then a secondary event resulting from special types of tissue damage rendering body components immunogenic. An example of this situation is kuru in New Guinea tribes.

Still another idea not yet tested and perhaps not yet testable has been put forward by Burch (1968) who advanced Burwell's (1963) contention that the primary function of the lymphocyte is to mediate control of growth and morphogenesis and postulated that lymphocytes either carry mitotic control proteins (MCP) on their surfaces or liberate MCP into the circulation, probably in the form of α-2 globulins. Every distinctive tissue in the body, perhaps 10^8 types, carries a tissue coding factor (TCF) on cell surfaces, a portion of which is identical with and therefore "recognizable" by the corresponding MCP. In the development of autoimmune disease, stem cells from which MCP cells arise are assumed to undergo mutation, and aberrant MCP is produced which instead of controlling normal mitosis destroys the corresponding target tissue.

A wide range of organ specific autoantibodies may be produced in experimental animals. However, tissue damage rarely occurs unless the antigen is chemically altered, immunization is repeatedly given over a long period of time, or a bacterial adjuvant is incorporated into the injection mixture. Thus encephalomyelitis in monkeys was produced by injection of cerebral tissue intramuscularly 46 to 85 times over a period of 5 to 9 months. The introduction of Freund's complete adjuvant has facilitated the production of encephalomyelitis and led to the production of a variety of experimental autoimmune diseases such as uveitis, orchitis, thyroiditis, and adrenalitis. Recently, detailed antigenic analysis by Eylar et al. has identified the complete amino acid sequence of encephalitogenic basic protein from myelin and elucidated the segment of the molecule that contains the sequences necessary for the production of encephalitis. Pursuit of this detailed analysis of antigen and manipulation of the host's immune response to favor development of tolerance and negative immunologic adaptation instead of cellular immunity has made it possible to prevent and even to treat effectively experimental allergic encephalomyelitis in monkeys. The future of such inquiry for practical approaches to autoimmune diseases seems bright indeed.

Since many forms of autoimmune disease are known to be transferred only by lymphocytes, but not by immune serum, it is postulated that cellular immunity may play a major part in the pathogenesis of autoimmune diseases both in man and in experimental animals.

New interest in the role of autoimmunity in the pathogenesis of hitherto unexplained diseases has resulted in the discovery of autoantibodies in many diseases. Whether these autoantibodies are mainly associated with the disease or whether they play a central role in the etiology of the disease in question is not always easy to determine. The same questions have been raised repeatedly in daily clinical practice as to whether the microorganism isolated from a patient is a causative agent of current illness. Adapting Koch's classical postulates, Witibsky et al. have proposed a similar criteria for establishing the autoimmune process as operating in the pathogenesis of the disease in question. Witibsky's postulates are:

1. The autoimmune response must be regularly associated with the disease.
2. The same disease must be produced in experimental animals by immunologic means.
3. The immunopathologic changes in natural and experimental autoimmune diseases should parallel each other.
4. Lymphocytes or serum from the patient can produce the disease in normal recipients.

The immune reaction, humoral and cellular, against self antigen initiates primary, secondary, and tertiary manifestations of immunologic injuries. The nature of the immunologic damages in these disorders must be viewed in the same way as are mechanisms of immunologic injury from exogenous antigen (Chapter 13). Thus, autoantigen-antibody complexes can produce indirect immunologic assault and directed immunologic injury. Anaphylactic reaction and intravascular coagulation can be predominant features in autoimmune disease. Inflammation and destruction of target tissues are often end results of many autoimmune processes.

The most recent work of Lerner and Dixon, which follows extensive work by Oldstone and Dixon, appears to fulfill Koch's classic postulates for the etiology of experimental lupus, the model of the prototype of one of the autoimmune diseases. In this extraordinary study the investigators have isolated and to some extent purified a virus immunologically related to the Moloney agent that is regularly present in the Scripps strain of New Zealand Black mice. With this agent in purified and concentrated form they have regularly been able to produce lupus in mice of strains like C57B1 which do not develop a lupus-like autoimmunity spontaneously. Thus they have regularly isolated "in pure culture" an agent that produced the lupus-like syndrome. In addition, clear serologic support for the etiology of the experimental lupus as a function of virus infection has been obtained. The pathogenesis of the lupus in this model also seems very clear; namely, it is due to antigen-antibody complex injury directed toward DNA. Whether the antigen operating initially as stimulus is of host or virus origin has not been established with certainty. The likelihood that human lupus and perhaps many other so-called autoimmune diseases are functions of infection, especially with viruses, received strong support from these studies of the Dixon group.

MECHANISMS OF MALIGNANT ADAPTATION

If it be true that immunity represents an adaptive process directed in a major way toward elimination of malignant cells from the body, it must also be true that the malignant process interacting with this adaptive process might itself be adaptive. Since high potential for malignant development has been present in all vertebrate species for at least 400 million years, survival advantage of the capacity for development of malignancy must be assumed. Thus immunity and malignancy may be incisively viewed as two interacting adaptive processes. Whenever such interacting adaptations are found in nature, multiple interfaces between the adaptive processes may be identified. This has certainly been true of the relationships between immunity and malignancy. The extraordinary interfaces between immunity and malignancy already described argue that there must be an essential relationship between the two processes. The possibility that this essential relationship exists in the pressure to malignant adaptation on one hand and effective immunologic defense against malignant adaptation on the other has been argued in earlier publications (Good and Finstad). As has been pointed out clearly by Prehn, however, this is not the only way or even the best way of thinking about the essentiality of the relationship between these interacting adaptive processes. Further investigations of these interfaces and adjustments of the adaptation to the benefit of man in manipulating his malignancies and in preventing the development of them seem indeed to hold promise for the future.

The idea that immunity might be effectively employed in the treatment of cancer was proposed by Himmelweit and Ehrlich at the turn of the century after Ehrlich had first stated clearly the immunosurveillance postulate. Numerous tumor lines have been developed by transplanting tumor cells successively from one animal to another. Enthusiasm for the possible use of the immune response to a tumor as a means of controlling cancer, however, was short-lived because it was soon realized that the rejection of these tumors was due to immunity directed against normal components of cellular antigens and may have little or no relation to inhibiting the malignancy of tumor cells arising *de novo* in the body.

The major step toward the modern concept of tumor immunology was not made until better inbred strains of mice were developed. Inbred pure (syngeneic) strains of mice provide a laboratory model in which transplantation immunity can be separated from tumor immunity.

Green in 1954 devised an immunologic theory of cancer in which he argued that carcinogen (chemicals) combines with a cell antigen and in doing so gives rise to a new antigen, a tumor specific antigen. This new antigen, being essentially foreign and not subject to tolerance, could provoke an immune response against both the new antigen and the one from which it was derived. By the unknown action of antibody or some equivalent immune response the antigen to which the carcinogen was initially bound is deleted, and in the process the cells escape from the attack of the immune system, become malignant, and thus establish themselves as cancer in the host. Prehn has postulated alternatively that immune responses directed toward the foreign antigens of the tumor might contribute in some essential way to the development or maintenance of the malignant process. Others have postulated that, by clumping tumor cells, immune responses contribute toward spread of cancer via metastases.

Tumor Specific Transplantation Antigens (TSTA)

A tumor specific antigen (TSA) may be defined as an antigen present in malignant cells but absent from the corresponding normal cells of the host. Malignant cells carry not only TSA but also other antigens as well, especially transplantation antigens (TA) and tissue antigens (Chapter 16) on their surfaces. The tumor specific antigen (TSA) that behaves like a transplantation antigen (TA) is called a tumor specific transplantation antigen (TSTA).

Therefore, it is necessary to exclude the effects of transplantation antigen (TA) in order to demonstrate unequivocally the tumor specific transplantation antigen (TSTA). For this purpose it is necessary to study the properties of TA in animals in which the tumor arises (the autochthonous host) or on transplantation to an animal with identical transplantation antigens, i.e., syngeneic inbred strain. A further problem is that syngeneic animals of the same inbred strain, over the course of many generations, and transplantable tumors on repeated passage may undergo spontaneous mutations affecting their antigenic properties. For these reasons, any demonstration of tumor specific immunity using tumors that had been maintained for long periods in many different individuals of the same strain or tissue culture should be interpreted with extreme caution.

It was not until the 1940s that work by Little, Snell, Gorer, and others firmly established the immunologic "rules of transplantation" by use of inbred strains of mice. Possibly the first milestone in the identification of tumor specific antigens is the report by Gross (1943), who also first demonstrated both RNA and DNA tumor viruses in mice. Gross observed that mice immunized against tumors from syngeneic (highly inbred) animals would not accept tumor transplants from these animals.

Gross's work was confirmed and extended in 1953 by Foley, who discovered that a chemically induced sarcoma produced immune response in inbred strains of mice. These findings have been confirmed and extended by Prehn and Main in 1957, by George and Eva Klein, and by others. Specific tumor immunity was demonstrated not only in chemically induced tumors but also in virus-induced tumors. The first well-controlled demonstration of tumor specific immunity is the report of Prehn and Main in 1957 in which they showed that mice immunized against a chemically induced tumor rejected a subsequent tumor graft, while retaining the skin graft of the same animal in which the tumor had originated. It was further shown that chemical carcinogens induce tumors with different TSTA in different mice of the same strain (Fig. 15-1). In other words, fibrosarcoma induced by methylcholanthrene (MCA) in mouse A has a different TSTA from MCA-induced fibrosarcoma in mouse B of the same strain. Even this clear-cut demonstration was not universally accepted because of the possibility of heterozygosity in the inbred strain used in the experiment. For this reason, Klein et al. used autochthonous tumor to demonstrate tumor specific immune response. Their model was to induce a sarcoma in the leg of a mouse and amputate the leg before the tumor spread. After the immunization provided by the tumor that had been re-

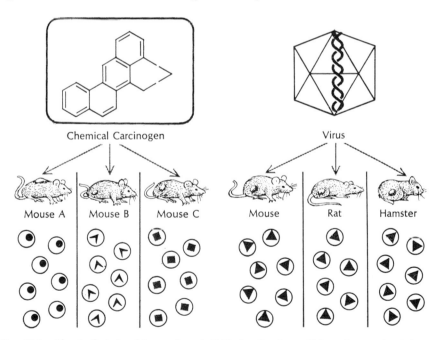

Fig. 15-1. Chemically induced tumors have individual antigenic specificity, whereas virus-induced tumors appear to carry antigens common to all tumors, even in different species. However, recent studies indicate that these rules are not absolute. [From Hellström, K. E., and Hellström, I. (1970): Hosp. Prac. 5:45.]

moved surgically, the mouse could be shown to have been immunized with its own tumor because it could resist transplantation of tumor cells from the autochthonous tumor.

An additional most interesting relationship has been proposed by Prehn. The most powerful, rapidly acting chemical carcinogens like methylcholanthrene (MCA) induce tumors that have great immunogenicity; more slowly acting, less powerful oncogens like plastic induce tumors of lesser antigenicity, and many spontaneously occurring tumors have very weak tumor specific transplantation antigens. These findings are compatible with the view that either the more slowly developing tumors have weak antigenicity because the more antigenic tumor cells have been selected out or, as is favored by Prehn, the more antigenic tumors are stimulated more vigorously by the immune response of the host and therefore develop more rapidly and express a greater vigor for malignant behavior.

Another major advance was made by Sjögren et al. who showed that tumor specific immunity could be induced in mice either with virus (polyoma virus) or with tumor induced by the same virus. Moreover, not only could this be done with single tumors, but mice immunized with cells from virus-induced tumor A would have resistance to tumor B. In other

Table 15-3. The Cross Reactivity of Various Tumor Specific Antigens

Chemical Carcinogens	
3-Methylcholanthrene 1,2,5,6-Dibenzanthracene 9,10-Dimethylbenzanthracene 3,4,9,10-Dibenzpyrene 3,4-Benzpyrene p-Dimethylaminoazobenzene	No cross reactivity
Physical Agents	
Films: Millipore filter Cellophane film Radiation: Ultraviolet Sr^{90}	
Viruses	
DNA Polyoma SV40 Adenovirus 12,18 Shope papilloma	Cross reaction within each group
RNA Mammary-tumor agent Leukemia (Cross reaction between groups) Gross Graffi Moloney Rich Rauscher Friend Rous (Schmidt-Ruppin)	

words, in contrast to the chemically induced tumors, these virus-induced tumors have cross-reacting or identical TSTA (Fig. 15-1 and Table 15-3).

Quite obviously, the cross reactivity or identity of TSTA in virus-induced tumors in animals has led to the speculation that a virus may be an etiologic agent in certain human cancers, e.g., Burkitt's lymphoma, osteogenic sarcoma, and neuroblastoma, in which antigens common to the tumors occurring in different human hosts have been demonstrated. Since viral infection can cause the host cells to acquire a new antigen without necessarily causing malignant change, such speculation requires further study. Recent discovery of carcinoembryonic antigen (CEA) in human colonic carcinomas indicates another mechanism by which human cancer can acquire common antigen. CEA is present in human colonic cancer and fetal gut epithelium but absent from normal human colon; hence it is called carcinoembryonic antigen. Reappearance of CEA in the colonic cancer cells may be interpreted as a sign of genetic *derepression* and does not necessarily imply virus induction of the cancer. A number of carcinoembryonic antigens have now been encountered. For example, α-fetoprotein has been shown to be a CEA.

It may be quite misleading to assume that chemically induced tumors are quite distinct antigenically from virus-induced tumors. If one assumes that a virus is widely distributed in a mouse population, the mouse population could then be expected to develop a high degree of immunologic nonresponsiveness to the virus and any new TSTA induced by the virus. Thus, if the action of chemical carcinogen is to activate latent virus, it is conceivable that the chemically induced tumors would have, in addition to the unique antigens, undetectable common antigen attributable to the latent virus. This possibility has been supported by the work of Old and his co-workers, who showed that a number of chemically induced tumors have, in addition to the individual TSTA, common antigenic determinants that cross react with tumors induced by Gross virus. Studies by Morton and Malmgren have also demonstrated that virus-induced mammary tumors of mice have individually distinct antigen in addition to common antigen.

Malignant Adaptation

In the preceding section we have reviewed the evidence for the existence of tumor specific antigen. The next obvious question is how is it possible for an antigenic tumor to escape the immunologic surveillance mechanism and establish itself in the host. In other words, what is the mechanism of malignant adaptation? It is conceivable that many tumors may arise and be destroyed by the host before they are ever recognized clinically. What kind of immune mechanism is responsible for the elimination of tumors?

In the 1950s Mitchison in England showed that the immunologic response to normal transplantation antigens is primarily mediated by lymph-ocytes and that one can transfer the immunity by immune lymphocytes. Winn showed that by neutralization of tumor cells the immune lympho-cytes directed against H-2 histocompatibility antigen can kill tumor cells that carry the same histocompatibility antigen. Klein et al. in 1960, using the same neutralizing system, showed that lymphocytes immune against tumor specific antigen can kill specifically corresponding tumor cells. A number of other experiments such as the colony inhibition test (Hell-ström) and direct cytotoxic test (Brunner) have established that cellular immunity can act to eliminate tumor cells *in vivo* and *in vitro*. Immune surveillance against tumor is believed to operate through cell-mediated immunity.

Although the exact mechanism(s) of malignant adaptation has not been fully elucidated, several possibilities of interaction between malignant cells and the host immune system have been proposed: (1) depression of the host immune function resulting in the failure of cell-mediated immu-nity to execute the surveillance function against the tumor cells; (2) changes in immunogenicity of tumor cells and deletion of modulation of TSTA of tumor cells in such a way that the host immune system is ren-dered unresponsive to TSTA; (3) production by the host of enhancing antibody that paradoxically interferes with the killer effects of immune lymphocytes; and (4) a "sneak in" mechanism by which a tumor due to a temporary immunologic lapse, as with a virus infection, or simply be-cause of the weak antigenicity of the tumor, gains a foothold and then keeps ahead of the host's immune defense line simply by its rapid growth and a numerical excess of tumor cells over immune lymphocytes.

Depression of Host Immune Function. Frequently an increased inci-dence of tumor development is associated with depression of the immune function of the host. For example, patients with congenital or acquired primary immunodeficiency disease have a higher incidence of malignant diseases of certain types than do members of the general population. An increased susceptibility to certain tumors has been noted in young animals. The incidence of malignancy is generally inversely related to advanced age (Fig. 15-2) when the immune system begins to get feeble. Immuno-suppression by both physical and chemical means has been accompanied by an increased incidence of certain forms of malignancy. An interesting coincidence is that all carcinogens (viral or chemical) have varying de-grees of general or specific immunosuppressive effects during the latent period in experimental animals. Therefore, it is tempting to speculate that malignant adaptation may always be preceded by some degree of de-pressed immune function.

Changes in Immunogenicity of Tumor Cells. *Deletion* of TSA was re-ported by Woodruff (1962) in spontaneously occurring mammary car-cinoma in mice. Possible mechanisms for the deletion of TSA are that (1)

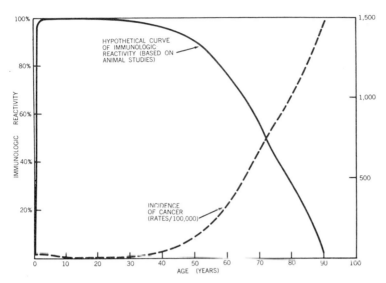

Fig. 15-2. The inverse relationship between the incidence of malignancy in man compared with the degree of immunologic reactivity during a normal life span. [From McKhann, C. F. (1970): In *Immunology*. Kalamazoo, Michigan, Upjohn Co., p. 28.]

antigen may be progressively diluted out by division of tumor cells—*antigenic dilution*—or (2) tumor cells may initially consist of mixed clones of cells with varying degrees of immunogenicity, and the most immunogenic clones are progressively eliminated by immune response of the host, leaving the less immunogenic clones free to proliferate—*immunoselection*. An unexpected event in which exposure to specific antibody suppresses the production of the corresponding TSA on the cell was first reported by Old et al. (1968) in one mouse system and is known as *antigenic modulation*. In this instance, the other antigens on the same cell increase in a compensatory fashion. In the absence of specific antibody the missing antigen reappears on the tumor. The possibility of early *immunologic paralysis* or *tolerance* as a means of malignant adaptation was suggested by Stjernswärd (1968). Finally, successful malignant adaptation may be inversely related to the capacity of a tumor to induce specific cell-mediated immunity in the host. For example, Oettgen et al. (1968) induced sarcoma in strain 13 guinea pigs with MCA. Extract of this tumor, together with Freund's adjuvant, was injected into the foot pads of guinea pigs of the same strain. Animals that developed delayed hypersensitivity to the extract of tumor were found to be resistant to subsequent transplantation of the same tumor.

Enhancement of Tumor Growth by Immune Response. A tumor which induces an immune response with antibody production may provide itself with a mode of self protection from the destructive action of *immune*

8

lymphocytes. Such antibody is called *enhancing antibody* because it appears to enhance the growth of tumor, or *blocking antibody,* since it blocks the killing effects of immune lymphocytes. Thus it appears that the immune response against TSA may adversely provide a favorable condition for malignant adaptation instead of eliminating malignant tissue. Immune responses, as has been pointed out, can be protective as well as harmful for the host, and TSA appears to confirm this observation. Enhancing effects of humoral immunity are found in transplantation of normal tissue as well as in malignant tissue (Chapter 16). The presence of blocking antibodies in experimental animals as well as in man has been demonstrated by Hellström et al., using the *tumor colony inhibition test* system. The colony formation in tissue cultures of tumor cells can be inhibited in the presence of specific immune lymphocytes—*colony inhibition.* Such colony inhibition can be blocked by addition of immune serum —blocking antibodies. Blocking antibodies appear to be IgG or a complex of IgG and TSA. Further, the Hellströms (1970) showed that when tumors regress, animals develop new antibodies which abrogate the blocking serum effect, and they called these *unblocking antibodies.*

Recently Prehn (1972) has noted a further paradoxical effect of immune response in tumor growth. The observations are the basis of his so-called *immunostimulation theory* of tumor development. The essence of this hypothesis is that, although specific immune reactivity may sometimes be adequate to control a neoplasm, a *lesser degree of immune reactivity* may promote the growth of nascent tumors. In other words, an immune reaction may at times produce better growth of tumor than would occur in the total absence of immune reactivity. Evidence for this theory has been provided in experimental animals (Prehn 1972). O'Connor (1970) also postulated stimulation as a factor in oncogenesis, especially in Burkitt's lymphoma.

"Sneak in" Mechanism. A number of investigators (Old et al., 1962) have shown that a very low dose of immunogenic tumor cells may survive and grow in an animal, whereas larger doses lead to the elimination of the tumor. This phenomenon has been ascribed to a delay in immunization of the host permitting the tumor implant to reach a rapid growth phase before the animal's immune defense reaches the capacity to eliminate the tumor. In other words, at any given time the immune response of the host may be inadequate to keep pace with a developing tumor. The "sneak in" phenomenon may have the best chance of resulting in tumor growth when tumor cells are weakly immunogenic or the host immune response has been temporarily weakened as during a virus infection.

IMMUNOTHERAPY OF CANCER

If the immunologic surveillance mechanism is a reality, then manipulation of the immune system would naturally provide a means of controlling cancer. Unfortunately no method has yet been established regularly to accomplish this goal. In general, attempts to treat cancer by immunologic means may be divided into two groups, those which aim at increasing the host's effective immune response to the tumor—*active immunization*—and those in which an extrinsic immunologic attack is mounted against the tumor—*adoptive immunization*. Theoretically, the increase of the host's immunologic response might be most effective for relatively early stages of cancer with good immunogenic TSA, whereas the extrinsic attack might be better applicable for advanced stages.

Nonspecific Stimulation of Cell-mediated Immunity and Immunofacilitation in Cancer Therapy

In 1959 Old et al. discovered that nonspecific stimulation of the immune system by administration of BCG to mice increases their immunologic reactivity to weak histocompatibility antigens. It was found that BCG could extend the latent period of certain chemically produced malignancies and prevent the development of other cancers. More recently Mathé used BCG and the synthetic polynucleotide, poly IC, together with chemotherapy to prolong remissions in leukemia. British investigators have shown in controlled clinical trials that using BCG with a combined chemotherapy regimen has clearly demonstrable advantage over the combined chemotherapy alone in treating acute myeloid leukemia. The mechanism underlying this influence of BCG is not yet clear, but nonspecific stimulation of cell-mediated immunity and consequent activation of macrophages has been shown by Mackaness to be one possibility (Chapter 12). BCG injected directly into the tumor has been shown by Rapp and associates regularly to induce regressions of transplantable chemically induced cancers in guinea pigs. This approach has been used by Klein and his associates and by Morton and his associates to induce dramatic regression of disseminated breast cancer or malignant melanomas in man. Mackaness believes that the stimulation of macrophages by BCG facilitates removal from circulation of antigen-antibody complexes that otherwise might act as blocking factors that favor tumor growth. In addition, of course, BCG stimulation can enhance cell-mediated responsiveness to tumor antigen and in this way could contribute to specific immune rejection of tumor. Hanna and his co-workers have emphasized the capacity of BCG to facilitate granuloma formation and have proposed that this granuloma reaction plays a crucial role in nonspecific induction of the tumor regression. Clinical experience with BCG injected into skin, administered by scarification, or even taken orally have been sufficiently encouraging as an approach to both prevention of tumors and elimination or regression of established tumors. Controlled clinical trials are under way to determine how much is to be gained from this modality of therapy along with surgery, irradiation, and chemotherapy in the treatment of human cancer.

In addition to BCG, considerable experimental work and some controlled and uncontrolled clinical experience has been obtained in evaluation of nonspecific facilitation of tumor immunity using another granuloma-producing organism Corynebacterium parvum, the influence of which was discovered by Halpern. Although certain similarities have been noted, the mechanism of action of C. parvum may be quite different from that of BCG. For example, BCG in some experimental tumor systems will act only when given in anticipation of the tumor to contribute to the prevention of establishment or elimination of the tumor. By contrast Currie and Bagshaw have shown that C. parvum can act to facilitate cure of the cancer only when given after chemotherapy has been employed. Thus, chemotherapy that will not cure a chemically induced malignancy by itself can lead to complete elimination of the cancer when the chemotherapy is used with C. parvum that is administered after the chemotherapy has been given.

Other means, too, have been found for facilitating immune elimination of cancer or enhancing resistance to cancer. For example, mixed bacterial vaccines and certain endotoxins in appropriate doses can lead to destruction of tumors and cancers and in addition can facilitate development and expression of tumor immunity. Extensive studies are in progress, both experimentally and clinically, to evaluate polynucleotides as immunopotentiators whose effect can be directed against tumor cells. Even small molecules like tetramisole and levamisole have been shown to be capable of potentiating immune response. It also has been claimed that they facilitate the elimination of tumors in experimental and clinical situations. Other pharmaceuticals like Tilerone have been found to be immunopotentiators, and claims have been made for such agents as huge doses of Vitamin A in this regard. Although there is still much noise in each of these systems, there is little question that immunopotentiation and immunofacilitation will be developed as approaches to management of cancer. How bright their future becomes depends upon continued insistence on a strong scientific approach to their development, analysis, and application.

Active Immunization of Host by Modified Tumor Antigen

Since the immunogenicity of antigen depends on a number of factors, it would be logical to attempt to induce a desired immune response by increasing the immunogenicity of tumor cells. For this purpose, various adjuvants have been used to enhance the immune response of the host. For example, Czajkowski et al. (1967) coupled the tumor cell to a highly antigenic foreign protein (rabbit gamma globulin) with bisdiazobenzidine, and injected this complex back to the original host. They claimed that 2 of 14 end stage tumor patients remained alive and were free from tumors for 4 years. Again in an experimental system Simmons and his associates have shown that modifications of the surface of the tumor cell with neuraminidase can alter host response to the tumor cells so that an already advancing tumor can be made to regress by this manipulation.

The potential power of being able to induce the host to look on tumor specific transplantation antigens as though they are strong transplantation antigens is illustrated by what happened with tumors inadvertently transplanted in immunosuppressed hosts. In immunosuppressed renal transplant recipients, tumor cells were inadvertently transplanted along with the kidney on several occasions. In at least 4 of these instances, the epithelial malignancies metastasized and became widely disseminated. All that was required to treat such metastatic and widely disseminated cancer was to stop immunosuppressive therapy. The host immune system, looking on the tumor allografts according to their strong allotransplantation antigenicity, was able to eliminate the entire disseminated cancer. This is, of course, a powerful antimalignancy treatment, and it encourages vigorous efforts both to understand and to learn to manipulate weak antigenicity and to make it possible to induce the host to look on weak TSTA as though they are strong antigens. This may be possible.

Adoptive Immunization

It is obvious that the above approaches depend on the presence of TSA against which host immunity could occur. Such a situation is unlikely to exist when the tumor is already established and advanced because the TSA may have been deleted or modulated or the host's immune system may have been crippled. Therefore, a logical approach is to transfer immunity directed against the established tumor by transplanting immunocompetent cells from an immunized donor of the same species, adoptively by using *allogeneic immunocompetent cells*. For this purpose spleen and lymph node cells from either normal or immunized animals which have been "immunized" against the tumors to be treated have been used. The animal bearing a tumor is given a lethal dose of either irradiation or cytotoxic drugs to eliminate hemopoietic cells and is also given an intravenous injection of immunocompetent cells (bone marrow, spleen, lymph node cells) from the donor to repopulate the recipient with fresh immunocompetent cells. A major limitation to this form of therapy is the concomitant induction of graft-versus-host disease, a disease due to the reaction of the donor's immune system against the recipient's tissues. Symes et al. (1968) gave stored human spleen cells to 4 patients with advanced tumors and obtained regression of the tumors, although all patients died eventually. A similar approach by transplantation of bone marrow from a histocompatible donor has been employed by Thomas et al. (1973) to treat leukemia patients who were refractory to all chemotherapeutics. In a few patients a long lasting remission of leukemia has been achieved. One patient has had a complete remission for more than three years. Of interest is the fact that in a few patients treated with this form of immunotherapy recurrence of leukemia clearly involved cells of the donor's karyotype, i.e., the donor's cells have acquired leukemic processes in the host's environment. This has occurred so far only with acute lymphatic leukemia and not with acute myelogenous leukemia. Thus the donor's cells have caught the leukemia.

Methods of either in vivo, or preferably in vitro, immunization are also being attempted. If either can be perfected it could add much to the immunologic approach to cancer therapy when coupled with transplantation of marrow, lymphoid tissue, or spleen.

SELECTED REFERENCES

Boorman, K. E., Dodd, B. E., and Loutit, J. F. (1946): Lancet *1*:812.
Brunner, K. T., et al. (1968): Immunology *14*:181.
Burch, P. K. (1968): *An Inquiry Concerning Growth, Disease and Ageing.* Edinburgh, Oliver and Boyd.
Burnet, F. M. (1970): *Immunological Surveillance.* New York, Pergamon Press, Inc.
Burnet, F. M., and Fenner, F. (1949): *The Production of Antibodies.* Melbourne, Macmillan and Co., Ltd.
Burwell, R. G. (1963): Lancet *2*:69.
Cinader, B., St. Rose, J., and Yoshimura, M. (1965): Int. Arch. Allerg. *27*:265.
Czajkowski, N. P., et al. (1967): Lancet *2*:905.
Dameshek, W., and Schwartz, S. O. (1938): New Eng. J. Med. *218*:75.
Dixon, F. J., and Maurer, P. H. (1955): J. Exp. Med. *101*:245.
Ehrlich, P., and Morgenroth, J. (1957): *The Collected Papers of Paul Ehrlich,* Himmelweit, F. (ed.). New York, Pergamon Press.
Eilber, F. R., and Morton, D. L. (1970): Cancer *25*:362.
Eylar, E. H., et al. (1969): Arch. Biochem. *129*:468.
Foley, E. J. (1953): Cancer Res. *13*:835.
Fudenberg, H. H. (1966): Arthritis Rheum. *9*:464.
Gold, P., and Freedman, S. O. (1965): J. Exp. Med. *122*:467.
Good, R. A. (1972): Proc. Nat. Acad. Sci. *69*:1026.
Good, R. A., and Finstad, J. (1968): Nat. Cancer Inst. *31*:41.
Gorer, P. (1937): J. Path. Bact. *44*:691.
Gross, L. (1951): Proc. Soc. Exp. Biol. Med. *76*:27.
Gross, L. (1955): Proc. Soc. Exp. Biol. Med. *88*:64.
Hellström, I., et al. (1970): Int. J. Cancer *7*:1.
Hellström, I., et al. (1971): Int. J. Cancer *7*:1.
Jerne, N. K. (1955): Proc. Nat. Acad. Sci. U.S.A. *41*:849.
Jerne, N. K., and Avengo, P. (1956): J. Immun. *76*:200.
Klein, E. (1968): N. Y. State J. Med. *68*:900.
Klein, G., et al. (1960): Cancer Res. *20*:1561.
Little, C. C. (1947): Biol. Rev. *22*:315.
Mariani, T., et al. (1960): Ann. N. Y. Acad. Sci. *87*:93.
Mathé, G. (1971): In *Progress in Immunology,* Amos, B. (ed.). New York, Academic Press, p. 899.
Medawar, P. B. (1959): In *Cellular and Humoral Aspects of the Hypersensitive States,* Lawrence, H. S. (ed.). New York, Hoeber-Harper, pp. 504-529.
Mitchison, N. A. (1955): J. Exp. Med. *102*:157.
Morton, D. L. (1971): J. Reticuloendothel. Soc. *10*:137.
Morton, D. L., and Malmgren, R. A. (1968): Science *162*:1279.
O'Connor, G. T.(1970): Amer. J. Med. *48*:279.

Oettgen, H. F., et al. (1968): Nature 220:295.
Old, L. J., et al. (1961): Cancer Res. 21:1281.
Old, L. J., et al. (1962): Ann. N. Y. Acad. Sci. 101:80.
Old, L. J., et al. (1968): J. Exp. Med. 127:523.
Prehn, R. T. (1970): Discussion in Immune Surveillance, Smith, R. T., and Landy, M. (eds.). New York, Academic Press.
Prehn, R. T. (1972): Science 176:170.
Prehn, R. T., and Main, J. M. (1957): J. Nat. Cancer Inst. 18:769.
Simmons, R. L., and Rios, A. (1971): Science 174:591.
Sjögren, H. O., Hellström, I., and Klein, G. (1961): Exp. Cell Res. 23:204.
Smith, R. T., and Bridges, R. (1958): J. Exp. Med. 108:227.
Snell, G. D. (1957): Ann. Rev. Microbiol. 11:439.
Stjernswärd, J. (1968): J. Nat. Cancer Inst. 40:13.
Symes, M. O., et al. (1968): Lancet 1:1054.
Tan, E. M., and Kunkel, H. G. (1966): J. Immun. 96:464.
Thomas, E. D., et al. (1973): Transpl. Proc. 5:917.
Thomas, L. (1959): In Cellular and Humoral Aspects of the Hypersensitive States, Lawrence, H. S. (ed.). New York, Hoeber-Harper, pp. 529-532.
Weigle, W. O. (1965): J. Exp. Med. 121:289.
Williams, R. C., Kenyon, A. J., and Huntley, C. C. (1968): Blood 31:522.
Winn, H. J. (1960): J. Immun. 84:530.
Witibsky, E., et al. (1957): JAMA 164:1439.
Woodruff, M. F. A., and Symes, M. O. (1962): Brit. J. Cancer 16:484.

FURTHER READINGS

Anderson, J. R., Buchanan, W. W., and Goudie, R. B. (1967): Autoimmunity. Springfield, Illinois, Charles C Thomas.
Burnet, F. M. (1959): The Clonal Selection Theory of Acquired Immunity. Nashville, Tennessee, Vanderbilt University Press.
Burnet, F. M. (1972): Aust. J. Exp. Biol. Med. Sci. 50:1.
Hellström, K. E., and Hellström, I. (1970): Ann. Rev. Microbiol. 24:273.
Landy, M., and Braun, W. (eds.) (1969): Immunological Tolerance. New York, Academic Press.
Mackay, I. R., and Burnet, F. M. (1963): Autoimmune Diseases. Springfield, Illinois, Charles C Thomas.
Möller, G. (ed.) (1971): Transpl. Rev. 7:3.
Schwartz, R. S. (ed.) (1970): Immunological Aspects of Neoplasia. New York, S. Karger.
Smith, R. T. (1968): New Eng. J. Med. 278:1207.
Smith, R. T. (1968): New Eng. J. Med. 287:439.
Smith, R. T., and Landy, M. (eds.) (1970): Immune Surveillance. New York, Academic Press.
Weiss, D. W. (ed.) (1971): Immunological Parameters of Host-Tumor Relationships. New York, Academic Press.

16
Immunobiology of Transplantation

The idea of replacing disabled organs or tissues with healthy ones appears to have been a dream of mankind since ancient times. For example, the famous Chinese surgeon, Pien Chiao, in the second century B.C., is reputed to have been operating painlessly and to have exchanged successfully the hearts of two patients. However, only during the past half century have the control of bacterial infection and perfection of surgical techniques made it possible to transplant almost any organ or tissue of the body if the problem of the formidable *histocompatibility barrier* could be solved. During the past 12 years a great deal of advancement has been made in this direction and now replacement of disabled organs, for example, the kidney, is not only a dream, but rather an accepted form of therapy.

The transplantation of living cells, tissues, and organs for experimental or therapeutic purposes has two inherent major problems: (1) preservation of the living organ or tissue until it is transplanted and (2) graft rejection by the recipient. It is a well-known fact that the destruction of grafts between two individuals other than identical twins or syngeneic mice is one of the most striking and reproducible of all immunologic phenomena found in all species of vertebrates so far studied.

A graft made between two sites on the same subject is called an *autograft*; a graft made between two subjects of identical genetic constitution, e.g., identical twins or inbred syngeneic animals, is called an *isograft*; a graft between two genetically nonidentical members of the same species is known as an *allograft*; a graft between members of different species is referred to as a *xenograft* (Table 16-1). When a graft is transplanted to its physiologic location, it is referred to as *orthotopic*, and when to another location, *heterotopic*.

One of the most successful and widely employed therapeutic allografts is the blood transfusion. The existence of blood groups in man was revealed by Karl Landsteiner in 1901. This discovery resulted in a fairly common clinical transfusion by 1920, and largely under the impetus of World War II, blood banks were instituted in the early 1940s when transfusion became a commonplace procedure. The discovery of the Rh blood group system in 1940 by Landsteiner and Wiener after the recognition of

Table 16-1. Terminology of Grafts

New Term	Donor & Recipient	Synonyms
Autograft	Same individual	Autogenous graft Autogeneic graft
Isograft	Individuals of identical genotype, e.g., isogeneic animals, identical twins	Isogeneic graft Syngeneic graft
Allograft	Individuals of same species but different genotype	Homograft Allogeneic graft
Xenograft	Different species	Heterograft Xenogeneic graft

Rh incompatibility as a cause of erythroblastosis fetalis by Levine opened a new field of immunobiology of the maternal-fetal relationship.

The discipline of tumor immunology has been intimately related to that of transplantation immunology. Nearly all studies of tumor immunity after 1900 were, in fact, examples of transplantation immunity but not recognized as such until the immunogenetic principles of transplantation biology were firmly established by use of properly inbred strains of mice. This is due to the fact, as we now know, that tumor cells carry histocompatibility antigens as well as tumor specific transplantation antigens which are stronger immunogens. Therefore, tumor specific immunity can be properly studied only in the inbred syngeneic strains of mice or in identical twins. For example, Ehrlich (1905) and Schöne (1912) first described the immunizing effects of an experimentally transplanted tumor and skin graft and the accelerated rejection of a second graft from the same donor in the same recipient. The analyses of the genetic background by Tyzzer (1909) and by Little (1914) of tumor susceptibility of Japanese waltzing mice were, in fact, reflections of susceptibility to allogeneic transplantation rather than of overcoming of tumor immunity.

The first important landmark was the demonstration that skin grafts between identical human twins are accepted, whereas those between genetically different persons are regularly rejected. With this as a point of departure, Gibson and Medawar studied skin allografts in burned patients, and Medawar (1944) analyzed experimentally the fate of skin allografts in rabbits. These studies established both the basic pathophysiology of allograft rejection and its immunologic principles. This important two-way exchange of information and ideas between the laboratory and the clinic has been the cornerstone of the recent accomplishments in transplantation as it has in all immunology. Despite the degree of success that has been achieved in renal transplantation, and to some extent in bone marrow, liver, and cardiac transplants in man, every clinical organ transplantation still may be considered as an "experiment" in transplantation immunology.

IMMUNOGENETICS OF TRANSPLANTATION

In many species of vertebrates a considerable number of genetic loci may be identified by the immunogenicity of their products in transplantation. They are thus termed *histocompatibility (or H) loci,* and their products *histocompatibility (or H) antigens.* H antigens are located mainly on the cell surface and are responsible for the uniqueness of an individual, which is clearly demonstrable in tissue rejection after transplantation. A brief account of the genetic theory of this phenomenon, its history and its present state, its laws and exceptions, will serve as an orientation for further understanding of the current status of transplantation in man.

Most of the genetic analysis of H antigens (H loci) has been performed in laboratory mice. Among the many H loci discovered in mice, the most important and the most thoroughly studied is the H-2 locus which is associated with the strongest H antigens. Methods used in the study of immunogenetics are combinations of both immunologic principles and genetic analysis, and the results of immunologic reactions are interpreted in genetic terms. Immune responses to H antigens obey the general rules of immune responses to any immunogen and involve humoral or cellular immune responses, or both.

Serologic Analysis

Serologic (humoral immunity) analysis of H antigens requires antiserum monospecific for the particular H antigens in question. Such monospecific antiserum can be obtained by repeated absorption to remove all nonspecific cross-reacting antibodies. If a serum contains only one monospecific antibody, its positive reaction with cells under test is simply interpreted as proof that the corresponding H antigen is present on the cells. This is not, however, usually the case. If a serum contains several antibodies, a procedure known as *absorption analysis* is necessary.

An example of absorption analysis is shown in Table 16-2. An antiserum directed against "x" of an unknown H antigen is prepared. The spectrum of antibodies will depend on the antigenic differences between H antigens of x cells and those of anti-x producer. Thus, an individual heterozygous for a number of H loci will, for example, induce only half of the antibodies in an individual homozygote for the same loci. The anti-x serum will react with x cells and give a variety of reactions (+ or −) with cells of, let's say, four other individuals. If the pattern of this reaction is 1(+) 2(+), 3(+), 4(−), then absorption of the antiserum with cells of individual 1 will modify the pattern of reaction as follows: 1(−), 2(+), 3(+), 4(−). This modification indicates that cells of individual 1 pos-

Table 16-2. Distribution of the Reactions (+ versus —) in Absorption Analysis of Anti-X Serum with Cells of Four Individuals

Test Cells from Individual		Anti-X Serum				
			Absorbed with Test Cells No.			
No.	Inferred Antigen(s)	Unabsorbed	1	2	3	4
1	A	+	—	+	—	+
2	B	+	+	—	—	+
3	AB	+	+	+	—	+
4	Neither A nor B	—	—	—	—	—

From Lengerová, A. (1969): *Immunogenetics of Tissue Transplantation.* New York, American Elsevier Publishing Company, p. 14.

sess some antigen which may be denoted A and which absorbs an antibody from the anti-x serum. Individual x must thus possess the same antigen A. If absorption with cells of individual 2 results in a pattern, 1(+), 2(—), 3(+), 4(—), the interpretation will likewise be that individuals 2 and x share in common a second antigen, B. An absorption pattern of 1(—), 2(—), 3(—), 4(—) from individual 3 indicates that cells of 3 must have both antigens A and B. Since unabsorbed serum does not react with cells of 4, these cells would have neither of the two antigens. This is an extremely simple example. In practice, one has to use multiple symbols, and sometimes the complexity of an antigenic system may exceed the analytical power of the traditional methods. This is particularly true with typing of leukocyte antigens in man, and attempts have been made to use computer techniques to permit interpolation and use of the information generated.

A number of test systems may be used for detection of antibody activities. Basically these employ the secondary manifestation of antigen-antibody interaction (Chapter 10), i.e., agglutination, hemolysis, plaque formation, complement fixation, mixed hemagglutination, immunofluorescence, and cytotoxicity.

Much of our information concerning the H-2 locus has been derived from serologic analysis. Largely due to the painstaking efforts of Snell and his collaborators, it is now known that various alleles at the H-2 locus are involved in determining no less than 24 different specificities (possibly up to 33 specificities) which collectively characterize this locus. Some of the known alleles and specificities of the H-2 system and the isogeneic strains that carry them are shown in Table 16-3.

Table 16-3.   Specificities and Strain Distribution of the Known H-2 Alleles

H-2 Alleles	| Alloantigenic Specificities (old symbols [letters] shown at top)	A	D^b	C	D	E	F	G	H	I	J	K	M	N	P	Q	S	V	Y	A^1	B^1	C^1	D^1	E^a	D^k	K^b	Inbred Strains
a		1	–	3	4	5	6	–	8	–	10	11	13	14	–	–	–	–	25	27	28	29	–	–	–	–	A, AKR.K, B10.A
b		–	2	–	–	5	6	–	–	–	–	–	–	14	–	–	–	22	–	27	28	29	–	–	–	33	A.BY, C3H.SW, C57BL/6, C57BL/10, C57L, CC57BR, CC57W, D1.LP, LP/J, ST/a, 129
c		–	–	3	4	?	–	6	–	8	–	*	–	13	–	*	–	–	–	*	27	28	29	–	31	*	–	D1.C
d		–	–	3	4	–	–	6	–	8	–	10	–	13	14	–	–	–	–	*	27	28	29	–	31	–	–	BALB/c, C57BL/Ks, B10.D2, DBA/2, ST.T6, WH, YBL/Rr, YBR/Wi, NZB
e		–	–	–	–	–	6	7	–	9	–	*	–	13	–	–	*	–	–	25	27	28	29	30	–	*	*	STOLI
f		–	–	–	–	–	?	7	8	9	*	–	11	13	–	–	–	–	22	–	27	–	–	–	–	*	*	A.CA, B10.M, RFM/Un
g		–	2	–	–	–	6	*	?	*	*	*	*	–	14	*	–	–	22	*	*	*	*	*	*	*	*	HTG
h		1	2	–	5	5	6	*	?	8	*	*	11	–	?	*	–	–	*	*	*	*	*	*	–	–	–	HTH, B10.A(2R)
i		–	–	3	4	5	6	*	8	?	*	–	13	13	*	–	–	22	?	?	*	*	*	*	*	–	33	HTI, B10.A(5R)
j		+	–	?	–	–	6	?	?	*	?	–	–	–	–	–	–	22	22	?	?	?	?	?	*	32	*	JK/St
k		–	–	–	–	–	–	–	8	–	11	–	–	–	–	–	–	–	25	25	27	28	29	30	–	32	–	AKR, B10.BR, CBA, CE, CHI, C3H, C57BR/a, C57BR/cd, C58, D1.ST, MA/J, RF/J, ST/bJ, 101
l		1	–	–	–	–	6	?	*	8	*	*	10	–	–	–	–	–	22	*	?	?	*	?	*	*	*	I/St, N/St(?)
m		1	–	?	5	5	?	?	8	8	*	*	–	13	13	–	–	*	–	*	27	28	29	30	–	*	*	AKR.M
n		1	–	–	5	5	6	*	8	8	*	*	10	–	14	*	–	–	*	*	*	*	*	–	–	*	*	F/St
o		–	*	–	–	–	6	*	*	*	*	*	*	–	–	16	–	*	*	*	*	*	*	31	*	*	*	HTO/Sf
p		1	–	–	5	5	6	?	–	8	*	–	–	13	–	–	17	–	–	25	27	28	29	30	–	–	*	P/Sn, C3H.NB
q		1	–	–	5	5	6	–	8	8	*	11	–	13	–	–	17	–	25	25	27	28	29	30	?	–	*	DBA/1, C/St, BUB
r		–	–	–	–	–	–	–	–	–	–	–	–	–	–	–	–	–	–	–	–	–	–	?	–	*	RIII/J, RIII/Wy, LP.RIII
s		–	3	–	5	–	6	7	–	–	–	–	–	13	–	–	–	19	–	–	28	–	–	–	–	*	A.SW, SJL
w		–	2	–	*	–	–	–	–	–	–	–	–	–	–	–	–	*	–	–	*	–	–	–	*	*	WB/Re, WC/Re

An asterisk indicates that no test has been made for the particular component; a negative symbol denotes the absence; a question mark indicates uncertainty; the numerical symbol indicates presence of the component concerned.

From Lengerová, A. (1969): *Immunogenetics of Tissue Transplantation.* New York, American Elsevier Publishing

Analysis of Cell-mediated Immunity to H Antigen

There are many instances in which cellular antigens fail to induce detectable antibody response, and therefore they are not susceptible to serologic analysis. Such antigens, however, tend to elicit cell-mediated immunity. At present, there is no generally applicable method for the quantitation of cell-mediated immunity, nor are the molecular bases for specificity and manifestation of cell-mediated immunity known. For this reason, analysis of cell-mediated immunity to H antigen is essentially qualitative. Several methods have been used for this purpose: (1) the inverse skin grafting method (Rapaport), (2) the third-man test, (3) the normal lymphocyte transfer test, (4) the irradiated hamster test, and (5) the mixed leukocyte culture (MLC) test. These methods are collectively called *histocompatibility (or tissue) matching* in contrast to *histocompatibility (or tissue) typing* in which the serologic methods are used. The MLC test is considered to be a final biologic matching procedure and is used most widely in selecting suitable donors in man. The genetic locus determining MLC antigens is separate from that determining the H-2 antigens and appears to reside between the D and K ends of the H-2 locus in the mouse and just distal to the HL-A locus on a somatic chromosome in man.

Genetic Laws of Tissue Transplantation

It is difficult to account for the products of histocompatibility genes in terms of the usual concept of phenotype. Unlike the phenotype of a certain specific gene, the phenotypic products of histocompatibility genes are *potential* histocompatibility antigens whose phenotypic manifestation depends upon the immune response of a recipient. Another important characteristic of the H antigens is that they are usually codominant; i.e., they are expressed in heterozygotes being inherited from both parents without dominance or interactions. A third characteristic feature of H antigens is that among the multiple H loci, dissimilarity at any single H locus is usually sufficient for rejection of graft.

From these three features of H genes and their products, the outcome of grafts between various genetic combinations of donor and recipient can be predicted. The rules governing the outcome of grafts were originally formulated by Little and revised by Snell and Stimpfling (1966). These are known as the five laws of tissue transplantation:

The First Law. Transplants exchanged between genetically identical individuals (isografts or syngeneic grafts) are expected always to be accepted permanently. Identical twins and members of the same highly inbred strain of laboratory animals are regarded as being genetically identical, grafts among them are called isografts and should be accepted. The exception to this rule is found in some inbred strains of mice where a one-way incompatibility between male and female has been demonstrated, i.e., a female rejects a graft from a male, probably because the H antigen is controlled by genes on the Y chromosome.

The Second Law. Transplants exchanged between homozygotes for different alleles at one or more H loci, e.g., between members of different inbred strains (allografts), are not successful. The exception to this rule is grafting tissue across very weak H loci differences.

The Third Law. Transplantation between homozygotes and heterozygotes for one or several histocompatibility loci (also called allografts) will follow one-way compatibility, i.e., grafts from either inbred parent strain to an F_1 hybrid recipient succeed while grafts in the reverse direction are regularly rejected (Fig. 16-1). Exception to this rule might occur if the products of some H loci are not codominant as postulated.

The Fourth Law. F_1 hybrids between two inbred strains are characterized by being universal recipients in the restricted universe of the two inbred strains and all possible hybrids derived from them. Exception to this rule might be derived from some non-codominant H genes.

The Fifth Law. Some grafts from either inbred parent may be expected to be accepted and some to be rejected in the F_2 generation. Similarly, grafts from one inbred parent to backcross progeny of F_1 hybrids to the opposite parent may sometimes be accepted, but the percentages of takes will be lower (Table 16-4).

These principles of immunogenetics of transplantation are based on the assumption that H genes are expressed in codominant fashion. How-

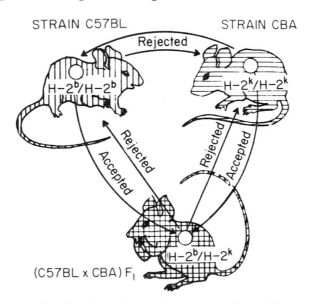

Fig. 16-1. Fates of skin allografts exchanged between mice of two different inbred strains, C57BL and CBA. [From Billingham, R., and Silvers, W. (1971): *The Immunobiology of Transplantation*. Englewood Cliffs, New Jersey, Prentice-Hall, Inc., p. 15.]

Table 16-4. Application of the Five Transplantation Laws to a Single Auto-somal H-locus with Two Alleles, a and b, Occurring with Same Frequency

| Genotype Combination | | Expected Result | Defined Generation with Similar Ratio of Takes |
Donor	Recipient		
aa	aa	Take (1)	{F₂ {(75% compatible) (5)
	ab	Take (3)	
	ba	Take (3)	
	bb	Rejection (2)	
ab	aa	Rejection (3)	
	ab	Take (4)	
	ba	Take (4)	
	bb	Rejection (3)	
bb	aa	Rejection (2)	{F₁ × aa {(50% compatible) (5) {F₁ × bb {(100% compatible)
	ab	Take (3)	
	ba	Take (3)	
	bb	Take (1)	

The numbers in parentheses correspond to the numbers of the law.
From Lengerová, A. (1969): *Immunogenetics of Tissue Transplantation*. New York, American Elsevier Publishing Company, Inc., p. 30.

ever, there are some indications that there might be exceptions to this rule of codominance. Further, these laws are only partially applicable to human transplantation for the obvious reason that here we are dealing with an outbred population.

IMMUNOLOGIC MECHANISMS OF GRAFT REJECTION

The most characteristic histologic feature of the rejection process is the presence of inflammatory cells of recipient origin in the immediate vicinity of a grafted tissue (Murphy, 1926). In initial grafts made to previously unsensitized recipients, infiltrating leukocytes are usually first seen by the second or third day and rapidly increase in number at the graft-host interface, though some infiltration into all parts of the grafts occurs. Vascular obstruction may follow in the late stage of the first set rejection when extensive death of graft cells takes place. In the second set rejection, where the recipient has been sensitized by a previous graft of the same donor origin, all the features of the process are accelerated and the rejection occurs with greater violence. The concentration of cells at the graft-host junction is often much greater, giving rise, for example, in rabbit skin grafts to a typical "black band" of cells that can be seen grossly on the stained histologic section (Medawar, 1944). A special form of graft called *white graft* (Rapaport and Converse, 1958) is referred to the course of certain second grafts which remain pallid and inert on their beds, never gaining a blood supply before becoming necrotic. Here, immunologically induced antibody-mediated vascular obstruction leads to an ischemic death of the graft with almost no visible inflammatory cells within it.

What is the meaning of the leukocytic infiltration to the grafted tissue? Murphy (1926) thought that "the round cell infiltration so characteristic of the reaction to foreign tissue grafts is a purposeful reaction and that these cells are the agent through which the mechanism exerts its force." Unable to demonstrate the formation of antibodies in any of his experiments, Murphy failed to realize that he was dealing with an immunologic phenomenon mediated exclusively by sensitized lymphocytes. That the cell-mediated immunity reaction is primarily responsible for the usual form of graft rejection was demonstrated when the state of transplantation immunity was shown to be transferable only by living cells but not usually by immune serum.

Decisive evidence that transplantation immunity is associated with delayed hypersensitivity or delayed allergy was presented by Brent et al. in 1958. They showed that guinea pigs sensitized by a skin allograft express the delayed hypersensitivity reaction to subsequent intradermal injection of living leukocytes (or cell extract) from the same donor—a *direct reaction*. A *transfer reaction* results when cells from regional lymph nodes of a sensitized recipient are injected intradermally into the original donor. This reaction is interpreted as a local passive transfer of the reactive state, a graft-versus-host reaction. Although cutaneous reactivity is not easily demonstrated in mice, this reaction can be reproduced in rabbits and man. Another evidence for the requirement of sensitized cells in graft rejection was provided by Weaver et al. (1955), who showed that allogeneic cells could survive in the recipient as long as they were contained in a filter chamber impermeable to host cells.

What is the specificity of the cells that gather around a graft at the time of its destruction? Najarian and Feldman in 1961 followed radioactively labeled lymphoid cells from specifically sensitized individuals after transfer to a second recipient about the time the latter received a graft from the original donor and showed that the transferred cells comprise a surprisingly small but significant proportion of the migrating cell population around the graft. Therefore, it appears that a relatively small number of sensitized lymphocytes which recruit bystander leukocytes may initiate a chain of reactions leading to inflammation and destruction of graft. Such sensitized lymphocytes are derived initially from the local or regional lymph nodes shortly after the graft has been made and can be found in the recipient's blood a day or two before the development of the lesion associated with rejection of graft. They are present in both the lymph nodes and the blood of mice as long as a year after rejection.

When animals are exposed to solid or dissociated cellular allografts of malignant or normal tissues, a variety of humoral antibodies also are formed. These have been identified as hemagglutinins, hemolysins, leukocyte agglutinins, and cytotoxins, depending on the manifestations of their secondary reactions. In mice all the evidence indicates that there is a group of isoantigens determined by the H-2 locus, and these isoantigens shared by erythrocytes and tissue cells manifest themselves as blood group antigens detected by one of the several reactions. Thus, the capacity of H antigens to evoke a humoral as well as a cellular immune response has served as the basis for tissue typing procedures (page 239).

ENHANCEMENT AND TOLERANCE

Enhancement

Cell-mediated immunity plays a major role in the rejection of grafts, but there is a question about the role of humoral antibodies against H antigen in graft rejection. Certainly, humoral antibody can exert a devastating effect on grafts of fully dispersed cells. However, the evidence incriminating humoral antibodies as major factors in the destruction of most solid tissue homografts is unsatisfactory. A notable exception to this assumption is the experiment of Hasek et al. (1961), in which passive transfer of large amounts of hyperimmune sera to recipient ducks resulted in overt lesions in established skin allografts within a few hours and the experiments of Milgrom et al. which show that renal allografts may be rejected by a humoral mechanism. Similarly, a heart graft in man may often be rejected largely by a humoral mechanism. The interesting well-known experiments of Algire et al. using Millipore chamber graft techniques further support the concept that in many grafts sensitized lymphocytes, not humoral antibodies, are primarily involved in the graft rejection. What then is the role of humoral antibodies directed against H antigens?

In certain tumors, and to a lesser extent in some normal tissues, it has been shown that the presence of a high titer of humoral antibodies may actually interfere with the rejection of a graft by sensitized lymphocytes. This apparently paradoxic phenomenon is known as *immunologic enhancement* or *immunologic facilitation*.

There are marked differences in induction of enhancement in different hosts, even within the same species. The route of immunization and other conditions influence development of the responsible antibodies. Nonviable tissue preparations provoke humoral immune response that can act to enhance allografts, whereas they usually fail to induce cellular immunity essential for most graft rejections. Syrian hamsters do not display measurable enhancement, and they also fail to produce demonstrable antibodies against H antigens. Since the enhancing principles have been located in the serum fractions as IgG globulins, it is tempting to assume that humoral antibodies are mainly responsible for the phenomenon of enhancement. These antibodies are called *enhancing antibodies*.

Can enhancing antibody be used to prolong normal tissue grafts? Dramatic results have been obtained recently by Stuart et al., who prolonged the survival of transplanted rat kidney for more than 200 days in histoincompatible recipients by infusion of enhancing antibodies. Whether these results can be reproduced in man remains to be seen.

Three possible modes of action have been studied: (1) enhancing antibodies may combine with the T antigens to prevent them from sensitizing the host—*afferent inhibition;* (2) the T antigens may reach the reactive centers of lymphoid cells, but the latter may be rendered incapable of making a cell-mediated immune response to them by some negative feedback influence of the antibody—*central inhibition;* and (3) enhancing antibodies may cover up the determinant site of T antigen so that the graft can evade the attack of sensitized cells—*efferent inhibition*—as shown by the Hellströms in their studies of blocking antibody. In recent experiments in rats and mice pretreating recipient organs or the whole animal with the Fab portion of IgG directed against H antigens has prevented graft rejection over very long periods. Further investigation is needed to analyze fully the role of enhancing antibodies in the adaptation to grafted tissue and their potential pragmatic use in overcoming transplantation barriers in organ or tissue transplantation.

Tolerance

Another fascinating phenomenon in transplantation immunobiology is that of tolerance. This term was used to describe a specific state of unresponsiveness to an antigen or antigens in adult life as a consequence of exposure to the corresponding antigen *in utero* or in the neonatal period —natural tolerance. Burnet and Fenner's "self marker" theory was developed to explain this phenomenon of natural tolerance (Chapter 15). When the phenomenon of tolerance was first discovered, it was generally believed that there is a critical period during the ontogenic development known as the *tolerance-responsive period.* In the light of subsequent findings, however, it became clear that tolerance can be induced in adult animals, that induction of tolerance is dependent on the dose and route of antigen administration as well as physicochemical characteristics of antigen, and that tolerance can be abolished or can be present only for a finite period unless antigen is replicated.

Another important concept in connection to the phenomenon of tolerance is that of "immunologically privileged" or favored sites in the body. For example, the anterior chamber of the eye, the cornea, the brain, the cheek pouch of the Syrian hamster, the testes, and fat pads are known to be sites in which grafts of living tissues from genetically dissimilar donors may be accepted or tolerated by the host, apparently disregarding the laws of transplantation. Although the existence of privileged sites is well established, further investigations are necessary to clarify the exact underlying mechanism. Recently Summerlin et al. (1973) showed that skin allografts can be made across the major H loci, as well as across species barriers, when the skin to be grafted is maintained for a period in organ culture *in vitro* prior to transplantation. Further, they showed that such allografts fail to initiate significant immune responses, humoral or cellular, directed against H antigens of the grafts. This phenomenon has not been fully investigated yet, but the application of such a simple procedure may be useful in the treatment of burn injury. Already the same principle can be extended to grafts of cornea and endocrine tissue, and Jacobs has done similar experiments with tumor grafts. The exact mechanisms of tolerance, the privileged site phenomenon, and the Summerlin phenomenon are not known. It seems likely that the explanation for this dramatic achievement may be quite simple. The culture conditions reduce the graft to a relatively simple state. Passenger leukocytes, a major source of host stimulation, and endothelial cells, a major target of the rejection response, are lost, and even the structural elements of the graft are reduced to progenitor cells under conditions of culture. After transplantation, the graft springs back, but now with host endothelium, and host passenger leukocytes return to the graft at a rate that keeps the dose to which the host is exposed below a critical level necessary for inducing the type of immune response effective in achieving graft rejection. However, when the grafts have been fully established, the cells of such grafts, e.g., the epidermal cells and fibroblasts of the skin, possess donor H antigens apparently in normal amounts.

GRAFT-VERSUS-HOST REACTIONS

When living tissues or organs are transplanted to a foreign host, the fate of graft will be either rejection or acceptance by the immune system of the host according to the five laws of transplantation (page 227). All the graft can do to the host is to invoke an immune reaction against the H antigens of the graft, since the host is immunologically competent and the graft is immunologically incompetent. The reverse situation, i.e., the graft containing immunocompetent cells when introduced into an immunologically incompetent recipient, results in a phenomenon known as *graft-versus-host* (GVH) reaction. This is due to the assault of immunocompetent cells in the graft against the host tissue: the graft in a sense attempts to reject the host.

Perhaps the earliest examples of what we now call GVH reaction can be found in the work of Murphy at Rockefeller Institute in 1916. He observed that inoculation of fragments of spleen or certain other tissues from adult chickens on chorioallantoic membranes of young chick embryos caused a striking enlargement of the spleen of the recipient and the development of whitish nodules on the membranes. He thought this striking phenomenon resulted from the stimulation of the host spleen by some unknown mechanism. The novel idea that GVH reaction might be due to the immunologic reaction of the graft against the host was first expressed in 1953 by Dempster and by Simonsen independently. The

GVH reaction can be reproduced experimentally. In this reaction the lymphocytes of the graft initiate immunologically a series of events that result in destruction of host tissues. Grafts might be able to react against their host under these conditions:

1. The graft must contain immunologically competent cells.
2. The host must be genetically different from the donor of the graft at H loci.
3. The host must be incapable of eliminating the graft.
4. The host must contain mesenchymal cells with which the donor lymphocytes interact.

One of the characterisitc forms of GVH reaction is known as runt disease and was initially observed by Billingham and Brent in 1956. Injection of allogeneic spleen cells into newborn mice resulted in retarded growth, frequent diarrhea, chronic emaciation, and stunted runts with sparse fur, hunched posture, and a peculiar mincing gait; hence the term *runt disease*. In the same year Simonsen produced a similar disease in newly hatched chicks by injecting allogeneic spleen cells. Subsequently, varieties of runt disease have been produced in many species, including mice, rats, hamsters, rabbits, guinea pigs, monkeys, and man. A variety of experimental situations in which GVH disease can develop are shown in Fig. 16-2.

Although runt disease in neonatal animals is a prototype of the GVH reaction, adult animals can be made to develop a GVH reaction which is called *homologous, allogeneic,* or *transplantation disease.* The GVH reaction can cause overt homologous disease in these situations:

1. Transfusion of large numbers of allogeneic lymphoid cells (e.g., several times the total number of host lymphoid cells) to adult animals.
2. Administration of normal parental strain lymphoid cells to a genetically tolerant F_1 hybrid.
3. Giving large numbers of lymphoid cells to adult animals previously rendered tolerant to H antigens of transfused lymphoid cells.
4. *Parabiotic intoxication* that is induced by uniting parabiotically unrelated partners of the same species.
5. *Secondary disease* in *radiation chimera.* When animals are given a transfusion of viable bone marrow cells after exposure to a lethal dosage of ionizing irradiation, the animal may recover from the immediate damages of irradiation, as the grafted bone marrow cells repopulate in the recipient—radiation chimera. Such animals may make apparent recovery only to develop so-called secondary wasting disease which is often fatal and is due to production by the marrow of stem cells that can develop to immunocompetent cells which in turn attack the host and initiate a GVH. The degree of severity depends upon the disparity of H antigens between the donor and

the recipient and the number of potentially immunocompetent cells transplanted.

6. Administration of immunologically competent lymphocytes to allogeneic hosts incapable of *mounting* an immune response against the foreign cells as in genetic defects of immune function or immunodeficiencies induced by immunosuppressive drugs including antilymphocyte globulin.

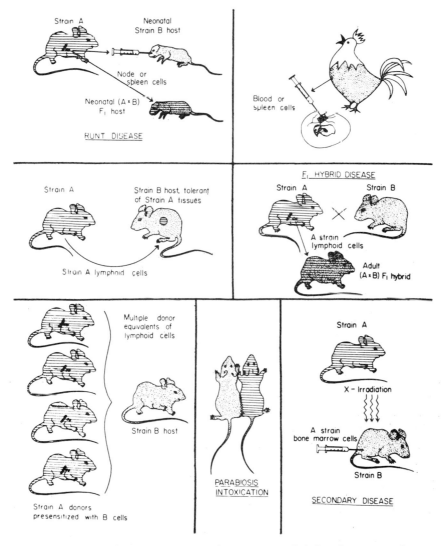

Fig. 16-2. A variety of different experimental situations in which homologous or graft-versus-host (GVH) disease syndromes can be produced. [From Billingham, R., and Silvers, W. (1971): *The Immunobiology of Transplantation*. Englewood Cliffs, New Jersey, Prentice-Hall, Inc., p. 150.]

One of the most important contributions from studies of GVH reactions is the demonstration that normal peripheral blood contains cells capable of causing GVH reaction when they are transfused into immunologically deficient recipients, especially infants with combined immunodeficiency disease (Chapter 19).

What is the underlying immunopathologic mechanism of the GVH reaction? When it was first established that splenomegaly is a result of the GVH reaction, it was generally assumed that proliferation of donor cells was responsible for the initial enlargement of both spleen and lymph nodes. However, subsequent critical studies have shown that the initial phase of hypertrophy of the lymphoid organs of the recipient is largely due to proliferation of the recipient's own cells. The cause of this massive proliferation is not clear, but the donor's cell-mediated immune reaction must initiate the sequence of events. Subsequently, damage to the host may be largely a consequence of the pathologic reaction of the host's own mesenchymal cells.

The relative paucity of demonstrable donor cells in the lymphoid organs of animals suffering from GVH disease may help to explain the difficulty of transferring this disease by lymphoid tissue transplant from the recipient animals.

Despite overwhelming evidence that the GVH reaction is basic to the pathologic mechanisms underlying various forms of homologous diseases, it is remarkable that only a few tissues are affected, and the damages to the parenchyma are usually trivial. The initial striking phase of hypertrophy of the spleen and the lymph nodes usually subsides and is followed by chronic involution. Hepatomegaly and hepatocellular damage are often early features of the disease. The gastrointestinal tract is often involved, and ulceration and bleeding are among the common features. Anemia occurs first with positive Coombs' test (antiglobulin test) and then aregenerative leukopenia, thrombocytopenia, and complete bone marrow failure may ensue. Skin lesions of varying degrees of severity, especially a morbilliform rash in man, are a prominent feature of the GVH reaction. Histologic sections of the skin reveal a prominent infiltration of mononuclear cells into the upper layers of the dermis; desquamation of epidermis may be seen in a later stage of the GVH reaction (Fig. 16-3).

Infection is often a terminal event in the graft-versus-host reaction. The damage to skin and bowel opens portals of entry to exogenous pathogens. Latent viruses may be activated, and the host's own immune functions abrogated. Thus, all manner of infections are expressed during the GVH. In a germ-free environment or in hosts protected against enteric pathogens, the fatal outcome of the GVH may sometimes be avoided.

Runt disease and secondary disease are systemic manifestations of the GVH reaction. A localized GVH reaction can be produced by inoculating immunologically competent cells into certain sites. The classical example

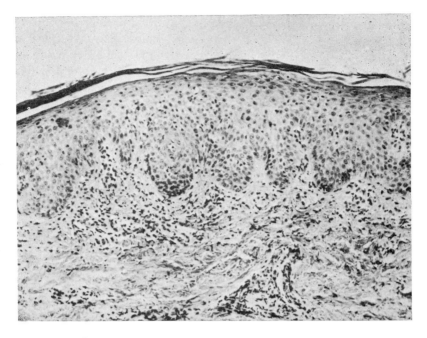

Fig. 16-3. Skin of a patient with graft-versus-host (GVH) reaction: a marked acanthosis with chronic inflammatory cell infiltration is seen in the area of the dermal papillae ($\times$ 40). [From Kersey, J. H., Meuwissen, H. J., and Good, R. A. (1971): Hum. Path. 2:392.]

is the white "pocks" that develop at the site of deposition of adult chicken splenic cells or peripheral leukocytes on the surface of the chorioallantoic membranes of allogeneic embryos. Another model for the localized GVH reaction has been described and extensively studied by Elkins (1966). Lymphoid cells from parenteral strain donors are injected beneath the kidney capsules of appropriate adult hybrid rats. A local reaction which is characterized by extensive proliferative activity of donor cells takes place for a period of 5 days or so and is followed by a local invasive destruction of kidney parenchyma that involves host cells. Intracutaneous GVH reaction is induced by injecting allogeneic lymphoid cells into the skin of guinea pigs, hamsters, sheep, men, and certain other species. Local manifestations of delayed skin reaction are initiated by donor's cells reacting against H antigens of the recipient. The intensity of this reaction—the normal lymphocyte transfer (NLT) reaction—provides a measure of the antigenic disparity between donor and host.

An assay procedure for GVH reaction using splenomegaly as an index has been devised by Simonsen and is known as the Simonsen assay. *Splenic index* is calculated for each experimental animal by dividing its relative spleen weight—the ratio of spleen weight to body weight—by the mean of relative spleen weights of control littermates. A standard number, e.g., 10^7, of allogeneic cells are injected intraperitoneally into newborn recipients incapable of rejecting the injected cells. Eight to 10 days later the animals are killed, and their body and spleen weights are recorded. Other assay systems utilize phagocytosis capacity of the reticuloendothelial system, weight gain, or chorioallantoic membrane "pocks" lesions in chickens.

Prevention or modification of a systemic GVH reaction in experimental animals has been achieved to a certain extent by (1) injection of syngeneic lymphocytes intravenously or intraperitoneally, (2) injection of allogeneic or xenogeneic antilymphocyte serum (ALS) (Chapter 17), (3) administration of various immunosuppressive drugs (Chapter 17), especially amethopterin (methotrexate), and (4) preincubation of donor's cells with immunosuppressive agents, especially ALS.

Systemic forms of the GVH reaction can be seen in man. Infants with hereditary thymic dysplasia may develop GVH reactions as a consequence of intrauterine transfusion of maternal blood or postnatal transfusion of allogeneic blood. Radiation chimeras achieved by total body irradiation followed by allogeneic bone marrow transplantation may result in GVH reaction.

HISTOCOMPATIBILITY TESTING IN MAN AND NEW CONCEPT OF IMMUNOGENETICS

In man two major histocompatibility systems are well established, the ABO system and the HL-A system. Landsteiner in 1901 observed that human blood showed individual differences characterized by agglutination reactions. Red cells of some of his co-workers agglutinated with the serum of some, but not all, of his associates. This observation led to the discovery of the ABO blood group system.

Division of individuals into four main blood groups is based on the fact that A and B antigens can be present singly or together or may be absent. These antigens can be identified by means of anti-A and anti-B agglutinins which can occur naturally in serum of individuals not possessing the corresponding antigen. This relationship of serum antibodies to cellular antigens is based on the rule of Landsteiner that corresponding antibodies and antigens cannot coexist.

It is interesting to note that at one time there were in use at least three different methods of designating the four blood groups of man. Two different nomenclatures used Roman numerals, I, II, III, and IV, and a third (Landsteiner's) used combinations of the letters A, B and O. In order to resolve the confusion, the Health Committee of the League of Nations in 1930 recommended the adoption of Landsteiner's ABO terminology as the sole method of designating human blood groups. However, it was not until the onset of World War II in 1940 (40 years after the discovery!)

that Landsteiner's nomenclature for human blood groups came to be accepted throughout the world.

Significance of ABO Antigens on Transplantation Immunity

Mammalian erythrocytes appear to be unable to provoke transplantation immunity, even though in some species they carry all histocompatibility antigens, particularly the major ones, i.e., they appear to be lacking transplantation antigens but possess histocompatibility antigens. These findings are in sharp contrast to the role of nucleated red cells of chickens on which transplantation antigens appear to be fully expressed. The basis for this apparent difference is not clear, but it is tempting to speculate that the loss of nucleus is accompanied by the loss of transplantation or histocompatibility antigens on the surface of red cells.

Human red cells to some degree represent an exception to this rule, and ABO antigens have long been recognized to be important not only in transfusion but also in the transplantation of other tissues and organs such as kidney and skin. Unlike the situation that exists in mice and rats, injection of mismatched red cells in man usually results in elucidation of transplantation immunity. This finding is in accord with the recent finding that ABO antigens on fixed tissue cells behave like "conventional" transplantation antigens. Despite the apparent effects of the ABO antigens in clinical transplantation, it has yet to be determined whether the immunity they induce is the same kind as that induced by H antigens associated with the nucleated cells of solid tissues.

Human Leukocyte Antigens (HL-A) and Tissue Typing

In 1946 Medawar showed that intradermal injections of leukocytes from rabbit D into rabbit R induced a state of transplantation immunity to subsequent grafts of the skin of D to R. This indicates that leukocytes, skin, and other organs share at least some important transplantation antigens. It was later observed that tolerance of skin allografts can be induced in very young rodents by inoculation with living leukocytes of the same allogeneic origin, a further indication that leukocytes must express all the transplantation antigens of the skin and perhaps of other tissues. Exceptions to this general relationship have now been encountered by the S antigens of mouse skin which behave as weak transplantation antigens. These findings, as well as the ease of obtaining leukocytes, made leukocyte typing important in histocompatibility testing. Since it was shown that the lymphocytes in man carry most (if not all) of the transplantation antigens (Friedman et al., 1961; Rapaport et al., 1962), a proper and precise typing of human lymphocytes would be expected to provide a useful means of selecting donor recipient for organ or tissue transplantation.

Dausset in 1958 demonstrated by serologic means the existence of leukocyte isoantigens in man, which he described as leukocyte group "Mac".

Payne and Hackel (1961) showed that these antigens are genetically controlled. Van Rood and van Leeuwen in 1963 refined the method of testing for leukoagglutinins and by use of cross absorption and computer analysis disclosed clearly the existence of a genetic locus in man controlling leukocyte antigens. This locus was initially designated as 4 with two possible alleles, 4a and 4b. The gene frequency for the alleles was estimated to be 0.38 and 0.62, respectively.

A method for assaying lymphocytotoxins on a microscale, which was developed by Terasaki and McClelland in 1964, circumvented many difficulties of the leukoagglutinin test. In 1965 Terasaki et al. used this method to characterize 154 samples of native human lymphotoxic antisera with respect to the strength, frequency, grouping, and the relevance of differences to kidney transplantation. The discriminatory capacity of a large panel of unabsorbed sera was sufficient to distinguish leukocytes of 9 pairs of duplicates from the leukocytes of 273 random persons. Two thirds of the 154 antisera could be classified into seven major groups. Two of these seven groups were shown to be associated with the LA-1 and LA-2 groups previously established by Payne et al. in 1964 by the leukoagglutinin method.

Van Rood et al. (1966) reported 5 new leukocyte antigens based on the study of 147 sera, and pointed out that there is good correlation between leukoagglutinin and lymphocytotoxin in the grouping of human leukocytes. However, the correlation between the normal lymphocyte transfer (NLT) test, skin graft survival, and the compatibility of leukocytes was poor.

Table 16-5. The HL-A System: Official Designation of the Fifth Histocompatibility Workshop, May, 1972

LA Locus (or 1st series)	4 Locus (or 2nd series)
HL-A 1	HL-A 5
HL-A 2	HL-A 7
HL-A 3	HL-A 8
HL-A 9	HL-A 12
W 23	HL-A 13
W 24	(HL-A) 14
HL-A 10	(HL-A) 17
W 25	(HL-A) 27
W 26	W 16
HL-A 11	W 20
W 19	W 21
W 29	
W 30	
W 31	
W 32	
(HL-A) 28	

Exchange of typing sera among the tissue typing laboratories and the results of several international workshops culminated in further definition of antisera and a standard nomenclature of human leukocyte antigens known as the HL-A system. More than 20 different leukocyte antigens have been recognized. Most of them belong to the HL-A system (Table 16-5). More than 30 different HL-A alleles have so far been identified, and perhaps more remain to be identified. Unlike the H-2 antigens of the mouse red cells, the HL-A antigens have not yet been shown to be present on human red cells.

Family studies have been especially helpful in analyzing the HL-A locus. Much of the advantage of these family studies is that the *haplotypes* of the parents can be deduced from the antigenic profiles of off-spring (Fig. 16-4). The term *haplotype* was introduced for the antigens of one HL-A unit of genetic information which corresponds to half the phenotype for a fully expressed codominant system. The chances of having an identical HL-A genotype between parent-child and sib-sib in various possible matings are shown in Table 16-6. Despite the refinements of the serologic method and more precise definition of a large number of antigens, the correlation of the HL-A system with the survival of a skin graft was not good. Further the successful kidney grafts from allogeneic donors have been poorly correlated with IIL-A typing except within mem-

Father	A	1, 2, 4	
	B	15, 1?	
Mother	C	4, 5	
	D	18	
Sib 1		15, 19	B
		18	D
Sib 2		15, 19	B
		4, 5	C
Sib 3		15, 19	B
		4, 5	C
Sib 4		1, 2, 4	A
		4, 5	C
Sib 5		1, 2, 4	A
		4, 5	C

Fig. 16-4. Illustrating the way in which family studies with typing sera provide evidence of the association of certain HL-A specificities. The father possesses antigens 1, 2, 4, 15, and 19. The mother lacks all of these except antigen 4. Consequently, the children can have inherited only the genetic determinants of antigens 1, 2, 15, and 19 from their father. Since the children have either antigens 1, 2, and 4 or 15 and 19, this indicates that all of these antigens are determined by the same genetic locus. Furthermore, it follows that antigens 1, 2, and 4 are determined by one chromosomal region (A), and 15 and 19 by the same region on the homologous chromosome (B). By a similar line of reasoning, one can work out the antigens determined by equivalent chromosomal regions (C) and (D) in the mother. [From Billingham, R., and Silvers, W. (1971): *The Immunobiology of Transplantation*. Englewood Cliffs, New Jersey, Prentice-Hall, Inc., p. 29.]

Table 16-6. Relation between the HL-A Genotypes of Parents and the Expected Frequency of Identical HL-A Leukocyte Groups in Parent → Child and Sib → Sib Pairs in the Family

Genotypes of Parents	Genotypes of Offspring	Donor-Recipient Combination	Grafts Expected to be Identical with Host at HL-A Locus (%)
ab × cd	ac ad bc bd	parent → child	0
		sib → sib	25
ab × ad	aa ab ad bd	parent → child	25
		sib → sib	25
aa × bc	ab ac ab ac	parent → child	0
		sib → sib	50

The HL-A alleles of the parents are designated a, b, c, and d.
From Billingham, R., and Silvers, W. (1971): *The Immunobiology of Transplantation.* Englewood Cliffs, New Jersey, Prentice-Hall, Inc., p. 30.

bers of a family. The extreme polymorphism of the HL-A system with more than 30 alleles in two separately segregating genetic systems and the influence of yet unidentified antigens are believed to account in a major way for the poor correlation. Recent evidence, however, suggests that there may be a separate locus which is primarily responsible for control of the expression of transplantation immunity.

Mixed Leukocyte Culture (MLC) Test

By 1963 it was clear that a large number of antigens, in addition to the well-known plant mitogen phytohemagglutinin (PHA), were capable of "activating" sensitive lymphocytes and inducing transformation and proliferation *in vitro*. It was also known that lymphocytes carry on their surfaces a number of important histocompatibility antigens. This background, together with incidental observation made by Schrek and Donnelly in 1961 that mitosis was noted in the mixed culture of leukocytes from two patients with hemochromatosis, led Bain et al. in 1963 to carry out further detailed study of mixed leukocyte culture in normal healthy persons, including twins. The results indicated clearly that the reaction, i.e., transformation, mitosis, and synthesis of new DNA by lymphocytes in the MLC, is related to the genetic differences and allograft immunity of the two individual donors.

It was further shown that no prior sensitization of the cells of donors was necessary for the MLC reaction. When the leukocytes from two individuals react against each other in a culture tube, it is difficult, if not impossible, to know the degree of the response of each population. Therefore, it is necessary to have one population of leukocytes in *static state* in terms of their proliferating activity while leaving the other intact and able to respond—*one-way MLC test of Bach*. For this purpose various means, i.e., leukocyte extracts, disrupted leukocytes, frozen cells, nitrogen mustard treatment, and irradiation, were tried without reproducible results. In 1966 Bach and Voynow used mitomycin for the purpose of one-way MLC with reproducible results. Incorporation of radioactively labeled thymidine into newly synthesized DNA was measured as an index of MLC reaction.

In an MLC test, the total of antigenic disparity between two individuals is measured without defining the kind and the numbers of antigens involved. A genetic analysis of the MLC test suggested that a single genetic locus with a minimum of 20 alleles is involved in the control of the antigens responsible for these leukocyte responses (Amos and Bach, 1968). This conclusion was based on the fact that 28.2 percent of 291 sibling pairs was nonstimulatory in the MLC test, and that 80 parent-child pairs and more than 600 unrelated pairs were always found to be stimulatory. It was further proposed that the locus controlling MLC reactivity is the same locus that determines the majority of HL-A antigens. The investigators called this locus the *major histocompatibility locus* of man. The correlation between MLC test and graft survival was good within the members of a family, but again it seemed poor when an unrelated donor was used. Likewise, the correlation between HL-A typing and MLC testing was good within the family, but poor among the unrelated.

New Concept of the Genetic Control of HL-A System, MLC Reaction, and Transplantation Immunity

The idea that a single genetic locus controls both the HL-A system and MLC reaction and that this locus is the major histocompatibility locus of man, must now be modified in light of recent findings. Amos and Bach in 1968 described an important exception to their proposed theory, i.e., one HL-A mismatched sibling pair failed to react in the MLC test. The possibility that this represented a rare instance of a recombination within the genetic material was considered. A clear example of a recombinant mismatched at HL-A, but matched in the MLC test, was observed in a family in which the recombinant sibling, mismatched at an antigen of the LA series whose cells were not stimulated in the MLC by the recipient's cells, was used as a successful bone marrow transplant donor (Gatti et al., 1968). This finding suggested strongly that HL-A and MLC, as well as HL-A mismatch and severe GVH reaction, could be dissociated. Based on the studies of families with "abnormal MLC" responses and dissociation of HL-A mismatches and MLC matches, Yunis and Amos (1971) proposed that there might be two other loci, one for the MLC reaction and one for graft survival, in addition to the HL-A loci and that these loci control transplantation immunity. This assumption was further supported by the report of Dupont et al. (1971), in which they proposed that the

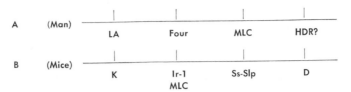

Fig. 16-5. Relative locations of histocompatibility loci in man (A) and in mice (B).

MLC reaction might be controlled by a third locus, which is closely linked to the locus that may control the four series of HL-A antigens. A tentative mapping of these loci that are involved in transplantation immunity is illustrated in Fig. 16-5A. More recently Bach et al. (1972) reported further evidence that separate loci control MLC reactions in mice and men and proposed a mapping of the loci (Fig. 16-5B).

Abundant evidence is rapidly accumulating to reenforce these developing new concepts. The new information explains the inadequacy to predict allograft survival from HL-A typing, except among siblings. It argues strongly for intensive additional research to facilitate matching of donor and recipient in the light of this new knowledge.

Already it has been possible, for example, to facilitate selection of a donor of bone marrow to be transplanted to an immunodeficient infant by matching with respect to the MLC test when a complete mismatch is present in the HL-A system (Chapter 35). The new studies also promise that in mice and men the chromosomal region of such complexity for histocompatibility analysis is also of major importance in the genetic control of the very antigens to which an individual can respond—*Ir system*. Serologic analysis in the mouse has revealed the presence of two separately segregating polyallelic systems between which the Ir and MLC genetic determinants are found. In man the location of the Ir region has not yet been established, but it is clear that the major MLC region lies outside the regions determining the composition of the LA and four histocompatibility antigens.

It is important for students and practicing physicians to watch closely the information developing from these genetic analyses of histocompatibility testing because susceptibility to some of the common and as yet poorly understood diseases of man like lupus erythematosus, leukemia, and Hodgkin's disease may become better understood from these investigations (Chapter 23).

SELECTED REFERENCES

Algire, G. H., Weaver, J. M., and Prehn, R. T. (1957): Ann. N. Y. Acad. Sci. *64*:1009.
Amos, D. B., and Bach, F. H. (1968): J. Exp. Med. *128*:623.
Bach, F. H., and Voynow, N. K. (1966): Science *153*:545.
Bach, F. H., et al. (1972): Science *176*:1024.

Bain, B., Vas, M., and Lowenstein, L. (1963): Fed. Proc. 22:428.
Billingham, R. E., and Brent, L. (1959): Phil. Trans. Roy. Soc. (Series B) 242:439.
Brent, L., Brown, J., and Medawar, P. B. (1958): Lancet 2:561.
Coons, H. A. (1971): Ann. N. Y. Acad. Sci. 177:5.
Dausset, J. (1958): Acta Haemat. (Basel) 20:156.
Dempster, W. J. (1953): Brit. J. Surg. 40:447.
Dupont, B., Nielsen, L. S., and Svejgaard, A. (1971): Lancet 2:1336.
Ehrlich, P. (1905): In The Collected Papers of Paul Ehrlich, Himmelweit, F. (ed.)
    (1957). New York, Pergamon Press.
Elkins, W. L. (1964): J. Exp. Med. 120:329.
Elkins, W. L. (1966): J. Exp. Med. 123:103.
Elkins, W. L. (1971): Progr. Allerg. 15:78.
Friedman, E. A. (1961): J. Clin. Invest. 40:2162.
Gatti, R. A., et al. (1968): Lancet 2:1366.
Gibson, T., and Medawar, P. B. (1943): J. Anat. (London) 77:299.
Glenny, A. T., and Hopkins, B. E. (1922): J. Hyg. (Camb.) 21:142.
Hellström, I., and Hellström, K. E. (1970): Int. J. Cancer 5:195.
Jacobs, B. B. (1970): J. Nat. Cancer Inst. 45:263.
Landsteiner, K. (1901): Wien. Klin. Wschr. 14:1132.
Landsteiner, K., and Wiener, A. S. (1940): Proc. Soc. Exp. Biol. Med. 43:223.
Levine, P., and Stetson, R. E. (1939): JAMA 113:127.
Little, C. C. (1914): Science 40:904.
Medawar, P. B. (1944): J. Anat. 78:176.
Medawar, P. B. (1946): Nature 157:161.
Milgrom, F., et al. (1966): JAMA 198:226.
Mitchison, N. A., and Dube, O. L. (1955): J. Exp. Med. 102:179.
Murphy, J. B. (1916): J. Exp. Med. 24:1.
Murphy, J. B. (1926): Monograph 21, New York, Rockefeller Institute for Medical
    Research, pp. 169-178.
Najarian, J. S., and Feldman, J. D. (1961): J. Exp. Med. 114:779.
Payne, R., and Hackel, E. (1961): J. Human Genet. 13:306.
Payne, R., et al. (1964): Cold Spring Harbor Symposium on Quant. Biol. 29:285.
Rapaport, F. T., and Converse, J. M. (1958): Ann. Surg. 147:273.
Rapaport, F. T., et al. (1962): J. Clin. Invest. 41:2166.
Rood, J. J. van, and van Leeuwen, A. (1963): J. Clin. Invest. 42:1382.
Rood, J. J. van, et al. (1966): In Histocompatibility Testing 1965. Copenhagen,
    Munksgaard, pp. 37-50.
Schöne, G. (1912): Die heteroplastische und homoplastische Transplantationen. Ber-
    lin, J. Springer.
Schrek, R., and Donnelly, W. J. (1961): Blood 18:561.
Simonsen, M. (1957): Acta Path. Microbiol. Scand. 40:480.
Simonsen, M. (1962): Progr. Allerg. 6:349.
Snell, G. D., and Stimpfling, J. H. (1966): In Biology of the Laboratory Mouse,
    Green, E. L. (ed.). New York, McGraw-Hill Book Co., pp. 457-491.
Stuart, F. G., Saitoh, T., and Fitch, W. (1968): Science 160:1463.
Summerlin, W. T., et al. (1973): Transpl. Proc. 5:707.
Terasaki, P. I., and McClelland, J. D. (1964): Nature 204:998.
Terasaki, P. I., et al. (1965): Vox Sang. 11:350.
Tyzzer, E. E. (1909): J. Med. Res. 21:519.
Voisin, G. A. (1971): Progr. Allerg. 15:328.
Weaver, J. M., Algire, G. H., and Prehn, R. T. (1955): J. Nat. Cancer Inst. 15:1737.
Winn, H. J. (1970): Transpl. Proc. 2:83.
Yunis, E. J., and Amos, D. B. (1971): Proc. Nat. Acad. Sci. U.S.A. 68:3031.

FURTHER READINGS

Billingham, R. E. (1968): Harvey Lect. 62:21.
Billingham, R. E., and Silvers, W. (1971): Immunobiology of Transplantation. Engle-
    wood Cliffs, New Jersey, Prentice-Hall, Inc.

Hamburger, J., et al. (1972): *Renal Transplantation: Theory and Practice.* Baltimore, The Williams & Wilkins Company.

Hraba, T. (1968): *Mechanism and Role of Immunological Tolerance.* New York, S. Karger.

Lengerová, A. (1969): *Immunogenetics of Tissue Transplantation* (North-Holland Publishing Company). New York, American Elsevier Publishing Company.

Marcus, D. M. (1969): New Eng. J. Med. *280*:994.

Medawar, P. B. (1957): Harvey Lect. *52*:144.

Najarian, J. S., and Simmons, R. L. (eds.) (1972): *Transplantation.* Philadelphia, Lea & Febiger.

17
Control of Immune Response

The adaptive immune response has emerged as a biologically unique system, incredibly intricate, involving the cooperation of various cell types and elaboration of both specific and nonspecific signals. Susceptible to external influences at every juncture, the adaptive immune response offers an almost infinite variety of possibilities and opportunities for modulation, deviation, or inhibition. As our knowledge of its underlying mechanisms increases, the number and kinds of methods for controlling adaptive immune response will surely be extended progressively to permit manipulation in both the laboratory and the clinic.

The manipulation of immunity by use of immunogens has been practiced for many years; prophylactic immunization (active and passive) against many forms of devastating bacterial and viral diseases and prophylactic treatment for hay fever are examples. More sophisticated use of immunogens is aimed at adjusting the overall specific immune response up or down, at selecting the kind of immune mechanism to be activated or inhibited (humoral or cellular), and at altering the balance of the kinds of antibody produced. General methods comprise (1) induction of tolerance, (2) feedback suppression of antibody formation, (3) adjuvant immunization, (4) immunodeviation, and (5) precise analysis of location and properties of control and activation of regional immunologic domains.

For the retention of an allograft, for example, it suffices either to suppress immune rejection or to induce tolerance; for the rejection of cancer we must try to break tolerance, overcome immunodeviation, and stimulate immune rejection. The methods of immunosuppression currently used are as crude as were the methods of surgery before Lister. It is obvious that more specific modulation rather than blunderbuss suppression of immune responses will become more and more possible in the future. This progress will surely utilize capacity for manipulation through skilled use of immunodeviation, negative feedback, and immunogens that are completely defined chemically, as well as through selective toxicity of antibodies and highly specific or more generally selective immunosuppression. It further seems certain that our pragmatic controls will soon use direct and indirect means to manipulate the genome and selectively manage gene action. We will be able to understand fully and manipulate the biologic language of the cell surface recognition and the signals from the cell surface to the nucleus that are involved in commanding cells to proliferate or express the potential of their differentiated state. Finally, we will find numerous ways of controlling the engagement of the major biologic amplification systems and effector mechanisms at will using both macromolecular and micromolecular pharmacology. With the coming of this day in the not too distant future much that now seems unmanipulable human disease will be susceptible to our therapeutic and prophylactic endeavors.

ACTIVE IMMUNIZATION—VACCINATION

One of the greatest triumphs of immunobiology in the past was the use of active immunization to control and prevent certain fatal, crippling, infectious diseases of man, such as smallpox and poliomyelitis. The term *vaccine* stems from the Latin word for cow, *vacca*, and refers to Jenner's discovery that he could use "variolation" with cowpox, vaccinia, to prevent smallpox. This term has been broadened to include the use of any biologic product prepared from microorganisms for the purpose of active immunization. The term *toxoid* refers to a toxin which has been rendered nontoxic while still retaining its immunogenicity. Such substances have been used with great success in preventing intoxications secondary to infection as in diphtheria and tetanus.

The total effectiveness of a vaccine is determined by the degree of protection afforded the host following natural or artificial challenge with a pathogenic organism. However, rise in antibody titer in the host can be used for the indicator of effective immunization. Depending on the pathogenetic mechanism of the disease in question, i.e., incubation time, type of organ, or tissue involved, the design of the immunization can be adapted to provide the best possible protection of the host. In general, an effective vaccine utilizes the same protective mechanisms seen following the natural infection. For example, increase in the production of IgA antibody in the respiratory tract would be the most effective way of providing protection against many respiratory infections, whereas increasing IgG antibody in the circulation would provide better protection against diphtheria toxin.

In general, live or attenuated vaccines induce more effective and longer duration of immunity than do the killed or inactivated forms of vaccines. This is believed to be due to the sustained stimulation of the immune response by living organisms. For the purpose of sustained stimulation by nonviable vaccines, inert material such as alum may be mixed with the immunogen—*alum precipitated vaccine*. If the interval between two live viral vaccinations is close, the immune response to the second vaccination may be inhibited. This phenomenon is called *interference*. For example, the immune response to the oral poliovirus immunization may be less effective during epidemics of enterovirus infections. The interference phenomenon is observed only with certain combinations of live viruses. It is interesting to note that Jenner was the first to recognize the possibility of virus interference when he admonished that vaccination must not be carried out while a person has a cold sore or fever blister because the virus of the latter may interfere with the acceptance and immunization provided by the former.

One of the important purposes of active immunization is to equip the growing infant with the immunologic experiences required to make a sufficiently rapid response to overcome the common and often life-threatening diseases which he will meet as he grows up. Fortunately in a number of the more important diseases, the provision of an immunologic education is relatively simple and minimally traumatic. The essential requirements are (1) that active immunization with suitably potent immunogens should be begun early, (2) that the booster immunizations should be repeated after suitable intervals so as to produce a good secondary response, and (3) that immunization should be repeated at appropriate intervals and timed in relationship to the infection against which it is intended to protect. Although it is known that young infants can make an adequate immune response to proper stimulations, it is also known that maternally transmitted antibody can inhibit the antibody response to immunogens such as poliomyelitis vaccine, or to diphtheria toxoid or pertussis vaccine. The degree of inhibition depends upon the level of preexisting antibody and the immunogenic potency of the preparations used for immunization.

Vaccination can cause small but significant numbers of side effects and complications. Therefore, the decision to use a vaccine must be made by weighing the risks of complications from vaccines against the morbidity and mortality of the disease itself. Routine vaccination against smallpox has been discontinued in the United States since 1972. Aside from the local irritation of the injected site which is associated with the development of an immune state, live vaccine can spread to involved eczematous areas of the skin or can cause fatal disease in immunodeficient children, e.g., paralytic poliomyelitis can occur as a consequence of the reversion of the attenuated virus to a virulent state. Immunization with live attenuated viruses or bacteria is dangerous for infants with an immunodeficiency disease. Here the vaccination may result in fatal complications because the host, lacking capacity to generate an immune response, may succumb to organisms in the vaccine, even though they are of low grade virulence for persons of normal immunologic potential. Postinfectious or postvaccinal encephalomyelitis is probably an example of a disease mediated by infection and/or immunologic process taking place in the central nervous system and can be a disastrous consequence of efforts at immunization.

The principles of active immunization now providing such effective protection against smallpox, measles, rubella, mumps, diphtheria, tetanus, pertussis, and tuberculosis will surely be extended to other diseases, such as varicella, herpes simplex, cytomegalic inclusion disease, and hepatitis. Additional bacterial vaccines can and should be developed to prevent common pathogens of infancy and childhood. Some of these new vaccines will utilize the oral and respiratory routes rather than the parenteral, e.g., typhoid vaccine and respiratory virus vaccine. Finally, effective vaccines that can prevent or modify human cancers will probably be discovered and developed in the future.

PASSIVE IMMUNIZATION—SEROTHERAPY

Passive immunization by means of specific antiserum is used either prophylactically when active immunization is not feasible or to reenforce the body's own immune response or to tide the patient over a period until the humoral immune response becomes effective. The dramatic success achieved by von Behring and Kitasato (1895) in preventing fatal complications of diphtheria infection by antitoxin opened a new era of serotherapy for infectious disease. However, this form of therapy has since been used less frequently due to the effective control of infectious diseases by active immunization and by antibiotic therapy. Nonetheless, serotherapy continues to be used in many situations as a supplement. In passive immunization, specific antibodies are passively transferred to neutralize toxins or viruses, to lyse bacteria, or to opsonize them for phagocytosis.

For therapeutic purposes, such large amounts of antibody are required that it is rarely possible to obtain a sufficient amount of immune serum from human beings, and therefore such sera have in the past often been made from the serum of immunized animals. Modern methods of plasma phoresis are changing these relationships, and more and more often passive immunization now utilizes preparations from the preimmunized human donors. The antibodies in the serum are concentrated by means of chemical fractionation, followed by enzymatic digestion and further purification.

Passive immunization has the disadvantage of being short-lived. If a given amount of human antibody is administered intravenously or intramuscularly into a patient, the antibody becomes diluted in the recipient's plasma and lymph. After this initial dilution, human IgG, for example, is gradually broken down, its half-life being approximately 24 days. When antibodies from an animal of a different species are used, an immune response in the recipient is directed against the foreign protein and results in rapid immune elimination of the foreign protein 10 to 14 days after the initial injection. When an immune reaction occurs against a foreign serum, it is sometimes accompanied by serum sickness. The latter occurs most commonly when crude antiserum or unrefined globulins are used. After development of immunity, further doses of antibody will be eliminated rapidly (immune clearance), and the recipient may run a considerable risk of various kinds of reactions such as anaphylaxis, vascular injury, and kidney damage. For this reason, passive immunization should always be preceded by meticulous precautions such as detailed past history and sensitivity testing. The diseases for which passive immunization is employed are also listed in the Appendix.

IMMUNOSUPPRESSION

To inhibit the immune response today we employ drugs capable of suppressing various aspects of the immune response (immunosuppressive drugs). Such agents may inhibit cellular and humoral immune responses and immunologic memory or facilitate induction of immunologic tolerance. Immunologically competent cells may be destroyed by irradiation or radiomimetic drugs, or these cells may be either removed via a chronic thoracic duct drainage or prevented from developing by thymectomy in certain species at birth. Apart from antilymphocyte serum, most immunosuppressive drugs were initially developed because they exhibited an inhibitory influence on growth of neoplastic cells (antimiotic). Many of their adverse side effects are due to their ability to inhibit cell division in rapidly regenerating organs such as bone marrow and intestinal epithelium, as well as in healing wounds. Immunosuppressive agents have been used in recipients for the prolongation of grafts, in patients with various forms of autoimmune or immunologically based diseases, and in bone marrow recipients to decrease severity of the graft-versus-host reactions.

Irradiation

Ionizing radiations damage immunologically competent cells during mitosis. Sublethal doses (300 to 600 R) of whole body radiation suppress immune response to many kinds of immunogens. Most experimental studies have been made on antibody production to red cell antigens in mice, rabbits, or guinea pigs. An increased survival of allogeneic skin grafts in rabbits and mice has been observed when the irradiation has been given one day before the grafting. Attempts to produce permanent survival of grafts by further increasing the dose of irradiation have not been effective and have led to death of the host from radiation damage to bone marrow and intestinal epithelium.

Within the first few hours after sublethal irradiation, the lymphoid tissues show arrest of mitotic activity and massive disintegration of lymphocytes. This is followed by phagocytosis of the debris which is completed within 24 hours. A period of inactivity is observed for a week or more, and then a period of mitosis and proliferation of lymphoblasts resulting in a complete regeneration of lymphoid tissue after 3 to 4 weeks. Little damage occurs in most macrophages, reticulum cells, and the epithelial elements of lymphoid tissues (e.g., Hassall's corpuscles). However, certain macrophages like the so-called dendritic macrophages or reticulum cells of the germinal centers are destroyed by irradiation. Heinecke in 1905 first described the radiosensitivity of lymphoid tissues. In 1914 Murphy showed that the survival of foreign grafts could be prolonged by pretreating recipients of allografts with ionizing radiation. Since then numerous investigations have confirmed and extended the initial observation of the effects of radiation on immune response. General features of the effects of irradiation of immune response are:

1. The primary humoral response is markedly depressed or abolished when immunogen is given 2 hours to 50 days after the irradiation, whereas it is increased or not affected at all if immunogen is given 2 hours to 3 days before irradiation.
2. When large amounts of protein antigens are given during the phase of immunologic depression 1 day after irradiation, long-lasting specific immunologic unresponsiveness may be induced.
3. Irradiation given 3 to 4 days after the immunization has little effect on the primary response.
4. Secondary response is not so much affected unless very large doses of irradiation are used.

A higher dose of irradiation causes death to the animals unless the deficient marrow is replaced by a transfusion of hematopoietic cells from isogeneic or allogeneic donors. Then animals populated by two genetically different cell lines may be produced. These are known as chimeras—in this instance irradiation chimeras—after the mythical monster which possessed a lion's head, a goat's body and a serpent's tail. The bone marrow that has been introduced may generate immunocompetent cells which in turn initiate an attack on host tissue resulting in overt graft-versus-host disease.

Cytotoxic Drugs

Drugs achieving chemical suppression of immunity may be divided according to influence by three classes of drugs: alkylating (radiomimetic)

Table 17-1. Cytotoxic Agents Frequently Used For Immunosuppression

---

Alkylating Agents
  Nitrogen mustard
  L-phenylalanine mustard (Melphalan)
  Cyclophosphamide (Cytoxan)

Antimetabolites
  Methotrexate (Amethopterin)
  6-Mercaptopurine (6-MP)
  Azathioprine (Imuran)

Others
  Actinomycin C
  Cortisone and analogs

---

agents, antimetabolites, and others (Table 17-1). *Alkylating agents* contain labile alkyl groups and react by transferring this group in place of important groups, e.g., amino, sulfhydryl, carboxyl, hydroxyl, and phosphate groups, resulting in alkylation of nucleoproteins. Biologic alkylation is quite complex, but the great body of evidence indicates that DNA is the main target of alkylating drugs. The electron donors in DNA are the nitrogen atoms of its purine and pyrimidine bases. As a result of alkylation, purines are ripped off the nucleic acid, a process known as *depurination*. When this occurs, the chain of the double helix falls apart. Another effect of alkylation is the formation of rigid links between the chains which block the capacity for DNA replication in dividing cells and stop mitosis. Because of their profound effects on cell growth, thousands of alkylating agents have been synthesized. The actions of these drugs are similar to those of X-rays; hence they are called *radiomimetic* drugs. The most promising agent at present is cyclophosphamide (Cytoxan), which suppresses immune responses more effectively than do doses of X rays of corresponding toxicity. The immunosuppressive effect of cyclophosphamide is short-lived and can be demonstrated only for a short period after the drug has been injected. The immune response and the lymphoid tissues recover promptly after injection is stopped. This drug is extremely active and exerts a powerful immunosuppressive action, especially in rodents. Recent studies have shown that a single large dose of cyclophosphamide can inhibit B-cells and antibody production while permitting an increase in cell-mediated immunity. Chromic administration of cyclophosphamide will depress both cell-mediated and humoral immune responses. Like other alkylating agents, cyclophosphamide can exert a carcinogenic action.

The *antimetabolites* are analogous to various DNA and RNA precursors and in excess are thus able to antagonize competitively the synthesis of DNA and RNA. These drugs were originally tested for their ability to suppress immune response because of their inhibitory effects on tumor cell division. Two kinds of analogs are well known, i.e., purine antagonists and folic acid analogs.

The prototype of purine antagonists is 6-mercaptopurine (6-MP), originally conceived as a simple analog of adenine. However, its biologic action is far more complex than its chemical formula suggests (Fig. 17-1). Two main steps are affected by 6-MP: purine biosynthesis and the utilization of inosinic acid. Purine synthesis in cells is controlled by a feedback mechanism in which purine ribonucleotides inhibit an enzyme, phosphoribosylpyrophosphate amidotransferase, essential for its first step. 6-MP is converted to a purine ribonucleotide, a fraudulent nucleotide that leads to a deceptive end product inhibiting *de novo* synthesis of purine. A second conversion product of 6-MP is thioinosinic acid. Thioinosinic acid, by substituting for inosinic acid, blocks the subsequent steps of pu-

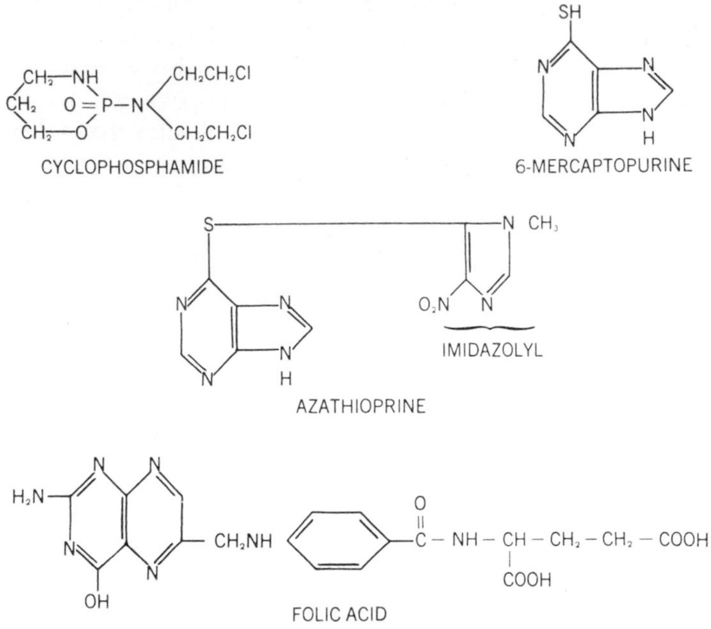

Fig. 17-1. Important chemical immunosuppressants.

rine synthesis, including the formation of adenine and guanine, the purines of nucleic acid. The cells affected by 6-MP thus manufacture substances able to disrupt their own synthetic processes.

Another purine analog of considerable importance is azathioprine. In this compound the H atom at position 6 of 6-MP is replaced by an imidazole ring (Fig. 17-1) resulting in a higher therapeutic effectiveness in mice and dogs. 6-MP and azathioprine are currently used as basic immunosuppressive drugs for kidney transplantation in man.

Folic acid, an essential vitamin, is converted to tetrahydrofolate by an enzyme, dihydrofolate reductase. Tetrahydrofolate converts deoxyuridylate to thymidylate, which is the rate-limiting nucleotide in DNA synthesis. Methotrexate (MTX), the principal folic acid analog, acts by inhibiting dihydrofolate reductase, the enzyme required to convert folic acid to its active form, tetrahydrofolate. Methotrexate actually binds the enzyme and has relatively little effect on RNA synthesis. Therefore, affected cells stop dividing. Such cells can, however, continue to synthesize RNA and protein resulting, for example, in megaloblastosis.

The biologic effects of cytotoxic drugs are a function of the administered dose. In high doses, lymphocytes may be killed directly, resulting in nonspecific general immunosuppression. When smaller doses are given, more actively proliferating cells are killed selectively. Since contact with an appropriate immunogen activates sensitive lymphocytes to proliferate, maximum immunosuppression may be obtained at lowest toxicity when the drug is given at the time of antigenic challenge. However, the optional time of immunosuppressive treatment in relation to the immunogenic stimulation can vary. Recently Santos (1972) classified all immunosuppressive agents according to the relationship listed in Table 17-2.

In addition to their toxic effect on cells essential to the body economy, immunosuppressive drugs of these classes have the drawback that they suppress the immune responsive nonselectively. Further, all of these agents are anti-inflammatory, as well as immunosuppressive, and much of their beneficial clinical influence, as well as their toxicity, relates to the latter effects.

In sufficiently large doses these drugs can suppress the secondary and even the tertiary immune responses. When large enough doses of antigen are used with the immunosuppressive agent, they induce specific unresponsiveness to the antigen even though immunity had previously been present.

Table 17-2.   Operational Classification of Immunosuppressive Agents

Class	Common or Generic Names	Trade Name
I (Active primarily when given before immune stimulus)	X-ray Melphalan, L-phenylalanine mustard Mitomycin C Phytohemagglutinin, PHA Cortisone Prednisone	Alkeran
II (Active primarily when given after immune stimulus)	Mechlorethamine, nitrogen mustard (HN2) Triethylenemelamine (TEM) Triethylenethiophosphoramide Chlorambucil Uracil mustard 6-Mercaptopurine, 6-MP Azathioprine 6-Thioguanine Methotrexate, amethopterin Actinomycin D, dactinomycin 5-Fluorouracil, 5FU Cytosine arabinoside, Ara-cytidine, Ara-C Vinblastine, vincaleukoblastine, VLB Vincristine, leurocristine, VCR	Mustargen Thio-tepa Leukeran Purinethol Imuran Cosmegen Fluorouracil Velban Oncovin
III (Active when given before or after immune stimulus)	Procarbazine Cyclophosphamide	Natulan Cytoxan

From Santos, G. W. (1972): In *Transplantation*, Najarian, J. S., and Simmons, R. L. (eds.). Philadelphia, Lea & Febiger, p. 208.

Often the physician must trade off the advantages of treatment for the disadvantages incurred by immunologic crippling and anti-inflammatory action. It is therefore of interest that several experimental models have shown that specific immunosuppression (immunologic tolerance) can be induced in animals treated with cytotoxic drugs together with appropriate amounts of immunogen as shown originally by Schwartz (1965). One mechanism of the development of such a tolerant state is presumed to be selective destruction of activated clones of immunocompetent lymphocytes.

Antilymphocyte Serum (ALS)

Destruction of white cells by immune sera was first described by Metchnikoff in 1899. He showed that guinea pig antisera prepared against spleen or lymph node cells from rabbits or rats agglutinated and killed polymorphonuclear leukocytes of the species used as original cell donors. Sporadic reports have since described effects of various antileukocyte antisera. Perhaps the first demonstration of immunosuppressive effects of ALS *in vivo* was made by Inderbitzen (1956) who showed that skin reaction to tuberculin and dinitrochlorobenzene could be suppressed. Waksman et al. in 1961 made systematic studies of the influence of ALS on a variety of cellular and humoral immune responses. Woodruff and Anderson in 1963 showed that ALS treatment prolongs graft survival in the rat. ALS has since been shown to be one of the most powerful, and in a sense, the only true immunosuppressant agent. ALS possesses some characteristics in common with Ehrlich's "magic bullet." Unlike the chemical immunosuppressants, ALS has the advantage of destroying certain lymphocytes selectively without causing major damage to other rapidly replicating cells in the body. Woodruff and Anderson reported the prolongation of allogeneic skin graft in rats up to 91 days (control 8 days) by combined treatment of rabbit anti-rat antilymphocyte serum combined with thoracic duct drainage. This initial exciting work has been confirmed repeatedly and extended by studies in mice, dogs, monkeys and man.

Despite the encouraging effects of ALS on graft survival, analysis of the potency of a given sample of ALS to suppress the allograft rejection is still difficult. Further, the exact mechanism by which ALS suppresses graft rejection is not known. Its primary action seems to be to destroy selectively the T lymphocytes because these cells are predominantly the circulating and recirculating lymphoid elements. By contrast the B-cells escape to some degree because they are more sessile and not so readily available to the action of the ALS in the blood. ALS has been shown to induce lymphopenia in a variety of species—mice, rats, monkeys, and man. An alternative hypothesis is that the antiserum acts as a competitive immunogen which, having a specific affinity for lymphocytes, preempts the available immunocompetent cells, leaving few free to respond to other

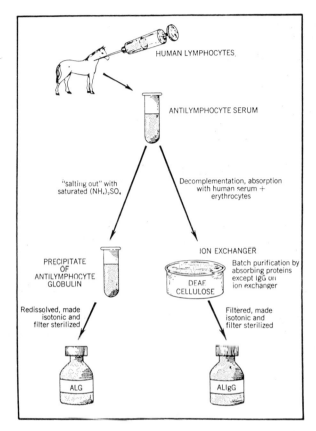

HUMAN LYMPHOCYTES

ANTILYMPHOCYTE SERUM

"salting out" with saturated $(NH_4)_2SO_4$

Decomplementation, absorption with human serum + erythrocytes

PRECIPITATE OF ANTILYMPHOCYTE GLOBULIN

ION EXCHANGER

DEAE CELLULOSE

Batch purification by absorbing proteins except IgG on ion exchanger

Redissolved, made isotonic and filter sterilized

Filtered, made isotonic and filter sterilized

ALG

ALIgG

Fig. 17-2. Schema for production of heterologous antilymphocyte antibody. [From Schwartz, R. S. (1970): *Immunosuppression in Immunology.* Kalamazoo, Michigan, The Upjohn Co., p. 52.]

immunogens. Another hypothesis is that ALS may coat the cell membranes of lymphocytes to prevent recognition of incoming immunogen. Perhaps all of these actions contribute to the immunosuppressive influence of ALS.

Although ALS is so profound a suppressant of the homograft reaction that it has been termed the magic bullet, its administration, particularly in man, has been accompanied by some dangerous side reactions. These are mainly consequent to the fact that it is a foreign protein, and anaphylaxis, serum sickness, renal injury (Masugi type and immune complex type), anemia, pain, edema, and fever occasionally occur with its use. Since ALS has been refined and freed of components other than the antibody against determinants on lymphocytes, adverse reactions other than those attributable to its primary antilymphocytic activity are now somewhat less frequent (Fig. 17-2).

Thymectomy and Thoracic Duct Drainage

In certain strains of mice, rats, rabbits, and hamsters removal of the thymus gland immediately after birth results in lymphopenia, deficiency of lymphoid tissue in spleen, prolongation of allogeneic skin grafts, and deficiency of antibody responses to certain antigens. Selective depletion of lymphocytes can be achieved by chronic thoracic duct drainage both in animals and in man. The results have been more effective when combined with one or more of the immunosuppressants discussed above.

IMMUNODEVIATION—ENHANCEMENT

Immunologic enhancement is the successful establishment or prolongation of allogeneic graft survival by administration of specific antibodies directed against the graft. The concept of enhancement was originally derived from the studies of tumor grafts. The possible mechanisms for this remarkable phenomenon have been discussed in Chapter 16. Although enhancement is a desirable goal for the transplantation of normal tissues, it is a threat to be avoided or thwarted for the control of tumors. Rejection and enhancement of grafts are the expressions of specific immune reactions to tissue alloantigens. The former is mediated principally by sensitized lymphoid cells; the latter reflects the influence of humoral antibody (Kaliss, 1969). The immune response of the vertebrate is biphasic, i.e., cellular and humoral, and these two phases vary in time. Enhancement appears to be dependent upon a relatively diminished effectiveness of cellular immunity and an increase in humoral antibody, probably antibody of high avidity and relatively low cytotoxic efficiency. The enhancing antibody appears to be 7S immunoglobulin, especially IgG α-2 globulins. The induction of enhancement can be passively transferred (Kaliss, 1956), and late hyperimmune sera are more efficient than are early ones.

INDUCTION OF TOLERANCE—UNRESPONSIVENESS

Specific immunologic tolerance may be defined as "a state of reduced or absent immune response to an immunogen or group of immunogens, which would ordinarily evoke a specific response as a consequence of prior exposure to same, or closely related immunogen." The existence of this type of tolerance was predicted by Burnet and Fenner in their theory of "self recognition" (Chapter 15). Although the first experimental evidences interpreted as immunologic tolerance were from allografts in mice, much earlier studies using pneumococcal polysaccharide antigens had been reported by Felton (immunologic paralysis). When tolerance is produced with simple protein antigens, its induction depends on dose of antigen and it is of relatively short duration unless additional antigen is given. The approach of tolerance induction to immunosuppression in treatment of human disease or prevention of unwanted immune reactions, as in graft rejection, has not yet been successful. Already, however, experimental results with defined antigens reveal an extraordinary promise.

Even an adult animal injected with a specific immunogen may be stimulated to produce either an immune response or an unresponsive state to subsequent injections of the same immunogen, depending upon the conditions under which the immunogen is exhibited. This immunologically unresponsive state is specific and differs from nonspecific immunosuppression in that it is directed toward the immunogen used. In the future, induction of tolerance will surely be one of the most powerful means of controlling the immune response.

The principles governing the establishment of immunologic unresponsiveness to any immunogen also apply to immunologic tolerance to histocompatibility antigens. Tolerance is more easily induced in neonatal animals because of their immunologic "immaturity," but it can also be induced in chemically immunosuppressed or irradiated adult animals. If a sufficient amount of antigen is available, tolerance can be induced and manipulated even in adult animals. The induction of immunologic unresponsiveness depends on the dose and nature of the immunogen. In general, more solubilized forms of antigens are more likely to induce unresponsiveness than are insoluble or cellular forms of immunogens. The duration of tolerance is proportional to the persistence of immunogen in the body. Tolerance is better induced when antigens are administered by the intravenous rather than by certain other routes. The degree of tolerance produced by a mixture of histocompatibility antigens is inversely proportional to the so-called strength of the antigen; i.e., it is relatively easy to induce tolerance to the weaker (H1, H3) than the stronger (H2) histocompatibility antigens.

At present the inhibition of allograft rejection relies on blockade of immune response by immunosuppressive agents. The present use of these agents is in the most part nonspecific and results in many undesirable side effects. Therefore, the ideal solution to problems of tissue transplantation is more likely in the future to be found in methods to induce and perpetuate the tolerant state.

IMMUNOLOGIC INTERVENTION

The immune response can be specifically inhibited by appropriate use of immunogens—induction of tolerance—or by passive administration of specific antibody. Suppression of antibody formation by passively administered antibody was shown by Gleny and Hopkins and later studied in detail by Uhr and Baumann in 1961. A great deal of information has since been accumulated as to the mechanisms involved in this dramatic influence (reviewed by Uhr and Möller, 1968).

Two theories attempt to explain the mechanism of antibody-mediated suppression of immune response. One is that passive antibody competes

Table 17-3.   Prevention of Rh Isoimmunization in Pregnant Mothers by Passive Antibody

| | Anti-Rh Response | | |
| | | Sensitized | |
Group	Total	No.	%
Passive antibody	3389	6	0.18
Control	1476	102	6.93

From Uhr, J. W., and Landy, M. (eds.) (1971): *Immunologic Intervention*. New York, Academic Press.

with immunocompetent cells for the immunogenic determinants by the formation of antigen-antibody complexes. Another theory suggests that passive antibody induces a reduction in the number of immunocompetent cells capable of responding to a given immunogen. Recent *in vitro* study by Feldmann and Diener (1970) indicates that *in vitro* effects of antibody-mediated suppression occur at the level of the immunocompetent cell.

The first practical application of this remarkable laboratory phenomenon was made in the prevention of Rh isoimmunization (Table 17-3). Thus the term *immunologic intervention* was used to describe the prevention of a naturally occurring immune response by immunologic means. Following the lead of an interpretation by Levine and Stetson of the experiment of Nature in which women different from their mothers at ABO determinants were noted to develop erythroblastosis less frequently than did women matched with mothers at ABO, Gorman predicted that antibody treatment of mothers with anti-Rh antibody might prevent sensitization and erythroblastosis fetalis. The first experiments were carried out by Stern and Berger who showed that Rh negative male volunteers given anti-Rh antibody along with Rh+ cells did not produce antibody to the latter. These findings extensively confirmed and extended by both Clarke et al. and Freda et al. led ultimately to the demonstration by Pollack et al. that anti-Rh antisera can be effectively used to prevent Rh sensitization and erythroblastosis in man.

Selective removal of lymphocyte subpopulations is another means of eliminating unwanted clones of lymphocytes and achieving immunologic intervention. It has already been shown that it is possible to reduce the number of peripheral lymphocytes (mostly thymus dependent cells) by chronic thoracic duct drainage and thus to prolong the survival of grafts. Selective intervention of immune responses *in vitro* can be achieved by removing antibody-forming cells using an antigen-coated affinity column. For example, a column coated with anti-θ antibody will combine selectively with mouse thymus derived cells bearing θ antigen on the surface and allow all other lymphocytes to pass through, resulting in a selective removal of thymus derived cell population. Similarly, a column coated with a specific antigen will combine with lymphocytes bearing specific antibody on the surface, resulting in selective removal of the particular clonal population of B-cells that have antibody at their surface. These methodologies have already been applied *in vivo,* and in the near future this form of immunologic intervention may be applicable to allografting of tissues, management of autoimmune disease, and perhaps even to the treatment of cancer. Solid immunoabsorption methodology, affinity chromatography can be adapted as a form of immunologic intervention to permit selective removal of antigen, antibody, or Ag-Ab complexes. It also has great potential for prevention and treatment of intoxication or immunologic injury.

AUGMENTATION OF IMMUNE RESPONSE

Immunologists have long been motivated to develop methods for stimulating the immune response. One of their earliest concerns was enhancement of humoral antibody responses. Consequently this focused on a search for methods of immunization that would insure sustained antibody production at a high level. Lewis and Loomis first noted that guinea pigs infected with tubercle bacilli often produced more antibody than did uninfected controls. Ramon (1926) and later Freund (1956) used various products together with specific antigen to increase the antibody response nonspecifically. The products have been termed *adjuvants.* Substances such as alum or other aluminum salts, bacteria endotoxins, and Freund's complete and incomplete mixture (i.e., water-in-oil emulsion with or without dead mycobacteria) are some of the more obvious adjuvants that are frequently used in experimental work. Other substances have been reported to have adjuvant effects. These include alginate, saponin, lanolin, phospholipids, methylcellulose, quaternary ammonium compounds, vitamin A, and silica. In addition, several bacteria, e.g., Bordetella pertussis, Corynebacterium rubrum, Corynebacterium parvum, BCG, and exotoxins from staphylococci and diphtheria bacilli have been used for their adjuvant effects. More recently Johnson et al. and Plescia and Braun have shown that polynucleotides such as poly AU and poly I also may act as adjuvants, and they have attempted to explain much of immune augmentation on the basis of the influence of the breakdown products of nucleic acids.

Despite the widespread and effective use of a great variety of adjuvants, the precise mechanism of their action is not known (Chapter 8). A meaningful dissection of this complex problem would not have been possible before (1) the recognition of the two components of immune system, i.e., cellular and humoral immunity, (2) the identification of the cooperation of T- and B-cells in regulating humoral immune response to certain antigens, and (3) studies of the role of macrophage in the degradation, processing, and concentration of immunogens.

Our goal is, of course, to regulate the various aspects of an immune response to suit the particular clinical situation, for example, enhancement of cellular immunity and suppression of humoral antibody against cancer cells, selective suppression of cellular immunity with increased synthesis of enhancing antibody for successful organ transplantation, or the development of methods to favor the synthesis of certain classes of immunoglobulins such as IgG at the expense of others such as IgE in hypersensitivity disorders.

Old et al. (1959) showed that BCG administration to mice resulted in enhancing cellular immunity to antigens of isogeneic solid tumors. More recently treatment with BCG using experimental chemically induced cancer systems in guinea pigs has been shown to be effective in completely eliminating cancers that have already metastasized. These findings have been extrapolated to therapy of human cancer, and in a few patients dramatic elimination of widely metastatic tumors seems to have been induced.

CELLULAR ENGINEERING

Bone marrow transplantation has been effectively used to reconstitute the immunologic apparatus in children born without either B- or T-cell immunity systems. Similarly, embryonic thymus transplants have reconstituted patients and animals born without a thymus whose immunity systems lack T-cells. In addition, a strange dialyzable factor obtained from sensitized lymphoid cells, the transfer factor of Lawrence, has been used in both animals and man to convert non-reactors to antigens to a capacity for specific reactivity. Transfer factor also has been used in the treatment of human diseases where deficiencies of cellular immunity can be demonstrated to be a significant component of the disease process.

Finally, leukocyte infusions are already being used temporarily to reconstitute or activate host factors, as for example in leprosy by liberation of lymphokines to reconstitute functions secondarily defective to the disease process. These approaches are potentially powerful new means of preventing or treating disease that cannot be managed by other means. How useful they will be as permanent components of the prophylactic or therapeutic armamentarium will be clarified only with time.

IMMUNOPHARMACOLOGY

The immune response with its multiplicity of cellular systems, obligatory cellular interactions, requirements for biologic amplification systems, mediators, and effector mechanisms is only now yielding the secrets of its organization to molecular analysis. It seems certain that a powerful macromolecular and even micromolecular pharmacology is already develop-

ing which can influence, alter, or inhibit crucial stages of these fundamental interactions. These forms of pharmacology first revealed in the
use of antihistamines to prevent symptoms of allergic disease and the use
of epinephrine to minimize dangerous symptoms deriving from immunologic events will be much more extensively developed in the future. Already on the horizon are many new compounds that can inhibit, modulate, or modify immunologic events and consequences of immunologic
events. It is certain that drugs will be developed selectively to interfere
with the development and expression of different components of cellular
and humoral immunity and different components of the complement cascade. Already we are beginning to see the development of endotoxoids
that can interfere selectively with complement activation and with inquiry
to the vascular endothelium. Thus it is already possible with this kind of
macromolecular pharmacology to prevent the Shwartzman reaction.
These are but the beginnings of an immunopharmacology that we can expect to develop apace. It seems certain that within a few years we will be
not only studying the components of the immune response more incisively
but also predicting and controlling the various components at will. The
possibility of this kind of manipulation of the fundamental basis of individuality is staggering to contemplate.

SELECTED REFERENCES

Feldmann, M., and Diener, E. (1970): J. Exp. Med. 131:247.
Felton, L. D. (1949): J. Immun. 61:107.
Finn, R., et al. (1961): Brit. Med. J. 1:1486.
Freda, V. J., Gorman, J. G., and Pollack, W. (1964): Transfusion 4:26.
Freund, J. (1956): Advances Tuberc. Res. 7:130.
Heinecke, H. (1903): Munchen. Med. Wsch. 50:2090.
Heinecke, H. (1905): Grenzgeb. Med. Chir. 14:21.
Inderbitzin, T. (1956): Int. Arch. Allerg. Appl. Immun. 8:150.
Johnson, A. G., Gaines, S., and Landy, M. (1956): J. Exp. Med. 103:225.
Kaliss, N. (1969): Int. Rev. Exp. Path. 8:241.
Kaliss, N., and Kandutsch, A. A. (1956): Proc. Soc. Exp. Biol. Med. 91:118.
Levine, P., and Stetson, R. E. (1939): JAMA 113:126.
Lewis, P. A., and Loomis, D. (1924): J. Exp. Med. 40:503.
Metchnikoff, E. (1899): Ann. Inst. Pasteur 13:737.
Murphy, J. B. (1914): JAMA 62:1459.
Old, L. J., Clarke, D. A., and Benacerraf, B. (1959): Nature (London) 184:291.
Plescia, O. J., and Braun, W. (1967): Advances Immun. 6:231.
Pollack, W., Gorman, J. G., and Freda, V. J. (1969): Progr. Hemat. 6:121.
Ramon, G. (1926): J. Med. Franc. 15:381.
Santos, G. W. (1972): In Transplantation, Najarian, J. S., and Simmons, R. L. (eds.).
    Philadelphia, Lea & Febiger, p. 208.
Schwartz, R. S. (1965): Progr. Allerg. 9:246.
Stern, K., and Berger, M. (1960): Abstract 13th AABB program 39.
Uhr, J. W., and Baumann, J. B. (1961): J. Exp. Med. 113:935.
Uhr, J. W., and Möller, G. (1968): Advances Immun. 8:81.
von Behring, E., and Kitasato, S. (1890): Deutsch. Med. Wschr. 16:1113.
Waksman, B. H., Arbouys, S. and Arnason, B. G. (1961): J. Exp. Med. 114:997.
Woodruff, M. F. A., and Anderson, N. F. (1963): Nature (London) 200:702.

FURTHER READINGS

Good, R. A. (1967): In *Immunopathology*, Miescher, P. A., and Grabar, P. (eds.). Vth International Symposium, New York, Grune & Stratton, Inc.

Hasek, M., Lengerová, A., and Vojtuskova, M. (1962): *Mechanisms of Immunological Tolerance*. New York, Academic Press, Inc.

Skinner, M. D., and Schwartz, R. S. (1972): New Eng. J. Med. 287:221.

Skinner, M. D. and Schwartz, R. S. (1972): New Eng. J. Med. 287:281.

Taliaferro, W. H., and Taliaferro, L. G. (1951): J. Immun. 66:181.

Taliaferro, W. H., and Taliaferro, L. G. (1964): *Radiation and Immune Mechanisms*. New York, Academic Press, Inc.

Uhr, J. W., and Landy, M. (eds.) (1971): *Immunologic Intervention*. New York, Academic Press, Inc.

Uhr, J. W., and Möller, G. (1968): Advances Immun. 8:81.

van Bekkum, D. W., and DeVries, M. J. (1967): *Radiation Chimeras*. London, Logos.

Weigle, W. O. (1967): *Natural and Acquired Immunological Unresponsiveness*. Cleveland, Ohio, The World Publishing Company.

Wolstenholme, G. E. W., and O'Connor, M. (1967): *Antilymphocytic Serum*. Boston, Little, Brown and Company.

18
Bulwarks of the Bodily Defense

Immunity, as a major contributor to survival, has proved to be a most complicated process, the understanding of which is only beginning to emerge. To understand fully the participation of immunity in the bodily defense one must consider cellular and molecular bases of immune reactions, the interrelations of the various cellular systems involved in immunity, the biologic systems by which these interactions can be amplified, and the effector processes that act together to achieve an effective defense. The mammalian host survives in a sea of bacteria, viruses, and fungi, many of which possess the capacity to invade and utilize bodily cells and fluids for their own nutrition and replication. The metabolic products of the microorganism are often toxic to Eutherian hosts, the placental mammals. Defenses against invasion by encapsulated extracellular pyogenic bacterial pathogens, facultative intracellular pyogenic bacteria, fungi, and viruses, as well as against invasion by neoplastic cells, represent major challenges for the immune reactions and their biologic amplification systems. Included among the latter must be the complement system, the kinin and kallikrein systems, production of lymphokines by T-cells, and release of histamine and other vasoactive amines. Cells of these have the function of engaging the effector mechanisms which include inflammation, phagocytosis by macrophages and microphages, coagulation of the blood, and reactivity of small vessels and lymphatics. As separate processes and as integrated systems of defense these effector mechanisms preserve the integrity of the individual.

Using evidence gathered in recent years from the study of patients with hereditary immunodeficiencies, immunodeficiencies associated with malignancies of the lymphoreticular apparatus, and from experimentally produced immunodeficiencies, we have been able to delineate some major bulwarks of the bodily defense. In this chapter we will suggest constellations of infection that may assist the practicing physician in recognizing certain immunodeficiencies and understanding new syndromes associated with infection. We further hope to provoke a new approach to the classification of pathogens of Eutherians and suggest new treatments for some infections of man.

267

DIFFERENTIATION OF THE TWO LYMPHOID SYSTEMS

Compelling evidence that the major roles in immunologic defense are to be divided into two separate systems of lymphoid cells, each of which employs different amplification systems to achieve its full potential in the bodily defense has been presented in Part I (Fig. 3-5). It seems clear that the hematopoietic tissues, e.g., yolk sac, fetal liver, and bone marrow contain a multipotent progenitor cell. Depending upon its movement this cell can respond to different microchemical environments and thereby differentiate along a variety of lines representing the definitive hematologic components. For example, these cells can differentiate to erythrocytes, granulocytes, megakaryocytes, eosinophils, or basophils, depending upon the microchemical environment in which the progenitor cell finds itself during the developmental process. Another direction of differentiation is to a lymphoid stem cell, which may develop in the yolk sac, fetal liver, or bone marrow. This lymphoid stem cell can be further differentiated into either of two separate populations of lymphoid cells, depending upon the nature of a second differentiative environment. One of these populations differentiated under thymic influence, probably actually within the microchemical environment of the thymus, represents a system of small lymphocytes, many of which are long lived, that percolate through the lymphoid tissues and in the lymph and blood. This system of cells in its fully differentiated forms has a strong propensity to reside in specialized areas or zones (thymus dependent zone) in the peripheral lymphoid organs, e.g., in lymph nodes and spleen and along the gastrointestinal tract. It represents an extraordinarily mobile system of cells, which can function as a veritable "flying squadron" capable of subserving the functions of cell-mediated immunity.

This lymphocytic system is to be sharply separated from a second system of lymphoid cells which in its fully differentiated form represents a more sessile population of cells responsible for production of circulating antibodies. This population of cells, too, tends to be located within rather specialized areas of the peripheral lymphoid organs (thymus independent zones). In fully differentiated form these cells represent veritable factories for production and secretion of the immunoglobulin molecules and the antibodies they represent. The site or sites in man where differentiation to the antibody-secreting, immunoglobulin-producing cells occurs (i.e., bursa equivalent) is not known, but in birds it appears to be confined to a peculiar lymphoepithelial organ located at the posterior end of the gastrointestinal tract, the bursa of Fabricius. The cells representing this line of differentiation possess an admirable machinery for protein synthesis and secretion and often have the appearance of plasma cells (Fig. 4-4). It seems no longer germane to argue whether lymphocytes or plasma cells synthesize antibodies. They both do, but when they are capable of executing this function they represent the end result of a specific line of differentiation which separates them distinctly from the line of differentiation of the population of long-lived small lymphocytes responsible for the cell-mediated immune response.

THYMUS DEPENDENT AND THYMUS INDEPENDENT AREAS OF PERIPHERAL LYMPHOID ORGANS

The population of small lymphocytes developing under thymic influence tends to reside in regions in the peripheral lymphoid organs and tissues that are rather specialized and that are separate (although overlapping of territories surely exists) from the regions in the lymph nodes and spleen that house the cells which produce antibodies (Fig 4-6). Such organization within the lymph nodes holds for mice, rabbits, guinea pigs, and man and thus represents an organization widespread in nature. In lymph nodes, the thymus dependent regions are located in the deep cortical or paracortical zones, whereas the far external cortical regions, the juxtamedullary areas, and the medullary cords represent thymus independent regions of the nodes. The germinal centers, which represent thymus independent structures, regularly appear within the thymus independent areas.

The populations of lymphoid cells in the peripheral lymphoid organs can be induced to proliferative expansion by antigenic stimulation. If appropriate antigens are chosen, the dual lymphoid populations can be expanded separately. For example, after intradermal injection of pneumococcal polysaccharide into the guinea pig or rabbit, which will bring about only antibody production, the lymphoid cells in the thymus independent regions proliferate and plasma cells develop in the medullary cords. By contrast, stimulation of the regional node at the base of the ear by topical application of 2,4-dinitrochlorobenzene (DNCB) or intradermal injection of DNP-bovine gamma globulin brings about proliferation of cells in the deep cortical region of the node without producing proliferative response in the far cortical regions or in medullary cords, and plasma cell formation is minimal or does not occur at all. In other words, appropriate antigenic stimulation which brings about either cell-mediated immunity or antibody formation, but not both, will stimulate independent proliferation and further differentiation of either the thymus dependent or thymus independent system of cells. However, most antigenic stimuli provoke both cell-mediated immunities and antibody production, leading to expansion of both populations of lymphoid cells.

EFFECT OF NEONATAL THYMECTOMY

In 1960 it was discovered that removing the thymus in rabbits or rodents in the immediate neonatal period will interfere with development of immunologic capacity. In mice, considerable strain differences have been observed in this influence, and the cleanest models have been obtained in both mice and rabbits when sublethal, total-body irradiation is given in the neonatal period to the thymectomized animals. Although some confusion was introduced by the fact that thymic influence was initially discovered with respect to antibody production, it soon became apparent that the major influence of thymic extirpation was on the ability to develop and execute the cell-mediated immune responses. Mice thymectomized as neonates or thymectomized and irradiated as neonates develop as immunologic cripples. Such animals cannot develop delayed allergy or reject allografts of skin. The lymphoid cells from their blood, thoracic duct, lymph nodes, or spleen will not initiate a graft-versus-host reaction, and they cannot resist infections with certain bacteria, fungi, and viruses. By contrast, such animals have normal amounts of each of the known immunoglobulins and can make antibodies as well as can normal animals when stimulated with appropriate antigens, e.g., Brucella, Salmonella, or flagella antigens.

Neonatally thymectomized mice and rabbits, however, are defective in producing antibodies to sheep red blood cells (SRBC), as well as to certain soluble protein antigens, but it has become clear that even with these thymus dependent antibody responses the actual production of antibody is achieved by thymus independent lymphoid cells and plasma cells. There is evidence that the thymus dependent lymphoid cells exert a helping role. By now it is certain that this helper function does not imply the existence of antigen sensitive cells which exchange information with antigen insensitive cells of the thymus independent system as was suggested first. In mice thymectomized at birth and in addition given near-lethal X-irradiation, the antibody production to SRBC is minimal, or absent. If such mice are given larger numbers of SRBC or are repeatedly stimulated with SRBC, antibody responses will usually occur and will achieve titers approximately equal to those of mice that have undergone sham operations and that possess an intact thymus dependent system of cells. Neonatally thymectomized and irradiated mice respond with antibody synthesis as do normal mice or those that have had sham operations to antigenic stimulation with Brucella or Salmonella antigens. It is now also clear that intact thymus dependent cells stimulated with antigen produce molecules that in some way prepare the B-lymphocytes for response to the thymic dependent antigens. The nature of these molecules is not yet clear.

THYMUS INDEPENDENT LYMPHOID SYSTEM

Plasma cell production, germinal center development, and lymphocyte concentrations in the far cortical regions are normal in mice from which the thymus has been removed (either in the neonatal period or in adulthood) that have also been subjected to near-lethal, total-body irradiation. Such animals are prone to infections with fungi, viruses, and pyogenic pathogens of otherwise low-grade virulence. When they become infected, they can often achieve marked elevations of immunoglobulin levels and seem very likely to develop autoimmune phenomena and amyloidosis.

Glick et al. (1956) had discovered that extirpation of the bursa of Fabricius early in life prevents development of normal ability to produce circulating antibodies against bacterial antigens. His experiments were elegantly confirmed by Wolfe and his collaborators with a variety of antigens and by Warner and Szenberg in Australia. The latter group, comparing hormonally bursectomized birds and hormonally and surgically thymectomized birds, had concluded that in chickens the bursa functions primarily to influence the development of the antibody-synthesizing capacity and that the thymus functions primarily in the development of homograft rejection capacity.

Already in 1962, Waksman and his associates in Boston were arguing that for the rat all antibody synthesis and all forms of cellular immunities were to be dissociated and that all cellular immunities were under thymic influence. An extensive series of experiments of Cooper et al. showed clearly that in chickens antibody and immunoglobulin synthesis develop under control of the bursa of Fabricius, whereas cell-mediated immunities, including ability to develop and express delayed allergy, solid tissue homograft rejection, and ability to initiate graft-vesus-host reactions, are dependent upon the thymus. The thymus dependent system of lymphoid cells in the chicken includes small lymphocytes in circulating blood and concentrations of small lymphocytes in the classic white pulp of the spleen and in the tiny little lymph nodes of these animals. By contrast, the bursal dependent system of lymphocytes and plasma cells includes the germinal center type follicles of the spleen, lymph nodes, and gut-associated lymphoid tissue and the plasma cells in all locations of the body.

Chickens exposed to near-lethal irradiation at hatching often grow up agammaglobulinemic, lacking both IgG and IgM immunoglobulins, and are unable to form antibodies even after repeated antigenic stimulation if the irradiation has been coupled with removal of the bursa of Fabricius. On the other hand, such chickens possess circulating lymphocytes that will initiate graft-versus-host reactions after intravenous injection into chick embryos, and they can develop and exhibit normal delayed allergic skin reactions and homograft rejections. Indeed, they can reject allografts, even to the degree of white graft rejection. By contrast, chickens irradiated and thymectomized in the newly hatched period grow up having normal concentrations of both IgG and IgM immunoglobulin. They make antibodies to numerous antigens only slightly less vigorously than do intact chicks and possess normal numbers of plasma cells and germinal centers in their spleen and lymph nodes. Such chickens, however, cannot develop delayed allergy, reject skin homografts, or launch a graft-versus-host reaction. In both neonatally thymectomized rodents and irradiated thymectomized chickens the lymphoid cells show deficient responses *in vitro* to phytohemagglutinin (PHA), to antigens with which the host has previously been stimulated, and to allogeneic cells. Chickens that have been irradiated and bursectomized at hatching possess circulating lymphocytes that respond normally to PHA, allogeneic cells, or antigens. Thus, in both groups of experimental animals the proliferative responses of peripheral blood lymphocytes to antigenic stimulation sort out with the cell-mediated, thymus dependent immune responses and are to be separated from the humoral immune responses.

To be absolutely certain that the development of capacity for immunoglobulin and antibody synthesis was dependent upon the bursa of Fabricius, it was desirable to avoid the unknown and to some extent unanalyzable influences of X-irradiation or of the hormones 19-nortestosterone and testosterone propionate. In short, Minnesota workers were able to demonstrate that complete *in ovo* removal of the bursa of Fabricius prior to the seventeenth day of embryonation often produced animals with both 19S IgM and 7S IgG hypogammaglobulinemia or agammaglobulinemia. These animals also lacked both plasma cells and germinal centers. If the bursectomy was completed after the seventeenth day but before the nineteenth or twentieth day of embryonation, the chicks were frequently dysgammaglobulinemic, lacking 7S IgG immunoglobulins but possessing apparently normal amounts of IgM immunoglobulin. Such chickens, when they could be studied 6 to 9 weeks after hatching, possessed normal or near normal numbers of plasma cells, made IgM antibodies normally, and showed both primary and secondary memory responses restricted to the IgM type of antibody; however, they lacked IgG and IgG antibodies, and germinal center development was extremely deficient.

THE GERMINAL CENTER

The above findings relate in still another way to the enigma of the germinal center. The germinal centers have been related to memory phenomena in immune responses by studies of Thorbecke et al. and to 7S IgG synthesis by phylogenetic analysis. In the latter studies, it was found that the development of capacity for germinal center formation was not present in phylogenetic forms immediately preceding the avians but may have appeared earlier in forms ancestral to modern lungfish and amphibians. The latter two groups are the most primitive vertebrates with the ability to synthesize immunoglobulins having both 19S and 7S types of heavy chains. In sharks, paddlefish, Mississippi dogfish (Amia calva), and marine teleosts 19S and 7S immunoglobulins and antibodies are to be found, but these immunoglobulins appear to possess a common heavy chain and thus do not represent antecedents of the two separate IgM and IgG immunoglobulins. Such animals have not been found to possess a germinal center type of organization. By contrast, the lymphoid tissues of both amphibians and lungfish seem to possess structures strikingly similar to the germinal centers found in mammalian lymphoid tissues, and these animals have two separate types of immunoglobulins with different heavy chains.

Consequently the germinal centers may be viewed as specialized sites in which apparently wasteful proliferation of lymphoid cells may occur in order, perhaps, to concentrate both antigen and antigen sensitive cells. This apparently wasteful proliferation, similar to that which occurs in the thymus and probably in cortical areas of bursal follicles, may be necessary to achieve dilution of some kind of derepressor and permit the lymphoid cells to arrive at a point in differentiation where a switch from IgM to IgG immunoglobulin synthesis can occur.

By clinical and experimental analysis it has been shown that germinal centers of man and rabbits contain antigen together with IgM or IgG antibodies and complement. These accumulations of immunoglobulins are capable of fixation of additional complement and thus of acting as antigen-antibody complexes. The latter are not contained within cells, but the immunoglobulin-antigen-complement complexes can be readily eluted, apparently from the surfaces of the dendritic reticulum cells.

In further experiments, it has been shown that bursectomy carried out, even after hatching, selectively prevents production of certain kinds of antibodies and responses to certain specific antigens but will not influence responses that have developed earlier. Among the later developing immune responses that can be inhibited by late extirpation of the chicken bursa is formation of certain antibodies of the anaphylactic type. Analysis of the questions raised by these experiments obviously will require much additional study, but the experiments indicate clearly that the final chapter in the story of the sequential influences of the bursa of Fabricius in development of the several types of immunoglobulin-producing cells has not yet been written.

THE MAMMALIAN BURSA EQUIVALENT

In analyzing the major bulwarks of bodily defense for Eutherians, we must of course be careful not to misinterpret or overemphasize these important studies in chickens. The lessons learned from the study of chickens, which present a definitive site of differentiation of the immunoglobulin-producing cells, have made it abundantly clear that the design of experimental models in mammals will be a crucial factor in obtaining equally penetrating results and avoiding misinterpretation of data suggesting the existence of a bursal equivalent in the mammal.

Studies with mice and rabbits irradiated and thymectomized in the neonatal period and of these same animals irradiated and thymectomized at more advanced ages indicate clearly that for mammals an equally sharp contrast exists between thymus dependent and thymus independent components of lymphoid tissue. Consequently, it has become a major challenge to determine the location in mammals of the differentiative influence that provides the focus for development of immunoglobulin- and antibody-producing cells. Although efforts to define the bursal equivalent in mammals have proceeded now for several years, full definition is not yet at hand. Studies in the rabbit have been interpreted to indicate that the bursal equivalent site, or a major component of the critical site, resides in certain gut epithelium-associated lymphoid tissue (GALT). By inference then, the lymphoid tissue of the appendix, Peyer's patches, and intestinal tonsils or sacculus rotundus could very possibly represent the bursal equivalent of other mammals and man or could be a special expanding site for cells of the B-cell system.

Like the chickens subjected *in ovo* to bursectomy, rabbits subjected in early life to complete extirpation of the GALT, or to irradiation plus extirpation, are very prone to infection and have a defective capacity for antibody response. Whether in other mammals and man this function is concentrated in the GALT is not known at present. From extirpation of the gut in sheep during embryonation, rather compelling evidence has been presented to indicate that in this mammal no area along the gastrointestinal tract plays a determinant role in development of the antibody-forming cells.

To us, it is not crucial that differentiation of the thymus independent cells be attributable to gut epithelium-associated lymphoid tissue in all or any mammals at all stages of embryonic development. Both phylogenetic and ontogenetic perspective reveals that several distinct sites have provided the differentiative influence for development of red blood cells. Yolk sac and fetal liver and bone marrow are the successive sites for this differentiative influence in ontogenetic development; the anterior kidney, gonad, and spleen play the same critical role in red blood cell differentiation during phylogenetic development before the bone marrow becomes the focus of this activity. Only quite late in phylogeny does the differentiative influence move to bone marrow. The important point from these analyses is that the differentiative influence for development of antigen-responsive lymphoid cells of the antibody-producing system and for immunoglobulin synthesis can be separated from the influence for development of cells subserving cell-mediated immunity. Studies to date indicate that this important dichotomy exists in all mammals and man, as well as in birds.

PRIMARY IMMUNODEFICIENCY DISEASES OF MAN

The genetically determined primary immunodeficiency diseases of man have so far provided the single most important evidence for the separate bulwarks of the bodily defense. They also serve as the prime support for the two-component immunologic model described here. Summarized in Figure 18-1 is an analysis of the levels of blockage in immunologic development thus far defined in the primary immunologic deficiencies of

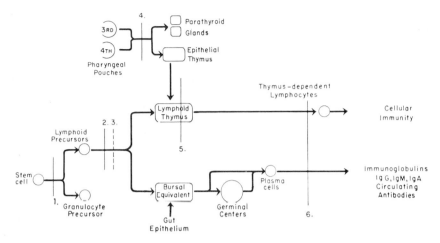

Fig. 10-1. Schematic diagram depicting points in immunologic development at which blocks might occur leading to various immunologic disorders. [From Hoyer, J. R., et al. (1968): In *Immunologic Deficiency Diseases in Man*, Good, R. A., and Bergsma, D. (eds.). Birth Defects Original Article Series, vol. 4, New York, National Foundation Press.]

man. It will be seen from the figure that patients have been described whose immunologic deficiency may be attributed to a block at the basic progenitor cell (block 1). In such patients not only lymphocytes and plasma cells fail to develop but also platelets, granulocytes, and red blood cells. The condition transmitted as an apparent autosomal recessive has thus far been extremely rare, and the patients have survived only a few days; consequently, they have not been sufficiently studied. The extreme nature of this lack of cells that serve as bulwarks against infection is implicit, however, in the rapid demise of these infants, even when maintained in the most protected environment.

Two genetic variants that reflect a block at the lymphoid stem cell stage (blocks 2 and 3 in our theoretical scheme) are now well known. In one of these groups the genetic fault is transmitted as an autosomal recessive characteristic. The defect, at least in some families, is associated with extreme deficiency of adenosine deaminase in the patients, and parents have values for this enzyme lower than normal but not so low as the patients. Both lymphocyte lines fail to develop normally, and plasma cells and small lymphocytes may be virtually absent from peripheral blood, bone marrow, and peripheral lymphoid systems. The thymus is almost entirely epithelial and represents an apparent early embryonic arrest in development. This condition has been called the Swiss-type agammaglobulinemia because Swiss investigators published the initial description and have been most actively involved in its analysis; it is also known as the lymphopenic agammaglobulinemia syndrome (Chapter 19). Since both systems of immunologic lymphoid cells are deficient and even lacking in the patients, development of the lymphoid system must be arrested sometime before the establishment of the cellular dichotomy. The considerable phenotypic variability that has been encountered within families in which the disease occurs may become more extreme as the disease is better defined and can be identified as one or more enzyme defects. Some patients with severe combined immunodeficiency disease do not have the deficiency of adenosine deaminase in the blood or tissue cells, even though they show clear evidence of a genetic defect transmitted as an autosomal recessive trait.

Similar to these patients and perhaps even more variable in the extremeness of expression of the lymphoid tissue deficit are patients suffering from a dual system of immunologic deficiency inherited as either a sex-limited or sex-linked recessive trait. These patients have similar deficiencies of their lymphoid and plasma cell systems in both central and peripheral lymphoid organs, their circulating lymphocyte counts are regularly low, and the numbers of small lymphocytes in the blood are clearly deficient. Like the patients with Swiss-type agammaglobulinemia, patients with sex-linked lymphopenic immunologic deficiency cannot survive, and death is attributable to infection with a variety of pathogens, including many different kinds of bacteria, viruses, fungi, and Pneumocystis. Neither parents nor patients with this syndrome lack adenosine deaminase, the enzyme that is lacking in patients having the autosomal recessive form of combined immunodeficiency. Recently, transplantation of bone marrow has restored complete immunologic competence of both thymus dependent systems of lymphoid cells in several patients with both autosomal recessive and X-linked lymphopenic immunologic deficiency.

A third type of immunodeficiency is the so-called DiGeorge syndrome (Chapter 19). Infants suffering from this disease fail to develop epithelial anlagen derived from the third and fourth pharyngeal pouches (block 4). These anlagen, after full differentiation, develop into thymus, parathyroids, and probably those clear cells of the thyroid responsible for calcitonin production. Infants with DiGeorge syndrome are generally brought to the pediatrician with hypoparathyroidism expressed as neonatal tetany. Thus, it is possible to recognize them, to analyze their immunologic deficiencies early, and to treat their deficiencies. Although they have normal immunoglobulin levels and nearly normal antibody responses to some antigens, children with DiGeorge syndrome lack a thymus dependent system and cannot cope normally with many kinds of infection. They have proved to be vulnerable to progressive infections with fungi, e.g., Candida. They cannot control infection with atypical acid-fast organisms of low-grade virulence and they often succumb to generalized infections with low-grade pyogenic pathogens, vaccinia virus, the virus of cytomegalic inclusion disease, or the measles virus. When exposed to opsonized bacteria, the granulocytes of patients with both lymphopenic immunodeficiency and the DiGeorge syndrome will phagocytize and kill the ingested organisms normally.

As was the case with children who suffer from the combined immunologic deficiency, it was the study of experimental models that led to the postulation that the deficiency of patients with DiGeorge syndrome might be cured if an appropriate thymic transplant could be achieved. Following directly this line of reasoning, Cleveland (1968) et al. transplanted a thymus from a human fetus to a patient with DiGeorge syndrome. The operation resulted in prompt establishment of immunologic function and provided evidence that the thymus is important in bodily defense. These findings have subsequently been confirmed in almost every detail by successful transplants of fetal thymus by August et al. (1968), Gatti et al., Biggar et al., and Fitzpatrick et al. (unpublished). Still more recently, Aiuti and associates have treated patients with the so-called Nezelof syndrome successfully by thymus transplantation. Two such patients having marked deficiency of T-cell numbers and functions were completely restored to full immunologic vigor by fetal thymus transplants. These remarkable feats of cellular engineering reveal a great potential for the future.

Another primary immunodeficiency of major importance in considering the bulwarks of bodily defense is the agammaglobulinemia first described by Bruton (1952) (Chapter 19). One form of this disease is sex-linked, is of very infrequent occurrence, and is associated with defects of immunologic function that are strikingly selective for the humoral immunities. These patients produce immunoglobulins very poorly or not at all and lack both plasma cells and germinal centers in their lymphoid tissues. They have normal or near-normal capacity to develop all of the cell-mediated immunities.

The patterns of infection that plague these children are dramatically different from those that prove fatal to children with DiGeorge syndrome or either form of lymphopenic immunologic deficiency syndrome. First of all, children with Bruton-type agammaglobulinemia are rarely sick during the first 6 months of their lives, since they are protected by antibodies derived from their mothers. By contrast, patients with lymphopenic agammaglobulinemia develop infections during the early weeks. Secondly, the infections in Bruton patients who have not been treated by injections of gamma globulin are predominantly those attributable to the high-grade, encapsulated, pyogenic pathogens. Pneumococci are the most frequent offenders; Haemophilus influenzae, streptococci, meningococci, and Pseudomonas aeruginosa also produce frequent infections. On the other hand, BCG vaccination, histoplasmosis, Candida infections, Brucella infections, and many virus infections evoke a vigorous immune defense in these patients. They can be immunized by vaccination with vaccinia virus. The reactions to vaccination develop, as do those of normal persons, into typical primary immune reactions. Upon subsequent exposure to vaccinia virus an accelerated immune reaction will occur and upon still a greater exposure an immediate reaction often is encountered. These immune reactions may develop in the absence of any demonstrable antibody titers for the virus. These patients can develop immunity to both chickenpox and measles; they develop the typical exanthema, and yet antibody responses to these agents may not be demonstrable.

In contrast to their extreme susceptibility to pneumonia, septicemia, meningitis, skin infections, conjunctivitis, and sinopulmonary infections with the encapsulated pyogenic pathogens, patients with Bruton-type agammaglobulinemia have little clinical trouble with recurrent viral or fungal infections or infections with Enterobacteriaceae, Klebsiella, or Serratia marcescens. They do, however, seem to be unusually susceptible both to infection with hepatitis virus and its progressive destructive effects and to Pneumocystis carinii. It is not so difficult to understand how defense against encapsulated pyogenic pathogens might require ability to form opsonins and a vigorous antibody response that could utilize the complement system for amplification of phagocytosis and even direct destruction of these organisms. By contrast, a major bulwark against fungus infections and infections by low-grade pyogenic pathogens, particularly the facultative intracellular pyogenic pathogens, is provided by cell-mediated immune responses which utilize the amplification mechanism of the activated or "angry" macrophages nonspecifically stimulated by a process set in motion by the thymus dependent lymphocytes. How the patients who lack gamma globulins and are unable to produce circulating antibodies, defend themselves so effectively against many viruses is far from clear, but from the study of the infections to which patients with Bruton-type agammaglobulinemia are most prone, together with study of patients with other immunodeficiencies, it is quite clear that a major bulwark of the bodily defenses against most viruses resides in the functions of the thymus dependent lymphoid system and in the biologic amplification system or systems that cell-mediated immunity can muster. Nonetheless, these patients also teach us that immunity to and recovery from some virus and Pneumocystis infections cannot be primarily attributed either to interferon or to cell-mediated responses. Much additional work needs to be done to meet the important challenge placed before us by this experiment of Nature in clinical immunobiology.

An example of the new definition of defense mechanisms that has been derived from clinical studies of immunologically deficient patients is represented by the children with the sex-linked recessive Wiskott-Aldrich syndrome (Chapter 19). These children suffer from a primary immunologic deficiency disease based upon failure to handle and respond normally to polysaccharide antigens. Rather paradoxically, there also develops in such patients a progressive deficiency of cell-mediated immunities that is apparently secondary to their difficulty in handling the polysaccharide antigens. These children also are born with profound deficiency of production of blood platelets. At present, the fact that they cannot survive seems to be due to their extreme susceptibility to infections with a wide variety of bacteria, viruses, and fungi to an extraordinary susceptibility to lymphoid malignancy and to their propensity to bleed excessively, especially during infectious episodes. Therapeutically, Bach et al. (1968) have achieved a long-lasting bone marrow transplant from a matched sibling which seems to have corrected, at least in part, some of the defects of a child with the Wiskott-Aldrich syndrome.

Until Thieffry et al. (1961), surveying immunologic parameters, discovered the association of ataxia-telangiectasia with the absence of IgA in the serum, the repeated sinopulmonary infections in patients with ataxia-telangiectasia were considered to be a function of the inadequate respiratory exchange consequent to the progressive neuromuscular disease in these patients. However, it is now clear that approximately 60 to 70 percent of patients with ataxia-telangiectasia lack IgA in the circulation, in their saliva, and in both nasopharyngeal and gastrointestinal secretions. A crude correlation was established between the IgA deficiency and susceptibility to frequent sinopulmonary infections in these patients. In the meantime, Heremans and Crabbé obtained evidence implicating IgE as a bulwark of defense of the gastrointestinal tract. Patients having ataxia telangiectasia have a deficiency of IgE as do other healthy members of their family. Further, they regularly have a defect of cellular immunity associated with deficient development of the thymus and thymus dependent lymphoid system. The basis of the increased susceptibility to infections of patients with ataxia-telangiectasia seems to be associated with the broad immunodeficiency of IgA, IgE, or cellular immunity and not with any particular defects. Why these patients do not develop gastrointestinal infections and sprue with greater frequency than they do remains an enigma. Very recently Waldmann and co-workers have found evidence that the liver in such patients is immature. As a reflection of this, alpha fetoprotein is present in large amounts in their serum. This finding is of special interest, since we earlier showed that the thymus of these patients is regularly embryonic in appearance.

SECONDARY IMMUNODEFICIENCIES

The secondary immunodeficiencies accompanying several malignancies of the lymphoreticular system provide additional support for interpretations concerning the major defense mechanisms against infections. Patients with Hodgkin's disease have long been known to express peculiar vulnerability to tuberculosis, to fungal infections, and infections with certain viruses, especially the pox and herpes viruses (Chapter 36). These patients likewise show a selective defect of immunologic functions which

10

worsens with progression and dissemination of the malignant disease. The immunologic deficiency of the patient with Hodgkin's disease is peculiar in that the use of intact cells from highly sensitized donors to transfer cellular immunity to this patient regularly fails, in contradistinction to regular transferability of this form of allergy to nonsensitive, but immunologically normal persons. On the other hand, untreated patients with Hodgkin's disease usually have at least normal levels of each of the known immunoglobulins. Although minimal deficiencies of primary antibody response in patients with Hodgkin's disease have been described, most untreated patients with this disease satisfactorily produce antibodies to many antigens. Further, they possess plasma cells and achieve plasma cell proliferation and germinal center formation after antigenic stimulation as do immunologically normal persons. Even though the thymus is quite normal in most patients with Hodgkin's disease, it must be concluded that their immunologic deficiency represents largely a perturbation of function of the thymus dependent lymphoid system.

In rather striking opposition to the set of immunodeficiencies observed in patients suffering from Hodgkin's disease are those encountered in patients with multiple myeloma (Chapter 36). In this malignant disorder, involving the thymus independent plasma cell line of differentiation, one sees great perturbation of immunoglobulin synthesis and humoral immune functions. Regardless of the cells and the type of immunoglobulins present in excess, deficiencies of antibody production and synthesis of each of the normal immunoglobulin classes are the rule. By contrast, cell-mediated immunities, like delayed allergy and allograft immunity, often show normal vigor. In contradistinction to the kinds of infections experienced by patients with Hodgkin's disease, patients with myeloma, just as the children with Bruton-type agammaglobulinemia, suffer from recurrent episodes of pneumococcal pneumonia, septicemia, and meningitis due most often to high-grade encapsulated pyogenic pathogens. Thus, patients with myeloma, which clearly represents a malignant deviation of the B-cell immunity system, have major deficiencies of function of the B-cell immunity system, but their T-cell immunity system not basically involved in their malignancy continues to function well.

Patients with chronic lymphatic leukemia (Chapter 36), too, experience profound and often progressive secondary immunodeficiencies. Like the children with lymphopenic agammaglobulinemia, adults with chronic lymphatic leukemia have dual-system immunodeficiencies even early in the course of their hematologic diseases. In most instances, however, this disease has been shown by a variety of new methods to represent a monoclonal expansion of B-lymphocytes. Usually the monoclonal expansion of B-lymphocytes involves IgM-producing lymphocytes which have *either* kappa *or* lambda light chains. A few cases have been shown to be monoclonal expansions of B-lymphocytes of the IgG or IgA class. A rare case of chronic lymphatic leukemia, on the other hand, has been found to be due to extensive expansion of a T-lymphocyte population. This seems to be true also in the Cesaris syndrome.

Surprisingly, children with acute lymphatic leukemia usually have normal immunoglobulin levels and usually can form circulating antibodies quite well. They are able to reject allografts of skin with vigor and to develop and express cell-mediated immunities as do normal persons. Of course, following prolonged antileukemic and immunosuppressive treatment they may develop iatrogenic hypogammaglobulinemia and immunologic deficiency. The cellular defects primarily associated with their malignant transformation include deficiency of red blood cells, platelets, and granulocytes. It is now known that the so-called lymphoblastic cells in acute lymphoblastic leukemia are generally not B-cells. At least some may be T-cells.

From study of the secondary immunodeficiencies of man and from the infections characteristically associated with each of these diseases we would conclude that the specific immunologic inadequacies and the constellations of infection that develop in patients with malignancies of the lymphoreticular apparatus provide firm support for the view that certain subcomponents of the immune response are especially concerned with defense of the body against a particular set of microorganisms. A corollary to this view is that one can begin to derive a classification of microorganisms in terms of the specific form of bodily defense which the mammalian organism has evolved to cope with potential invasion and injury by specific groups of pathogens. Since analysis of both microorganisms and constellations of infection is only beginning, the ultimate usefulness of this approach as compared, for example, to Gram's staining cannot yet be appreciated. Its basis in fundamental ecologic interrelationships makes this an attractive basis for classification. A most dramatic example of the impact of this new view of the microbial universe has been revealed in a study of host-parasite relations in the fatal or chronic granulomatous disease of childhood. In this disease both B-cell and T-cell immunity systems are intact, but the phagocytic mechanism is defective. Certain bacteria can be engulfed normally by phagocytes, but the organisms are not killed with the usual vigor after phagocytosis. This defect of killing capacity is due to an enzyme deficiency that interferes with the normal production of H_2O_2 by the phagocytes of such children. Such defective microphages and macrophages can kill the catalase-negative organisms like pneumococci and streptococci but cannot kill the catalase-positive staphylococci, Klebsiella-aerobacter, paracolon bacilli, Serratia marscescens, or fungi. Consequently, children who have the "Achilles heel" represented by this inborn error of metabolism, have one life-threatening infection after another due to staphylococci, Klebsiella-aerobacter, Serratia marscescens, or fungi because a major bulwark of the bodily defense is lacking or defective and a certain population of microorganisms is not destroyed during phagocytosis.

BIOLOGIC AMPLIFICATION SYSTEMS AND EFFECTOR MECHANISMS

The cell-mediated immunities do not utilize in obvious ways the complement system. The classic complement system consists of interacting proteins, polypeptides, and enzymes and represents an extraordinary biologic amplification mechanism for those humoral immune responses that are based on production of IgM and IgG immunoglobulins (Chapter 11).

Antibodies execute biologic effects by combination with antigens and by activation of other biologic systems. The means by which immunity is ultimately expressed is of great interest to clinicians. A whole galaxy of cellular products that are involved in cellular and humoral responses has been described in recent years. These factors may be produced by, or be called into play by, lymphocytes reacting with specific antigen in cell-mediated immune responses (Fig. 18-2). Whether there are many such factors, e.g., the migration inhibition factor (MIF), cytotoxic factor, macrophage stimulation factor, chemotactic factor, or a recruitment factor such as transfer factor or *in vitro* transfer factor, or whether these observations reflect a number of different biologic assays for one or several mediators will only be determined by comparative biochemical studies and comparative bioassays. Perhaps from these studies will come further understanding of other mechanisms of bodily defense afforded by cell-mediated immune reactions.

The details of the intimate relationship of lymphocytes to histiocytic cells and macrophages in inflammation also will require further intensive

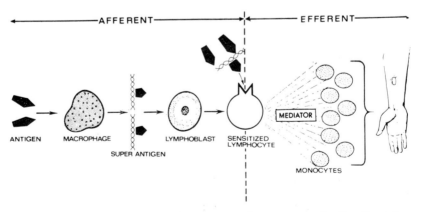

Fig. 18-2. Schematic representation of biologic amplification system of cell-mediated immune response. The macrophage ingests and processes antigen to produce a "super antigen" capable of sensitizing lymphocytes which then initiate chemotactic mediator(s). Monocytes are summoned into an area by such mediator(s). [Modified from Chilgren, R. A., et al. (1969): Lancet 1:1286.]

analysis. There can be no doubt, however, from the studies of Mackaness and his associates (1969) that activation of macrophages represents one means by which cell-mediated immunities can alter the capacity of the body to rid itself of microorganisms. These investigations show that specific cellular immunity associated with delayed allergy can bring into play extraordinary amplification mechanisms in the bodily defense by activating histiocytic cells or macrophages to increased vigor in destroying a number of different facultative intracellular bacterial pathogens. The changes induced in the macrophage population that bring about increased capacity for killing Listeria monocytogenes, BCG organisms, and other facultative intracellular bacterial pathogens include (1) increase in size and mobility of the phagocytic cells, (2) increase in numbers and size of the cytoplasmic organelles, e.g., lysosomal particles, and (3) increase in phagocytic activity and increase in number of monocytic phagocytes through induced proliferation. These changes of the macrophage, in addition to their recruitment in inflammation, occur only after stimulation by lymphoid cells which have themselves been aroused by contact with a specific antigen to which cell-mediated immunity has been induced. This nonspecific change in an effector cell population represents another extraordinary biologic amplification system which, like the complement system, can be brought to bear by specific immunologic reactions. In this instance, however, it is cellular immunity rather than IgG or IgM dependent humoral immunity which activates the nonspecific host response to achieve the increased destruction of the microorganisms. Other major biologic amplification systems involved may be in cell-mediated immunity.

It seems likely that this mechanism stands as a major bulwark not only against the facultative intracellular bacterial pathogens but also against fungi. Could this also be the means by which cellular immunity defends against certain viruses? It can be said almost without argument that virus-neutralizing antibodies represent one major element of defense against both recurrent and continuing virus infection. It also seems almost axiomatic that interferon represents an important nonspecific bulwark of defense that can be brought to bear to facilitate recovery from virus infection. While the biologic importance of these mechanisms is accepted, it is most provocative that defense against many virus infections, as seen through the clinical experiments of nature, involves cell-mediated immunity in a most fundamental and essential way. Progressive vaccinia, overwhelming Hecht's pneumonia as a reflection of rubeola infection, fatal varicella infection, progressive inclusion body virus disease, and perhaps a host of other infections like generalized fungal infections, BCG infections, and progressive destructive infection by other facultative intracellular pyogenic pathogens seem to relate more to cell-mediated immune deficiencies than to ability to produce circulating antibodies and immuno-

globulins. The modus operandi of the bodily defense and of the amplification resources used in the cellular defenses against viruses has not yet
been clarified. The role of "angry" macrophages and other means of cellular destruction that might be brought to bear on host cells containing
virus or against viruses directly needs much further analysis. It seems
certain that clinical experience will play a crucial role in achieving this
understanding. Further, the establishment of the clinical significance and
the importance in the body economy of interactions, obligatory or not, of
the two separate cellular immunity systems in achieving most effective
antibody production requires further assessment.

Studies of the genetic perturbations of the biologic amplification systems and the significance of these disturbances as a basis for increased
susceptibility to infection is only beginning to be recognized (Chapter
20). In these experiences, as in study of specific immunologic deficiency,
evidence of specialization within the systems for major roles of defense
against particular sets of pathogens has already been forthcoming. An
inherited abnormality of granule morphology and doubtless of lysosomal
function, as yet poorly defined, appears to underlie the increased suscepti-

Table 18-1. Constellations of Infection

Pathogens	Primary Bodily Defense Mechanism
Pneumococcus Haemophilus influenzae Streptococcus Meningococcus sp. Pseudomonas aeruginosa Hepatitis virus Pneumocystis carinii	Humoral immune responses
Rubeola Varicella Vaccinia Cytomegalic inclusion disease virus Mycobacterium tuberculosis Candida albicans Histoplasma	Cellular immune responses
Staphylococcus Klebsiella sp. Aerobacter aerogenes Serratia marcescens Candida albicans Aspergillus Nocardia	Leukocyte bactericidal function

Three groups of microorganisms are arranged according to the primary mechanism
of host defense against each pathogen. These constellations of infection have been
assembled mainly from clinical experience with patients suffering from immunodeficiency diseases and chronic granulomatous disease of childhood.

bility to infection observed in the Chediak-Higashi syndrome (Chapter 21). Similarly, abnormalities in capacity of polymorphonuclear leukocytes and monocytes to kill phagocytized fungi or bacteria normally underlie the lethality of fatal or chronic granulomatous disease of childhood (Chapter 21). In table 18-1 are summarized certain constellations of infection that relate to particular deficiencies of the bodily defense.

It is certain that, just as study of the defects of the two individual components of the lymphoid system and the one defect of phagocytic function have yielded evidence of major bulwarks of body defense against particular organisms, studies of additional human diseases based on deficiencies of development of the complement system, kallikrein-kinin system, inflammatory functions, and phagocytic activities will provide further evidence of crucial components of the defense mechanisms geared to cope with major threats from the microbial universe. Already, for example, from study of the inherited defects of the complement system, we can see evidence for the crucial role of the third component of complement and the membrane attack of the C5-9 portion of the complement system. Further, we see evidence that the early complement components protect against lupus erythematosus and vascular disease (Chapter 20). These are only beginnings, and continued studies of the rare patients with unusual susceptibility to disease by modern tools of immunobiology, biochemistry, and molecular biology will yield major dividends in understanding how, in health, we maintain our individuality and defend ourselves against such a versatile population of organisms that might find invasion of our bodies attractive. Thus clinical disease in the future will be found to reflect deficiencies of the chemotactic process, lymphokine production, bactericidal functions of complement, mobilization and function of phagocytic cells, and interactions and communications between the two immunity systems, the biologic amplification systems, and the major effector processes.

IMMUNOLOGIC SURVEILLANCE AGAINST MALIGNANCY AND AUTOIMMUNITY

Although a mountain of evidence has been accumulated to indicate both the reality and importance of immunologic surveillance against cancer, only a brief summary of clinical evidence of the nature of this bulwark against internal invasion will be given here. The incidence of cancer in patients with each of the different kinds of primary immunologic deficiency is far in excess of that in members of the general population. In those with Bruton-type agammaglobulinemia, leukemias predominate. This complicating disorder has occurred 6 times among 70 patients with this disease. This incidence is between 1000 to 10,000 times the frequency of occurrence in the general population and does not seem to extend to other malignancies. These children lack only humoral immunities. Carcinomas, epitheliomas, solid tissue sarcomas, and Hodgkin's disease have not yet been found in them. On two occasions thymus involvement occurred early in the course of the leukemia, and apparently the disease either began in the thymus or involved the thymus dependent lymphoid system in a major way early in the course of the disease. In this regard, it is of interest that Gorer (1958) presented evidence in experimental animals that circulating antibodies can represent a major form of immunity against leukemias but do not seem to be nearly so important for immunity against tumors. The inordinate susceptibility to leukemia of children with a genetically determined lack of antibody-producing capacity further argues that the humoral immune mechanism may represent a major bulwark against occurrence of malignancy involving dispersed hematopoietic or lymphoid cells.

The malignancies observed in patients with the late-occurring immunologic deficiency, whose deficiency involves both cellular and humoral systems, have included gastric and colonic carcinomas, epitheliomas, reticulum cell sarcomas, lymphomas, and leukemias. Indeed, nearly the whole range of those malignancies that occur with greatest frequency in man have turned up in such patients. Similarly, patients with ataxia-telangiectasia have had malignancies of a wide range of types, including lymphosarcomas, reticulum cell sarcomas, Hodgkin's disease, and carcinomas. Numerically the lymphoreticular malignancies dominate these listings. In the Wiskott-Aldrich syndrome, in which the inherited deficit seems to involve the afferent limb of the immune response, the malignancies appear to be quite uniformly reticulum cell sarcomas and lymphomas. The incidence of successful malignant adaptation in these three groups of patients has exceeded 10 percent and may reach even higher levels as reporting becomes more complete. Malignancy has also occurred in lymphopenic agammaglobulinemia. Thus, in most forms of primary immunodeficiency of man, malignancy occurs with inordinate frequency; this finding is concordant with the view that the immunologic system stands as a major bulwark against malignant adaptation. Here, however, as with the infectious diseases, we see evidence that bodily defense must be highly selective. In children with the primary immunodeficiencies, for example, all malignancies are not occurring with inordinate frequency. Neuroblastomas, Wilms' tumors, retinoblastomas, for example, do not seem to be occurring too frequently in children suffering from the primary immunodeficiencies. Instead, leukemias, lymphosarcomas, gastric carcinoma, and colonic carcinomas are more prevalent. Why? The most likely reason is that, as with microbial infections, many mechanisms of bodily defense stand against invasion by malignant cells just as many forms of defense stand against bacterial, virus and fungus infections. Dissection of these mechanisms in the future will be based on studying and correcting the deficiencies in those individuals and families where the defenses against particular forms of cancer are defective. The deficiency of DNA repair based on a missing enzyme in xeroderma pigmentosum and increased susceptibility to induction of transformed cells in Down's syndrome, familial myelogenous leukemia, and Klinefelter's syndrome represents evidence for "intracellular defenses" perhaps as important or more important than the immunologic defenses against cancer.

Recent studies of patients receiving immunosuppressive therapy to prolong or prevent allograft rejection have indicated that they have a susceptibility to transplantation of cancer as well as to the development of primary malignancies. During the past several years more than 75 primary malignancies have been encountered among patients under effective immunosuppression, often including antilymphocyte serum. This incidence of cancer again exceeds that expected for persons of the same age in the general population. The kinds of primary malignancies observed under these conditions include the full gamut of malignancies that are frequent in man, e.g., lymphomas, reticulum cell sarcomas, leukemias, anaplastic carcinomas, epitheliomas, and Hodgkin's disease. Here again, however, lymphoreticular malignancies have occurred with the greatest frequency. This experiment of Nature in a test situation again provides substantial evidence that an intact immune systems stands as a major bulwark of defense against cancer.

In clinical medicine further support for this view derives from evidence of the flagging of immunologic vigor that occurs with aging. This loss of immunologic vigor is reciprocal to the increasing incidence of cancer with aging in both man and animals. Further, once a malignancy has developed in a person, the chances of a second primary cancer developing seem in some studies to be greater than normal. This finding is consistent with observations that cell-mediated immunities may become progressively deficient with the extension of malignancy in man. Further, evidence recently accumulated by the Hellströms argues strongly that the lymphoid cells of patients with neuroblastoma exhibit an immunity to the tumor tissue which is somehow neutralized by an antibody or antibody-like substance circulating in the serum of these patients (Chapter 15).

From studies in experimental cancer biology, the immunologic bulwark against the internal invasion represented by cancer has gained abundant support, and it has even appeared reasonable to postulate an essential relationship between malignancy, the lymphoid system, and immunity. Basically, the reflection of this bulwark argues that for cancer to succeed, immunologic surveillance of vigor of the immune mechanism must be compromised. The failure of immunologic surveillance may be generalized or local and may represent a highly specific deficiency of a more broadly based one.

It seems eminently clear that major bulwarks of the bodily defense stand as well against neoplastic invasion from within as they do against micro-bial invasion from without. The dissection and resolution of the specific details of the nature of the bulwarks against specific forms of internal invasion and the extension of analysis of the defenses against external invasion by microorganisms will surely continue to depend heavily on those extraordinary experiments of Nature represented by genetic faults that reveal specific deficits and their biologic implications so clearly.

SELECTED REFERENCES

August, C. S., et al. (1968): Lancet 2:1210.
Bach, F. H., et al. (1968): Lancet 2:1364.
Bruton, O. C. (1952): Pediatrics 9:722.
Cleveland, W. W., et al. (1968): Lancet 2:1211.
Cooper, M. D., et al. (1966): J. Exp. Med. 123:75.
Gatti, R. A., et al. (1968): Lancet 2:1366.
Glick, B., Chang, J. S., and Jaap, R. C. (1956): Poult. Sci. 35:224.
Gorer, P. A. (1958): Ann. N. Y. Acad. Sci. 73:707.
Hellström, E., et al. (1968): Proc. Nat. Acad. Sci. U.S.A. 60:1231.
Heremans, J. H., and Crabbé, P. H. (1968): In Immunologic Deficiency Diseases in Man, Good, R. A., and Bergsma, D. (eds.). Birth Defects Original Article Series, vol. 41. New York, National Foundation Press, pp. 298-307.
Mackaness, G. B. (1969): J. Exp. Med. 129:973.
Thieffry, S., et al. (1961): Rev. Neurol. (Paris) 105:390.
Thorbecke, G. J., et al. (1967): In Germinal Centers in Immune Responses, Schindler, R., and Congdon, C.C. (eds.). Berlin, Springer-Verlag, pp. 259-269.
Waksman, B. H., Arnason, B. G., and Jankovic, B. D. (1962): Exp. Med. 116:187.
Waldmann, T. A., and McIntire, K. R. (1972): Lancet 2:1112.
Warner, N. L., and Szenberg, A. (1964): In Thymus in Immunobiology, Good, R. A., and Gabrielsen, A. B. (eds.). New York, Hoeber-Harper, pp. 395-411.

19
Immunodeficiency Diseases

The delineation and treatment of immunologic defects require a conceptual framework for understanding the immune response in man, just as the specific diagnosis and therapy of anemia require knowledge of iron metabolism, hemoglobulin synthesis, and erythrocyte production. The complexity of the immune system is reflected in the multiplicity of its disturbances and derangements. More than 20 types of deficiency in immunity that have been described form a complex of syndromes which superficially appear to fit no pattern.

CLASSIFICATION OF IMMUNODEFICIENCY DISEASES

The classification of primary and secondary immunodeficiency diseases shown in Tables 19-1 and 19-2 is based on the current concept of cellular basis for the development of adoptive immunity (Fig. 18-1, page 275). Stem cells from bone marrow have the capability for differentiating into two defined lymphoid cell populations. T-cells are responsible for cellular immunity and are dependent on the thymus for their differentiation. They may become cytotoxic for certain target cells, and upon stimulation they release several effector substances primarily aimed at stimulating macrophages, enhancing inflammation, or destroying foreign cells. The second population, B-cells, functions to synthesize antibody. They are for the most part independent of thymus function. Many of the immunodeficiency syndromes conform well to the model. However, some of the syndromes cannot be explained or understood on the basis of our current framework and are included in the group called common variable immunodeficiency.

Recent demonstration of adenosine-deaminase deficiency in infants with defective cellular immunity (Giblett et al., 1972) has provided for the first time the possibility of classifying immunodeficiency diseases in molecular biologic terms. A standard method for evaluation of cellular and humoral immunity in patients has been recommended by the World Health Organization (WHO) Committee (Fudenberg et al., 1971).

INFANTILE X-LINKED AGAMMAGLOBULINEMIA

Male infants with agammaglobulinemia usually remain relatively well during the first 6 months of life, probably because of passive protection

Table 19-1. Classification of Primary Immunodeficiency Diseases

Type	Cellular Defect		Genetics
Infantile X-linked agammaglobulinemia	B	Recurrent infection with extracellular pyogenic pathogens	X-linked recessive?
Selective immunoglobulin deficiency (IgA)	B°	Bronchitis, sinusitis, malabsorption, steatorrhea, or remain healthy	Unknown (autosomal recessive?)
Transient hypogammaglobulinemia of infancy	B	Recurrent infection with extracellular pyogenic pathogens	Familial (genetic?)
X-linked immunodeficiency with hyper-IgM	B°	Recurrent infection, thrombocytopenia, aplastic and hemolytic anemia	X-linked?
Immunodeficiency with low IgM	B	Recurrent infection	
Thymic hypoplasia (pharyngeal pouch, or DiGeorge syndrome)	T	Usually die in infancy, frequent virus, fungus, or pneumocystis infection	No evidence
Episodic lymphopenia with lymphocytotoxin	T	Recurrent infection, lymphopenia	?
Immunodeficiency with normal globulinemia or hyperimmunoglobulinemia	B T†	Recurrent pneumonia	?

	B T S		
Immunodeficiency with ataxia-telangiectasia	B T	Frequent sinopulmonary infection in cases with low IgA	Autosomal recessive
Immunodeficiency with thrombocytopenia and eczema (Wiskott-Aldrich syndrome)	B T	Frequent infection with virus, fungi, and pyogens	X-linked recessive
Immunodeficiency with thymoma	B T	Recurrent infections with pyogens, sometimes with virus, fungi	?
Immunodeficiency with short-limbed dwarfism	B T	Short-limbed dwarfism, lymphopenia	Autosomal recessive?
Immunodeficiency with hematopoietic hypoplasia	B T S	Rarely survive beyond first few weeks of life	
Severe combined immunodeficiency (a) Autosomal recessive (b) X-linked (c) Sporadic	B T S B T S B T S	Recurrent infection, failure to thrive	
Variable immunodeficiency	B T	Recurrent infection primarily with both viral and bacterial pathogens	Autosomal recessive?

B: B-cells T: T-cells S: stem cells

* Involve some but not all B-cells.
† Encountered in some but not all patients.

Table 19-2.   Examples of Secondary Immunodeficiency Syndromes

---

Defective Cellular Immunity
1. Malignancy, e.g., Hodgkin's disease
2. Infection or granuloma, e.g., leprosy, sarcoid, rubella, measles
3. Obstruction of lymph flow, e.g., intestinal lymphangiectasia
4. Aging
5. Chronic lymphatic leukemia
6. Nutritional deprivation
7. Surgery

Defective Humoral Immunity
1. Decreased synthesis of immunoglobulins, e.g., lymphoreticular malignancy, malnutrition
2. Increased catabolism of immunoglobulins, e.g., nephrotic syndrome, myotonic dystrophy
3. Increased loss of immunoglobulins, e.g., enteropathy, exfoliative dermatitis, burns
4. Increased synthesis of pathologic immunoglobulins coupled with decreased synthesis of normal immunoglobulin and antibodies, e.g., multiple myeloma, macroglobulinemia
5. Monoclonal malignant deviation of the B lymphoid cells as in chronic lymphatic leukemia, certain lymphosarcomas, with defective production of normal immunoglobulin antibodies and deficiency of T-cells

---

afforded by maternal γ-globulin. Undue susceptibility to infection becomes evident during the second half of the first year of life. However, depending on the environment in which the child is reared, the onset of frequent infection may sometimes be even further delayed. These children almost invariably contract infection with pyogenic organisms, principally pneumococci, streptococci, Pseudomonas, meningococci, and Haemophilus influenzae. The infections are usually readily controlled with antimicrobial chemotherapy. These infants rarely survived beyond infancy before the era of antibiotics. Purulent sinusitis, pneumonia, septicemia, meningitis, and skin abscesses are the most common types of infection. They may be persistently recurrent until proper prophylactic therapy is undertaken. Untreated, many of these children develop chronic progressive bronchiectasis and ultimately die of the pulmonary complications if they survive the innumerable acute septic infections. Agammaglobulinemic children do not seem to have increased susceptibility to many common viral diseases or the exanthems of childhood. They usually sustain measles, mumps, varicella, and rubella in quite ordinary fashion. The enterobacilli are not usually invasive in affected children. Deaths from Pseudomonas aeruginosa sepsis and pneumonia, as well as from Pneumocystis carinii have frequently occurred, however, in agammaglobulinemic infants and young children with this form of disease. Some patients having pneumocystis infection have been successfully treated with pentamidine isethionate.

Many affected boys develop arthritis, particularly of the larger joints.

This complication disappears once replacement therapy with gamma globulin has been begun. Other collagen-like diseases have been observed in children with agammaglobulinemia. A syndrome resembling dermatomyositis has been reported in these patients. Biopsy and autopsy material show lymphocytes infiltrating around the small blood vessels. Similar involvement of the central nervous system has been observed with progressive, ultimately fatal neurologic disease. Neither steroids nor immunosuppressive agents have proved useful in ameliorating the downhill course of this complication, which may be due to the effects of an unidentified or slow virus. Adenovirus type 12 and ECHO virus type 9 were cultured from several organs from two patients at the time of death.

Hemolytic anemia, drug eruptions, atopic eczema, poison ivy, allergic rhinitis, and asthma have been observed with a high frequency in agammaglobulinemic patients. However, a wheal and flare reaction associated with active atopic immunity usually cannot be elicited.

The study of large number of kindreds with multiple occurrences of congenital agammaglobulinemia has revealed an X-linked pattern of inheritance. In addition to the occurrence of the disease in brothers, the diagnosis has been established in boys whose sisters subsequently had male offspring with the disease.

The serum of children with congenital agammaglobulinemia regularly contains less than 100 mg of IgG per 100 ml. Serum IgA and IgM concentrations are usually less than 1 percent of normal adult values, and both IgA and IgE are absent or very low. The isohemagglutinin levels are low or nil. A positive reaction to the Schick test in the presence of a history of diphtheria-pertussis-tetanus immunization will be elicited. Antigenic stimulation with any of a number of antigens fails to provoke an antibody response. With sensitive methods of antibody measurement, low levels of antibody to certain animal viruses and phage particles can sometimes be demonstrated. In other patients, however, the sensitive immunologic methods have failed to detect antibody in serum even after intensive immunization. The small amount of gamma globulin present in the serum may not be inert.

It is not uncommon to observe either leukopenia or striking leukocytosis in patients with agammaglobulinemia at the time of severe pyogenic infections. Lymphocyte counts are normal (more than 2000 cells/mm^3). Delayed hypersensitivity reactions of both the tuberculin and the skin contact type are usually intact, although they may be quantitatively reduced in some patients, perhaps as a consequence of their infections. The former can be universally demonstrated with intradermally injected Candida antigen, with killed vaccinia virus after vaccination, or with tuberculin after infection with BCG, and the latter with dinitrochlorobenzene (DNCB) applied to the skin as a patch test after suitable stimulation with a vesicant dose of DNCB. The response of peripheral blood lymphocytes to phytohemagglutinin (PHA) is normal, and these cells make normal amounts of macrophage inhibitory substances. Allograft rejection is also intact.

The sine qua non of the diagnosis of X-linked agammaglobulinemia is the demonstration that plasma cells are not to be found in lymph nodes stimulated with antigen. The basic defect in the disease is, in fact, the absence of plasma cells from the lymph nodes, spleen, intestine, and bone marrow. It has been pointed out that without careful quantitative studies bone marrow is a poor site to ascertain whether or not plasma cells are present in normal numbers in young children. Lymph node biopsy after antigenic stimulation has been the best means of establishing the diagnosis. With newer methodologies for quantitating numbers of B-cells in the circulation by fluorescent microscope studies, the absence of lymphocytes that have immunoglobulin in receptor distribution at their surface by fluorescent microscope studies may be a more quantifiable and readily available diagnostic test. Studies of biosynthesis of immunoglobulin have shown that the lymphocytes of patients with X-linked infantile agammaglobulinemia cannot synthesize γ-globulins.

In addition to the absence of plasma cells from the usual sites, the lymph nodes show characteristic features, including deficient numbers of cells and absence of germinal centers in the far cortical areas of the node and well-developed lymphocyte accumulations in the deep cortical areas

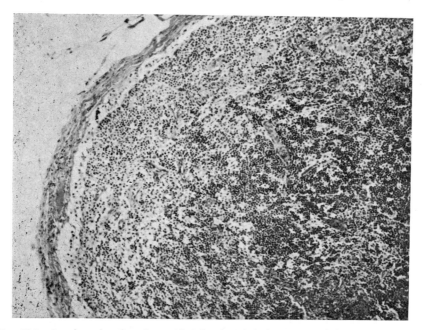

Fig. 19-1. Lymph node of patient with infantile X-linked agammaglobulinemia showing the absence of germinal centers.

(Fig. 19-1). Hypoplasia of the tonsils seen on examination of the oropharynx is an important clue to the diagnosis. Roentgenograms of a lateral view of the nasopharynx will reveal that the paucity of adenoid tissue results in a widened airway. Hyperplasia of the reticulum cells may be apparent after antigenic stimulation in patients with agammaglobulinemia and may become so striking as to produce persistent lymphadenopathy in older children. The thymus gland is normal.

The injection of gamma globulin has proved to be effective in preventing the severe recurrent pyogenic infections in these patients. The effective prophylactic dose of gamma globulin has been established empirically. Raising the serum level of gamma globulins approximately 200 mg/100 ml, usually prevents invasive bacterial infections. To achieve the desired level, a newly diagnosed patient is given 1.8 ml, or 300 mg, of gamma globulin per kilogram of body weight, usually in three divided doses of 0.6 ml (100 mg) per kilogram. This raises the serum concentration by about 300 mg/100 ml. Since the half-life of the gamma globulin injected is 24 to 30 days or more in these patients, they must receive γ-globulin injections every 3 weeks to 1 month in a dose of 0.6 ml (100 mg) per kilogram to maintain the desired level of approximately 200 mg/100 ml. Smaller doses are less effective.

We have not found it necessary to give prophylactic antibodies to these patients who are receiving monthly injections of adequate doses of gamma globulin. Antibiotic therapy is used only to treat specific infections that may supervene, and these respond satisfactorily to such therapy.

Standard gamma globulin fractions cannot be given intravenously; severe pyogenic and cardiovascular reactions follow intravenous injection in many recipients, particularly those who are acutely ill. The noxious effects have been attributed to aggregation of small amounts of gamma globulin during preparation procedures.

Barandun et al. noted in dose response studies that patients with antibody deficiency syndromes tend to have a high incidence of and greater susceptibility to adverse reactions to intravenously injected gamma globulin. After intravenous administration 93 percent of such recipients had such reactions, whereas only 13 percent of control subjects exhibited untoward effects. When such reactions have been experienced, the patient remains in a tolerant or refractory state to further intravenous challenge for 4 or 5 days. The more pronounced the reaction, the more lasting this strange tolerance.

During intravenous infusion, reactors first experience tachycardia and respiratory distress, facial flushing, a sensation of pressure in the chest, and flank pain. These initial symptoms are followed by chills, fever, pallor, and malaise. In more serious reactions nausea, vomiting, and circulatory collapse occur.

Several approaches to rendering gamma globulin safe for intravenous use have been attempted. In Western Europe a preparation of pepsin-treated gamma globulin, marketed as Gammavenin, has been used. The half-life of the $F(ab')_2$ fragment of this digestant is very short, less than 1 day. Treatment of gamma globulin with plasmin has resulted in less drastic alteration in the size of the molecules but permits complete dis-aggregation. Swiss workers have treated gamma globulin by reducing the pH of the solution to 3.5 to 4.0 and incubating it at 37° C for 24 hours. This "acid-treated" gamma globulin has been used extensively in Switzer-land. It has, however, a tendency to reaggregate on storage. Successful prophylaxis has been achieved with plasmin-digested gamma globulin administered intravenously, but this preparation has not yet been ap-proved for routine use.

Commercial gamma globulin preparations contain only trace amounts of IgA and IgM. No preparation of these immunoglobulins is currently available for clinical use. To circumvent this difficulty whole plasma in-fusion by a "buddy system" has been successfully used to achieve pro-phylaxis against infection. The buddy system employs a single donor or very few donors known to be free of Australia antigen and to have no history of hepatitis. Their plasma can then be obtained by plasmaphore-sis, and one unit can be infused every month to control susceptibility to infection.

SELECTIVE IMMUNOGLOBULIN DEFICIENCIES

The development of immunoelectrophoretic techniques led to a more precise definition of immunoglobulin defects in several situations in which the hypogammaglobulinemia involved one or two of the immunoglobu-lin groups while levels of the others were normal or elevated. Six combi-nations of the deficits of the three major immunoglobulins are obviously possible, although only two of these have been reported extensively. There have been many attempts to classify these abnormalities, and at present it is more confusing and less helpful to abide by one or another system of designations of dysgammaglobulinemia than to describe the immunoelectrophoretic stigmata of the defect under discussion. It has been estimated that about 1 in 200 random hospital admissions in major medical centers now represent some form of selective immunoglobulin deficiency.

The isolated absence of IgA from the serum occurs in a significant but small proportion of the normal population. IgA deficiency has been asso-ciated with steatorrhea and nontropical sprue. Such patients lack IgA-producing cells in the lamina propria of the intestinal tract where such cells are normally found in greatest abundance. Many patients with con-nective tissue disease and 70 to 80 percent of patients with ataxia-telan-giectasia lack serum and secretory IgA.

Although familial lack of IgA is well documented, the mode of inheritance of the defect is not clearly established. Several patients with absence of IgA have circulating anti-IgA antibodies which may result in rapid catabolism of IgA and plasma transfusion reactions.

Selective IgM deficiency has been associated with septicemia in the few cases reported. Selective IgG subclass deficiencies have also been found in patients with chronic progressive bronchiectasis. A high incidence of collagen disease has been noted in patients with such selective immunoglobulin defects, particularly those with IgA deficiency. Isolated deficiencies of IgE have been found in family members of patients with ataxia-telangiectasia. This deficiency has usually not been associated with increased susceptibility to infections. However, in several patients deficiency of IgE and numerical and functional defects of lymphocytes in the circulation seem to have been associated with frequent respiratory disease.

When selective deficiency of IgA is coupled with ability to form IgE, a greater propensity to respiratory disease is observed than when IgA and IgE are both lacking.

TRANSIENT HYPOGAMMAGLOBULINEMIA OF INFANCY

The human fetus is capable of forming antibodies *in utero* when adequately stimulated after the twentieth week of gestation. Intrauterine infection with syphilis, cytomegalovirus, rubella virus, or Toxoplasma results in antibody synthesis by the fetus. These antibodies are mainly IgM and occasionally IgG or IgA.

In normal circumstances the full-term human newborn infant is endowed with maternal IgG so that umbilical cord serum contains a quantity of gamma globulin similar to that of the maternal serum. Infants born of agammaglobulinemic mothers have no discernible gamma globulin in cord serum. Virtually no maternal IgA and very little maternal IgM traverses the placenta into the fetal circulation. The cord blood contains less than 1 percent of maternal serum levels of IgA, IgD, IgE and IgM. At the very most about 10 percent of the maternal IgM level is reached in cord blood.

The transplacental passage of gamma globulin begins in the third or fourth month of fetal life. Although amniotic fluid contains 20 to 30 mg/100 ml of IgG, there is no direct evidence that this gamma globulin enters the human fetal circulation in significant amounts. It is noteworthy that a sizable amount of maternal gamma globulin leaks from the fetal circulation into the fetal intestinal lumen and provides the newborn infant with intestinal immunity, which can render early oral poliomyelitis immunization ineffective if the mother has a high titer of poliomyelitis antibody.

The transplacental passage of IgG appears to involve an active transport system in the placenta which recognizes some specific structural attribute of the Fc fragment of the IgG molecule. Studies with radio-iodinated proteins injected into pregnant women near term confirm this conclusion.

There is no substantial evidence that maternal colostral antibody is absorbed in significant quantity from the intestine of the newborn infant. There is evidence, however, that breast feeding provides the infant with intestinal immunity and that the IgA molecules in breast milk survive passage into and through the gastrointestinal tract.

The newborn infant upon stimulation after birth starts synthesizing IgM antibodies, and IgM levels rise rapidly; by the end of the first year of life, the infant has normally close to 75 percent of normal adult IgM levels. The newborn infant can also synthesize IgA by the third week of life. The level of this group of globulins tends to rise more slowly and reaches up to 75 percent of normal adult values by the end of the second year. Thereafter, the level rises very slowly throughout childhood. The maternal IgG is slowly catabolized, so that the infant's serum IgG level reaches its low point of approximately 200 to 300 mg/100 ml by the end of the second month of life when infants begin to synthesize significant amounts of IgG. Serum levels of IgG rapidly rise toward normal adult values by the end of 1 year of age (Fig. 22-3, page 356).

No plasma cells can ordinarily be found in the normal newborn infant. As the infant matures immunologically, a concomitant maturation of the lymphoid tissue with organization of follicles and the appearance of plasma cells occur ordinarily during the second or third month of life. In certain infants there is an abnormally prolonged delay in the onset of gamma globulin synthesis, which has been designated *transient hypo-gammaglobulinemia* of infancy. This abnormality appears with equal frequency in males and females. These infants usually recover from this incapacity between 18 to 30 months of age. However, before the onset of normal immunoglobulin synthesis, infants with transient hypogamma-globulinemia may display an undue susceptibility to infections of the skin, meninges, or respiratory tract, usually owing to infections with high-grade encapsulated organisms. Recurrent otitis media, bronchiolitis, and bronchitis are the most common infections in such infants. Multiple cases in a single family have been observed. Lymph nodes display very small or no germinal centers and few, if any, plasma cells. Cellular immunity is intact. The rapid onset of normal B-cell function in these infants suggests that this disease is analogous to allotypic suppression of antibody formation in rabbits. However, no evidence has yet been forthcoming to document this possibility. A search for Gm agglutinators in affected infants and their mothers has not revealed a consistent abnormality. In a few families persistently lower than normal levels of IgG immunoglobulin reflect presence of the disorder even into older childhood. Treatment of these children may in some instances require gamma globulin administration. However, through a negative feedback influence the parenterally administered gamma globulin may contribute to persistence of the immunodeficiency. Thus, it has been our policy to use gamma globulin sparingly in such infants and to treat their intercurrent infections with antibiotics. Stimulation of the immunoglobulin-producing apparatus by killed antigens seems in some instances to hasten development of capacity for antibody production and synthesis.

X-LINKED IMMUNODEFICIENCY WITH HYPER-IgM

One of the common partial immunoglobulin defects is characterized by a deficiency of IgA and IgG and increased amounts of IgM in the serum. The IgM levels range from 150 to 1000 mg/100 ml in these patients. Despite the enormous elevations of the IgM levels, the IgM does not exhibit an M component. The IgM in such patients appears to be composed of normally distributed molecules with antibody activity, associated with the macroglobulins, and to have a normal distribution of κ and λ chains. Several, but not all, of these patients have had an elevation of the serum IgD and IgM subunits. In addition to their undue susceptibility to infection, many of these patients acquire thrombocytopenia, neutropenia, renal lesions, and aplastic and hemolytic anemia, presumably manifestations of autoimmune processes. Administration of exogenous IgG has not been generally noted to decrease IgM levels, although Hitzig and Schlapfer reported that it did ameliorate the severe neutropenia in a boy whom they studied. In a recent report the IgM level was decreased by administration of exogenous IgG in some patients.

The defect can apparently be inherited as an X-linked phenomenon. In one instance, four boys of one kindred and two boys of another were reported to have this defect, and identical twins have been affected. Several of the cases have been found in adult females and older girls in whom the defect appears to be a primary acquired form, but, of course, has a different hereditary basis.

Patients with this syndrome sometimes develop a malignant infiltrative process of IgM-producing cells which proves fatal. Although it usually starts in the gastrointestinal tract, ultimately all the viscera are involved.

Hyper-IgM with immunodeficiency has frequently been associated with congenital rubella.

CONGENITAL THYMIC APLASIA (DIGEORGE SYNDROME)

Far less is known of the ontogeny and perinatal physiology of cellular immunity in man than of the immunoglobulins in the fetus and newborn. DiGeorge observed that a congenital anomaly may result from the failure of embryogenesis of the entodermal derivatives of the third and fourth pharyngeal pouches (Fig. 18-1, page 275). This leads to aplasia of the parathyroid and thymus glands. This abnormality has not shown a famil-

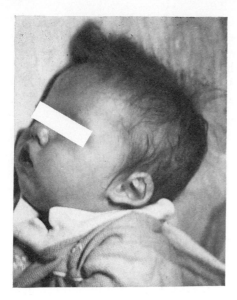

Fig. 19-2. Characteristic ears and face of
an infant with DiGeorge syndrome.

ial incidence and does not appear to be hereditary but seems rather to be
the consequence of some intrauterine accident. All infants with this
syndrome thus far studied have manifested neonatal tetany. The hypo-
calcemia tends to ameliorate with age during the first year of life. Hyper-
telorism, a shortened lip philtrum, low-set ears, notched pinnae, and nasal
clefts are some of the characteristic features (Fig. 19-2). In addition,
anomalies of the great blood vessels are almost always present; tetralogy
of Fallot and right-sided aortic arch are the most commonly encountered
defects.

Infants with thymic aplasia who survive the neonatal period exhibit
untoward susceptibility to viral, fungal, and bacterial infections which
ultimately may be overwhelming. At autopsy, although parathyroids and
thymus may be lacking entirely, some parathyroid tissue and a miniature
thymus gland may be found in an ectopic position upon careful sectioning
of the neck organs. Nephrocalcinosis has been encountered in over half
the cases. The lymphoid tissue, bone marrow, spleen, and gastrointestinal
tract have normal numbers of plasma cells, and cortical germinal centers
are present, if not exuberant, in the lymph nodes. The subcortical thymus
dependent region exhibits moderate to severe depletion of lymphocytes
so that the reticulum cells appear to be unusually prominent in this area
(Fig. 19-3). The lymphoid sheaths of the spleen are also depleted of
lymphocytes.

Antibody responses to some primary stimuli may be normal. Serum
concentrations of immunoglobulins are normal. However, delayed hypersensitivity is not manifested to common antigens such as Candida or strep-

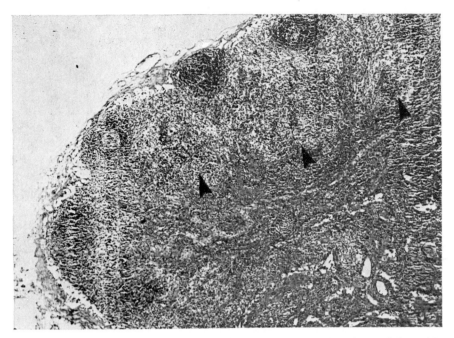

Fig. 19-3. The lymph node of a patient with DiGeorge syndrome. The subcortical thymus dependent region (arrows) shows a marked depletion of lymphocytes.

tokinase. Sensitization to dinitrofluorobenzene (DNFB) is unsuccessful or yields a weakly positive result. Skin allograft rejection has been absent or abnormally delayed. Lymphocyte transfer tests and macrophage-immobilizing factor synthesis are abnormal. The peripheral blood lymphocytes respond poorly, if at all, to *in vitro* stimulation by phytohemagglutinin allogeneic cells and antigen to which the host has been sensitized.

All these deficits of *in vitro* and *in vivo* lymphocyte function have been dramatically reversed by transplants of fetal thymic tissue into children with this syndrome. Increase in lymphocyte populations of the thymus dependent area, return of normal skin allograft rejection, return of normal responses to intradermal antigens and to DNFB, and normalization of phytohemagglutinin response *in vitro* have been documented. That some of these corrections have become apparent as early as 48 hours after the transplants argues that lymphocytic recognition mechanisms in these infants may have developed intact and that the small amount of fetal thymus tissue provides some critical element permitting their prompt responses.

More recently, it has been appreciated that an incomplete form of the syndrome may result in a clinically more benign course. Death may occur later in childhood from cardiac anomalies rather than from infectious complications. However, even in the more severe forms of the defect, some T-cell function may be acquired with time.

Correction of the defect by thymus transplantation leads to progressive fall from the high percentage of B-cells in the circulation (85 to 95 percent) regularly seen in the untreated patient to normal 40 to 50 percent and reciprocal increase in numbers of T-cells and vigor of the T-cell responses.

EPISODIC LYMPHOPENIA WITH LYMPHOCYTOTOXIN

A few children have been described in whom T-cell function is episodically but profoundly depressed by a circulating lymphocytotoxin which is complement dependent. Recurrent lymphopenia, hyperimmunoglobulinemia, and absent T-cell function are hallmarks of the syndrome. It is familial and is associated with D group chromosomal abnormalities. If death from infection does not occur, rapidly progressive lymphoreticular malignancy is ultimately observed.

IMMUNODEFICIENCY WITH NORMAL GAMMA GLOBULIN OR HYPERIMMUNOGLOBULINEMIA

In 1957, Giedion and Scheidegger reported the case of an infant with recurrent bacterial infections. His serum lacked IgA and IgM but contained normal concentrations of IgG. Because he was unresponsive to a variety of antigenic stimuli, Giedion and Scheidegger designated this entity immunoparesis. Only a few other cases have been studied, and very little is known about the histopathology of this disease, nor has an explanation for the supposed "inert" gamma globulin been forthcoming.

Although specific immunologic paralysis is a well-studied laboratory phenomenon, only a few clinical analogs of the experimental model are well documented. Perhaps the most striking of these is Hecht's giant cell pneumonia due to persistent measles infection. No antibody to measles virus can be detected in these patients. Kempe ascribed cases of progressive and generalized vaccinia to specific immunologic paralysis to vaccinia virus.

More recently Seligman and others have observed patients with normal or increased amounts of all gamma globulins who cannot produce antibodies to stimuli that regularly elicit responses in normal children. The basis of this strange deficiency is not at all clear at this writing, but the possibility that continuing infection may be depressing responsiveness to antigen in these children has been considered.

HEREDITARY ATAXIA-TELANGIECTASIA

Hereditary ataxia-telangiectasia is apparently transmitted in recessive mode. Affected infants are first noted to be ataxic and develop choreoathetoid movements and pseudopalsy of eye movements during infancy.

The telangiectasias usually appear later, at 5 or 6 years or even not until adolescence. They invariably involve the conjunctival and other body areas, such as the face, ear pinnae, eyelids, and antecubital and popliteal spaces. Progressive sinopulmonary infection also appears irregularly and may occur either early or late in the course of the disease. Death from chronic respiratory infection or from lymphoreticular or other malignancies is common in the second or third decade of life.

About 80 percent of patients with ataxia-telangiectasia lack both serum and secretory IgA. In some patients antibody to IgA and rapid catabolism of injected radioactively labeled IgA are noted. Patients and family members frequently lack IgE or have a deficiency of it.

All patients with ataxia-telangiectasia exhibit a defect in cellular immunity. The thymus gland is dysplastic or hypoplastic, and there is depletion of the thymus dependent areas. Delayed hypersensitivity, *in vitro* response of blood lymphocytes to phytohemagglutinin, and allograft rejection are blunted.

Lambrechts and Snoijink have proposed that this disease may be in some way based on isoimmunization of the mother to antigens common to the lymphoid system, skin, and brain.

WISKOTT-ALDRICH SYNDROME

The Wiskott-Aldrich syndrome is characterized by eczema, thrombocytopenia, and recurrent infections. Inheritance of the syndrome is X-linked. Affected boys rarely survive beyond the first decade of life, as death from overwhelming infection, hemorrhage (Fig. 19-4), or lymphoreticular malignancy shortens life expectancy. Both gram-positive and gram-negative bacteria, as well as viruses and fungi, cause severe infections. There appears to be a progressive deterioration of thymus dependent cellular immunity with concomitant changes in the histopathology of lymph nodes which show progressive depletion of the paracortical area in older surviving patients. Serum IgM concentration is usually low, but IgG and IgA levels are normal or elevated. Isohemagglutinins are regularly absent from the serum. This observation suggested a specific inability to respond to polysaccharide antigens. This has now been demonstrated quite conclusively with A and B substances, pneumococcal polysaccharide, and Salmonella Vi lipopolysaccharide. No unifying hypothesis explains the disparate elements of this disease.

Nevertheless, most aspects of the syndrome have been ameliorated by bone marrow transplantation or by the administration of transfer factor obtained from dialysates of normal donor lymphocytes in a few instances. The effect of transfer factor may last for as long as 1 year. Recent evidence suggests that this influence may not be as specific as originally thought.

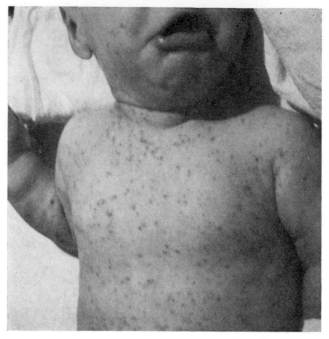

Fig. 19-4. An infant with Wiskott-Aldrich syndrome. A marked petechial hemorrhage occurs all over the body surface due to thrombocytopenia and malfunction of platelets.

IMMUNODEFICIENCY WITH THYMOMA

Agammaglobulinemia is observed with considerable frequency in patients with thymoma. These patients may also have a progressive deterioration of their T-cell function. The broadly based immunodeficiency observed was taken as an experiment of Nature raising the critical question concerning the role of thymus in the body economy. The thymic abnormality in these patients regularly is a stromal epithelial thymoma. The question raised by these patients led to the experimental analysis which established that the thymus plays a crucial role in both the development and the maintenance of the immunologic apparatus.

IMMUNODEFICIENCY WITH SHORT-LIMBED DWARFISM

Short-limbed dwarfism and one of its forms, cartilage-hair hypoplasia, are associated with T-cell defects in particular. Lymphopenia and diminished *in vitro* responses of lymphocytes to PHA and specific antigens have been noted. Several patients have had fatal or very severe varicella or vaccinia infections. In some cases the association of short-limbed dwarfism with broadly based combined immunodeficiency, skin abnormality, and abnormal thymus development has been described. These defects are apparently inherited as autosomal recessives.

SEVERE COMBINED IMMUNODEFICIENCY

In 1950, Glanzmann and Riniker described two unrelated infants who succumbed to overwhelming infection during the second year of life after having experienced through their entire life a succession of serious infections. The latter included pulmonary disease, diarrhea, thrush, and persistent morbilliform rash. They noted persistent and profound lymphopenia in these two infants and thus called the disease essential lymphocytophthisis. More than 200 cases of this disease have by now been described. It may prove to be one of the most common genetically determined defects in immunity. It has been estimated that 10 percent of extraneonatal infant mortality is caused by this syndrome, but this figure seems too high to the authors.

In the early European descriptions, it appeared that the disease was transmitted as an autosomal recessive phenomenon; consanguinity among approximately one-third of parents of affected children was documented. Further studies of affected families in America and Europe strongly suggest that another form of this disease is transmitted as an X linked trait. The latter conclusion is based on (1) documentation of affected males in up to three generations, (2) the appearance of the disease in both sons of two mothers who were identical twins, and (3) the appearance of the disease in two sons with the same mother but different fathers. The fact that the phenocopy can arise from two different modes of inheritance, both autosomal and X-linked recessive, probably accounts for the 3:1 ratio of males and females observed among the reported cases. The new evidence that reveals in some patients a deficiency of adenosine deaminase indicates further that the autosomal recessive inheritance may actually pertain to two separate genetically determined abnormalities.

For purposes of clinical description, it is easier to lump the two genetic types because there is no discernible difference in their clinical course nor, for that matter, can they yet be separated by pathologic study. Infection begins early in life, usually between 3 and 6 months of age, and a rapid succession of debilitating infections brings about early demise during the first 2 years of life. Almost all infants with this disease have loose, watery, chronic diarrhea. Frequently, stool cultures grow out Salmonella or enteropathic Escherichia coli strains. Pulmonary infection is also almost universally encountered. Abscesses of the lung containing Pseudomonas aeruginosa are a common cause of death, as is pneumonitis due to Pneumocystis carinii. Extensive moniliasis of the mouth or diaper area that persists beyond the neonatal period is often a first sign of the disease. Thrush is usually present even before any antibiotic therapy is instituted. Furthermore, these infants are incapable of limiting and terminating the most benign viral infections. Death has resulted from generalized chickenpox, measles with Hecht's giant cell pneumonia, and in a few instances from cytomegalovirus and adenovirus infections. Vaccination results in progressive, ultimately fatal vaccinia infection. BCG inoculation has also resulted in progressive "BCGosis." Live poliovirus immunization leads to persistent and aberrant infection with this virus. In one case, for example, the vaccine strain of poliovirus was readily isolated from the lungs in association with a fatal pulmonary complication. In summary, these infants are prey to all kinds of viral, bacterial, fungal, and protozoan infection. This susceptibility is usually manifested by skin, pulmonary, and gastro-intestinal infection. Ultimately, the infants fail to thrive, and the lack of weight gain causes the appearance of runting, which may be aggravated by protein-losing enteropathy.

In 1958, the Swiss workers pointed out that agammaglobulinemia is a prominent feature of this disease entity. Serum concentrations of immunoglobulins are very low, and the IgG may exhibit restricted heterogeneity. No antibody synthesis can be detected. Acute phase-reacting proteins rise in the usual manner with infection. C1q, a component of the complement system, has been reported to be low in most patients, but this is not an invariable finding. Interferon synthesis is normal.

Leukopenia is usually encountered because of the low lymphocyte counts, usually less than 2000/mm^3. The lymphocyte count may be variable and decline from initial normal neonatal levels (greater than 3000/mm^3) to more profoundly lymphopenic levels. A single lymphocyte count, nonetheless, is not a reliable index of the disease, as normal lymphocyte counts can be observed. Electron microscopy reveals that these blood lymphocytes are mostly very immature forms resembling lymphoblasts. Granulocytes and platelets are normal, although normal leukocytosis may not occur in the presence of overt infection. Eosinophilia is common, and abnormal granulation has been reported in the eosinophils.

The bone marrow is uniformly deficient in plasma cells, lymphocytes, and lymphoblasts. Bone marrow of normal infants contains up to 20 percent cells in the lymphocytic series. The primary defect in some forms of this disease may well be the failure of formation of an immunopotential cell that originates from the marrow. Lymph node biopsy, when feasible, exhibits a complete lack of germinal centers, plasma cells, and a gross deficiency or absence of lymphocytes. Only the stroma of the node is seen to contain occasional mast cells and eosinophils or, rarely, small collections of lymphoid cells without apparent organization.

None of the parameters of delayed sensitivity can be elicited in the most extreme cases. These infants are unresponsive to Candida antigen in the presence of overt, chronic Candida infection. They cannot be sensitized to dinitrofluorobenzene (DNFB). The peripheral blood lymphocytes are completely unresponsive to phytohemagglutinin or allogeneic stimulation. Skin grafts are accepted with no microscopic or macroscopic signs of rejection. At autopsy, lymphoid tissue is extremely deficient in the spleen, tonsils, appendix, or intestines. The thymus gland is found with difficulty and is usually located high in the neck, the gland usually having failed to descend in the normal manner into the anterior mediastinum. It regularly weighs less than 1 gm and is composed of primordial spindle-shaped cells, which occasionally form swirls or rosettes. No Hassall's corpuscles and few, if any, lymphocytes are present. The hypoplasia and dysplasia of the thymus gland are the uniformly characteristic feature of

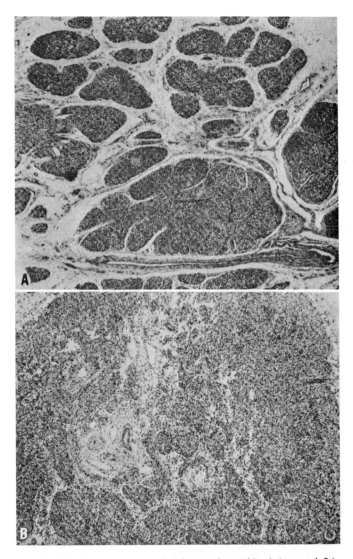

Fig. 19-5. A. Hypoplastic thymus gland of infant with combined immunodeficiency disease. B. Lymph node of infant with combined immunodeficiency disease. Marked depletion of lymphocytes in paracortical area and absence of germinal centers.

this entity (Fig. 19-5). The thymus of these children is not to be confused with so-called accidental involution of the thymus. In the latter, by contrast, Hassall's corpuscles can almost always be found, even though their size and number may be decreased. Much fatty tissue is usually found to occupy the region around the gland and the blood vessels are much larger than those that supply the underdeveloped thymus of children with severe combined immunodeficiency disease.

Very little inflammatory reaction is seen in extensively infected tissue, such as lung, skin, or intestines. Intravascular coagulation has been noted in a few infants who died of a complicating hemolytic-uremic syndrome.

Gamma globulin therapy is of no avail in averting the fatal outcome of the defect. Attempts to restore immunologic competence with thymus grafts, fetal hematopoietic cells, and bone marrow transplants have in the past uniformly failed to achieve this end. Although transitory beneficial effects have been accomplished, fatal graft-versus-host disease resulted following bone marrow or whole blood transfusion. A characteristic maculopapular rash starting on the face heralds the onset of graft-versus-host disease about 7 days after the administration of immunocompetent cells.

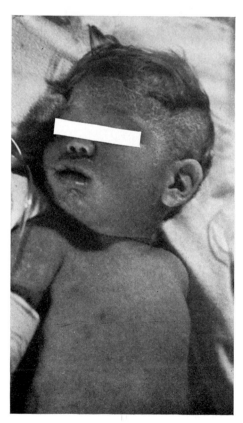

Fig. 19-6. Typical rash of graft-versus-host reaction 18 days after transplantation of bone marrow from mother.

The rash spreads rapidly to involve ultimately all skin surfaces, including the palms and soles (Fig. 19-6). Thrombocytopenia, leukopenia, jaundice, and anasarca follow in quick succession, and the bone marrow aplasia leads to death from massive hemorrhage by the second or the third week. On the basis of experimental observations, it has been reasoned that transplants of bone marrow cells as a source of immunopotential stem cells would restore immunologic competence to these infants and that it would be necessary to circumvent the difficulties of graft-versus-host disease by administering bone marrow cells histocompatible with the recipient according to the major histocompatibility determinants (HL-A). This remarkable feat has now been achieved in 25 children suffering from severe combined immunodeficiency. Transplants of histocompatible bone marrow from sibling donors equip such infants with both T- and B-cell populations and function. The lymphoid chimerism when immune function is reconstituted can be demonstrated. Despite HL-A identity between bone marrow donors and recipients, some degree of graft-versus-host reactivity is almost invariably noted, but its course is less severe and it does not have a fatal issue. In one of these cases, the donor and recipient were ABO-incompatible, and the recipient developed an immunologically based aplastic crisis which was treated with a second bone marrow transplant that in turn switched the blood type from A to O and established erythrocyte and leukocyte chimerism in the recipient. Thus far, such transplants usually cannot succeed across the major barrier of HL-A differences. With the developing understanding of genetic control of major histocompatibility determinants in man, however, it has been possible, in one instance, to overcome a "full-house" HL-A mismatch and achieve dramatic immunologic reconstitution using as a donor for the bone marrow an uncle matched with the recipient at the MLR locus of Yunis and Amos. Even in the first successful marrow transplant, it is now clear that the two marrow transplants which corrected the inborn immunodeficiency and later the aregenerative pancytopenia were derived from a donor mismatched with the recipient at the LA locus or at genes controlling the first segregant series but matched with recipient at the MLR locus. Since the MLR locus plays such an important role in controlling graft-host reaction and since marrow transplantation will be much developed in the future as a basis for cellular engineering, it is essential that simplified and reliable means for defining MLR compatibilities be developed.

Some infants with severe combined immunodeficiency have normal levels of one or all immunoglobulins. This form of lymphopenia with normal immunoglobulins has often been designated Nezelof's syndrome, after the investigator who termed the defect *aplasie lymphocytaire normoplasmocytaire et normoglobulinemie.* Indeed, abundant numbers of plasma cells are found in the spleen, intestine, lymph nodes, and elsewhere at autopsy, along with thymic dysplasia and lymphoid depletion. The clinical course of these infants may be slightly less malignant, but death by the third year of life has been the rule. A high incidence of Coombs'-positive hemolytic anemia has been encountered together with other autoimmune phenomena. Antigenic stimulation with phage particles, and bacterial toxins may not result in a normal or even detectable antibody response and only one of these infants had a satisfactory antibody response to poliovirus. It appears that the immune response in these infants is grossly abnormal despite normal immunoglobulin levels. Recently two cases which appeared to be variants of the Nezelof syndrome were treated by Aiuti and Gatti by giving transplants of fetal thymus. Within one day T-cell immunity functions began to appear, and cellularity of the blood and both T- and B-cell numbers and functions were fully restored. Thus in this syndrome, as in the DiGeorge syndrome, fetal thymus transplants have contributed maximally to the cellular engineering necessary to permit normal immune functions.

Several such infants have been reported in whom absence of T-cells and deficiency of T-cell functions have occurred together with general B-cell deficiency but with the presence of one or another immunoglobulin, e.g., IgM, IgA, or IgG in the serum. It seems likely from family studies and variability among siblings in a particular kindred that there exists considerable variation of phenotypic expression in both autosomally inherited and X-linked forms of the disease. Recent studies suggest that the enzyme adenosine-deaminase may be absent in some of the involved children and reduced values of this enzyme present in both parents of children with one form of this disease. This surprising observation encourages hope that severe combined immunodeficiencies soon will be defined in molecular terms.

Reticular Dysgenesis of DeVaal. In yet another form of stem cell immunodeficiency there is total myelopoietic failure, so-called reticular dysgenesis. The few infants with this disease have died within the first week of life of overwhelming staphylococcal sepsis. In addition to the characteristic thymic dysplasia, lymphopenia, and lymphoid depletion, there is severe neutropenia, thrombopenia, anemia, and depletion of myeloid precursors from the marrow. This disease, which is transmitted as an autosomal recessive, may represent the only true stem cell defect.

COMMON VARIABLE IMMUNODEFICIENCY

Most patients with immunodeficiency do not readily fall into any of the aforementioned defined syndromes. Such patients are said to have "acquired" or "late-onset" agammaglobulinemia or any of several forms of so-called dysgammaglobulinemia. Deterioration of T-cell function is often observed. The acquisition of agammaglobulinemia has now been documented in several cases, but close observation of these situations has not revealed the cause for the sudden depression of gamma globulin synthesis. In other cases deficiency of immunoglobulins expressed in very mild perturbations at first may extend to more profound defects and clinical disease over a period of years. The variability of the disease from time to time in the same patient and from patient to patient in the same family has led us to emphasize the variability in the name we use for the syndrome.

Primary acquired hypogammaglobulinemia has been found equally in males and females. Although there is no clear-cut establishment of the genetic influence, multiple cases in a single kindred have often been reported. In some families the data have indicated dominant inheritance of a general abnormality of immunologic function which may or may not be expressed as dysgammaglobulinemia, hypogammaglobulinemia, or agammaglobulinemia. In other instances clear evidence of autosomal recessive inheritance has been presented.

Cruchaud et al. reported agammaglobulinemia in one of identical twins. There has been a high incidence of other immunologic abnormalities in relatives of patients. These have included lupus erythematosus, hemolytic anemia, and other apparent autoimmune manifestations and phenomena, e.g., positive rheumatoid factor, thrombocytopenic purpura, antithyroid antibodies, and even pernicious anemia.

Undue susceptibility to pyogenic infection, particularly recurrent sinusitis and pneumonia, is also the prominent clinical feature of this form of immunodeficiency. Patients with chronic progressive bronchiectasis should be prime suspects for the diagnosis.

A prominent and frequent complication of common variable immunodeficiency which is rarely, if ever, seen in the X-linked disease, is a spruelike syndrome. Diarrhea, steatorrhea, at times protein-losing enteropathy, and a whole range of malabsorption abnormalities afflict more than half of affected adults. An intestinal biopsy is rarely rewarding in these cases because, more often than not, the characteristic flattening of the villi seen in nontropical sprue is absent, and biopsy material appears to be quite normal. In some cases nodular lymphoid hyperplasia has been reported. Bacterial counts of the succus entericus in these patients are not consistently different from the normal. Some of these patients have improved on a gluten-free diet, and others after elimination of milk from the diet. Recent studies in Seattle by Ochs et al. have emphasized that the sprue syndrome in these patients may often be caused by infection with Giardia lamblia. Often these organisms cannot be demonstrated by examination of stools but must be demonstrated by smears of the mucus of the ileum obtained by biopsy of the small bowel. Treatment with metronidazole (Flagyl) then may give dramatic relief of the malabsorption. It has been our experience, however, that the sprue-like syndrome may persist in this disease in many patients thoroughly treated with metronidazole.

11

Another distinguishing feature of the variable form is the frequent occurrence of noncaseating granulomas. The lungs, spleen, skin, liver, and bone marrow are most frequently involved. No microorganisms have ever been consistently found in these lesions. Steroid therapy has been helpful. Several patients have splenomegaly or hepatosplenomegaly and lymphadenopathy. In some the complications of hypersplenism have developed. This syndrome has affected multiple members of at least one kindred. Many patients with variations of this disease develop pernicious anemia very early in life as compared to the time of development of this autoimmune disease in the general population. When this complication occurs, the usual autoantibodies associated with pernicious anemia may be absent.

Quantitation of immunoglobulins in the sera of patients with acquired agammaglobulinemia usually reveals levels of IgG under 500 mg/100 ml. These levels, however, are almost always higher than those encountered in the sera of children with X-linked disease. Both IgA and IgM may also be detected in significant quantity in the sera of these patients. The IgG may exhibit restricted heterogeneity and abnormal balance of the subclasses.

Lymph nodes usually have few plasma cells, but unlike the absence of follicles noted in X-linked agammaglobulinemia, hypotrophy of the follicles or striking follicular hyperplasia may be evident. *In vitro* culture of lymphocytes from patients with primary acquired agammaglobulinemia reveals decreased RNA and DNA synthesis after stimulation by PHA or allogeneic cells. Lymph node transplants have survived and functioned for a time in some of these patients, and rejection of allografts of skin has often been very slow. From *in vitro* and *in vivo* studies it does not appear that an inhibitory factor causes this disease.

An unusually high incidence of "autoimmune" disease, such as pernicious anemia and hemolytic anemia, is noted. Although patients with lymphoma or chronic lymphocytic leukemia may present with or develop hypogammaglobulinemia, the progression of primary agammaglobulinemia is associated with a late development of lymphoreticular malignancy only in about 5 to 10 percent of the cases. Further, epithelial cancers, especially of the stomach and large bowel, also occur far too frequently in these patients to be explained by chance association.

B-lymphocytes may be observed in the circulation in normal, near normal, or only moderately reduced numbers in this disease. Such B-cells are absent in the X-linked form of agammaglobulinemia. Also the lymph node cells as studied by modern tools of molecular biology reveal capacity to synthesize immunoglobulin that is associated with deficiency in capacity to secrete these molecules. By contrast, the cells of many patients with Bruton's type agammaglobulinemia can neither synthesize nor secrete significant amounts of immunoglobulin. Further, the immunoglobulin found in the cells of some patients with common variable immunodeficiency, like cells of the bursa of Fabricius, produces immunoglobulin that lacks the galactase residues associated with secretion of the molecule.

SECONDARY DEFECTS IN IMMUNITY

Decrease in normal B-cell function may occur secondary to lymphoid malignancy, particularly chronic lymphatic leukemia. The catabolism of immunoglobulins increases in the nephrotic syndrome and myotonic dystrophy to produce hypogammaglobulinemia. Increased loss of immunoglobulins accompanies exfoliative skin disease and exudative enteropathy of any cause. In myeloma patients there is an increase in the catabolic rate of all immunoglobulins as a consequence of the high levels of myeloma globulin and decreased synthesis of "normal" immunoglobulins.

T-cell deficiency may be secondary to malignancy of the lymphoid system as in Hodgkin's disease or chronic lymphocytic leukemia. It may also accompany infections in leprosy where the thymus dependent regions of the node are congested with nonlymphoid histocytic cells filled with the acid-fast organisms.

Virus and parasitic infections can produce temporary or longer lasting defects of T-cells and T-cell functions. As has been shown experimentally, perturbations or depressions of B-cell function may be secondary to infections, especially with viruses, for example, oncogenic viruses.

Pestilence and famine go hand in hand through history. Nutritional deprivation and chronic deprivation of essential nutriments, including vitamins, minerals, proteins, and calories, have been associated with immunodeficiency. Recent studies have linked severe chronic protein and protein-calorie malnutrition early in life with immunodeficiency, failure to develop immunoglobulins normally, agammaglobulinemia, hypogammaglobulinemia, and the antibody deficiency syndrome. Later occurring extreme deficiencies as in kwashiorkor have been associated with defects of both cellular and humoral immunologic vigor.

Moderate chronic, but not acute, protein deprivation may interfere experimentally with primary, secondary, and tertiary antibody responses while leaving intact cell-mediated immunities. More severe protein or protein-calorie malnutrition will interfere with both the T-cell and B-cell immunologic functions. With the widespread malnutrition throughout the world today perhaps the most common form of immunodeficiency disease may be that associated with chronic malnutrition (Chapter 14).

SELECTED REFERENCES

Classification of Immunodeficiency Diseases

Fudenberg, H., et al. (1971): Pediatrics 47:927.
Giblett, E. R., et al. (1972): Lancet 2:1067.
Good, R. A., and Bergsma, D. (eds.) (1968): Immunodeficiency Disease in Man. New York, National Foundation Press.

Infantile X-linked Agammaglobulinemia

Barandun, S., et al. (1962): Vox Sang. 7:157.
Bruton, O. C. (1952): Pediatrics 9:722.
Fudenberg, H. H., German, J. L. III, and Kunkel, H. G. (1962): Arthritis Rheum. 5:565.
Fudenberg, H. H., and Hirschhorn, K. (1965): Med. Clinc. N. Amer. 49:1533.
Gitlin, D., et al. (1959): In Cellular and Humoral Aspects of the Hypersensitive States, Lawrence, H. S. (ed.). New York, Hoeber Medical Division, Harper & Row, p. 375.
Good, R. A. (1954): Amer. J. Dis. Child. 88:625.
Heiner, D. C., and Evans, L. (1967): J. Pediat. 70:820.
Holland, N. H., and Holland, P. (1966): Lancet 2:1152.
Hong, R., and Good, R. A. (1967): Science 156:1102.
Janeway, C. A., and Rosen, F. S. (1966): New Eng. J. Med. 275:826.
Marshall, W. C., Weston, H. J., and Bodian, M. (1964): Arch. Dis. Child. 39:18.
Ochs, H. D., Ament, M. E., and Davis, S. D. (1972): New Eng. J. Med. 287:341.
Peterson, R. D. A., Page, A. R., and Good, R. A. (1962): J. Allerg. 33:406.
Porter, H. M. (1957): Pediatrics 20:958.
Robbins, J. B., et al. (1965): New Eng. J. Med. 272:708.
Rosen, F. S., and Janeway, C. A. (1966): New Eng. J. Med. 275:769.
Schaller, J., et al. (1966): Lancet 2:825.
Stiehm, E. R., Vaerman, J. P., and Fudenberg, H. H. (1966): Blood 28:918.

Selective Immunoglobulin Deficiencies

Bachmann, R. (1965): Scand. J. Clin. Lab. Invest. 17:316.
Bloom, B. R., and Merrill, W. C. (1966): Progr. Allerg. 10:151.
Crabbe, P. A., and Heremans, J. F. (1967): Amer. J. Med. 42:319.
Gryboski, J. D., et al. (1968): Pediatrics 42:833.
Nell, P. A., et al. (1972): Pediatrics 49:71.
Rockey, J. H., et al. (1964): J. Lab. Clin. Med. 63:205.
Schaller, J., et al. (1966): Lancet 2:825.
Schur, P. H., et al. (1970): New Eng. J. Med. 283:631.
South, M. A., et al. (1968): Amer. J. Med. 44:168.
South, M. A., et al. (1966): J. Exp. Med. 123:615.
Stocker, F., Ammann, P., and Rossi, E. (1968): Arch. Dis. Child. 43:585.
Strober, W., et al. (1968): J. Clin. Invest. 47:1905.
Tomasi, T. B. Jr. (1968): New Eng. J. Med. 279:1327.
Vyas, G. N., Perkins, H. A., and Fudenberg, H. H. (1968): Lancet 2:312.

Transient Hypogammaglobulinemia of Infancy

Gitlin, D., et al. (1964): J. Clin. Invest. 43:1938.
Rosen, F. S., and Janeway, C. A. (1966): New Eng. J. Med. 275:709.
West, C. D., Hong, R., and Holland, N. H. (1962): J. Clin. Invest. 41:2054.

X-linked Immunodeficiency with Hyper-IgM

Barth, W. F., et al. (1965): Amer. J. Med. 39:319.
Burtin, P. (1961): Rev. Franc. Etud. Clin. Biol. 6:286.
Gleich, G. J., Condemi, J. J., and Vaughan, J. H. (1965): New Eng. J. Med. 272:331.
Goldman, A. S., et al. (1967): J. Pediat. 70:16.
Hitzig, W. H., and Schlapfer, A. (1964): In International Society of Haematology: Abstracts of the 10th Congress. Copenhagen, Munksgaard, p, 23.
Hobbs, J. R., Russell, A., and Worlledge, S. M. (1967): Clin. Exp. Immun. 2:589.
Hong, R., et al. (1962): J. Pediat. 61:831.
Huntley, C. C., Lafferty, J. W., and Lyerly, A. (1963): Pediatrics 32:407.
Rosen, F. S., and Bougas, J. A. (1963): New Eng. J. Med. 269:1336.
Rosen, F. S., et al. (1961): Pediatrics 28:182.
Stiehm, E. R., and Fudenberg, H. H. (1966): Amer. J. Med. 40:805.

Congenital Thymic Aplasia (DiGeorge Syndrome)

August, C. S., et al. (1968): Lancet 2:1210.
Cleveland, W. W., et al. (1968): Lancet 2:1211.
DiGeorge, A. M. (1968): In *Immunologic Deficiency Diseases in Man,* Bergsma, D. (ed.), Birth Defects Original Article Series 4:116. New York, National Foundation Press.
Gatti, R. A., (1972): J. Pediat. 81:920.
Good, R. A., et al. (1969): Lancet 1:946.
Huber, J., Cholnoky, P., and Zoethout, H. E. (1967): Arch. Dis. Child. 42:190.
Kempe, C. H. (1960): Pediatrics 26:176.
Kretschmer, R., et al. (1968): New Eng. J. Med. 279:1295.
Lischner, H. W., Dacou, C., and DiGeorge, A. M. (1967): Transplantation 5:555.
Lischner, H. W., Punnett, H. H., and DiGeorge, A. M. (1967): Nature (London) 214:580.
Steele, R. W., et al. (1972): New Eng. J. Med. 287:787.
Taitz, L. S., Zarate-Salvador, C., and Schwartz, E. (1966): Pediatrics 38:412.

Episodic Lymphopenia with Lymphocytotoxin

Kretschmer, R., et al. (1969): New Eng. J. Med. 281:285.

Immunodeficiency with Normal Gamma Globulin or Hyperimmunoglobulinemia

Barandun, S., et al. (1959): Helv. Med. Acta 26:163.
Giedion, A., and Scheidegger, J. J. (1957): Helv. Paediat. Acta 12:241.
Gilbert, C., and Hong, R. (1964): Amer. J. Med. 37:602.
Kempe, C. H. (1960): Pediatrics 26:176.
Mitus, A., et al. (1959): New Eng. J. Med. 261:882.
Williams, R. T. (1966): Clin. Exp. Immun. 1:223.

Hereditary Ataxia-Telangiectasia

Aisenberg, A. C., and Leskowitz, S. (1963): New Eng. J. Med. 268:1269.
Ammann, A. J., et al. (1969): New Eng. J. Med. 281:469.
Ammann, A. J., and Hong, R. (1971): J. Pediat. 78:821.
Bellanti, J. A., Artenstein, M. S., and Buescher, E. L. (1966): Pediatrics 37:924.
Boder, E., and Sedgwick, R. P. (1958): Pediatrics 21:526.
Eisen, A. H., et al. (1965): New Eng. J. Med. 272:18.
Epstein, W. L., et al. (1966): Int. Arch. Allerg. 30:15.
Fireman, P., Boesman, M., and Gitlin, D. (1964): Lancet 1:1193.
Lambrechts, A. F., and Snoijink, J. J. (1971): *Ataxia-telangiectasis, morbus lympholyticus congenitalis.* Tilburg, Netherlands, Nordic Immunological Laboratories.
Naspitz, C. K., Eisen, A. H., and Richter, M. (1968): Int. Arch. Allerg. 33:217.
Oppenheim, J. J., et al. (1966): Brit. Med. J. 2:330.
Peterson, R. D. A., Blaw, M., and Good, R. A. (1963): J. Pediat. 63:701.
Peterson, R. D. A., Cooper, M. D., and Good, R. A. (1966): Amer. J. Med. 41:342.
Peterson, R. D. A., Kelly, W. D., and Good, R. A. (1964): Lancet 1:1189.
Schalch, D. S., McFarlin, D. E., and Barlow, M. H. (1970): New Eng. J. Med. 282:1396.
Smeby, B. (1966): Acta Paediat. (Stockholm) 55:239.
Strober, W., et al. (1968): J. Clin. Invest. 47:1905.
Young, R. R., Austen, K. F., and Moser, H. W. (1964): Medicine 43:423.

Wiskott-Aldrich Syndrome

Aldrich, R. A., Steinberg, A. G., and Campbell, D. C. (1954): Pediatrics 13:133.
Bach, F. H., et al. (1968): Lancet 2:1364.
Baldini, M. G. (1969): New Eng. J. Med. 281:107.

Blaese, R. M., et al. (1968): Lancet *1*:1056.
Cooper, M. D., et al. (1968): Amer. J. Med. *44*:499.
Hermans, P. E., et al. (1966): Amer. J. Med. *1*:78.
Krivit, W. E., and Good, R. A. (1959): Amer. J. Dis. Child. *97*:137.
Levin, A. S., et al. (1970): Proc. Natl. Acad. Sci. U.S.A. *67*:821.
ten Bensel, R. W., Stadlan, E. M., and Krivit, W. (1966): J. Pediat. *68*:761.

Immunodeficiency with Thymoma

Good, R. A., and Zak, S. J., (1956): Pediatrics *18*:109.
Jeunet, F. S., and Good, R. A. (1968): In *Immunologic Deficiency Diseases in Man,*
    Good, R. A., and Bergsma, D. (eds.). New York, National Foundation Press.
Josse, J. W., and Zack, S. I. (1958): New Eng. J. Med. *259*:113.
Korn, D., et al. (1967): New Eng. J. Med. *276*:1333.

Immunodeficiency with Short-limbed Dwarfism

Gatti, R. A., et al. (1969): J. Pediat. *75*:675.
Gotoff, S. P., et al. (1972): J. Pediat. *80*:1010.
Lux, S. E., et al. (1970): New Eng. J. Med. *282*:231.

Severe Combined Immunodeficiency

Becroft, D. M. O., and Douglas, R. (1968): Arch. Dis. Child. *43*:444.
Berry, C. L., and Thompson, E. N. (1968): Arch. Dis. Child. *43*:579.
Biggar, W. D., Good, R. A., and Park, B. H. (1972): J. Pediat. *81*:301.
DeVaal, O. M., and Seynhaeve, V. (1959): Lancet 2:1123.
Gatti, R. A., et al. (1968): Lancet 2:1366.
Glanzmann, E., and Riniker, P. (1950): Ann. Paediat. (Basel) *175*:1.
Hitzig, W. H., et al. (1971): J. Pediat. 78:968.
Hoyer, J. R., et al. (1968): Medicine 47:201.
Jacobs, J. C., et al. (1968): Lancet *1*:499.
Meuwissen, H. J., et al. (1969): New Eng. J. Med. *281*:691.
Rosen, F. S. (1968): New Eng. J. Med. 279:643.
Schaller, J., Davis, S. D., and Wedgwood, R. J. (1966): Amer. J. Med. *41*:462.
Stiehm, E. R., et al. (1972): New Eng. J. Med. *286*:797.

Common Variable Immunodeficiency

Buckley, R. H., Wray, B. B., and Belmaker, E. Z. (1972): Pediatrics *49*:59.
Gleich, G. J., et al. (1966): J. Clin. Invest. *45*:1334.
Grant, G. H., and Wallace, W. D. (1954): Lancet 2:671.
Hobbs, J. R. (1968): Lancet *1*:110.
Hobbs, J. R., Russell, A., and Worliedge, S. M. (1967): Clin. Exp. Immun. 2:589.
Kempe, C. H. (1960): Pediatrics *26*:176.
Mitus, A., (1959): New Eng. J. Med. *261*:882.
Prasad, A. S., and Koza, D. W. (1954): Ann. Intern. Med. *41*:629.
Rosen, F. S., et al. (1961): Pediatrics *28*:182.
Sanford, J. P., Favour, C. B., and Tribeman, M. S. (1954): New Eng. J. Med.
    250:1027.

20
Deficiencies of Complement Components

A number of examples of isolated, genetically determined deficiencies of individual complement components have been reported. Such deficiencies have been encountered in most of the common laboratory animals used in complement work, and it is interesting that in each species the component found missing has so far been different from that in other species.

In man since the report of the first case in 1960, a number of families are known to have an isolated deficiency of C2. A number of other deficiencies have been described in man. Indeed isolated, apparently genetically determined deficiencies of individual complement components have now been described in man for C1q, C1r, C1s, C1 esterase inhibitor, C2, C3, stabilizer of C3, C5, C6, and C7. It is certain that as time passes more abnormalities or deficiencies of each of the complement components, inhibitors, and stabilizers will be encountered and associated with diseases.

C2 DEFICIENCY

Several families of C2-deficient humans have been described since the first report by Silverstein (1960). The original subjects were all described as healthy but there are now at least 6 patients in whom C2 deficiency has been associated with serious disease. One case had glomerulonephritis and later developed a lupus-like syndrome, 2 cases had lupus, 1 case has an almost lifelong history of a Henoch-Schönlein type of purpura, and 1 patient suffered from dermatomyositis. The relationship of these conditions to the C2 deficiency is not yet clear, but renal vascular diseases occur far too frequently in patients with C2 deficiency to be explained by chance alone. Persons deficient in C2 had 0.5 to 4 percent of the normal amount of C2 in their serum. This deficiency may explain why the serum of C2-deficient subjects can show positive immune adherence reactions and in full concentration, as in the blood, will kill bacteria normally when the antibody normally present in the serum is used. At high levels of antibody or dilutions of serum a cytolytic defect for bacteria is apparent. Patients with C2 deficiency also seem to be unusually susceptible to infection.

In both the C4-deficient guinea pigs and the C2-deficient humans there is evidence that the alternate pathway of complement activation is intact and that this may account both for the relatively benign nature of these deficiencies and for the vascular disease associated with deficiencies of C2 in man. It is now clear that C2 deficiency in man may not be clinically benign as had originally been thought and that the apparent vigor of both man and laboratory animals lacking early C components may be an artifact of the special environment in which the susceptible strain is raised. In other words, the immunologist in whom C2 deficiency was first discovered is not an appropriate test system for the importance of this component.

C3 DEFICIENCY

Two common genetically determined allotypes of C3 have been identified. The genes are designated C3^s and C3^f according to the relative electrophoretic mobilities of their gene products. Seven other electrophoretically distinct but rare alleles have also been recognized. All the variant forms, as well as the common allelic products, appear to have normal hemolytic activity and occur in roughly equal proportions in the sera of heterozygotes.

One patient has been studied in whom the serum C3 concentration is approximately half of normal, 69 mg/100 ml. The 7 affected siblings are clinically well. Hemolytic titers are normal or slightly reduced. Immune adherence and bactericidal activity are normal. Enhancement of bacterial phagocytosis is about half normal. Genetic typing of C3 in members of this child's family revealed the presence of apparent homozygotes among the members with half normal levels. A likely explanation is that the affected individuals are hemizygous and that they have inherited an allele which is silent. Two matings in the family were informative in this regard in that the expressed allele could only have been inherited from a normal parent. The abnormality in this child predicts that the homozygous deficiency state can potentially exist but has not yet been found.

In another patient, three members in three generations were found to be heterozygotes for C3. However, the C3^f was relatively decreased in concentration compared to C3^s. The seemingly hypomorphic form of C3^f was designated C3^{f3}. When C3^f and C3^s were isolated from normal serum, labeled with ^{125}I, and injected into the propositus and normal controls, it was found that individuals with C3^{fs} synthesized the f variant at 40 percent of the normal rate.

DEFICIENCY OF C3b INACTIVATOR AND INCREASED CATABOLISM OF C3

Alper et al. have studied a patient who presented with increased susceptibility to pneumonia and other infections. In this patient a C3 stabilizer or inhibitor of C3, C3b inactivator was absent or grossly deficient from the blood. Consequently the extremely low concentrations of C3 lead to the inordinate susceptibility to infection. An additional kindred having a similar deficiency of C3 has recently been studied, and again marked susceptibility to infection has been the clinical manifestation.

C3b inactivator was described as an inactivator of fixed C3 by Tamura and Nelson (1967) and as an activator of the reactant for bovine conglutinin (KAF) by Lachmann in 1968. The two are certainly the same, and the material has been purified and characterized to the extent that a monovalent antiserum is now available against it.

KAF is apparently an enzyme existing in active form in whole serum and awaiting the generation of its substrate. Inactivation of C3b presumably is proteolytic and is irreversible. It is not clear that a fragment of any size is released during this reaction, but the KAF-treated C3b becomes exquisitely sensitive to the action of further proteolytic enzymes which appear to bring about the split into C3c and C3d. At the present time, there are no other substrates upon which KAF is known to act.

In the clinical case the protein is absent by antigenic analysis and by the failure to detect any activity in either the conglutinating or hemolysis-inhibiting functional assays in samples taken from a patient.

It has been postulated that the homeostatic control provided by KAF is required to prevent spontaneous activation of the complement and C3 bypass mechanism. Consequently the factors involved, such as C3 proactivator, are depleted and the exhaustion of the bypass mechanism in this way leads to failure of antibacterial immunity. These findings again indicate that the complement system is vital to life.

C5 DYSFUNCTION

An infant described by Miller and his associates was found to be unduly susceptible to gram-negative sepsis and to have Leiner's disease. Her resistance to infection could be bolstered by infusions of plasma. *In vitro* her serum, as well as that of her mother and grandmother, did not promote phagocytosis of zymosan particles. A reagent which failed to restore the patient's serum to normal *in vitro* was serum from C5-deficient mice. Although the serum was hemolytically normal, isolated C5 from the patient's mother was shown to have only 10 percent of normal hemolytic activity. Immunochemical studies showed the patient to have immunochemically identifiable C5 in serum in normal amounts, but this protein did not function as does normal C5. An additional family with this disease has also been discovered and studied by the same investigators. All the evidence obtained thus far indicates that the C5 present in these patients' serums, although seemingly quite normal chemically, is functionally inactive. It is the abnormality of this protein molecule that accounts for the skin infections, bowel infections, and propensity to sepsis experienced by these children and corrected by treatment with normal plasma.

DEFICIENCY OF C$\overline{1}$ INHIBITOR—HEREDITARY ANGIONEUROTIC EDEMA

The inhibitor of the activated first component of complement (C$\overline{1}$ inhibitor) was described by Levy and Lepow (1959) and recently identified by Pensky and Schwick as being identical to the alpha-2 neuraminoglycoprotein. This protein inhibits a number of plasma enzymes: C$\overline{1}$ (C1 esterase), kininogenase, plasmin, activated Hageman factor, activated thromboplastin antecedent, PF/dil, and C1r, the component that brings about the activation of C1 or C$\overline{1}$. The inhibition is stoichiometric and the inhibitor acts as a competitive substrate which is split, but its major products are not released nor are they biologically active. That the clinical syndrome of hereditary angioneurotic edema is characteristically associated with the deficiency of this inhibitor was first shown by Donaldson and Evans (1963)—a finding widely confirmed. The deficiency is incomplete, however, and affected subjects may have as much as 25 percent of the normal level of activity. Affected individuals are regularly heterozygous, and the defect is transmitted as an autosomal dominant.

Patients with hereditary angioneurotic edema suffer episodes of acute nonpainful edema in the subcutaneous tissues or in the mucosa of the respiratory or alimentary tracts (Fig. 20-1). The swellings are usually sin-

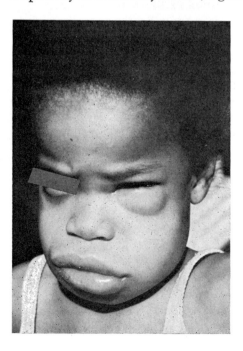

Fig. 20-1. Shown is a girl during an attack of hereditary angioneurotic edema involving the lips and eyelids.

gle but may be multiple and usually are self-limited after 2 to 3 days. The condition may be distressing, particularly if the abdominal tract is affected because of associated pain and can be life threatening when the larynx and trachea are involved. Initiation of the attacks appears to involve the coagulation pathway rather than the complement system per se, and the main mediator is believed to be a kinin-like C2 fragment split from C2 by the action of C$\overline{\text{I}}$ and C4 in solution. Individual attacks appear to be precipitated by the local exhaustion of the reduced amount of C$\overline{\text{I}}$ inhibitor, probably as a consequence of the activation of any of the enzymes with which the C$\overline{\text{I}}$ inhibitor can react. Once local exhaustion of inhibitor has occurred, activation of C$\overline{\text{I}}$ can occur apparently autocatalytically, and unrestrained breakdown of C4 and C2 can occur. The attacks can be successfully treated by the administration of fresh plasma as a source of inhibitor and can be largely prevented by the prophylactic use of epsilon-amino-caproic acid and its analogs which act by preventing the activation of plasma proteases and therefore show an inhibitor-sparing effect.

C1r DEFICIENCY

Recently Pickering et al. reported a case of C1r deficiency associated clinically with increased frequency of infections and a renal vascular disease suggestive of lupus erythematosus. The low hemolytic C1 activity of the patient's serum could be restored by the addition of purified C1r to the serum. Bactericidal activity and immune adherence of serum were found to be impaired. The alternate pathway for the activation of the terminal portion of the complement cascade was found to be intact. In an additional family studied by Moncado et al. and Day et al. two siblings lacked C1r. Both showed marked susceptibility to infection and a propensity to severe vascular disease, as well as rheumatoid and renal diseases. C1r was absent from their sera and purified C1r corrected the serum abnormality. Three additional siblings in this large family had died and in two, increased susceptibility to infection and/or renal vascular disease resulted in death. Recently the renal disease of our first case of C1q deficiency developed to a terminal illness. Renal transplantation carried out to correct the kidney failure also apparently corrected the complement deficiency. This finding suggests that C1r can be synthesized in the kidney. As an experiment of Nature this family provides evidence for the survival advantages of C1r and the classical complement cascade. It also argues for the participation of the alternate complement pathway in the pathogenesis of a renal vascular disease suggestive of lupus.

Pondman has described isolated deficiency of C1s and in this case as in those with C1r deficiency, lupus, or a disease strikingly like lupus was lethal. Marked deficiency of C1q is quite regularly seen in children with severe combined immunodeficiency disease. Somewhat low levels of C1q have also been encountered in some children with agammaglobulinemia syndromes. Correction of the C1q concentrations in patients with severe combined immunodeficiency diseases has been achieved by successful marrow transplantation that has corrected the immunodeficiency. In each instance the correction of C1q concentrations has coincided with evidence of a successful marrow engraftment.

Leddy and co-workers have recently studied a case of deficiency of C6. This young adult female is thus far well. A patient with C7 deficiency has recently been defined and this patient has rheumatoid disease.

Complement component deficiencies in experimental animals, C5 deficiency of mice, C6 deficiency in rabbits, and C4 deficiency of guinea pigs have been described (Chapter 11). Although initial studies seemed to indicate that animals with these deficiencies were clinically well, this conclusion may be reflective of the protected environment of modern laboratory animal husbandry. C5-deficient mice, for example, are at least 10 times more susceptible to lethality in experimentally induced infection with pneumococci than are normal mice.

SELECTED REFERENCES

C2 Deficiency

Alper, C. A., and Rosen, F. S. (1971): Advances Immun. *14*:252.
Agnello, V., DeBracco, M. M. E., and Kunkel, H. G. (1970): J. Immun. *108*:837.
Ruddy, S., et al. (1970): Immunology *18*:943.
Silverstein, A. M. (1960): Blood *16*:1338.

C3 Deficiency

Alper, C. A., and Propp, R. P. (1968): J. Clin. Invest. *47*:2181.
Alper, C. A., et al. (1969): J. Clin. Invest. *48*:553.
Alper C. A., and Rosen, F. S. (1969): J. Clin. Invest. *48*:2a.
Johnston, R. B. Jr., et al. (1969): J. Exp. Med. *129*:1275.

Deficiency of C3b Inactivator and Increased Catabolism of C3

Alper, C. A., et al. (1970): J. Clin. Invest. *49*:1975.
Lachmann, P. J. (1971): Immunochemistry 8:81.
Mueller-Eberhard, H. J. (1969): Ann. Rev. Biochem. *38*:389.
Tamura, N., and Nelson, R. A. (1967): J. Immun. 99:582.

C5 Dysfunction

Miller, M. E., et al. (1968): Lancet 2:60.
Miller, M. E., and Nilsson, U. (1970): New Eng. J. Med. *282*:354.

Deficiency of C1 Inhibitor—Hereditary Angioneurotic Edema

Donaldson, V. H., and Evans, R. R. (1963): Amer. J. Med. *35*:37.
Fong, J. S., and Good, R. A. (1970): J. Lab. Clin. Med. 76:836.
Levy, L. R., and Lepow, I. H. (1959): Proc. Soc. Exp. Biol. Med. *101*:608.
Pensky, J., and Schwick, H. G. (1969): Science *163*:698.
Pickering, R. J., et al. (1971): J. Pediat. 78:30.
Schultze, H. E., Heide, K., and Haupt, H. (1962): Naturwissenschaften 49:133.

Clr Deficiency

Day, N. D., et al. (1972): J. Clin. Invest. *51*:1102.
Pickering, R. J., et al. (1970): J. Exp. Med. *131*:803.
Shin, H. S., Smith, M. R., and Wood, W. B. Jr. (1969): J. Exp. Med. *130*:1229.

21
Deficiency of Phagocytic Functions

Phagocytosis and intracellular processing of microbes that have penetrated the barriers of skin and mucous membranes are primary and essential functions for host resistance against microbial disease. The discovery of Metchnikoff clearly established this fact, and his studies on the biology of phagocytic cells serve as a foundation for current investigations of the phagocytic system.

Phagocytic cells can be divided into two compartments, i.e., circulating phagocytes and fixed phagocytic cells of the reticuloendothelial system. Polymorphonuclear leukocytes, monocytes, eosinophils, and basophils comprise the circulating compartment. Splenic macrophages, liver Kupffer cells, pulmonary alveolar macrophages, lymph node macrophages, and the microglia cells of the brain are fixed phagocytic cells and comprise the reticuloendothelial system (Chapter 12). Circulating phagocytic cells are readily available for migration to sites of bacterial invasion and function in defense against local or fixed infections in tissues. Fixed phagocytic cells of the reticuloendothelial system, on the other hand, protect against circulating infectious agents in the blood and lymph. Circulating phagocytic cells reach maturity in the bone marrow, circulate in the blood for a short time, and enter tissue spaces by *diapedesis* through capillary walls in response to inflammatory stimulation (Chapter 13). The polymorphonuclear leukocytes are short-lived in tissue as well as in blood; however, mononuclear cells, the M-cells, from the blood are capable of cell division and may differentiate into tissue macrophages with a long life span. Tissue macrophages that can also migrate limited distances within the connective tissues comprise an additional compartment and represent, at least in part, the extension of circulating phagocytes to the connective tissues. Whether all of the tissue phagocytes were derived from the circulating compartment is moot and needs further study.

For decades, clinicians have noted that adequate numbers of phagocytic leukocytes are necessary for vigorous host defense, since neutropenia, either congenital or as a result of malignancy or chemotherapy, invariably results in increased susceptibility to infection and poor response to antibiotic therapy. In recent years, methods that have been developed to permit the study of various parameters of leukocyte function have been applied to analysis of patients with increased susceptibility to infection. Several clinical conditions have been found in which abnormality of leukocyte bactericidal function is associated with recurrent severe bacterial disease. Chronic granulomatous disease of childhood and Chediak-Higashi syndrome are examples of such diseases. In both of these conditions, the leukocytes have defective bactericidal capacity, and patients suffer recurrent severe bacterial disease. Patients with leukocyte myeloperoxidase deficiency and patients with absent glucose 6-phosphate dehydrogenase have leukocytes with abnormal bactericidal function but suffer less generalized susceptibility to infection. Disorders of leukocyte chemotaxis and defective opsonic activity of serum have also been reported to be associated with recurrent bacterial infections.

FATAL (CHRONIC) GRANULOMATOUS DISEASE OF CHILDHOOD

Fatal granulomatous disease of childhood was first described by Berendes et al. as a distinct clinical entity of unknown etiology. This disease is characterized by recurrent infection with low-grade pathogens, formation of granulomata which ultimately become suppurative, and normal humoral and cellular immunity. The onset of increased infections occurs early in life (one patient died at six days of age), the disease is generally chronic (the oldest survivor at present is 25 years old), and the outcome is fatal—the result of overwhelming infection or infection destroying a vital organ.

Since the original report, similar cases have been presented and various names, e.g., progressive septic granulomatous disease and congenital dysphagocytosis, have been used. We now use the term *chronic granulomatous disease* (CGD) clinically for purposes of relieving parental apprehension.

Eighty-three years after Metchnikoff's theory of phagocytosis (1883), Holmes et al. (1966) clearly demonstrated in CGD patients that a defect in phagocytic function is a major cause of the inadequacy in host defense against invading organisms. Thus, major advances in the theory of phagocytosis, as well as the understanding of the pathogenesis of CGD, were made, and this disease became a unique experiment of Nature for the study of phagocytosis.

Clinical Features

The hallmark of this disease is the occurrence, in combination, of septic purulent infection by low-grade pyogenic organisms (Table 21-1) and the formation of granulomata in response to these infections.

The early presenting clinical problems are recurrent infection of the skin, persistent purulent rhinitis, and lymphadenopathy in a well-nourished infant of otherwise normal appearance (Table 21-2).

Table 21-1. A Classification of Bacteria according to the Bactericidal Capacity of Leukocytes from Patients with Fatal Granulomatous Disease

A. Bacteria that are not killed (catalase positive)
  1. Coagulase-positive Staphylococci
  2. Escherichia coli
  3. Aerobacter aerogenes
  4. Paracolon hafnia (Klebsiella)
  5. Serratia marcescens

B. Bacteria that are killed (catalase negative)
  1. Lactobacillus acidophilus
  2. Streptococcus viridans
  3. Diplococcus pneumoniae
  4. Streptococcus faecalis

Table 21-2. Clinical Features of Fatal Granulomatous Disease

  1. Recurrent infections with low-grade pathogens starting early in life
  2. Chronic suppurative granulomatous lesions of the skin and lymph nodes
  3. Hepatosplenomegaly—parenchymatous granuloma and liver abscess
  4. Progressive pulmonary disease—granulomatous infiltration, abscess, empyema
  5. Granulomatous septic osteomyelitis
  6. Pericarditis
  7. Normal cellular and humoral immune response
  8. Familial occurrence

The skin lesion is characterized by granulomatous eruption and surrounding impetigo; it progresses slowly to suppuration. The healing process is also extremely slow, resulting in a granulomatous nodular appearance, and the granulomatous nodules may persist for months. These lesions of the skin may be found in any part of the body, the face and neck being the more frequent sites.

Purulent rhinitis and otitis are characteristic clinical features of this disease. They occur frequently and represent recurrent clinical problems. With adequate local and systemic antibiotic therapy, the lesions of the external nares clear up rather quickly, only to recur within a few days after the treatment is discontinued.

Lymphadenitis is another common clinical feature and occurs in the majority of patients during the course of the disease. This is characteristically chronic first, granulomatous, then suppurative, and very often requires surgical drainage. Swelling and induration of cervical, axillary, and inguinal lymph nodes are most frequently seen, but involvement of hilar and mesenteric lymph nodes may also occur.

In the common form of this disease the family history usually reveals strong evidence of X-linked recessive inheritance.

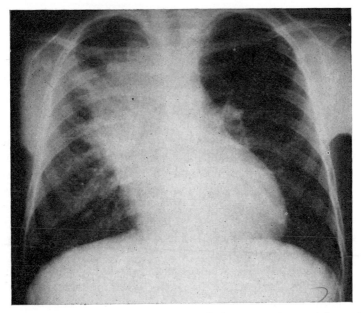

Fig. 21-1. Roentgenogram of the chest of a child with chronic granulomatous disease. Chronic progressive infiltration of lung parenchyma took place despite massive antibiotic therapy. Surgical resection of lesions is often necessary to prevent further destruction of lung parenchyma and to contain the spreading infection.

On physical examination, hepatosplenomegaly occurs in the majority of patients. An increased anteroposterior diameter of the chest is present in those patients with chronic fibrotic lungs.

The most prominent pulmonary lesions include an extensive infiltration of the lung parenchyma and prominent hilar adenopathy demonstrable on roentgenograms (Fig. 21-1). In addition, bronchopneumonia, often combined with lobar pneumonia, pleural effusion, pleural thickening, pulmonary abscess, and atelectasis of the right middle lobe may be seen. An extensive reticulonodular infiltration often leads to pulmonary insufficiency and death.

The pneumonia characteristically begins as a hilar infiltration; it is bronchial and may be unilateral or bilateral or may be basilar. In spite of extensive antibiotic treatment, these lesions may regress slowly over a period of weeks to months or may frequently progress to involve an entire lobe. An unusual manifestation of pulmonary involvement is the so-called encapsulated pneumonia. This pneumonia is characteristically seen on a roentgenogram as a homogeneous, discrete, and relatively round lesion; it may occur singly or in groups of two to three infiltrates. The size and contour of the lesions may change within a few days or remain unchanged for a period of weeks or months. Discoid atelectasis, thickening of the bronchi, air bronchogram, "honeycombing" and loss of lobar volume are occasionally observed. When underlying reticulation of the lungs persists, the pulmonary function may be correspondingly impaired.

Hepatic abscess, mesenteric lymphadenitis, osteomyelitis, often of multiple bones, and oophoritis are frequently noted. Anemia is often seen and may be an early sign of parenchymal infection.

Laboratory Findings

The intensive search for the organisms that are usually associated with the production of parenchymal granulomatous infiltration (mycobacteria, fungus) has usually been of no avail. Indeed, organisms considered to be true bacterial, viral, or fungal pathogens have rarely been isolated from the lesions. The organisms frequently associated with the lesions are low-grade pyogenic pathogens. It is striking that those organisms infecting the patients and causing clinical illness can now be grouped together as the catalase-producing organisms.

Immunologic study has revealed normal or slightly elevated circulating immunoglobulins, normal response to active immunizations, and normal cellular immunity.

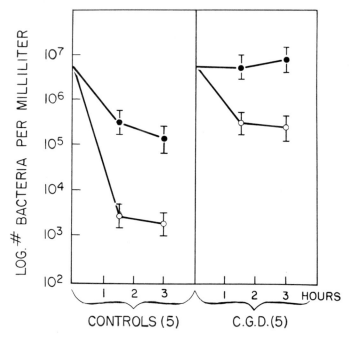

Fig. 21-2. Bactericidal test of leukocytes. Staphylococcus aureus 502A was incubated with leukocytes, and the number of surviving bacteria was determined by colony count at intervals. ●: no antibiotics were added. ○: penicillin and streptomycin were added at 15 min. of incubation. CGD = Chronic granulomatous disease. The number of patients or controls is shown in parentheses.

The clinical dilemma involved in pathogenesis, i.e., the apparent deficiency of host defense against infection despite normal immunity, provoked an extensive search for a deficiency of bodily defense. The first major breakthrough in this clinical dilemma was made by Holmes et al. who reported that the leukocytes of CGD patients failed to kill ingested bacteria (Fig. 21-2). It is interesting to note that ingested bacteria are actually protected from antibiotics. It has been established that CGD leukocytes are unable to kill a number of organisms usually associated with the lesions but are able to kill catalase-negative organisms, e.g., pneumococci and streptococci, which cause little clinical difficulty in these patients (Table 21-1).

The demonstration of the bactericidal defect in the leukocytes of CGD patients led Holmes et al. to study the metabolic response of leukocytes during phagocytosis. It was clearly shown that the leukocytes of CGD patients have deficiencies of the metabolic stimulation that in normal subjects is regularly associated with phagocytosis (Table 21-3). Concurrent with the diminished bactericidal capacity are decrease in respiratory response, hexose monophosphate pathway activity, and H_2O_2 synthesis in the phagocytosing leukocytes. The failure of normal H_2O_2 formation leads to deficient halogenation of ingested catalase-positive organisms in CGD leukocytes. Iodination requires the myeloperoxidase present in lysosomal granules plus hydrogen peroxide, and this combination is bactericidal in a cell-free system. It is now clear that it is the major bactericidal capacity associated with this metabolic function that cannot be exercised by patients with CGD.

The leukocytes of CGD patients have a deficiency of NADH oxidase and fail to reduce nitroblue tetrazolium (NBT) dye during phagocytosis. Holmes et al., however, did not find the NADH oxidase deficiency. Glutathione peroxidase of the leukocytes was, however, found to be deficient

Table 21-3. Metabolic Changes of the Leukocytes of CGD Patients during Phagocytosis*

A. Not increased (abnormal response)
   1. Oxygen consumption
   2. Hydrogen peroxide production
   3. Hexose monophosphate pathway activity

B. Increased (normal response)
   1. Glucose uptake
   2. Lactate production
   3. Lipid turnover
   4. Krebs cycle activity

* See Karnovsky, M. L. (1968): Seminars Hemat. 5:156, for review of leukocyte metabolism.

in some of the rare female patients with a similar phagocytic defect. The glucose 6-phosphate dehydrogenase (G-6-PD) of leukocytes from the male patients has been reported to be much less stable at 4° C and 38° C than is the G-6-PD of normal leukocytes. This abnormality does not seem to be due to an abnormality of the G-6-PD enzyme itself, but seems attributable to some modifying factor that is abnormal in the patients' cells.

Electron microscopic evidence indicates that phagocytosis of bacteria by CGD leukocytes is not accompanied by the same vigorous degranulation which occurs in normal leukocytes. However, other evidence that granule lysis is normal in the patient's leukocytes has been presented.

At present writing no satisfactory explanation at the enzymatic level for the metabolic abnormalities observed in any patients with this syndrome has been forthcoming. However, the diminished hydrogen peroxide production by CGD cells appears to be of major importance in the bactericidal defect. The enzyme responsible for the transfer of hydrogen ion from reduced pyridine nucleotide to NBT dye seems to be localized in the granules of the cytoplasm. This enzyme is present and normal in the granules of the leukocytes from CGD patients. The failure of NBT dye reduction by the leukocytes of CGD patients may, in fact, be due to an anomaly in the rupture of the specific granule containing this enzyme. Delayed granule rupture and delayed release of myeloperoxidase may also be factors in the bactericidal defect.

Inheritance

At present, at least four separate groups of patients with the leukocyte bactericidal defect have been identified. The first is the group described by Berendes et al. and subsequently studied by others; this group represents the classic form of this disease. Male offspring are selectively involved and the mothers and grandmothers, as well as approximately half the sisters, are identifiable as carriers. In the bactericidal test and the NBT test, the leukocytes of carriers (of the defect) show abnormalities intermediate between those of CGD patients and normal controls.

In the second group the defect appears to be inherited as an autosomal recessive trait, but thus far only female patients have been proved to be affected. These patients present a clinical picture similar to those of the first group, but the disease may not be as severe. Holmes et al. reported that leukocyte glutathione peroxidase is deficient in two of these patients and the parents in one family had glutathione peroxidase values approximately one-half that of normal activity. Clinically these patients differ significantly from those with either of the first two forms of CGD.

The third group is represented by the cases originally described by Ford and studied by Rodey et al. The latter reported that a defective bactericidal activity of leukocytes was found in females with lipochrome histiocytosis. Levels of glutathione peroxidase in the leukocytes of these patients were normal. The finding by carrier-revealing criteria for the X-linked disease that the mother was not a carrier in these cases does not support the idea of X-linked inheritance. The family history is compatible with an autosomal recessive inheritance.

The fourth form is represented by the case of Cooper et al. in which a complete absence of glucose 6-phosphate dehydrogenase was associated with defective bactericidal activity of the patients' leukocytes. The mode of inheritance of this defect is not clear.

Diagnosis

The history and physical examination will reveal the characteristic clinical features of chronic granulomatous disease. By use of a simple screening test it is now possible to make a prompt presumptive diagnosis. In this test, the total absence of reduced NBT dye in the leukocytes of patients is observed in each of the aforementioned four groups. This initial screening test should be followed by a more elaborate functional and metabolic study of the leukocytes. The demonstration of a defect in bactericidal function of leukocytes establishes the diagnosis.

Treatment

The new knowledge of fatal granulomatous disease is useful in making the diagnosis at an early stage of the disease. The recognition that the bacteria associated with the lesions are pathogenetic permits an appreciation of the significance of low-grade pyogenic pathogens in each infection. This knowledge of the causative organisms facilitates the prompt use of appropriate antibiotics and chemotherapy at an earlier time than was previously possible. In spite of this progress in diagnosis and treatment, this disease continues to have a high mortality rate due to overwhelming or uncontrollable infection.

Treatment with gamma globulin, leukocyte transfusion, vitamin A to facilitate degranulation, methylene blue to initiate pentose pathway activity in leukocytes, and "prophylactic" antibodies has been tried without clinical benefit. Early surgical drainage, excision of extending lesions, and, at times, even radical surgery can be helpful in clinical management of the infections.

Close supervision of patients, early recognition of the characteristic symptoms and signs of each infection, and the prompt initiation and appropriately prolonged treatment with antibiotics constitute the most effective present day treatment. The ultimate cure of this disease should be possible in the future when the new approach of "cellular engineering" permits safe transplantation of bone marrow from a healthy donor. In the meantime Baehner et al. have advocated prolonged prophylactic antibiotic therapy with a broad spectrum antibiotic. We have obtained results approximately equivalent to those obtained by Baehner by using the combination mentioned above and still avoid the use of prophylactic antibiotics largely on theoretical grounds.

MYELOPEROXIDASE DEFICIENCY

Graham, using a benzidine method for staining leukocyte myeloperoxidase, observed that leukocytes from patients with severe acute infections had a marked depletion of cytoplasmic myeloperoxidase (MPO). In addition to this early report of reduced myeloperoxidase activity in leukocytes during acute infection, 5 persons from 3 families have been described who show complete absence of myeloperoxidase. The leukocytes of one of these patients who suffered recurrent acute Candida albicans infections were completely incapable of killing intracellular Candida albicans. Unlike the leukocytes from children with CGD, however, it was found that O_2 consumption during phagocytosis by this patient's leukocytes was normal and there was normal hexose monophosphate shunt activity. However, as in CGD leukocytes, there was little iodination of intracellular bacteria and diminished bactericidal activity. That these patients have little difficulty with the catalase-positive bacteria has been demonstrated by the increased activity of the H_2O_2-producing metabolic pathway of their leukocytes. It has been shown that the patients of this group have an apparently compensatory increase in ability to form H_2O_2 in their phagocytizing leukocytes.

Davis, Brunning, and Quie recently have described a patient with presumed acquired leukocyte myeloperoxidase deficiency. A man with myelomonocytic leukemia was hospitalized with Candida infection and pneumonia. His peripheral leukocytes and bone marrow leukocytes showed no myloperoxidase activity, and studies revealed a bactericidal deficiency. Although not measured in this patient's leukocytes, increased levels of H_2O_2 that have been demonstrated in the leukocytes from another patient with MPO deficiency suggest cellular adaptive compensating mechanisms. The myeloperoxidase-H_2O_2 iodide system is sensitive to the heme protein inhibitor, azide; however, azide-insensitive systems compensate in MPO-deficient leukocytes by greatly increasing H_2O_2 production and increasing nonenzymatic bactericidal activity of H_2O_2. Azide profoundly inhibits the bactericidal capacity of normal leukocytes, an indication that the myeloperoxidase system is highly significant for efficient bactericidal activity in normals. Fortunately, patients with myeloperoxidase deficiency have compensating mechanisms and produce large quantities of H_2O_2.

CHEDIAK-HIGASHI SYNDROME

Patients with the Chediak-Higashi syndrome, like patients with CGD, suffer frequent and severe pyogenic infections. Unlike CGD, however, the diagnosis of this syndrome is relatively simple, since the patient's

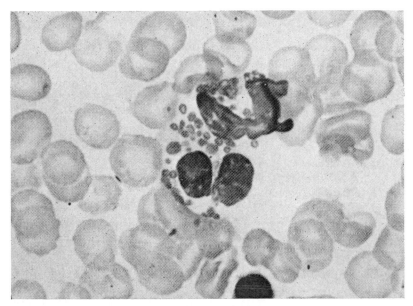

Fig. 21-3. Abnormal giant granules in the cytoplasm of neutrophils (Wright-Giemsa stain X1200). (Courtesy of Dr. Richard D. Brunning, Associate Director of Special Hematology, University of Minnesota Health Science Center, Minneapolis, Minnesota)

phagocytic cells contain characteristic large cytoplasmic inclusions. (Fig. 21-3).

On the basis of electron photomicrographs and histochemical evidence, it appears that phagocytic cells in patients with the Chediak-Higashi syndrome are engaged in autophagocytic activity, which accounts for the large inclusions in the cytoplasm. Peripheral neutropenia in these patients secondary to increased intramedullary destruction of granulocytes and hypersplenism, which, in turn, may result from the process stimulating autophagy are additional problems. Blum et al., on the basis of striking elevations in serum muramidase activity and increased numbers of granulocytic precursor in the bone marrow, suggested an accelerated rate of granulocyte turnover in these patients.

Recent studies have demonstrated defective bactericidal activity in the leukocytes of patients with the Chediak-Higashi syndrome. In these studies, leukocytes from patients with the Chediak-Higashi syndrome phagocytized Staphylococcus aureus at normal rates, but there was defective intracellular bacterial killing. Streptococci and pneumococci also were killed at a slower rate than in the leukocytes of controls. It was observed that the cytoplasmic inclusions that identify Chediak-Higashi leukocytes remained intact after phagocytosis and although seemingly incorporated into the phagocytic vacuole did not discharge contents into the vacuoles as efficiently as is normal.

The "resting" metabolic state of leukocytes from patients with the Chediak-Higashi syndrome was characterized by hexose monophosphate shunt activity two times normal. Oxygen consumption and H_2O_2 formation increased during phagocytosis. A defect in intracellular killing of bacteria despite normal hexose monophosphate shunt suggests that there may be two phases of intracellular killing. The early phase of bactericidal activity may be dependent on lysosomal factors (which are compromised in the Chediak-Higashi syndrome) and continued killing of intracellular bacteria, depending on the respiratory oxidative response with H_2O_2 formation. In contrast, the leukocytes of patients with CGD have little activation of respiratory metabolism and no increase in intracellular hydrogen peroxide, so there is a persistent intracellular killing defect. The basic abnormality of the Chediak-Higashi anomaly in man, as well as in experimental animals, may be attributable to diffusion distances in the gigantic granules.

It was found that the specific activity of beta-glucuronidase and myeloperoxidase in the phagocytic vesicles from 2 patients with the Chediak-Higashi syndrome was approximately one-half the activity found in leukocytes from patients with CGD and normals. Interestingly, there was no difference in activity of acid or alkaline phosphatase and the levels of activity of all enzymes were similar to those of normal leukocytes when whole cell homogenates were used. These observations confirm previous histochemical studies that the giant granules in Chediak-Higashi leukocytes contain peroxidase and beta-glucuronidase and not alkaline phosphatase and do not disrupt normally during phagocytosis so that their enzymes are not discharged appropriately into phagocytic vacuoles.

DEFECTIVE CHEMOTAXIS

Chemotaxis of leukocytes is defined as directed movement of the cells in response to chemical substances. These chemical substances can be generated from serum. For example, complement component C3 yields a split product in the presence of streptokinase and plasminogen, which stimulates chemotaxis of polymorphonuclear leukocytes. Antigen-antibody complexes also induce chemotactic factor formation from C5 and the trimolecular complex of C567. The latter is heat stable and stimulates chemotaxis of polymorphs (Chapter 11). In addition, chemotactic factors are produced by bacteria. These are active in very small concentrations *in vitro* and presumably play an important biologic role *in vivo*.

Recently, impairment in the response of phagocytic cells in chemotactic factors has been demonstrated in such diverse clinical conditions as diabetes mellitus, rheumatoid arthritis, and the Chediak-Higashi syndrome. In diabetes, the chemotaxis of leukocytes was improved by incubation in insulin. In rheumatoid arthritis, defective chemotaxis was believed to be secondary to phagocytized immunoglobulin complexes. In the Chediak-

Higashi syndrome there may be inability of cell diapedesis due to large inflexible cytoplasmic inclusions.

Miller found a defective response to chemotactic stimulation in leukocytes from 2 children with recurrent severe infections and neutropenia. The peripheral leukocytes and leukocytes from the bone marrow had normal phagocytic and bactericidal activity but did not respond to chemotactic stimulation. These children were severely neutropenic, even though bone marrow leukocytes were present in adequate numbers. Rebuck skin windows failed to demonstrate a typical inflammatory response even after infusion of fresh plasma, suggesting a primary defect of neutrophil function rather than lack of plasma factor. He called this disease the lazy leukocyte syndrome.

Patients with cirrhosis of the liver have increased susceptibility to severe, disseminated bacterial infections, and recent findings suggest that defective leukocyte chemotaxis may contribute to this susceptibility. De-Meo and Andersen found that sera from 22 cirrhotic patients contained an inhibitor of chemotaxis of the patients' own leukocytes and also of normal leukocytes. The patients also had subnormal concentration of the complement component C3; therefore, two aspects of their defense system seem to be compromised, i.e., attraction of leukocytes to infected tissue and opsonization of circulating bacteria.

DEFICIENCY OF OPSONINS

Miller and Nilsson reported a deficiency of opsonin in a 3-month-old female infant suffering from severe diarrhea and recurrent infections with Staphlyococcus aureus and gram-negative species. Using a method for determining opsonic capacity of serum that involved phagocytosis of yeast particles preincubated in serum, it was observed that the patient's serum and serum from her mother and other family members failed to opsonize yeast. If yeast particles were incubated in normal serum, the patient's leukocytes were capable of normal phagocytosis and there was normal intracellular bacterial killing by the patient's leukocytes. When Miller found that normal serum restored full opsonic capacity to the patient's serum, he searched for the component that might be missing from the serum. The complement component C5 in addition to C1423 was found to be necessary for opsonization and phagocytosis of yeast and the addition of purified C5 to the patient's serum fully restored opsonic activity. That C5 also may be involved in enhancement of bacterial phagocytosis or perhaps other aspects of host bacterial defense mechanisms was suggested by a striking clinical response of staphylococcal lesions coincident with therapy with fresh frozen plasma that contained active C5.

Jacobs and Miller very recently have reported a second family with deficient serum opsonic capacity and with dysfunction of the fifth component of complement. The affected child in this family had the following

clinical features originally described by Leiner in 1908 and usually diagnosed as Leiner's disease: (a) seborrheic dermatitis, (b) severe diarrhea
with severe wasting, and (c) recurrent systemic infections. The patient's
serum was studied in several ways, and Miller found that inability of
serum to opsonize yeast for phagocytosis by polymorphs was the only
way dysfunction of the fifth component of complement could be detected.
For example, there was normal opsonization and uptake of pneumococci,
and immunochemical measurements revealed normal levels of C5. Dramatic clinical improvement occurred when the patient was given fresh
plasma, and the patient has been maintained in good health on frequent
transfusions with fresh plasma. The plasma used for therapy in this condition must be stored less than 5 days in the blood bank, since C5 is extremely labile.

It is evident that assay of yeast phagocytosis should be carried out on
the sera of infants presenting with clinical features of Leiner's disease,
and if dysfunction of C5 is revealed, transfusions of fresh plasma are indicated.

CHRONIC MUCOCUTANEOUS CANDIDIASIS

A great deal of interest has been generated recently in patients with
abnormal immunologic response to Candida albicans and this subject has
been reviewed. Clinical manifestations of chronic mucocutaneous candidiasis are prolonged, chronic, and recurrent lesions of the mucous membranes, the skin and the fingernails, and the toenails (Fig. 21-4). Patients
usually are not susceptible to other infectious agents, but there is frequent
association with endocrine disorders. Endocrinopathies such as hypopara-

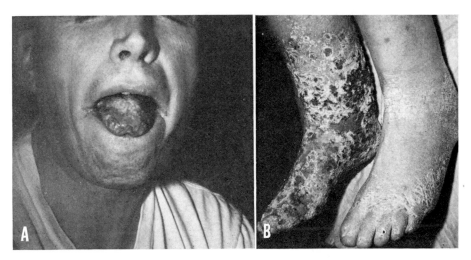

Fig. 21-4. Lesions of chronic mucocutaneous candidiasis involving mucous membranes of mouth
(A) and skin of feet (B).

thyroidism, pernicious anemia, hypothyroidism, and hypoadrenalism may occur after Candida infection or in association with chronic mucocutaneous candidiasis. The endocrinopathy may either precede or follow the development of Candida infections. Autoimmunity may play a role in pathogenesis of both Candida lesions and the dysfunction of endocrine organs.

Usually evidence for some disorder of cellular immunity can be found in patients with chronic mucocutaneous candidiasis. Failure of response to Candida skin test antigen is regular, and some patients have a generalized cutaneous anergy and do not respond to a wide variety of unrelated antigens.

Delayed hypersensitivity to Candida antigen fails to develop despite high titers of circulating antibodies to several Candida antigens. The role of these antibodies in the pathogenesis of the lesions or the abnormal hypersensitivity response is not clear but has been suggested especially in those instances where response to unrelated antigen is normal.

Normal serum brings about clumping of Candida when low levels of antibody to Candida surface antigens are present. When IgG antibodies are present in high titers, which is the case with serum from patients with chronic mucocutaneous candidiasis, clumping does not occur, and furthermore, when anti-Candida antibodies are added to normal serum, clumping of Candida is prevented. Although normal human serum has been reported to be fungicidal, this probably is not true, and it is strictly fungistatic. The role of these specific antibodies undoubtedly is protective because they are opsonic and in the presence of these antibodies rapid uptake of Candida by polymorphonuclear leukocytes and mononuclear cells occurs. Phagocytosis of Candida by polymorphs or macrophages is necessary for fungal killing. Complement is necessary for phagocytosis and from the observations of Miller, it appears that complement component C5 as well as components C1423 are required.

It is interesting that sera with low levels of antibody are more effective as opsonins for Candida than are sera with high levels of antibody. For example, when polymorphonuclear leukocytes from normal persons or from patients with mucocutaneous candidiasis are incubated with Candida and serum from a patient with chronic mucocutaneous candidiasis, prompt phagocytosis of the organisms takes place, but delayed killing of the intracellular Candida, directly proportional to the level of anti-Candida antibody, is seen. A logical explanation for this paradox is that the yeasts are coated with a thick coat of protein in the phagocytic vacuoles of the polymorphs, and it may require time for leukocyte cathepsins to expose the organism to fungicidal components of the phagocytic cell.

It is believed that abnormal lymphocyte function may be directly related to pathogenesis in chronic mucocutaneous candidiasis. Absence of migratory inhibitory factor has been demonstrated in several patients. In addition, transfer factor, the dialysate from extracts of lymphocytes from patients sensitive to Candida skin test material, has been used in treatment of mucocutaneous candidiasis, and dramatic results have been reported in some cases. It has recently been suggested by Kirkpatrick and others that combinations of antibiotic therapy to reduce the load of organisms and transfer factor therapy may be especially helpful in treatment of this awful disease. Several clinical investigators have suggested that the form of chronic mucocutaneous candidiasis that responds to treatment with transfer factor is the granulomatous form.

The possibility that the persistence of the mucocutaneous candidiasis is in some cases consequent to an immunodeviation, or blocking of effective cellular immunity, is certainly worth considering.

SECONDARY DEFICIENCY OF PHAGOCYTOSIS

Several pharmacologic agents have been found to interfere with the phagocytosis function. These include narcotics, phenobarbital, steroids, chloramphenicol, sulfonamides, iron, phenylbutazone, and alcohol.

Phagocytosis is impaired in patients with splenic deficiency syndrome, e.g., congenital asplenia and sickle cell disease, and in patients with liver disease, rheumatoid arthritis, severe bacterial infection, and burns. Patients with congenital or acquired neutropenia have a propensity to develop overwhelming bacterial infection because they lack a most important population of phagocytes. Impairment of the phagocytosis function has been reported in newborns, and these defects are associated with a deficiency of the phagocytosis-promoting capacity (opsonins) of the serum. The defect of opsonins in sickle cell anemia has been shown to be due to the absence of a normal alternate pathway to the complement system. Recently, a new syndrome with defective phagocytosis has been reported by Constantopoulos et al. in two cases and found to be associated with *tuftsin* deficiency. One parent in each family showed tuftsin deficiency but had no evidence of phagocytic defects. Tuftsin (named after Tufts University) is a tetrapeptide (L-threonyl-L-lysyl-L-prolyl-L-arginine) that is made in the spleen and reported to exhibit all the properties that characterize peptide hormones.

JOB'S SYNDROME

Davis, Schaller, and Wedgwood used the term Job's syndrome to describe patients with characteristically "cold" staphylococcal abscesses of the skin, subcutaneous tissue, or lymph nodes. The lungs, liver, or abdominal cavity may be involved also, requiring repeated surgical procedures and prolonged antimicrobial therapy. Eczematoid skin lesions, chronic nasal discharge, and otitis media occur during infancy and recur throughout life. Lymphadenopathy with lymphadenitis and suppuration are recurrent in these patients; despite large abscesses containing copious quantities of pus, little local inflammatory reaction of tissue surrounding the lesions is seen. Each episode is accompanied by systemic signs of infection, i.e., fever, leukocytosis, and increased sedimentation rate. Davis et al. postulated a "defect in local resistance to staphylococcal infection," since Staphylococcus aureus were recovered from all lesions in children with Job's syndrome. The staphylococci successfully breach the anatomic barriers of the body surface in these patients, establish residence, and multiply without stimulating local erythema, heat, or pain. It is this association of repeated invasion of the skin by staphylococci with "cold" abscesses that contain viable bacteria that makes this appropriately named syndrome an intriguing subject of laboratory investigation.

Bannatyne, Skowron, and Weber presented evidence that Job's syndrome might be a variant of CGD of childhood. They reported a 5-year-old girl with red hair and fair skin with recurrent suppurative infections due to Staphylococcus aureus. Lesions included respiratory infections, liver abscess, and chest abscess. Death of the child occurred at 5½ years of age as a result of subphrenic abscess. These investigators studied polymorphonuclear leukocyte bactericidal function in the patient and in the patient's parents and siblings and found an intracellular bactericidal defect. We believe that this patient probably had a variant form of chronic granulomatous disease as it is presently defined and did not have Job's syndrome. Patients with classic Job's syndrome have been repeatedly studied in our laboratory, and no defect of phagocytic function has been demonstrable.

Another patient studied by Pabst et al. was a 9-year-old girl with "cold" staphylococcal abscesses involving the forehead, kidney, and abdomen unaccompanied by pain or local signs of acute inflammation. Biopsy of normal skin and tissue surrounding the abscesses showed a striking accumulation of eosinophils, increased numbers of basophils, and a decided scarcity of neutrophils. The serum immunoglobulins were normal except for an extremely high concentration of IgE. This observation of an association of increased serum IgE, subcutaneous eosinophilia, minimal inflammatory response, and diminished local resistance to staphylococcal infections is extremely intriguing but is as yet unexplained.

SELECTED REFERENCES

Quie, P. G. (1972): Curr. Probl. Pediat. *11*:11.

Fatal (Chronic) Granulomatous Disease of Childhood

Berendes, H., Bridges, R. A., and Good, R. A. (1957): Minn. Med. *40*:309.
Cooper, M. R., et al. (1970): Lancet 2:110.
Good, R. A., et al. (1968): Seminars Hemat. 3:215.
Holmes, B., and Good, R. A. (1972): J. Reticuloendothel. Soc. *1Ω*:216.
Holmes, B., Page, A. R., and Good, R. A. (1967): J. Clin. Invest. 46:1422.
Holmes, B., et al. (1966): Lancet *1*:1225.
Rodey, G. E., et al. (1970): Amer. J. Med. 49:322.

Myeloperoxidase Deficiency

Davis, A. T., Brunning, R. D., and Quie, P. G. (1971): New Eng. J. Med. 285:789.
Graham, G. S. (1920): New York J. Med. 20:46.
Lehrer, R. I., and Cline, M. J. (1969): J. Clin. Invest. 48:1478.

Chediak-Higashi Syndrome

Blum, R. S., et al. (1968): New Eng. J. Med. 279:1009.
Dent, P. B., et al. (1966): Lab. Invest. 15:1634.
Root, R. K., Rosenthal, A. S., and Balestra, D. J. (1972): J. Clin. Invest. 51:649.
Stossel, T. P., Root, R. K., and Vaughan, M. (1972): New Eng. J. Med. 286:120.
White, J. G. (1966): Blood 28:143.
Windhorst, D. B., Zelickson, A. S., and Good, R. A. (1968): J. Invest. Derm. 50:9.

Defective Chemotaxis

Clark, R. A., and Kimball, H. R. (1971): J. Clin. Invest. 50:2645.
DeMeo, A. N., and Andersen, B. R. (1972): New Eng. J. Med. 286:735.
Mowat, A. G., and Baum, J. (1971): New Eng. J. Med. 284:621.
Mowat, A. G., and Baum, J. (1971): J. Clin. Invest. 50:2541.

Deficiency of Opsonins

Jacobs, J. C., and Miller, M. E. (1972): Pediatrics 49:225.
Miller, M. E., and Nilsson, U. R. (1970): New Eng. J. Med. 282:354.

Chronic Mucocutaneous Candidiasis

Lehrer, R. I. (1972): J. Clin. Invest. 51:2566.
Miller, M. E. (1970): Med. Clin. N. Amer. 54:713.
Quie, P. B., and Chilgren, R. A. (1971): Seminars Hemat. 8:227.

Secondary Deficiency of Phagocytosis

Constantopoulos, A., Najjar, V. A., and Smith, J. W. (1972): J. Pediat. 80:564.
Ellis, E. F., and Smith, R. T. (1966): Pediatrics 37:111.
Forman, M. L., and Stiehm, E. R. (1969): New Eng. J. Med. 281:926.
Gladstone, G. P., and Walton, E. (1971): Brit. J. Exp. Path. 52:452.
Johnston, R. B. Jr., et al. (1969): J. Exp. Med. 129:1275.
Mandell, G. L., Rubin, W., and Hook, E. W. (1970): J. Clin. Invest. 49:1381.
McCall, C. E., et al. (1971): J. Infect. Dis. 124:68.
Solberg, C. O., and Hellum, K. B. (1972): Lancet 2:727.
Strauss, R. R., Paul, B. B., and Sbarra, A. J. (1968): J. Bact. 96:1982.
Wurster, N., et al. (1971): J. Clin. Invest. 50:1091.

Job's Syndrome

Bannatyne, R. M., Skowron, P. N., and Weber, J. L. (1969): J. Pediat. 75:236.
Davis, S. D., Schaller, J., and Wedgwood, R. J. (1966): Lancet 1:1013.
Pabst, H. F., et al. (1971): Proc. Soc. Pediat. Res., Atlantic City, N. J.

22
Immunobiology of Fetus and Newborn

Widespread interest in the homograft reaction that developed after the Second World War led a number of investigators to wonder about the anomalous position of the mammalian fetus, contained in the maternal uterus somewhat in the manner of a homograft, albeit a successful one in contrast to the usually unsuccessful experimental homografts. The paternal component of the fetus' genetic constitution should render it foreign and unacceptable to the mother, and the means by which it avoids rejection might be of considerable theoretical and practical interest.

The fetus presents several unique features as compared with the usual homograft:

1. Its genetic constitution is, to be sure, half incompatible with that of the mother, but is also half compatible in that fraction which is derived from the mother. Whether this unusual property is used in some way to preserve the pregnancy is a question.

2. The initial immaturity of the conceptus and the wide developmental range through which even fetuses of shortest gestation pass *in utero* raise questions both as to the antigenic maturity of fetal tissues and as to the fetus' own capacity to achieve an immune response, in this case against those antigens of the mother not represented in the fetus' genetic make-up.

3. The mammalian fetus is unlike a homograft in that the fetus maintains a certain degree of separation from the mother of such a nature as to largely preclude the free exchange of cells between mother and fetus, though permitting exchange of other elements.

MATERNAL-FETAL IMMUNOLOGIC INTERACTIONS

These questions have invited experimentation of a highly diverse nature in a wide variety of animals. The results are often in apparent conflict, and certainly at the moment no unified explanation of maternal-fetal immunologic relationships is possible. Nevertheless, a picture appears to be emerging from the accumulating fragments of information. The picture resembles in some ways that of hormonal control of mammalian reproduction, which shows a remarkable diversity between species, albeit with basic similarities in all. In immunology, a similar diversity is already well established in some areas, for example, in the methods by which maternally derived passive immunity is transmitted to the offspring. Interesting problems can be posed by the search for new understanding of maternal-fetal immune relationships; new ideas on the mechanisms of antigenic recognition, instruction of lymphocytes for antibody production, tolerance, and immunologic paralyses are changing and enlarging our current understanding.

In outbred populations every pregnancy represents a natural parabiotic union and mutal exposure of mother and fetus to each other's potentially foreign tissues and cells. This situation exists, since the fetus inherits from its father a variable number of transplantation antigens that are foreign to the mother and fails to inherit from the mother all of her antigens. Consequently, ever since the principles of transplantation immunology were established, an explanation has been sought for the empirical fact that, unlike homografts transplanted to most sites in the body, naturally implanted embryos in the uterus normally fail to incite an effective level of sensitization on the part of their mothers. Some idea of the magnitude of the homograft problem posed by pregnancy may be gained from the fact that females of many species, including mice and rats, can easily deliver several times their own weight of offspring during their reproductive lifespan.

With the exception of parthenogenesis, the only situation in which a fetus cannot confront its mother with any foreign antigens is when its parents belong to the same inbred strain, in which case it receives similar genetic endowments from both.

Not only are fetuses incapable of eliciting effective levels of sensitivity from their mothers, but they are also totally resistant to, and thus able to override with impunity, an extant state of specific resistance evoked experimentally in the mother. For example, in heterospecific matings (those in which the parents are genetically disparate) preimmunization of the female against the alien tissue antigens of her consort fails to prejudice either the implantation or the normal development of zygotes. An experiment performed by Lanman and his associates demonstrated this in a particularly forceful manner. The success of foster pregnancies in rabbits was impaired by skin grafting the surrogate mothers to produce hyperimmunization against the tissue antigens of both parents of subsequently transferred blastocysts.

Various hypotheses, which have been advanced to acccunt for this virtually unqualified success of fetuses as homografts, must be considered to explain the success of pregnancy in the presence of immunogenetic disparity of mother and offspring.

1. Complete separation of the maternal and fetal circulations is an important contributory factor.

2. The fetus, and especially its membranes in direct contact with maternal immunocompetent cells, is antigenically immature or does not express histocompatibility antigens.
3. The immunologic reactivity of the mother is weakened during pregnancy.
4. The uterus is an immunologically privileged site.
5. A physiologic barrier exists between mother and fetus.
6. The mother is indeed regularly immunized by the fetus, but an immunodeviation also occurs which protects the fetus from the destructive consequences of that immunization.

After reviewing the extensive studies in this field, the authors are struck with the lack of satisfactory explanation of this fundamental question in immunobiology. Perhaps a combination of factors already studied, such as the barrier provided by the placenta, lack of expression of histocompatibility antigens by the trophoblastic cells, and capacity of the mother to achieve an immunodeviation as observed by the Hellströms, explains the success of the fetus as an allograft. But it seems entirely possible that none of these represents the real explanation and that more work is needed to understand the basis for this phenomenon. Perhaps substances produced locally in or by the placenta interfere with an expression or execution of effective antigenic stimulation. Whatever its basis the answer when obtained may give a crucial lead to controlling large tissue and organ allografts.

TRANSPLACENTAL PASSIVE IMMUNIZATION OF FETUS

The earliest record of antibody in cord blood appears to be that of Fischl and Von Wunscheim (1895) who found diphtheria antitoxin in fetal blood in a number of instances. Diphtheria antitoxin was shown to be present in the sera of all infants of Schick negative mothers, whether immunized or not, at levels at least equaling, and often exceeding, those of the mothers. It was absent from the sera of all infants of nonimmunized Schick positive mothers but was present in the sera of some immunized Schick positive mothers. In most instances the level in the infant was actually higher than that of the mother. A close correspondence of maternal and infant titers of antistreptolysins and antistaphylolysins exists by the second half of pregnancy.

Antibodies against the enteric group of organisms have been shown always to be present in massive amounts in the maternal sera but in low titers in the cord sera. It appears from these results that the antibodies to the common enteric pathogens are transmitted from mother to fetus much less readily than, for example, antitoxins. Antibodies against virus appear to be readily, if somewhat erratically, transmitted.

The transmission of antileukocyte antibodies, cold agglutinins, antiplatelet antibodies, antithyroid antibodies, antinuclear antibody from a mother with systemic lupus erythematosus, antipenicillin antibodies, and antibodies to vitamin B-12 intrinsic factor has been reported. Consequently, infants may suffer from thyrotoxicosis due to transfer of LATS to the fetus or from B-12 deficiency due to transfer of antibodies against intrinsic factor to the developing infant.

It is well known that antibodies to the blood group substances, including both naturally occurring isoagglutinins of the ABO system and immune antibodies to antigens of the other blood group systems, are transmitted from mother to fetus. However, the facility with which these antibodies are transmitted varies greatly, some being transmitted at very low levels or not at all and others being readily transmitted and capable of attaining titers in the cord blood comparable to those in the maternal circulation. In general, immune antibodies are transmitted much more readily than the naturally occurring isoantibodies. Moreover, complete agglutinins, detectable by the saline agglutination method, are transmitted at very low levels or not at all, but incomplete agglutinins, detectable only by titration in colloid media or by the indirect Coombs' technique, are readily transmitted. These differences appear to depend largely on the distribution of antibody activity between the various immune globulins, since it has been shown that IgM antibodies are not transmitted in man and that only 7S IgG antibodies are present in cord sera. Since the complete blood group agglutinins are associated with IgM and the incomplete agglutinins with the IgG, this finding goes a long way toward accounting for the major differences in transmission. IgA and IgE, like IgM, are not transferred from healthy mothers to healthy fetuses.

Study of maternal-fetal incompatibility for the genetic Gm characters of the heavy chains of IgG by Fudenberg and Fudenberg (1964) revealed an instance of a Gm(a−) mother of four children by a Gm(a+) father, who developed anti-Gm(a) antibody during the third trimester of pregnancy with her fourth, and first (a+), child. This was taken as evidence of fetal synthesis of Gm (a+) IgG and of its transplacental leakage. Evidence of transplacental leakage was provided also when the mother's titer of anti-B isoagglutinin increased sharply at the same time, the fetus being group B. It was suggested that the transmission to the fetus of such maternal IgG antibodies to a fetal antigen could be important in the etiology of transient hypogammaglobulinemia of infancy. Steinberg and Wilson (1963) found anti-Gm antibodies in the sera of 8 infants who lacked a Gm factor and had never been transfused. In all 8 cases it was found that the mothers had been positive for the Gm factor, the probability of this occurring by chance being very small. It was concluded that the antibodies must have been formed against the maternal gamma globulin passively acquired during gestation. The authors never detected these antibodies in the cord blood and found them only after the infants were 7 weeks of age.

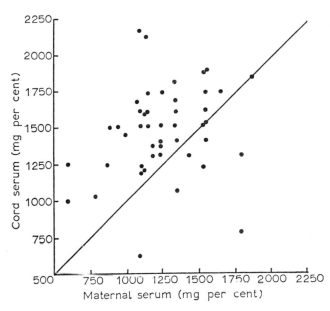

Fig. 22-1. The relation between the IgG-globulin concentrations in maternal and cord sera [From Kohler, P. F., and Farr, R. S. (1966): Nature (London) 210:1070].

Kohler and Farr (1966) compared the IgG concentrations in 46 pairs of normal maternal–cord sera using the agar plate technique of precipitation with an antiserum specific for IgG heavy chains. They found the mean cord concentration to be 1512.5 mg/100 ml (SD 323, range 640 to 2250) and the mean maternal concentration to be 1260.1 mg/100 ml (SD 286, range 600 to 1875) (Fig. 22-1). Thus, the mean concentration in the cord sera significantly exceeded that in the maternal sera (P<0.01) confirming earlier work with less precise methodologies.

Gitlin and Boesman (1966) followed the changes in alpha-fetoprotein, albumin and IgG in the fetal serum from 6½ weeks' gestation to birth. The alpha-fetoprotein had a molecular weight similar to that of albumin and was not found in the maternal serum. It increased in amount in the fetal serum to a maximum at 13 weeks and then declined rapidly to a minimum of less than 2 percent of the maximum at 34 weeks. It was still detectable in the serum of the newborn infant. The albumin concentration reached a plateau at 22 to 24 weeks and remained at this level. The IgG concentration was less than 0.2 gm/100 ml up to 22 weeks and then increased to the neonatal level by 26 weeks.

TRANSPLACENTAL PASSAGE OF CELLULAR ELEMENTS

It has been customary to think of the placenta as a perfect barrier between maternal and fetal circulations that allows the passage of some substances in one direction or the other and excludes others. In recent years it has become increasingly apparent, in the human at least, that leakages of blood from one circulation to the other occur with sufficient frequency to be regarded as normal events. The active immunization of pregnant Rh negative women by their Rh positive fetuses reflects the probability of leakage of fetal red cells into the maternal circulation, and this has been demonstrated to occur both during gestation and at parturition. Fetal red cells have been demonstrated in the maternal blood in a substantial proportion of pregnancies, though in the majority the proportion of fetal cells is so small as to be accounted for by a leakage of a fraction of a milliliter of blood. Leakage can also occur in the other direction, from mother to fetus, and at parturition the passage of platelets and leukocytes to the fetus has been demonstrated.

Red Blood Cells

The occasional passage of large numbers of red blood cells from the fetus into the mother was recognized over 20 years ago by relatively crude techniques. Fetal cells could be detected only when there were enough fetal cells to form small agglutinates with appropriate antisera and when the transplacental hemorrhages were larger than 50 to 100 ml. The development by Jones and Silver (1958) of the sandwich technique in which the isolated minor cells are coated with an incomplete antibody and then with antihuman gamma globulin made it possible to detect small minor fetal cell populations. When relatively large numbers of marker cells coated with incomplete antibody are added to the minor cells rosettes form when the two populations of red cells react. This technique can be used to follow the survival of Rh positive cells injected into Rh negative subjects. Rh positive cells can be detected in a concentration of 1 in 5000 among Rh negative cells.

About the same time, Kleihauer et al. described a technique that has since revolutionized the study of transplacental hemorrhage. The principle of this technique is the differential elution of adult (HbA) and fetal (HbF) hemoglobulin, using a citric phosphate buffer on a blood smear; after treatment, the adult cells appear as ghosts, and the fetal cells stand out as dark refractile bodies (Fig. 22-2).

Various modifications of this technique have been suggested. Considerable attention to detail is required in applying the technique, and a certain amount of experience is needed in the interpretation of individual cells, but in careful hands it gives reliable results. It is the most reliable method for detecting fetal cells at the level of about 1 in 30,000 adult cells, which corresponds to a transplacental hemorrhage of about 0.25 ml fetal blood.

One of the main drawbacks of the acid-elution technique is that about 2 percent of normal adult men and women and as many as 6 percent of

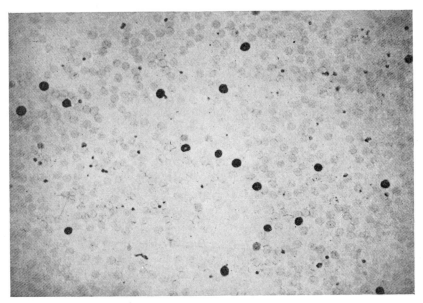

Fig. 22-2. Ghosts of maternal red cells produced by Kleihauer technique. Fetal red cells containing HbF remain uneluted and appear normal (shown as dark).

pregnant women have small proportions of red cells containing HbF. When such numbers are found during or following pregnancy, it is impossible to say whether there are cells of fetal origin in the smear. From the point of view of preventing Rh immunization, women with such findings are probably best regarded as having had a moderate fetal hemorrhage and should be given appropriate doses of anti-D gamma globulin. In patients with thalassemia major, whose red cells contain a large proportion of HbF, transplacental hemorrhages cannot be detected by the Kleihauer technique. Other techniques using fluorescent antibodies have since been introduced but have not gained widespread popularity.

Fetal White Cells and Platelets

The formation of leukoagglutinins during pregnancy and the observation that in most pregnancies the maternal antibodies react with the infant's leukocytes carrying antigens inherited from the father suggest that fetal white cells also may cross the human placenta. At least two pregnancies seem to be needed for the production of leukoagglutinins. Similarly, lymphocytotoxic antibodies are frequently found in maternal serum, especially after multiple pregnancies.

Direct evidence of fetal white cells in the maternal circulation has been obtained by Walknowska et al. (1969) using a cytogenetic approach. Cells with 46/XY karyotype were detected in the circulation of mothers who gave birth to male infants.

Direct evidence that platelets cross the human placenta is lacking, but it is well known that thrombocytopenia occurs in infants born to mothers whose serum contains isoantibodies against platelets.

Antigen Introduced into the Mother

A large number of red cell antigens have now been described; the degree to which they stimulate antibody activity varies greatly. The antigens A and B of the ABO blood system are unique in that anti-A and anti-B "naturally occurring" antibodies are present in subjects lacking the corresponding antigens. Fetal A antigens entering group O or B mothers cannot induce a primary immunization because anti-A is already present. Of all the antigens of the Rh blood group system, D is very much more immunogenic than any other, to the extent that anti-D causes about 99 percent of all cases of hemolytic disease of the newborn not due to anti-A or anti-B. The antigens c, C, and E are the next most strongly antigenic of the Rh system, while the remaining dozen Rh antigens only rarely immunize. Of all the other blood group systems, only antigen K of the Kell system is strongly immunogenic, but occasional cases of hemolytic disease due to maternal immunization against k, Jk^a, M, S, s, and Fy^b have been observed. Race and Sanger list more than 30 inherited blood group antigens; these rarely induce maternal immunization.

Leukocytes carry some, but not all, of the red cell antigens; those of the ABO, MN, and P systems have definitely been detected, but those of the Rh system have not. In addition, leukocytes have antigens not found in red cells. These antigens are detected by using the sera from people who have received multiple blood transfusions or from multiparous women. The sera of the multiparae contain monospecific antibodies more often than do the sera of transfused people; in the latter, antibodies of a variety of specificities tend to be found. Techniques of agglutination, cytotoxicity, and complement fixation are used in studying these antibodies.

The identification of leukocyte antigens is an expanding field of activity, especially since it was realized that some of the antigens are identical with the histocompatibility antigens and are concerned in the rejection of organ transplants. In transfusion practice, leukocyte antigens appear to be much more frequent causes of isoimmunization than are the other relatively poor immunogenic red cell antigens, such as K.

Platelets carry some red cell antigens, some antigens found on leukocytes, and, in addition, antigens which may only be found on platelets. The terminology for platelet antigens is still rather confused; so far six have been identified that are probably primary platelet antigens. They can be detected by thromboagglutination, by complement fixation, or by the mixed antiglobulin technique.

Fetal plasma contains many antigenic substances which might be expected to set up maternal reaction. In particular, the plasma of secretor infants contains the A, B, and H antigens and it may be that these water-soluble antigens are of prime importance in enhancing the production of immune anti-A and anti-B. The Lewis blood group substances Le^a and Le^b may also be present in fetal plasma.

If a sufficient number of immunologically competent cells from adult donors are injected into very young (fetal or perinatal) homologous avian or mammalian hosts, runt disease or transplantation disease may result. Soon after it had been shown that peripheral blood contains immunologically competent cells among its small lymphocyte moiety, attention was drawn to the possibility that runt disease might sometimes occur naturally if enough maternal leukocytes gained access to a genetically appropriate fetus.

Since 1965 a few cases of XX/XY mosaicism in the blood of infants or abortuses with only XX cells in the epithelium have been reported which appear to be due to prenatal entry of maternal (XX) cells into the circulation of male fetuses. In some of these, symptoms highly suggestive of runt disease have been described.

HEMOLYTIC DISEASE OF THE NEWBORN

Humoral immunity of the mother resulting in the production of maternal antibodies to fetal antigens occurs in both man and other animals and gives rise to fetal and neonatal diseases of varying severity and importance when the maternal antibodies are transmitted to offspring possessing the corresponding antigens. It has been realized for a long time that this might happen, but the first clear demonstration of the natural occurrence of such a disease came in 1936 with the discovery of Rhesus disease in man. This discovery led rapidly to an appreciation of its great importance and to the discovery of a number of other similar diseases in man and of comparable diseases in animals, notably in the horse and the pig. All result from the production by the mother of antibodies to fetal blood cell antigens inherited from the father and from the transmission of these antibodies to the young before or after birth. Most relate to antigens borne by the red blood cells and are grouped under the title of hemolytic disease of the newborn.

Rh Hemolytic Disease

The first significant step in the discovery of hemolytic disease of the newborn in man was taken by Levine and Stetson when they recorded the case of a woman, who had borne two previous children, giving birth to a stillborn fetus. In consequence of serious hemorrhage she was given blood transfusions from her husband, both donor and recipient being of group O and apparently compatible. A transfusion reaction occurred, and it was found that the woman's serum contained an isoagglutinin which agglutinated her husband's red cells and those of 80 percent of group O donors. The reactions were independent of the M, N, and P factors, and the iso-antibody was as active at 37° C as at 20° C. The next step was the announcement by Landsteiner and Wiener (1940) that the sera of rabbits immunized with Rhesus monkey blood agglutinated the corpuscles of 39 of 45 group O donors. The following year, Levine et al. showed that hemolytic disease resulted from Rh blood group incompatibility between mother and child.

Following the discovery of Rh incompatibility, the 85 percent of people in the American population whose blood was agglutinated by anti-Rh serum were said to be Rh+, and the remainder Rh—. The Rh antigens, like those of other blood groups, are inherited in a mendelian manner. It soon became apparent that a number of distinct antigens were involved in the system and that three closely linked pairs of alleles, Dd Cc Ee, now thought to belong to one complex locus or cistron, were necessary to account for them, the dominant D being responsible for the Rh+ antigen. Some 30 antigens belonging to the system have been recognized, and there is some doubt if so simple a symbolism can continue to be adapted to represent the increasing complexity of their genetics. However, since the majority of cases of hemolytic disease are due to the offspring inheriting the D antigen from the father, who may have it in a double or a single dose (DD = homozygote; Dd = heterozygote), while the mother lacks it (dd = homozygote), the simpler notation of Rh+ (Dd or DD) and Rh— (dd) is adequate in practice in most cases for serologic purposes. It should be added that the Rh genes are inherited independently of the ABO genes and of the genes of all other known blood groups.

An Rh— woman may become immunized and produce anti-Rh antibodies in one of two ways: (1) by transfusion with Rh+ blood (or injection with material containing Rh+ red cells), or (2) by pregnancies with Rh+ fetuses. Transfusion is the more effective way. A single transfusion of Rh+ blood stimulates the formation of anti-Rh antibodies in at least 50 percent of cases. Even if antibody is not produced in response to a single transfusion, the subject is usuallly sensitized and is likely to produce antibody on any subsequent stimulation. An Rh— woman who has had an Rh+ transfusion has about an 80 percent chance of producing antibody during her first subsequent pregnancy with an Rh+ infant. However, some subjects do not produce antibody even after repeated transfusion.

Pregnancies with Rh+ fetuses alone, without previous transfusion, can induce the formation of antibodies in Rh— women, although in the majority of cases they fail to do so. It is rare for antibody to be produced during a first such pregnancy, the incidence being less than 1 percent. The probability of antibody being produced for the first time is greatest with the second Rh+ pregnancy and declines steeply with subsequent pregnancies. As a rule the production of anti-Rh antibody requires a minimum of two antigenic stimuli from Rh+ fetuses.

Transfusion, on the other hand, is highly efficient and in the majority of cases achieves sensitization on the first occasion and may even result in the production of large amounts of antibody. Once sensitization has occurred, a subsequent pregnancy with an Rh+ fetus is an efficient means of inducing the formation of antibody and does so in the majority of cases, as witness the 80 percent chance of a previously transfused Rh— woman producing antibody with her first subsequent Rh+ pregnancy. Sensitization by pregnancy, when it occurs, is most frequent with first Rh+ pregnancies, as is shown by the decline in the probability of antibody production from the second Rh+ pregnancy onward.

The commonest time for the appearance of antibody induced by pregnancy is immediately post partum. When antibody is already present in the serum, it generally shows a rise in titer after delivery, reaching a peak in 1 to 3 weeks. Since the Rh antigens are not present in solution in body fluids, as are the A and B antigens and those of some other blood groups, but are confined to the red blood cells, it is thought that immunization by pregnancy must involve the passage of fetal corpuscles into the maternal circulation. That the passage of red blood cells occurs most frequently at parturition is indicated by the rarity of immunization during a first pregnancy and by the postparturient rise in titer.

Rh+ red cells of an ABO blood group that is incompatible with the recipient are much less likely to induce Rh— immunization than are Rh+ red cells that are ABO compatible. Thus injections of Rh+ ABO incompatible cells induced the production of anti-Rh antibody in only 15 percent of recipients, whereas similar injections of Rh+ ABO compatible cells induced anti-Rh antibodies in nearly 70 percent of recipients. This effect is apparent also in immunizations of pregnancy, for hemolytic disease occurs more often when the parents are ABO compatible than when they are incompatible. ABO incompatibility appears to afford the greatest protection when the recipient is group O and will therefore have isoantibodies to both A and B antigens. The reasons for the protection afforded by ABO incompatibility, although not fully understood, appear to relate to the difference in the distribution of the antigens present on the red blood cells after contact with circulating antibody than when no antibodies are present in the circulation.

Natural antibodies produced without apparent stimulation by antigen, such as anti-A and anti-B isoagglutinins which are normally present in the sera of persons lacking the corresponding antigen on their red blood cells and such as are found with some other blood groups, do not normally occur in the Rh system. The antibodies result from stimulation with Rh antigens of persons who lack them and are always immune antibodies. The antibody produced against Rh+ cells in Rh— subjects is usually only anti-D, although the sensitizing red cells may have borne other Rh antigens which the subject lacked. The Rh antibodies found in pregnant women are anti-D in 95 percent of cases. Stimulation with Rh antigen generally results in the production of γM-antibodies first, then γG-antibodies as well, and finally only γG-antibodies. Sera contain antibodies which attach to Rh+ red cells but which do not agglutinate them in a saline medium, in addition to those that do agglutinate in saline. The former antibodies have come to be known as "incomplete." Incomplete antibodies will agglutinate the red blood cells if the latter are suspended in serum or suitable colloidal solutions. A sensitive test for such antibodies is the antiglobulin test known as the Coombs' test. The red blood cells after exposure to serum suspected of containing incomplete antibody are washed and exposed to an antihuman γ-globulin serum, prepared in a rabbit or other suitable animal, which reacts with any incomplete antibody attached to the red blood cells and agglutinates them. Antibodies that are γM-globulins usually are of the complete type and agglutinate incompatible red blood cells in saline, whereas γG-antibodies are usually incomplete. Occasionally γA anti-D antibody may be produced, and it can be either complete or incomplete. It appears that only γG globulin is transferred across the fetal membranes to the human infant *in utero*. Since γG anti-Rh antibodies are mostly incomplete, it is these that are most frequent in cord blood and are by far the most important in causing hemolytic disease.

The severity of Rh disease can vary widely with, at the one extreme, slight and transient neonatal symptoms and, at the other extreme, death before or after birth or permanent damage to infants who survive. The rate of stillbirth of Rh+ infants, excluding the first, of Rh— mothers with anti-Rh antibodies in their sera is about 29 percent. The overall stillbirth rate in pregnancies with Rh antibodies in the sera is approximately 12 percent. Intrauterine death may occur sometimes before the twentieth week but usually takes place in the last trimester. Many stillbirths exhibit the condition of hydrops fetalis and are grossly edematous. Infants born alive may be only moderately anemic and develop jaundice within a few hours. Jaundice becomes profound in severe cases, and the tissues of the brain may become stained with bilirubin and permanently damaged by the condition known as kernicterus. However, in the first affected infant the disease tends to be less severe than in subsequent ones. The hemolytic process resulting from the reaction of the maternal antibodies with the infant's red cells is maximal at the time of birth, since the transmission of immunity does not continue after birth. Knowledge of the nature and causes of the disease have led to great advances in the prediction of its incidence and severity and in its treatment by postnatal exchange transfusion and intrauterine transfusion, as well as in its prevention by administration of antibody directed at the babies' Rh($+$) red blood cells when they enter the maternal circulation, but it is still a serious hazard to infant survival.

Prevention of Rh Hemolytic Disease by Immunologic Intervention

The sensitization of Rh— mothers can be effectively prevented by immunologic intervention (Chapter 17). A recent report by a WHO scientific group indicated the effectiveness of this method on the basis of total information available from several thousands of women and many subsequent Rh positive pregnancies. Despite differences in the trials, the results have been remarkably uniform. At six months the incidence of detectable anti-Rh antibody has been about 0.5 percent, and a further 1 to 2 percent of women have formed anti-Rh by the end of the next Rh positive pregnancy. By comparison, when no anti-Rh immunoglobulin has been given, the incidence of detectable immunization is about 8.5 percent at six months and a further 8.5 percent at the end of the next Rh positive pregnancy, i.e., a total of 17 percent.

All Rh negative women who are not already immunized to Rh and who give birth to an Rh positive infant should receive a dose of anti-Rh antibody. Anti-Rh immunoglobulin should be given as soon after delivery as convenient, and within 72 hours whenever possible. It can be given either intramuscularly or, if suitably prepared, intravenously. When the intramuscular route is used it is well to avoid injection into adipose tissue to insure rapid and complete absorption of antibodies.

Assuming that the administration of anti-Rh to recently delivered Rh negative women becomes a routine procedure and that the treatment proves to be not less than 90 percent effective in suppressing immunization, some of the consequences can be predicted. Suppose that the incidence of hemolytic disease due to anti-Rh is 5 per 1000 live births, that 60 percent of affected infants require exchange transfusions, that the overall mortality in live-born infants with hemolytic disease due to anti-Rh is 0.3 per 1000 live births, and the incidence of intrauterine deaths due to Rh immunization in pregnant women is 1 per 1000. If all Rh negative women at risk were treated after delivery with anti-Rh and if such treatment had been in use for 20 years or more, then the overall death rate should have fallen from 1.3 to 0.13 per 1000 pregnancies. Similarly, the number of exchange transfusions required should have fallen from approximately 3 per 1000 to approximately 0.3 per 1000 live births. Since there are, approximately, one billion people in the world belonging to populations in which the incidence of the Rh negative phenotype is about 15 percent, the number of exchange transfusions performed annually should have fallen by tens of thousands, and thousands of deaths should have been prevented. In addition, it would be possible in the future to reassure hundreds of thousands of Rh negative women by telling them that their chances of having diseased infants through becoming immunized to Rh would be negligible.

ABO Hemolytic Disease

Apart from anti-D antibody, antibodies to a number of other blood group antigens have been known to cause hemolytic disease. These include other antigens belonging to the Rh group and antigens of the ABO, MNSs, Kell, Duffy, Kidd, Diego, and a number of the rare or so-called "private" groups. The most important are the A and B antigens of ABO group. Hemolytic disease due to the isoantibodies to these antigens differs in several respects from that resulting from anti-D.

Naturally occurring isoantibodies anti-A and anti-B are normally present in the sera of persons lacking the corresponding antigens; thus group O blood will have both antibodies, group A or group B blood will have one or the other antibody, and both are absent in group AB sera. The antigens occur in solution in body fluids and in most tissues and are borne by the leukocytes and platelets, as well as by the red blood cells. About 80 percent of the population have the antigens in solution in their saliva, gastric juices, and other secretions and are known as secretors. The secretor character is inherited as a Mendelian dominant. These two respects in which the ABO system differs from the Rh system have important bearings on hemolytic disease.

The naturally occurring isoantibodies are usually IgM and do not reach the fetus. The antibodies formed in response to immunization by transfusion or pregnancy are most often of the 7S IgG class, and it is only these which reach the fetus. People of groups A or B form IgM antibodies predominantly, whereas group O people form both IgM and IgG antibodies. The immune 7S IgG antibodies are mainly incomplete agglutinins, but a serum with a potent IgG agglutinin is almost invariably also hemolytic. Incomplete agglutinins are transmitted readily to the fetus, whereas complete agglutinins are transmitted at a low rate, presumably because they tend to be mainly IgM. Hemolysins appear to reach the fetus less readily than incomplete agglutinins but more readily than complete agglutinins.

The antibodies reach the fetus more readily when the mother is group O than when she is group A or group B, and also more readily when she is subgroup A_2 than when she is subgroup A_1. Maternal anti-A antibody does not react with the corpuscles of infants of subgroup A_2, possibly because the antigen on the corpuscles is not sufficiently developed at birth, and in consequence hemolytic disease due to ABO incompatibility is confined to group B and subgroup A_1 infants, subgroup A_2 being spared. The disease is almost confined to the infants of group O mothers because their production of IgG antibody tends to be greater than with group A or group B mothers.

The proportion of ABO incompatible infants in the population is about

20 percent, but as the disease is almost confined to group A or group B infants of group O mothers only about ¾ of these, or 15 percent of all infants, are at risk. Although antibody may reach the fetus in a large proportion of those at risk, the effect in most cases is subclinical or only mildly clinical. Cases sufficiently severe to require treatment are only about 1 in 3000 births, or 10 percent of the number requiring treatment for Rh disease. It is doubtful that ABO incompatibility ever causes intrauterine death, but severe cases do occur and can cause kernicterus and neonatal death, though the latter is very rare. ABO disease, unlike Rh disease, may affect the firstborn, and often unaffected infants may be born after affected ones. Probably the A and B substances in the tissues of the fetus are mainly responsible for protecting it against the incompatible antibodies.

Neonatal idiopathic thrombocytopenia appears to be a disease resembling hemolytic disease in that it is due to the transmission of antiplatelet antibodies (auto- or iso-) from the mother to the fetus. These antibodies when present during pregnancy can result in thrombocytopenia of the mother only, or of both mother and child, or of the child only. Cases of the latter are very rare.

IMMUNE FUNCTION OF NEWBORN

The normal infant is born without active immunity, and the passive immunity it acquires mainly, probably exclusively, before birth begins to wane from the time of birth. Its resistance to disease during the neonatal period depends on these two phenomena and their interactions with each other. Any interval between the decline of passive immunity below an effective level and the development of a sufficient capacity for active response to antigenic stimulation could constitute a period of special vulnerability. Maternal passive immunity obviously can provide the infant only with protection against those antigens to which the mother has had immunologic experience. The child may meet with other challenges before it is itself fully competent to deal with them.

It is apparent from these considerations that in newborn infants the half-life of maternal antibody passively acquired is in the range of 24 to 30 days and that it is considerably longer than the half-life of immune globulin in the normal adult which is about 18 days (Fig. 22-3). Thus passive immunity in the neonatal period is more persistent and provides protection over a somewhat longer period than it would in adult life.

The decline in concentration of gamma globulin during the first month is exponential, with an apparent mean half-life of 20 days or, in the case of one individual infant followed throughout this period, of 25 days, neither half-life being corrected for growth increment in fluid volume. Thus there appeared to be little autogenous gamma globulin produced during this period. Breast-feeding, as compared to bottle-feeding, did not affect the

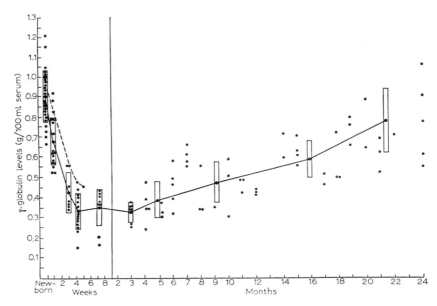

Fig. 22-3. Changes in serum gamma globulin levels from birth to 2 years of age. Note the changes at 2 months. The dots represent the individual values. The solid line connects the mean values, which are at the mean ages of the groups, separated by vertical lines from 2 months to 24 months of age. The bars across the mean values show the range of 1 standard deviation. The broken line connects the values of a single case followed from birth to 5½ weeks of age [From Orlandini, O., Sass-Kortsak, A., and Ebbs, J. H. (1955): Pediatrics 16:579].

exponential nature of the decline in concentration of gamma globulin as it would have done if significant augmentation of the gamma globulin had resulted. The gamma globulin levels of newborn infants as a group are slightly higher than those of their mothers at the time of parturition. After birth the gamma globulin level of the infant falls in a logarithmic fashion for a variable period, lasting in most infants between 1 and 2 months. The half-life of gamma globulin during this period ranges between 19 and 44 days. Sometime between 3 weeks and 4 months of age, varying greatly from infant to infant, logarithmic decline in gamma globulin concentrations ceases, and a brief period of steady state is followed by relatively rapid gamma globulin accumulation. The IgM and IgA are regularly absent from the sera of the newborn, and these begin to appear in the circulation in detectable quantities between the second and fourth months of life. The stage at which autogenous gamma globulin becomes appreciable was shown very clearly by infants born to a mother who suffered from agammaglobulinemia for at least 8 years before the birth of the first and whose gamma globulin level was between 5.6 and 12.8 mg/100 ml. The infants' levels at birth were similar to those of their mother, and they did not show significant rise in gamma globulin until approximately 25 to 42 days of age in the one and 21 to 28 days of age in the other. Their capacity to form antibodies to certain antigens could be demonstrated only after the levels began to rise. In a subsequent infant born to an agammaglobulinemic mother, whom we studied, a much earlier increase of gamma globulin occurred following intensive immunization in the neonatal period.

It appears that the normal human infant, sheltered from antigenic stimulation *in utero,* and possibly with passively acquired maternal antibodies that block stimulation by the common antigens for an interval after birth, does not produce appreciable quantities of immune globulin until it is several weeks old. Given appropriate antigenic stimulation it is equally clear, however, that competence can develop much earlier and the infant at birth, or even the fetus, can produce antibody and that such antibody probably is at first exclusively IgM and only later switches to IgG. It is possible, therefore, to use a single determination of IgM as a nonspecific indicator of infection or antigenic stimulation *in utero.* It is well established that the presence of a sufficient level of passively acquired specific antibody can interfere with active immunization at all ages. There is evidence that in the newborn the presence of maternal passive immunity can interfere similarly with active immunization. It was suggested that active immunization of the neonatal infant depends upon both the potency of the antigen and the level of passive immunity to it that has been acquired from the mother.

Antibodies and Serum Proteins of Colostrum and Milk

Comparatively little attention has been paid to the immunology of human colostrum and milk compared to that which has been paid to bovine lacteal secretions. Much more information is required, not only about the antibody levels of maternal serum and unsuckled colostrum but also about the distribution of activity in each between the various components, γM, γA, $\gamma_1 G$ and $\gamma_2 G$, before a clear picture can be obtained of the immunity provided by human colostrum and milk. Even if little or no antibody is transmitted to the infant's circulation after birth, this immunity could be of great importance for neonatal health through its effect on enteric infections in the alimentary tract. In cultures where sanitation is not so well developed as in the western world enteric infection is a great threat to survival, and diathetic immunization invoking the local immunity system of the breast may be much more important than we have realized to date.

Results obtained thus far suggest that there are large differences in the extent to which a given antibody is secreted in the colostrum and milk in man but that secretion tends to favor antibodies to enteric organisms. Moreover, the amounts of immune globulins in human colostrum are small compared to those present in ungulates, and a large proportion of the immune globulin present may be IgA. It may be that antibodies borne on this fraction of the immune globulins function mainly in the lumen of the alimentary canal rather than in the circulation.

There is no reason to doubt that very small amounts of intact proteins, including immune globulins, may be transmitted from the gut to the circulation of the newborn infant, as they can be in the adult, for it is known that people can be anaphylactically sensitized and desensitized by proteins absorbed by the alimentary tract. The weight of evidence at present is against the transmission of passive immunity to the circulation of the human infant after birth, though there is a much more credible case for thinking that colostral antibodies can afford significant protection against enteric infections operating in the alimentary tract in the human.

In addition to the impairment of humoral immunologic vigor, infants have been shown to have impaired phagocytic function especially attributable to deficits of opsonic capacity of the serum, although bactericidal function of phagocytes is nearly normal. Newborn infants with congenital neutropenia or isoimmune neutropenia may have additional major defects in the defense mechanism.

FETAL AND NEONATAL INFECTIONS

Infection of the fetus due to transplacental egress of rubella virus from the infected mother usually causes abortion or induces teratogenic effects in the fetus if this occurs during the first 3 to 4 months of life. Even when the mother has only a subclinical infection, the virus can still concentrate and replicate in the fetus. Invasion by rubella virus occurs maximally in the early phase of fetal development when the organs concerned are still rapidly dividing and differentiating; it is not surprising, therefore, that the virus damages fetal tissues, and the result is teratogenesis. A rapid linear decline in the severity of teratogenic action due to rubella virus occurs during the first 16 weeks gestation. Virus-neutralizing antibody, which may be either actively produced by the fetus itself or passively acquired from the mother after infection, does not appear to have much protective effect, as fetal infection can still occur when this antibody is present in large amounts in the circulation. This lack of protection may also apply to other intrauterine infections, which are most frequently due to influenza viruses and cytomegaloviruses.

Natural infection of newborn and premature babies during the first weeks of postnatal life with adenoviruses types 1, 2, and 3 and the enteric cytopathogenic ECHO viruses (types 9, 18, and 20) leads to only very feeble antibody responses at 2 weeks of age, although titers rise as high as 1/128 by 4 weeks in some cases.

It has been noted that even prematurely born infants appear to be highly resistant to infection with serum hepatitis virus, as they develop no recognizable symptoms. Infection with serum hepatitis, mumps, and influenza viruses is rare in newborn and very young infants.

Infection with poliomyelitis virus in infancy or early childhood is notable for its frequent lack of serious symptoms, which are usually confined to disturbances in the gastrointestinal tract (the site of infection), and there are few cases of paralysis. Before artificial immunization became effective, the incidence of paralysis in older children increased with age, and this trend continued to adulthood. A protective role of maternal antibody to poliomyelitis virus in the neonate is well established.

Pagano et al. (1964) administered Type 3 attenuated poliomyelitis vaccine (Cox strain) by mouth to 74 premature babies (794 to 2040 gm). A smaller proportion of infants who were born with high titers (at least 1/2048) of maternal antibody were excreting poliomyelitis virus 3 weeks later than babies born with lower levels of maternal antibody. By 3 to 5 months of age, 90 percent of all infants began actively to synthesize their own neutralizing antibody; when re-exposed to the vaccine at this age, their feces were only infective for a brief period, an indication that the babies were resistant to infection. The great theoretical advantage of the Sabin oral vaccine lies in the establishment of a mild intestinal infection by the attenuated virus at the site where natural infection would normally take place. There may be preferential multiplication of one type of poliomyelitis virus (usually Type 2) when a trivalent vaccine is given orally. About 75 percent of babies fed monovalent poliomyelitis vaccine (Sabin Type I) within the first few days of life became immune as was revealed by cessation of excretion of homotypic virus challenge. No advantage was gained by giving oral vaccine at 3 months instead of 6 weeks of age. During the first 10 weeks after birth a mild poliomyelitis infection could be established in the intestinal tract with oral vaccine, but after 10 weeks of age this was more difficult to achieve. The reason may lie in the slow onset of local production of specific IgA antibody by the cells of the lamina propria lining the intestine. In any case, all infants were shown to be resistant on re-exposure to the attenuated virus at a later date.

Fungal infections such as thrush and candidiasis may be acquired by the newborn from the birth canal during delivery, as thrush rarely occurs in babies born by cesarean section. Except for oral and cutaneous manifestations of candidiasis, fungal infections of the newborn are rare, although thrush and monilial dermatitis can be common during the first week of life.

The two main routes of infection that may lead to disease in the newborn are the placenta or ascending infections of the genital tract. In the latter instance, bacteria may invade the fetus and lodge in the lung. As many as 16 percent of perinatal deaths may be due to bacterial infections acquired in the birth process or immediate neonatal period. By far the most common are bacterial infections which ascend the genital tract; these are usually pathogenic strains of Escherichia coli or staphylococcus. Premature babies tend to be more prone to these infections than are full-term infants. From their mothers all newborn babies acquire bacteria that are present on the neonate's skin and in the upper respiratory and gastrointestinal tracts within a few hours of birth. However, only a few newborn children manifest symptoms of bacterial infection.

The pattern of neonatal infections in this era of antibiotics has changed somewhat. Streptococcus pyogenes is no longer the important pathogen it once was. Staphylococcal infections still occur quite frequently, but neonatal infections with enteric pathogens are now the greatest problem. Rickettsial diseases, psittacosis, and typhoid fever are relatively severe in older people but produce only mild symptoms in children. Newborn children are quite susceptible to infection with gram-negative bacteria, possibly because they receive little or no maternal antibody to such organisms and lack crucial opsonins in their sera.

While maternal antibodies transmitted to the fetus *in utero* from the maternal circulation may protect the newborn from immediate exposure to bacteria carried by the mother, this is not the case when children are born in hospitals. In fact in hospital nurseries it is likely that the newborn baby may acquire his first resident strain of staphylococcus, not from his mother but from the nurses. Outbreaks of diarrhea in newborns are sometimes due to Proteus or Pseudomonas but are more commonly due to Salmonellae or one of at least ten different serotypes of Escherichia coli of which the most common are strains O-55:B5, O-111:B4, and O-26:B6. These pathogenic strains of Escherichia coli are usually responsible for nursery epidemics of gastrointestinal disease. Their pathogenicity probably lies not in any greater ability to disseminate more extensively than relatively avirulent strains but in their ability to multiply rapidly at the site of infection.

Mycobacterium tuberculosis most frequently becomes established at the primary site of invasion—the lung. There used to be a high incidence of fatalities following tuberculosis infection of infants in the first 6 months and again during adolescence, but tuberculosis has now been almost completely eradicated in Europe and the United States, although there is still a fairly high incidence among the people from developing countries. In such countries, BCG vaccination is usually performed routinely soon after birth. In Europe, vaccination with BCG is now restricted to contacts of patients with tuberculosis and optionally to adolescents leaving school.

Vaccination with BCG on the first day of life is both practicable and effective. Even prematurely born babies (the smallest was 1800 gm body weight) react well to BCG vaccination, and the only adverse effect has been adenitis. One reason for the effectiveness of vaccination at birth may be the complete absence of maternal antibodies to the mycobacterium. The newborn is, therefore, able to launch an active response without hindrance. Mycobacterium tuberculosis, like most bacteria, will induce humoral antibody formation directed against its polysaccharide antigen and a delayed type of hypersensitivity to its protein antigens; resistance is probably largely dependent on thymus derived small lymphocytes and the phagocytes they utilize in the biologic amplification of their influence. Isoimmune neonatal neutropenia due to maternal isoimmunization can cause cutaneous and occasionally systemic infection in the newborn.

SELECTED REFERENCES

Maternal-Fetal Immunologic Interactions

Anderson, J. M. (1971): Lancet 2:1077.
Beer, A. E., and Billingham, R. E. (1971): Advances Immun. 14:1.
Beer, A. E., and Billingham, R. E. (1973): Science 179:240.
Billingham, R. E. (1964): New Eng. J. Med. 270:667.
Lanman, J. T. (1965): J. Pediat. 66:525.

Transplacental Passive Immunization of Fetus

Brambell, F. W. R. (1966): Lancet 2:1087.
Fischl, R., and von Wunscheim, O. (1895): Z. Heilk. 16:429.
Fudenberg, H. H., and Fudenberg, B. R. (1964): Science 145:170.
Nathenson, G., Schorr, J. R., and Litwin, S. D. (1971): Pediat. Res. 5:2.
Solomon, J. B. (1971): Foetal and Neonatal Immunology. Amsterdam, North-Holland/American.
Thomaidis, T., Fouskaris, G., and Matsaniotis, N. (1967): Amer. J. Dis. Child. 113:654.

Transplacental Passage of Cellular Elements

Jones, A. R., and Silver, S. (1958): Blood 13:763.
Kadowaki, J. I., et al. (1965): Lancet 2:1152.
Kleihauer, E., Braun, H., and Betke, K. (1957): Klin. Wschr. 35:637.
Race, R. R., and Sanger, R. (1968): Blood Groups in Man, 5th ed., Oxford, Blackwell Scientific Publications.
Wiener, A. S. (1948): Amer. J. Obstet. Gynec. 56:717.

Hemolytic Disease of the Newborn

Landsteiner, K., and Wiener, A. S. (1940): Proc. Soc. Exp. Biol. 43:223.
Levine, P., and Stetson, R. (1939): JAMA 113:126.
Levine P., et al. (1941): Amer. J. Obstet. Gynec. 42:925.
Mollison, P. L. (1967): Blood Transfusion in Clinical Medicine, 4th ed. Oxford, Blackwell Scientific Publications.
Race, R. R., and Sanger, R. (1968): Blood Groups in Man, 5th ed. Oxford, Blackwell Scientific Publications.
WHO Technical Report Series No. 468 (1971): Prevention of Rh Sensitization. Report of a WHO Scientific Group, Geneva.

Immune Function of Newborn

Alford, C. A., et al. (1967): New Eng. J. Med. 277:437.
McCracken, G. H. Jr., and Eichenwald, H. F. (1971): Amer. J. Dis. Child. 121:120.
Yeung, C. Y., and Hobbs, J. R. (1968): Lancet 1:1167.

Fetal and Neonatal Infections

Benirschke, K. (1960): Amer. J. Dis. Child. 99:714.
Boxer, L. A., Yokoyama, M., and Lalezari, P. (1972): J. Pediat. 80:783.
Eichenwald, H. F., and Kotsevalov, O. (1960): Pediatrics 25:829.
Eichenwald, H. F., and Shinefield, H. R. (1962): Advances Pediat. 12:249.
Hardy, J. B. (1968): Postgrad. Med. 43:156.
Krugman, S., et al. (1961): Amer. J. Dis. Child. 101:23.
Overall, J. C. Jr., and Glasgow, L. A. (1970): Fetal Neonat. Med. 77:315.
Pagano, J. S., Plotkin, S. A., and Cornely, D. (1964): J. Pediat. 65:165.
Rendle-Short, J. (1964): Lancet 2:373.
Sever, J. L. (ed.) (1969): J. Pediat. 75:1111.

23
Immunodermatology

Skin, a tissue easily accessible and technically exploitable, has long been favored by basic and clinical investigators for studies of allergic diseases and transplantation immunity. Because of gross differences in the timing and the histopathology of test responses to various allergens, skin provides a convenient indicator of allergic states and functions as an aid in the identification of allergies.

Many of the allergic diseases that do not express themselves primarily in the skin can be correlated with skin test responses. Other allergic states can produce pathologic changes in the skin secondarily. On the other hand, skin can actually be a primary target against which the host may react immunologically.

ALLERGIES OF THE SKIN

The skin is a convenient and sensitive indicator of allergic states. It is possible to expose a homogeneous group of experimental animals to a given antigen or to an antigenic determinant and to induce the formation of predictable antibodies. On re-exposure, the resulting antigen-antibody complexes will elicit changes that are similar to, or identical with, changes reported in clinical immunologic entities of the skin.

In a clinical setting, on the other hand, a clear and reproducible cause-and-effect relationship between sensitization and cutaneous reaction does not always exist. Allergic contact dermatitis is the obvious exception. In "endogenous" allergic disorders, the immunologic sequence is often obscure. The attempt to trace the disease to one of a multitude of possible antigens is rarely successful. When antigen is elusive, the antibody cannot be identified. The clinical diagnosis of immunologic entities of the skin remains a difficult and often treacherous task.

Antigen, antibody and sensitized cells are essential components of immunologic disease in skin and elsewhere but do not, per se, determine the nature and extent of the resulting changes. The immunologic diseases of the skin are often multifactorial. Moreover, each of the many factors involved may be controlled to some degree by genetics, age, sex, food, emotions, and even by circadian rhythms.

Drugs are attractive instruments for the study of cutaneous sensitiza-

tion. Chemicals have contributed greatly to our understanding of immediate, as well as of delayed, sensitization. It has been demonstrated that
prefeeding guinea pigs with nitrophenols prevents subsequent attempts
to induce sensitivity to the chemical. Can the same protection be accomplished in man? There is no answer. Patients are often unable to provide
informative clues, since they take not only a "drug" of which they are
aware but also a multitude of chemicals with colors and flavors—foods,
stabilizers, and antioxidants. Even a particular drug is rarely the final
culprit; "haptens" emerge during biotransformation of the drugs or
chemicals that may have scant resemblance to the drug that has been
taken or applied. The relationship between disease and drug in the pathogenesis of presumably immunologic reactions in the skin is poorly understood, but it is known that interactions occur and assume various forms:
(1) the disease may simulate a drug reaction; (2) a drug may, without
sensitizing, alter the immunologic behavior toward agents involved in
the disease for which it is given; and (3) the disease may influence the
immunologic reaction to the drug.

Roughly estimated, there are between 30 and 40 million atopic persons
in the United States who must have one, two, or more positive skin tests
to common allergens. Nevertheless only some 10 million people have hay
fever, and not more than 4 million have bronchial asthma. If skin tests
are done, their statistical hazard is apparent. The burden of proof that
a cause-and-effect relationship exists between positive skin reactions and
clinical symptoms lies with the physician.

The variation from patient to patient in the final step of the immunologic sequence of the release of chemical mediators, and their action upon
target tissue have been considered integral parts of the make-up of the
host. Numerous authors have tried to define the kinetics of the antigen-
antibody complexes as they act on cellular membranes, which in turn
release chemical mediators, or of the action of chemical mediators as they
act on target tissue.

Systemic empirical removal of potential allergens from the patient's
environment or intake is often still the most powerful tool available to
the physician in manipulating allergic diseases of the skin.

ALLERGIC CONTACT DERMATITIS

Allergic eczematous contact dermatitis is a form of delayed hypersensitivity reaction. Patients with eczema are classified on a basis of clinical
pattern and etiology, although an appreciable proportion (20 percent or
more) defy classification. Until the end of the nineteenth century all eczema was believed to be of endogenous origin, but in 1896 Jadassohn
showed that he could produce a reaction at will by the simple application of iodoform to the skin of a surgical patient who had shown an adverse reaction to it. Extensive human and animal studies resulted in the

segregation of cases of exogenous or contact dermatitis from all the other types, which were grouped as endogenous. Evidence was at the same time being provided, largely by physicians in industrial medicine, that dermatitis could be caused by chemical injury or irritation of the skin, irrespective of allergic sensitization.

A dermatitis can be produced by contact between any part of the skin surface and a noxious substance. There are two distinct mechanisms possible. One involves purely chemical damage (the so-called irritant, primary irritant, or toxic dermatitis), and the other is dependent on a specific immunologic reaction (called allergic contact dermatitis). The two mechanisms may be combined in one patient, and a single substance may be capable of acting via either mechanism separately. Allergic contact dermatitis is the only type of dermatitis for which the causative agent and its effects have been subjected to extensive experimental analysis, partly because skin testing can identify the agent and partly because it can be reproduced and studied in animals. No satisfactory test procedure can be used to prove causes of irritant or toxic contact dermatitis in man, and the diagnosis is usually made on the basis of the history and clinical symptoms.

The causative agents in allergic contact dermatitis vary enormously (Table 23-1). The most frequent in men are substances encountered in the course of their work, especially chromates, formalin, synthetic resins, turpentine, and other chemicals; in women, nickel-plated stocking suspenders and other clips and fasteners on clothing are by far the most common sources. In addition, cosmetics, rubber, articles of clothing, and various cleaning agents often cause contact allergic reaction. In both sexes topically applied medicaments form a big group of contact sensitizers.

Contact with poison ivy and poison oak often results in probably the most important practical examples of delayed contact sensitivity. Many people come into contact with these widely distributed plants each year and presumably absorb the active principle, urushiol (a mixture of pentadecylcatechols). These substances are presumed to be absorbed through the skin. Studies of their distribution, metabolic rate and method and time of elimination might contribute to the elucidation of the mechanism of induction of delayed contact sensitivity.

Allergic eczematous contact sensitivity, once established, often persists for many years. However, loss of sensitivity after a few years is not uncommon and seems to vary somewhat with different allergens. Continued exposure or lack of exposure to the allergen does not appear to be a decisive factor. Under experimental conditions, early spontaneous loss of contact sensitivity has been observed.

The keystone of effective management of allergic eczematous contact dermatitis is the discovery and elimination or avoidance of the causal

Table 23-1.   Examples of Characteristic Localizations of Allergic Eczematous Contact Dermatitis and Common Causal Allergens Suggested by Each Site

Localization	Suggested Causes
Scalp	Lotions, scalp tonics, hair creams, hair sprays, hair straighteners, hair dyes, wavesets
Ears	Earrings of nickel, white gold, other metals, scalp preparations (see above), plastics in earphones, hearing aids, perfumes
Trunk, various sites	Clothing, brassieres, girdles, underwear, night clothes, sweaters, bathing materials, bath salts, soaps, perfumes, massage creams
Thighs, legs, ankles	Dye and materials of trousers, underwear, socks; match boxes, cigarette lighters, coins, and other metallic objects carried in trouser pockets; volatile and airborne substances, dusts inside trousers; garters (rubber, elastic, dyes, metal clasps)
Feet (particularly dorsa of great toes), sides and dorsa of feet, sometimes soles (often with little interdigital involvement)	Shoe leather dyes, tanning agents, shoe polishes, chemicals in shoe materials, rubbers, foot powders, sock and stocking dyes and finishes

Adapted from Baer, R. L., and Harber, L. C. (1971): In *Immunological Diseases*, Samter, M. (ed.). Boston, Little, Brown and Co., p. 937.

agent. This is possible through clinical observation, including clues from localizations and periodicity of the eruption and a detailed and well-focused history. If necessary, this can be combined with patch tests. As with other laboratory procedures, however, the results of such tests must be closely correlated with the history and clinical course before they are accepted as being significant, since positive results of patch tests may be totally unrelated to the presenting symptoms.

Symptomatic topical and systemic therapy should be instituted as quickly as possible, whether or not the etiologic factor has been discovered. For toxicologic reasons, attempts to abolish specifically an existing sensitivity by oral or parenteral hyposensitization procedures generally are impractical.

Topical treatment with protective ointment and lotions still seems the best treatment in most instances. Topical or systemic adrenal steroids can suppress contact allergic reactions. The basis of their influence is probably their anti-inflammatory activity. Antibacterial therapy should not be used for prophylaxis but only when bacterial infection has been demonstrated.

ATOPIC ECZEMA (ATOPIC DERMATITIS)

The condition known as atopic eczema has a marked hereditary element and usually starts in early childhood. The eczematous condition appears characteristically more prominent on the face and in the distal flexures. Histologically vascular dilatation and noticeable infiltration of the dermis with lymphocytes, occasional macrophages, and plasma cells are found. The condition is invariably vesicular and often secondarily infected. Children with this disease seem predisposed to develop asthma in adolescence or early adult life. Patients with this disease readily develop skin-sensitizing (reaginic) antibodies in their serum to a wide range of different allergens. There is also a high incidence of elevated levels of IgG antibodies in patients with this condition. On the other hand they have a lowered resistance to the viruses of herpes simplex and vaccinia, especially in involved skin, and are susceptible to secondary infections. Although there is a high incidence of skin-sensitizing IgE antibodies in the serum of patients with atopic eczema, the latter do not appear to play a crucial role in the pathogenesis of the disease. This is indicated by the observation that atopic eczema occurs in children with agammaglobulinemia who do not produce skin-sensitizing antibodies in demonstrable amounts. It is possible that small amounts of antibody below the level of usual methods of detection play a role, but this seems doubtful, since in agammaglobulinemic children with atopic eczema the wheal and erythema skin reactions, often positive in immunologically vigorous children with atopic dermatitis, are lacking.

Little is known about the etiology of atopic eczema; however, the evidence at hand seems to indicate that this syndrome is associated with a number of functional abnormalities of the antibody-producing mechanism, probably of hereditary origin. The high incidence of skin-sensitizing antibodies and of patients with a raised level of IgG in the serum, associated with a marked susceptibility to infection, would indicate that there could be a functional overproduction of certain antibodies and a reduced production of other types of antibodies. The hypothesis that atopic eczema is the result of a malfunctioning antibody-producing mechanism or dysgammaglobulinemia is supported by the regular occurrence of this skin condition in the Wiskott-Aldrich syndrome. This syndrome, which consists of eczema, thrombocytopenia, and frequent severe infections, is a sex-linked recessive disease in which there is a high mortality from infection. Although normal levels of IgG are found in the serum, the patients regularly show reduced levels of IgM and extraordinarily high levels of IgA and IgE. Their clinical symptoms are those of immunodeficiency syndromes because they are unable to produce antibodies to polysaccharides and some other antigens normally. Consequently, their sera have low levels of isohemagglutinins and heterolysins. If the cause of this disease is really immunodeficiency and an imbalance of the immunologic response, it may be that a similar imbalance of lesser degree underlies the development of atopic eczema in apparently immunologically vigorous children. Unfortunately in this syndrome treatment is often unsatisfactory, empirical, and nonspecific. Again, topical corticosteroids are resorted to when conventional empiricism fails.

PEMPHIGUS, PEMPHIGOID AND BEHCET'S SYNDROME

The association of autoantibodies directed against different parts of the epidermis in the serum of patients with various bullous diseases is well documented. The significance of these antibodies is not entirely clear.

Immunologic studies of pemphigus and bullous pemphigoid (pemphigoid) have shown that their pathogenesis is almost certainly due to auto-aggressive (autoimmune) phenomena. Beutner and Jordan (1964) provided the earliest evidence for this theory by demonstrating antibodies against epithelial components in the sera of patients with these two diseases. These antiepithelial antibodies are detected by immunofluorescent assay techniques. In the indirect immunofluorescent test, the antibodies present in sera from patients with pemphigus or pemphigoid are specific for each disease and produce typical immunofluorescent patterns. In pemphigoid, a disease with subepidermal bullae, the antibody binds specifically to the basement membrane of skin or esophagus and not to basement membranes of intestine or kidney tubules. (Fig. 23-1). In pemphigus, an intraepidermal bullous disease, the antibody binds to the surface of epithelial cells in the prickle cell layer so that the immunofluorescence outlines the boundaries of the cells in this zone (Fig. 23-2, Table 23-2).

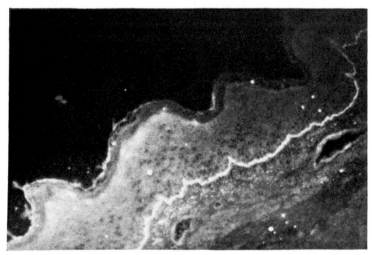

Fig. 23-1. Indirect immunofluorescence staining of guinea pig oral mucosa using the serum of bullous pemphigoid, ×400. Staining of basement membrane zone is evident. [Courtesy of Dr. R. E. Jordan, Department of Dermatology, Mayo Clinic, Rochester, Minnesota.]

Table 23-2.   Patterns of Indirect Immunofluorescent Staining in Bullous Dermatoses

	Intra-epithelial	Epithelial Basement Membrane	Epidermal Nuclei
Pemphigus vulgaris	+	–	–
Bullous pemphigoid	–	+	–
Dermatitis herpetiformis	–	–	–
Erythema multiforme bullosum	–	–	–
Pemphigus erythematosus	+	–	+

Adapted from Beutner, E. H., Chorzelski, T. P., and Jordon R. E. (1970): *Autosensitization in Pemphigus and Bullous Pemphigoid.* Springfield, Illinois, Charles C Thomas.

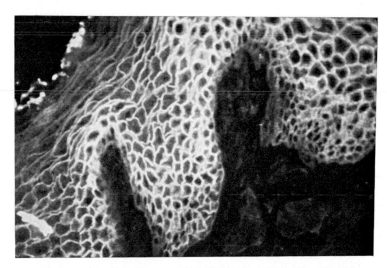

Fig. 23-2.   Indirect immunofluorescence staining (IgG) of guinea pig oral mucosa using the serum of a patient with pemphigus vulgaris, ✕ 400. Staining of intercellular area is evident. [Courtesy of Dr. R. E. Jordon, Department of Dermatology, Mayo Clinic, Rochester, Minnesota.]

Autoantibodies are present in the sera of patients with pemphigus vulgaris, pemphigus foliaceus, and pemphigus vegetans. These antibodies are directed against the intercellular substance of the stratum spinosum (prickle cell layer) of the epidermis. This is the site in the epidermis where these diseases develop, as pathologically they are associated with degenerative processes involving the intercellular bridges between the cells of the prickle cell layer of the epidermis. This causes loss of contact between the cells and results in the formation of the bullae.

In pemphigus, bullae develop intraepidermally after loss of coherence between individual squamous cells. This process is termed *acantholysis*. Acantholysis is preceded by dissolution of the intercellular cement substances, apparently the first histopathologic event detectable by electromicroscopy. Wherever acantholysis is to take place, the cement substance is partially or entirely dissolved. The indirect immunofluorescent test demonstrates antiepithelial antibodies of the IgG class bound to areas corresponding to this cement substance. Direct immunofluorescent tests of diseased skin reveal IgG and complement bound to the pericellular areas. Normal epidermis from patients with pemphigus contains neither gamma globulin nor components of complement in these areas.

The difference between the various types of pemphigus is related to the level in the epidermis at which the immunologic reaction occurs. In pemphigus vulgaris the process occurs deeper in the epidermis, and the prognosis in this variant of the disease is worse than in the other two forms. In pemphigus foliaceus the epidermal cells involved in the immune reaction are more superficial. Pemphigus vulgaris can be controlled by treatment with corticosteroids and immunosuppressives, and under these conditions the level of circulating antibody diminishes.

Bullous pemphigoid is a far less serious disease and is associated with separation of the basement membrane from the epidermis. This disease is also associated with autoantibodies in the serum directed against a constituent of the epidermis. However, whereas in pemphigus vulgaris the antibodies are directed against the intercellular substance of the prickle cell layer, in bullous pemphigoid the antibodies are directed against the basement membrane of the epidermis, again the site of the primary lesion in this disease. One hint as to the relation of these antibodies to the pathogenesis of the disease is that in some cases they are not demonstrable in the serum until the disease has been present for some time, although γ-globulins and complement can be demonstrated bound to the epidermis. Antibodies may not be present in demonstrable amount in the circulation at this stage of the disease, although skin lesions are present. Bullous fluid from patients with pemphigoid reveals clear evidence of activation of the complement systems and especially evidence for activation of both classic and alternate pathways. In pemphigus, too, studies of the bullous fluid reveal evidence for activation of the biologic amplification systems. This is not surprising, since "pemphigoid" antibodies have been shown to be capable of complement fixation.

Dermatitis herpetiformis, a disease often indistinguishable from bullous pemphigoid histologically, can be distinguished sharply by immunologic methods, since the former has not so far been found associated with the development of autoantibodies against any components of the epidermal basement membrane. However, direct immunofluorescent techniques have been used to demonstrate that IgA, not IgE, is deposited in dermatitis herpetiformis skin lesions, especially at the tips of the dermal papillae.

The pathologic significance of these autoantibodies has been a matter for intense discussion. The intradermal injection of serum from a patient with pemphigus vulgaris back into his own skin does not cause the development of a bulla. The only lesion which is found is the typical wheal and flare of a local anaphylactic reaction in the skin. It is well known that one can induce autoantibodies in the serum of experimental animals without causing any disease in the target tissue to which they are directed.

Circulating antinuclear factors, antibodies directed against thyroid microsomal and gastric parietal cells, and disturbance of immunoglobulin levels have been encountered in the serum of patients with dermatitis herpetiformis. In some, the skin lesions are reported to be improved by a gluten-free diet. It has been postulated that in this disease and in celiac disease circulating antibodies to the reticulum of the small bowel may occur. In dermatitis herpetiformis the disturbance may spread to involve also the dermal reticulum. Whether the IgA deposition present in dermatitis herpetiformis skin lesions represents antibody to dermal reticulum remains to be determined. The dramatic response of patients with dermatitis herpetiformis to sulfapyridine remains at best incompletely explained. It is clear, however, that improvement of skin lesions by sulfone treatment may not be associated with improvement of the malabsorption syndrome of the bowel and that improvement of the malabsorption syndrome by a gluten-free diet may leave the skin lesions unimproved.

Another disease of the skin and mucous membranes associated with the development of autoantibodies in the serum is the so-called *Behcet's syndrome*. Symptoms consist of ulcer formation in the mouth and on the genitals, urethritis, arthritis, and in some cases encephalitis. Histologically the lesions show mainly nonspecific inflammation in the dermis. Autoantibodies against cells derived from oral mucous membranes are found in the sera of patients with focal oral ulceration, as well as in those with the complete disease complex of Behcet's syndrome. The antibodies do not appear to be organ specific but cross react with fetal skin and colon. In at least one form of Behcet's syndrome, that with herpetiform lesions, an infective agent has been suggested, since inclusion bodies consistent with viral etiology have been found in the nuclei of cells within the lesions. Moreover, the disease sometimes seems to respond to treatment with tetracycline. Mycoplasma have also been suggested as causative factors in other forms of this disease. No real proof, however, of viral or mycoplasma etiology has been established. It may be, therefore, that in Behcet's syndrome, as in bullous disease of the skin, the production of autoantibodies is secondary to exposure to antigen as a result of infection possibly of viral origin. Better methodologies for isolation of occult viruses or demonstration of their presence in tissues still needs to be applied in these patients.

LUPUS ERYTHEMATOSUS

Development of immunohistochemical techniques, capacity to define complement profiles, and study of circulating antigen-antibody complexes have aided in the analysis and immunologic dissection of the pathogenesis of lupus erythematosus (LE), a multisystem disease that affects many organs or a single organ and in which immunopathologic mechanisms seem clearly to be operative. Investigators using immunofluorescent techniques have observed that the deposition of antibodies and complement occurs in various tissues, namely, kidney, spleen, and skin, in a distribution characteristic of an indirect immunologic assault. The limitations of the immunofluorescent techniques have led to a search for other methods to label antigens and antibodies for serologic, histologic, and ultrastructural studies in LE.

Vazquez and Dixon, applying immunofluorescence to the analysis of lupus erythematosus, demonstrated gamma globulin at the sites of renal and splenic lesions. The renal lesions of LE have been extensively studied for the localization of immune globulins, complement, and fibrinogen. In systemic lupus erythematosus, immune globulins and complement are localized on the epithelial side of the glomerular basement membrane. When resolution by immunofluorescence is adequate, the antibody deposits appear irregular and granular. Somewhat similar patterns are seen in poststreptococcal nephritis and the glomerulonephritis of quartan malaria. These deposits are also similar to the deposits produced in antigen-antibody complex serum sickness and in the Dixon model of experimental chronic nephritis. No deposition of these immunologic components is noted in renal glomeruli of pyelonephritis or essential hypertension. By contrast, a linear pattern of deposition of gamma globulin and complement is associated with intrinsic basement membrane antigens. This type of immunohistopathology is exemplified by Goodpasture's syndrome (Chapter 25). In lupus, electron microscopy has revealed electron-dense deposits on the epithelial side of the glomerular membrane in a "lumpy bumpy" distribution. These are thought to be deposits of antigen-antibody complexes. Soluble antigen-antibody complexes are not so well cleared by the reticuloendothelial system as are less soluble complexes. Thus deposits in this location suggest that soluble antigen-antibody complexes are the basis of the most characteristic lesions.

Burnham et al. first applied immunofluorescence techniques to the study of skin lesions in lupus erythematosus and demonstrated localization of gamma globulin at the basement membrane in the dermal-epidermal junction. Numerous immunofluorescent studies have demonstrated that all three immunoglobulins (IgG, IgA, IgM) and complement may be bound at the dermal-epidermal junction in LE. This is not evidence that the globulins are antibodies to skin but is compatible with the view that an indirect immunologic assault may be occurring in the skin as in the kidneys. The findings of Tan and Kunkel (1966) support this view. Apart from the globulin in the dermal-epidermal junction, they found large aggregates of various sizes and shapes, mainly within the capillaries of the upper dermis, which contained desoxyribonucleic acid, globulin, and complement. In some sections, globulin also lined the endothelium of the dermal arterioles and was present within the nuclei of epidermal cells. Bound antibody, eluted from LE skin lesions at acid pH, however, revealed reactivity with epidermal basement membranes in addition to nuclei.

No antibody to skin was found by indirect immunofluorescence in the sera of these patients. This absence strengthens the conviction that most of this globulin was deposited in the skin as complexes or had formed complexes with soluble material diffusing from damaged skin. The development of anti-basement membrane antibodies may be secondary to the deposition of such complexes.

The globulin in skin of systemic lupus erythematosus differs from the antibodies to epithelium found in bullous pemphigoid because in systemic lupus erythematosus no antibody that combined with the basement membrane was found in the serum. IgG is present consistently enough at the dermal-epidermal junction of even clinically normal skin in systemic lupus erythematosus so that these deposits can be regarded as a diagnostically useful test. Such deposits, however, occasionally occur in other diseases, e.g., rheumatoid arthritis and dermatomyositis, and have rarely been found in clinically normal persons. In discoid LE, on the other hand, IgG deposition occurs at the dermal-epidermal junction in skin lesions but is not found in clinically normal areas. Thus the γ-globulin deposits in the skin, like the autoantibodies in pemphigoid or the "lumpy bumpy" deposits in the kidney, are not absolutely diagnostic, but they are most useful, along with other criteria, in indicating the pathogenetic basis of the lesions.

The presence clinically of "large vessel vasculitis" is relatively uncommon in lupus erythematosus. Vascular depositions of IgG and complement are observed irregularly in other forms of necrotizing vasculitis. In the skin lesions of LE and even in the absence of frank vasculitis, immunoglobulin-complement deposits may be seen in skin vessels. Changes in the dermal-epidermal zone in cutaneous LE have been studied by electron microscopy. In early lesions changes in all components were minimal. The half desmosomes and tonofibrils were quite normal. However, although the basement membrane appeared normal by electron microscopy, projections of basal cells themselves were irregular and have the appearance of microvilli. In more advanced lesions irregular electron-dense deposits along the basement membrane similar to those in the renal lesions are identifiable.

The morphologic changes detected suggest that immunopathologic events occurring at the dermal-epidermal zone play an important role in the pathogenesis of cutaneous lupus erythematosus. Circulating antigen-antibody complexes may be deposited at the dermal-epidermal zone. Several reports have implicated DNA-anti-DNA complexes at the basement membrane in the pathogenesis of nephritis in systemic LE. The presence of complement at the site of the lesions supports its participation. Both primary and alternate complement pathways can be shown to have been activated in systemic lupus erythematosus. Studies of the kinetics of the complement components reveal that the complement system is being excessively utilized in systemic lupus erythematosus. Chemotaxis of leukocytes, seen in early cutaneous LE lesions, can lead to the release of cathepsins, contents of leukocyte granules, and other permeability factors, which in turn can cause destruction of the elastic lamina of arteries, alteration of the basement membrane, and dissolution of the basement membranes. Low levels of all serum complement components have been noted regularly in systemic lupus erythematosus and even in some patients with extensive cutaneous systemic lupus erythematosus. The LE cell test, so useful as a diagnostic clinical hematologic test, is based on the demonstration of engulfed nuclei by granulocytic cells (Fig. 23-3). When LE

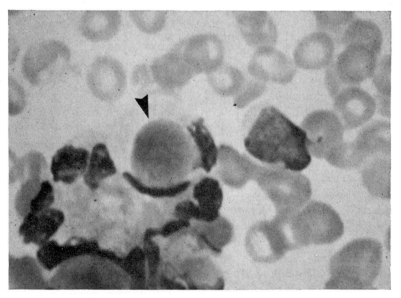

Fig. 23-3. A typical LE cell (arrow) found in the positive LE test, a useful diagnostic clinical test for lupus erythematosus. Opsonized, denatured nuclei are engulfed by neutrophilic granulocytes. [Courtesy of Dr. R. Brunning, Associate Professor, Department of Laboratory Medicine, University of Minnesota Medical School.]

cells are stained with antigamma globulin reagents, the engulfed nucleus regularly stains brilliantly. The gamma globulin on the nucleus of the LE cell is directed toward nuclear protein constituents. The antinuclear factor most diagnostic of LE is, of course, the anti-DNA antibody.

The fluorescent antinuclear-antibody test involves the identification of gamma globulin on nuclei of cells. Various sources of cell nuclei are used, the common ones being human leukocytes, tumor tissue, and mouse or rat liver or calf thymus cells. Depending on the techniques used, a positive preparation can appear as one of the following morphologic types: homogeneous (diffuse), speckled, "nucleolar," and outlined

Table 23-3. Disorders Associated with Antinuclear Antibodies

Collagen-Vascular Diseases
  Systemic lupus erythematosus
  Rheumatoid arthritis
  Juvenile rheumatoid arthritis
  Progressive systemic sclerosis
  Polymyositis
  Sjögren's syndrome

Hepatic Disease
  Chronic active liver disease

Lymphoproliferative and Myeloproliferative Disorders
  Hyperglobulinemic purpura of Waldenström
  Waldenström's macroglobulinemia
  Lymphoma
  Chronic leukemia

Pulmonary Disease
  Chronic bronchitis
  Tuberculosis
  Histoplasmosis
  Fibrosing alveolitis

Miscellaneous Disorders
  Chronic discoid lupus
  Hashimoto's thyroiditis
  Pernicious anemia
  Ulcerative colitis
  Chronic membranous glomerulonephritis
  Lepromatous leprosy
  Neoplasms
  Drug reactions
  Myasthenia gravis
  Recurrent thrombophlebitis
  Infectious mononucleosis
  Idiopathic autoimmune hemolytic anemia
  Apparently healthy individuals

Adapted from Freedman, S. O. (ed.) (1971): *Clinical Immunology.* New York, Harper & Row Publishers, Inc. p. 211.

(shaggy or membranous). The homogeneous type of staining is the common one in both systemic and discoid lupus erythematosus; it reflects antibody to nucleohistone. Speckled fluorescence, the next most common pattern, reflects antibody to a saline-soluble protein of the nucleus and is seen in patients with Raynaud's disease and in the early stages of scleroderma, in addition to those with systemic lupus erythematosus. Antibody to nuclear RNA may be the basis for the "nucleolar" pattern, which is usually seen in scleroderma and occasionally in L.E. The outlined staining pattern reflects a high titer of anti-DNA antibodies and may be seen in patients seriously ill with systemic lupus erythematosus.

The antinuclear-antibody test is thought to be more sensitive but less specific than the LE cell test (Table 23-3). Positive LE tests occur rarely, if at all, in patients with negative antinuclear-antibody tests. Therefore, the latter can be considered an excellent screening procedure.

Numerous antibodies to a variety of nuclear constituents have been described in the sera of man. Of the many nuclear antigens reacting with antinuclear antibodies in serologic tests, however, only anti-deoxyribonucleic acid (DNA) is useful diagnostically for lupus. Although DNA-anti-DNA complexes have been implicated in production of the renal vascular lesions in lupus, the role of antinuclear antibodies in production of disease has not been established.

Treatment of lupus erythematosus is still difficult and in some cases unsatisfactory. When the lesions do not involve the kidney, low doses of adrenal steroids as needed are sufficient to control symptoms and mild hematologic manifestations. When renal lesions are present, more vigorous therapy is indicated because the disease so often progresses to terminal renal failure.

Very large doses of adrenocorticosteroids or lower doses of adrenocorticosteroids coupled with immunosuppressive drugs like azathioprine (Imuran) or cyclophosphamide, used over long periods, have been shown to alleviate the most severe hematologic manifestations, improve renal function, and even reverse the immunohistochemical and histologic lesions in the kidney and skin.

DERMATOMYOSITIS AND SCLERODERMA

Dermatomyositis is a disease having a very characteristic and even specific skin rash, trophic changes in the extensor surfaces, and inflammation in the muscles. The rash is constant in location and appearance but varies in intensity. A purplish pink (heliotrope) rash occurs over the eyes and bridge of the nose. A most characteristic feature is the development of erythematous trophic scarring lesions often seen on the knuckles of hands (Fig. 23-4). Long-standing skin and muscle disease often leads to subcutaneous and cutaneous calcification. In a few cases with muscle weakness, the presence of dermatomyositis is not immediately ascertained,

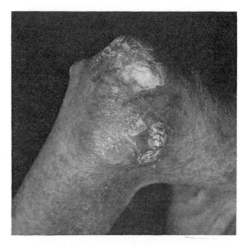

Fig. 23-4. Erythematous trophic scarring lesions of dermatomyositis. These lesions are often seen on the knuckles of the hands, the elbows, and the ankles.

but the later appearance of cutaneous calcifications suggests the ongoing unrecognized disease. Diagnosis of dermatomyositis, although it is usually a most characteristic clinical disorder, is sometimes difficult because some 10 percent of adults with this disease also show features of scleroderma. In fact, cases exhibiting features of both diseases are often referred to as *sclerodermatomyositis.*

The principal changes in muscle in both dermatomyositis and polymyositis include focal or extensive degeneration or regeneration of muscle fibers, interstitial collections of chronic inflammatory cells (lymphocytes, some plasma cells, and occasional histiocytes), fibrosis, and variation in muscle fiber size. Children with dermatomyositis have a high incidence of vasculitis in muscle, skin, gastrointestinal tract, fat, and small nerves. The prominence of lymphocyte accumulation in the muscle lesions might be considered evidence of immunologic assault, but inflammatory cells also occur in response to muscle necrosis.

Inflammatory lesions sometimes are completely lacking in biopsy specimens, a finding often attributable to sampling error. No clear evidence of involvement of immunologic mechanisms has been brought forward in this disease. Complement levels are normal or high, and no significant immune complex, gamma globulin, or complement deposits have been located in lesions of this disease. The disease, however, occurs very frequently in agammaglobulinemic children, a finding that suggests that it indeed may in some way be based on an immunologic perturbation. Gamma globulin levels, however, are normal in the blood of patients with this disease.

Dermatomyositis is frequently associated with malignant neoplasms. The latter association found in nearly 50 percent of adult cases is almost never encountered in children with this disease. Scleroderma may occasionally be confused with dermatomyositis and a *mixed connective tissue disorder* associated with features of dermatomyositis, vasculitis, scleroderma, and Raynaud's phenomenon.

Dysphagia occurs in about 35 percent of patients with dermatomyositis and may sometimes be related to the dilatation and loss of esophageal peristalsis that are also seen in scleroderma. Arthralgia is common in dermatomyositis, but frank manifestations of rheumatoid arthritis usually do not occur. Vasculitis is common in systemic lupus erythematosus, the prototype of both collagen-vascular and autoimmune disease. However, typical dermatomyositis usually does not develop in lupus erythematosus. These rather localized small vessel lesions, however, seem to be quite characteristic of dermatomyositis, and the lesion is not the usual diffuse vasculitis seen in lupus.

Adrenocorticosteroid therapy is a generally accepted treatment for dermatomyositis. Prednisone is most commonly used, starting with 80 mg daily for an adult and perhaps 40 mg in children. Persistent therapy with moderate doses of steroids seems to give the best results.

The empirical evidence that steroids are beneficial is equivocal, and the rationale for treatment is equally obscure. If they are truly beneficial, their effect could be the result of their anti-inflammatory influence on the vascular lesions. More specific immunosuppressive treatment (azathioprine and methotrexate) has been used in many cases and in our experience is rarely beneficial. Over and over again we have tried to confirm the dramatic success reported for amethopterin, but no evidence of benefit has been observed.

Scleroderma (systemic sclerosis) is another generalized disorder of the connective tissue. This disease is characterized by marked swelling, inflammation, and accumulation of collagen in the affected skin and tissues but shows little histologic evidence of involvement of the lymphoid tissues. The synovial membranes of affected joints may show a mild degree of infiltration by lymphocytes and plasma cells. Serologic abnormalities are common. In about one half of the cases, the serum gamma globulin is elevated, and positive lupus erythematosus cell tests are frequently seen. Antinuclear factor is present in the sera of the majority of patients with scleroderma. Nucleolar and speckled patterns of nuclear fluorescence are said to be an important distinguishing characteristic of the antinuclear factor of scleroderma. Skin lesions are frequently associated with dysphagia due to esophageal inflammation and dysfunction and with Raynaud's phenomenon. Iridocyclitis, uveitis, and inflammation of the parotid, lacrimal, and submaxillary glands are sometimes encountered. Treatment of scleroderma is far from satisfactory.

Recently Sharp et al. described a clinical syndrome called *mixed connective tissue disease*, which is characterized by a combination of features similar to those of systemic lupus erythematosus, scleroderma, and polymyositis. Most of these abnormalities are reported to be responsive to corticosteroid therapy. All the patients with mixed connective disease had hemagglutinating antibody to an extractable nuclear antigen (ENA) which consists mainly of protein and ribonucleic acid (RNA).

ERYTHEMA MULTIFORME

Erythema multiforme is an acute inflammatory condition with a wide range of clinical manifestations, largely of unknown pathogenesis. The clinical spectrum of the disease varies greatly; there may be a few asymptomatic macules or a generalized bullous eruption involving the mucosal surfaces and severe constitutional signs and symptoms which may be lethal. It is now evident that exposure to a great number of unrelated agents, such as drugs, bacteria, viruses, and fungi, among others, can precipitate erythema multiforme. The present belief is that erythema multiforme is a reaction pattern of the skin in which a number of physical and chemical factors, as well as immunologic factors, can precipitate the disorder.

The operation of an immune mechanism in erythema multiforme is suggested by the following evidence. A period of 10 days to 3 weeks elapses between initial exposure to a drug and development of erythema multiforme. But on re-exposure the time interval may be only a few days and may be as short as several hours. This time sequence is similar to the latent periods following the induction and elicitation of antigenic stimuli in allergic reactions. Erythema multiforme can be precipitated by re-exposure to the suspected antigen in those cases in which the latter has been identified. The extremely small dose of drug that can precipitate the disease suggests that it does not result from a primary effect of the drug. The histopathologic changes in small blood vessels are similar to those seen in allergic vasculitis, except for a predominance of a lymphocytic infiltration.

Attempts have been made to demonstrate antibodies in the skin by immunofluorescent staining techniques. In contrast to other vesicobullous diseases of the skin in which immunologic factors are believed to play a role, such as pemphigus and pemphigoid, no circulating antibodies to epidermal or basement membrane antigens have been demonstrated, although they have been looked for. Nor has it been possible by direct immunofluorescent staining to demonstrate bound immunoglobulins or complement in the epidermis or in the basement membranes. However, the earliest lesion of erythema multiforme is perivascular and inflammatory, an implication that if immunologic factors play a role, blood vessels or their surrounding structures must be the target organ. No immunofluorescent studies of these dermal structures have been reported.

Erythema multiforme exudativum (Stevens-Johnson syndrome) was described first by von Hebra as a separate form of dermatosis. In 1922, Ste-

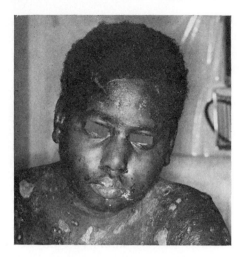

Fig. 23-5. A boy with Stevens-Johnson syndrome, a severe form of erythema multiforme exudativum involving mouth and eyes.

vens and Johnson reported two children with a similar diffuse eruption, fever, conjunctivitis, and stomatitis. Ginandes in 1935 proposed that the term erythema exudativum multiforme (Hebra) be retained and that Stevens-Johnson syndrome be used to describe the more severe form of erythema exudativum multiforme with ocular and oral involvement (Fig. 23-5). Recently Stevens-Johnson syndrome has been associated with mycoplasma infection in some patients.

Steroid therapy is sometimes beneficial for the symptomatic treatment of erythema multiforme.

ERYTHEMA NODOSUM

Erythema nodosum usually appears suddenly without warning as multiple, painful red nodules distributed bilaterally on the pretibial areas. The lesions clinically are round and raised, with a firm center and vague irregular borders; they do not coalesce or suppurate, but the leg may swell. With time, individual lesions evolve like a bruise, changing color gradually and healing without a scar in 3 to 4 weeks, although the entire bout may last 6 to 8 weeks as new crops of nodules appear. Erythema nodosum recurs in about 30 percent of cases. Often the disease is accompanied by malaise, fever, and arthralgia, especially of the knees. Concomitant phlyctenular conjunctivitis is seen occasionally. Erythema multiforme may be associated in a small percentage of cases. It affects predominantly women; however, the sex incidence is equal before the age of puberty. All age groups are susceptible, but the disease occurs mostly in young adults. The diagnosis usually is readily made, but aberrant nodules on the arms, face, and trunk tend to be more edematous and confusing.

Erythema nodosum is generally considered to be a hypersensitivity response, and evidence to date suggests that it is produced by antigen-antibody-complement deposits. The following points seem important in considering the pathogenesis. The onset is explosive; the eruption occurs deep at the junction of the dermis and subcutis, and the lesion heals spontaneously without ulceration or scarring. This suggests a transient acute process without intravascular coagulation or tissue infarction. Erythema nodosum has appeared in conjunction with tuberculosis, streptococcal respiratory disease, fungus infections, the lepromatous form of leprosy, and therapy with certain drugs. It also commonly occurs in patients with chronic ulcerative colitis. The association with all of these diseases in which delayed allergy plays such an important role led to the view that erythema nodosum is a manifestation of cell-mediated immunity. Turk's analysis, especially in lepromatous leprosy, however, links the pathogenesis to antigen-antibody-complement complexes.

COLD URTICARIA AND HYPERSENSITIVITY REACTIONS TO PHYSICAL AGENTS

Physical agents such as cold, pressure, and different wave lengths of light can modify the tertiary structure of skin proteins in such a way that the body may not be able to recognize its own tissue proteins as "self" and they become antigenic, in much the same way as if a foreign chemical group were attached to the molecule. The body can react with either an urticarial reaction or with delayed hypersensitivity to the application of ice to the skin if a patient has been sensitized in this way. In patients with cold urticaria, skin-sensitizing antibodies (reagins) can be demonstrated in their sera. If these are transferred to the skin proteins whose tertiary structure has been modified by cold, occasionally abnormal circulating IgG molecules are capable of being precipitated in the cold, and the complexing of these molecules in the periphery will induce a reaction that has been described as urticarial, but is not a true anaphylactic reaction. If these IgG proteins are transferred to the skin of another individual and cold is applied, a similar reaction will develop. In some instances true reagins presumably of IgG class have been shown to be associated with cold urticaria. In other patients no antibodies have been demonstrable, and the mechanism of the urticaria remains obscure.

In some patients the application of pressure directly to the skin will produce a reaction similar to the Arthus phenomenon, with erythema and swelling developing in 4 to 6 hours. This condition must not be confused with dermatographism in which histamine is released into the skin within a few minutes of drawing a hard object across the surface of the skin. The latter reaction is probably due to the direct release of pharmacologic agents from cellular damage as a result of the trauma. Although it has many features in common with the Arthus reaction, there is no direct evidence that pressure urticaria is immunologically induced.

Ultraviolet light can induce either delayed hypersensitivity or urticarial reactions in sensitive subjects—*solar urticaria.* Urticarial sensitivity can be transferred locally by skin-sensitizing IgE antibodies. Certain chemical substances attached to the body's protein are recognized as antigens when activated by light of particular wavelengths. These drugs are chlorpromazine, chlortetracycline, sulfonamides, and chlorpropamide. The drugs bind to skin protein and are activated when light of the correct wavelength is delivered to the skin. The response is usually a cell-mediated type of immune reaction taking 24 to 48 hours to develop with erythema, induration, and vesiculation. After a heavy exposure to light the reaction in the skin may persist for a week or more before resolution. A most fascinating light sensitivity reaction has been described in lupus erythematosus; a peculiar antigenically distinct nucleohistone is released from cells of both experimental animals and man with lupus after treatment with ultraviolet light.

Photoallergic reactions must not be confused with *phototoxic reactions.* The former are based on immunologic mechanisms and can be elicited only in a small number of individuals who have been previously sensitized by exposure to the photosensitizer and to light; the latter are based on a nonimmunologic mechanism and can be elicited in the majority of individuals on the first exposure.

ANAPHYLACTOID PURPURA

Anaphylactoid purpura is also called Henoch's purpura, Schönlein's purpura, Henoch-Schönlein syndrome, and peliosis rheumatica. This syndrome consists of nonthrombocytopenic purpura, arthralgia, abdominal pain with gastrointestinal hemorrhage, and, occasionally, renal disease.

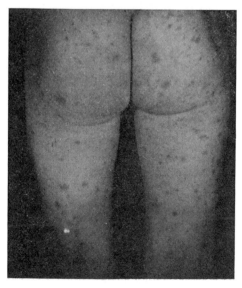

Fig. 23-6. Anaphylactoid purpura involving buttocks and lower extremities.

The disease usually begins abruptly, primarily in children and young people, frequently after an upper respiratory infection. The purpura involves the buttocks and lower extremities and resolves in 2 to 3 weeks, with frequent recurrences before eventual spontaneous remission (Fig. 23-6). Although the term Schönlein's purpura has been used to describe patients with primarily joint involvement and the term Henoch's purpura when gastrointestinal symptoms predominate, this distinction seems unjustified, since most patients have symptoms in both systems, and all the clinical manifestations undoubtedly result from the same pathologic process.

This entity was first reported more than 160 years ago. Schönlein described the arthritic component in 1837 under the name *peliosis rheumatica*. In 1874 Henoch further defined the syndrome and identified abdominal pain, gastrointestinal hemorrhage, and renal involvement as frequent manifestations. Osler, who established the disease as a specific clinical entity, believed that purpura, like serum sickness, resulted from an anaphylactic reaction. Frank, and later Glanzmann, expanded Osler's ideas and introduced the term *anaphylactoid purpura*.

The etiology is unknown. A close relationship between Henoch's purpura and acute glomerulonephritis is suggested by age of onset, sex ratio, seasonal trends, incidence of preceding upper respiratory infection, and similarities in the latent period before the onset of symptoms. Some cases have been provoked by ingestion of specific foods, for example, chocolate.

Hypersensitivity is still believed to be the most likely cause of this syndrome, however, and bacterial products and foods remain the prime etiologic suspects. Recent studies of the skin lesions and focal glomerular lesions have led to the implication of antigen-antibody complexes deposited focally in small blood vessels as the basic pathogenetic mechanism. The triad of rash, abdominal pain, and joint involvement is classic but does not necessarily occur in every patient. This disease is characterized by widespread diffuse vasculitis. The vascular inflammation is similar in all lesions reported, differing only in degree. This uniformity is in striking contrast to the remarkably variable clinical findings.

The renal pathology has been studied extensively. Vernier et al. examined 9 kidney biopsies from 8 children with Henoch's purpura. Their findings refuted the association between an acute glomerulonephritis and Henoch's purpura. The acute lesion of Henoch's purpura is characterized by focal and local glomerular proliferation and capillary occlusion by fibrinoid deposition. Older lesions appear as segmental hyaline deposition with frank scarring. Irreversible renal damage can occur from the extensive lesions, but more often only a small portion of the glomeruli are involved, and healing occurs with good function and no recurrence.

Because the glomerular disease of anaphylactoid purpura resembles in some ways the renal lesions of systemic lupus erythematosus (SLE), some investigators classify Henoch's purpura with the diffuse vascular fibrinoid diseases (collagen vascular diseases) rather than with purpuric disorders, glomerulonephritis, or other forms of vasculitis. The most striking differences between the renal lesions of anaphylactoid purpura and lupus are found in immunohistochemical analysis. Mesangial deposits of gamma globulins and complement are found in Henoch-Schönlein renal disease, but the "lumpy bumpy" irregular deposits along the epithelial side of the basement membrane are lacking. However, both the skin lesions and the focal glomerular lesions in anaphylactoid purpura may be initiated by antigen-antibody deposits.

Anaphylactoid purpura thus may result from an imunologic mechanism analogous to that associated with the LE and other immune complex diseases. Vernier et al. have reported additional information to support an immune origin of anaphylactoid purpura. The leukocyte-platelet thrombi occasionally found in anaphylactoid purpura are a characteristic morphologic finding in tuberculin hypersensitivity, in reactions to soluble antigen-antibody complexes, and in both the Shwartzman and Arthus reactions. These authors postulate that an antigen, or an antigen-antibody complex, is phagocytized by capillary endothelial cells and that this phagocytic capacity is enhanced by histamine. Polymorphonuclear leukocytes attach to these damaged endothelial cells, producing the thrombus observed histologically. Focal endothelial damage leads to focal edema and hemorrhage with subsequent thrombosis and production of the clinical disease.

Prognosis for the acute disease is excellent, particularly if renal disease is minimal (or not evident after one week of illness) and gastrointestinal involvement is mild. Rarely, patients may have profuse hemorrhage from the gastrointestinal tract, develop an intussusception, or progress rapidly to renal failure and death. No specific therapy is available. Symptomatic treatment for arthritis, rash, edema, fever, and abdominal discomfort is helpful. Treatment with prednisone may often bring dramatic improvement of symptoms, including those of the central nervous system.

TOXIC EPIDERMAL NECROLYSIS (THE SCALDED SKIN SYNDROME)

The possible mechanism of the "scalding" in one form of toxic epidermal necrolysis (TEN) is becoming clear. Although some cases of this syndrome remain unexplained, there are two definite etiologic factors— drugs and infection with Staphylococcus aureus, usually phage group II. Melish and Glasgow found that injection of living staphylococci of phage group II into newborn mice caused scalding, whereas mice more than 7 days old developed localized abscesses without scalding.

The terms *exfoliation* and *exfoliative toxin* have been used to describe the epidermolytic toxin, but a better term would be *epidermolytic toxin*, since the skin suffers epidermolysis. It is tempting to extrapolate from mice to man and to suggest that the human disease is due to epidermolytic toxin. The clinical and histologic similarities between mouse and human diseases are striking. The susceptibility of newborns to this bacterial toxin is largely unexplained, but the immunologic incompetence of newborns might be related. Toxic epidermal necrolysis has been reported in patients suffering graft-versus-host disease after bone marrow transplantation from allogeneic donors, and its association with streptococcal as well as staphylococcal infection in recent epidemics suggests a hypersensitivity rather than a toxic mechanism in this disease.

DERMATITIS HERPETIFORMIS

There is now considerable evidence to implicate an immunologic mechanism in the pathogenesis of dermatitis herpetiformis; circulating antinuclear factors, antibodies directed against thyroid microsomal and gastric parietal cells, disturbances of immunoglobulin levels, and deposition of IgA, IgG, and IgM in the skin have all been encountered. It is interesting to note that in some patients the skin lesions are reported to be improved by a gluten-free diet. It has been postulated that both dermatitis herpetiformis and celiac disease have circulating antibodies to the reticulum of the small bowel, and in dermatitis herpetiformis the disturbance spreads to involve also the dermal reticulum. The dramatic response of patients with dermatitis herpetiformis to sulfapyridine remains incompletely explained.

VITILIGO

Vitiligo, the local depigmentation of skin, is associated frequently with hypogammaglobulinemia, immunodeficiency, autoimmune phenomena, and autoimmune diseases. Frequently antithyroid and antiparietal cell autoantibodies are present in the circulation in patients with vitiligo. Recently Gatti described several patients having vitiligo and selective absence of IgA in their serum. Summerlin et al. have studied this relationship in more detail and have found the isolated absence of IgA to be a frequent concomitant of vitiligo and, unlike the case with usual selective absence of IgA, the IgA-possessing B-cells are absent or deficient in the circulation. These findings suggest that vitiligo itself may be due to an autoimmune phenomenon induced by an antigen in the diet or derived from the intestinal flora that cross reacts with antigens on or in the melanin-producing cells of the skin.

AUTOANTIBODIES TO KERATIN

Keratin is an antigen likely to induce formation of autoantibodies. Recently Krogh (1969), using a sensitive red cell immune adherence test, found in most human sera antibody-like IgG and IgM that reacted specifically with the stratum corneum. Since keratin is relatively insoluble in physiologic solutions and is mainly confined to degenerated cells or dead squames, the antibodies to keratin are almost certainly harmless. They could be beneficial and opsonic to keratin if the latter entered the body, as might happen within a ruptured hair follicle.

SELECTED REFERENCES

Allergies of the Skin

Battisto, J. R., and Chase, M. W. (1965): J. Exp. Med. 121:591.
Ishizaka, K. (1969): Hosp. Prac. 4:70.

Allergic Contact Dermatitis

Fellner, M. J., et al. (1969): JAMA 210:2061.
Gell, P. G. H., and Benacerraf, B. (1961): J. Exp. Med. 113:571.
Good, R. A., et al. (1957): J. Clin. Invest. 36:894.
Jadassohn, J. (1896): Verh. Deutsch. Derm. Ges. 5:103.
Walker, F. B., Smith, P. D., and Maibach, H. I. (1967): Int. Arch. Allerg. 32:453.

Atopic Eczema

Krivit, W., and Good, R. A. (1959): Amer. J. Dis. Child. 97:137.
Meara, R. H. (1962): Proc. Roy. Soc. Med. 55:558.
Peterson, R. D. A. (1965): J. Pediat. 66:224.
Rostenberg, A., and Solomon, L. M. (1968): Arch. Derm. (Chicago) 98:41.
Tips, R. L. (1954): Amer. J. Hum. Genet. 6:328.

Pemphigus, Pemphigoid, and Behcet's Syndrome

Bean, S. F., et al. (1971): Amer. J Dis. Child. 122:137.
Beutner, E. H., Chorzelski, T. P., and Jordon, R. E. (1970): *Autosensitization in Pemphigus and Bullous Pemphigoid.* Springfield, Illinois, Charles C Thomas.
Beutner, E. H., and Jordon, R. E. (1964): Proc. Soc. Exp. Biol. Med. 117:505.
Jordon, R. E., Sams, W. T. Jr., and Beutner, E. H. (1969): J. Lab. Clin. Med. 74:548.
Kalbian, V. V., and Challis, M. T. (1970): Amer. J. Med. 49:823.
Kay, D. M., and Tuffanelli, D. L. (1969): Ann. Intern. Med. 71:753.

Lupus Erythematosus

Burnham, T. K., Neblett, T. R., and Fine, G. (1693): J. Invest. Derm. 41:451.
Dubois, E. L. (ed.) (1966): *Lupus Erythematosus.* New York, McGraw-Hill, Inc.
Landry, M., and Sams, W. M. Jr. (1972): Lancet 1:821.
Tan, E. M., and Kunkel, H. G. (1966): Arthritis Rheum. 9:37.
Vazquez, J. J., and Dixon, F. J. (1957): Lab. Invest. 6:205.

Dermatomyositis and Scleroderma

Beck, J. S., et al. (1963): Lancet 2:1188.
Rodnan, G. P. (1963): Bull. Rheum. Dis. 13:301.
Sharp, G. C., et al. (1972): Amer. J. Med. 52:148.
Sullivan, D. B., et al. (1972): J. Pediat. 80:555.
Whitaker, J. N., and Engel, W. K. (1972): New Eng. J. Med. 286:333.

Erythema Multiforme

Ashby, D. W., and Lazar, T. (1951): Lancet 1:1091.
Bell, W. E., Riegle, E. V., and Golden, B. (1971): Clin. Pediat. 10:184.
Cameron, A. J., Baron, J. H., and Priestley, B. L. (1966): Brit. Med. J. 2:1174.

Ginandes, G. J. (1935): Amer. J. Dis. Child. 49:1148.
Lynch, F. W. (1955): South. Med. J. 48:279.
Stevens, A. M., and Johnson, F. C. (1922): Amer. J. Dis. Child. 24:526.
von Hebra, F. (1866): *On Diseases of Skin, Including the Exanthemata*. London, The Sydenham Society 1:285.

Erythema Nodosum

James, D. G. (1961): Brit. Med. J. 1:853.
Löfgren, S. (1967): Scand. J. Resp. Dis. 48:348.
Sams, W. M., and Winkelmann, R. K. (1968): South. Med. J. 61:676.
Turk, J. L., and Waters, M. F. R. (1969): Lancet 2:243.

Cold Urticaria and Hypersensitivity Reaction to Physical Agents

Houser, D. D. et al. (1970): Amer. J. Med. 49:23.
Muller, S. A. (1961): Arch. Derm. 83:930.
Sams, W. M., Epstein, J. H., and Winkelmann, R. K. (1969): Arch. Derm. 99:390.
Sherman, W. B., and Seebohm, P. M. (1950): J. Allerg. 21:414.

Anaphylactoid Purpura

Frank, E. (1915): 52:454.
Glanzmann, E. (1920): Jahrb. Kinderh. 91:391.
Henoch, E. (1874): Berlin Klin. Wschr. 11:641.
Mauer, A. M. (1966): In *Disease-a-Month*, October. Chicago, Year Book Medical Publishers, Inc.
Norkin, S., and Wiener, J. (1960): Amer. J. Clin. Path. 33:55.
Osler, W. (1895): Amer. J. Med. Sci. 110:629.
Schönlein, J. L. (1837): Allgemeine und specielle Pathologie und Therapie 2.45.
Vernier, R. L., et al. (1958): Amer. J. Dis. Child. 96:306.
Vernier, R. L., et al. (1961): Pediatrics 27:181.

Toxic Epidermal Necrolysis

Levine, G., and Norden, C. W. (1972): New Eng. J. Med. 287:1339.
Melish, M. E. and Glasgow, L. A. (1970): New Eng. J. Med. 282:1114.
Peck, G. L., Herzig, G. P., and Elias, P. M. (1972): Arch. Derm. (Chicago) 105:561.
Thomas, F. B. (1972): Lancet 2:484.

Dermatitis Herpetiformis

Fraser, N. G., Ferguson, A., and Murray, D. (1968): Brit. Med. J. 4:30.
Holubar, K., Doralt, M., and Eggerth, G. (1971): Brit. J. Derm. 85:505.
Marks, R., and Whittle, M. W. (1969): Brit. Med. J. 4:772.
Seah, P. P., et al. (1971): Lancet 1:834.
Van de Staak, W. J. B. M., et al. (1970): Dermatologica 140:231.

Vitiligo

Brostoff, J., Bor, S., and Feiwel, M. (1969): Lancet 2:177.
Editorial (1971): 2:1298.
Gatti, R. A. (1972): Lancet 1:91.
Summerlin, W., et al. (in press): In *Immunodeficiency Diseases in Man*, Good, R. A., et al. (eds.). New York, National Foundation.

Autoantibodies to Keratin

Krogh, H. K. (1969): Int. Arch. Allerg. 36:416.

24

Immunopathology of Collagen Disease

The prototype of the collagen or mesenchymal diseases in many ways is disseminated lupus erythematosus, a disorder that has been discussed at some length in the chapter on immunodermatology (Chapter 23). Lupus erythematosus is a multisystem disease involving regularly in most instances the hematologic system, skin, kidneys, heart, central nervous system, gastrointestinal tract, and lymphatic tissue.

SYSTEMIC LUPUS ERYTHEMATOSUS

In systemic lupus, damage to tissues appears to be consequent in large part to autoimmune phenomena which injure the small vessels largely because antigen-antibody complexes capable of activating the complement system by both the efficient primary and the alternate pathways are present in the circulation. The complex mechanism that activates the primary pathway in this disease also activates the alternate pathway by a kind of feedback amplification. These antigen-antibody complexes also probably activate other biologic amplification systems, e.g., the kinin system and blood coagulation. The site of injury seems to be primarily the small vessels as in kidney, skin, spleen, brain, joints, and heart, but large vessels may also be damaged.

The etiologic basis of lupus in general is unknown and the possibility of persistent injury attributable to virus infection must be considered. In some instances, as in sensitivity to the hydantoin and other anticonvulsive agents in children and the antihypertensive drug hydralazine in adults, the etiologic agent or at least the triggering agent is known. Treatment of the latter form of the disease, which otherwise may be fatal, is accomplished when the offending sensitizer is recognized and its intake eliminated. Treatment of the disease of unknown etiology is not so satisfactory and requires long-term therapy with adrenal steroids, often in very high doses, or smaller doses of adrenal steroids coupled with immunosuppressive or anti-inflammatory agents, e.g., azathioprine or cyclophosphamide. In this disease, many kinds of autoantibodies may be found, including autoantibodies directed to components of the surface of erythrocytes,

platelets, and leukocytes. Antibodies against factors essential to blood coagulation may cause hemorrhagic diathesis which can be fatal. The most
extraordinary experimental models of lupus erythematosus are available
in the NZB and NZB × NZW inbred strains of mice (Chapter 15). Here
genetic factors and virus infection interact to play major roles in etiology
of the disease. Recently electron microscopic studies have presented morphologic evidence suggesting that viruses may also play an important role
in human lupus. Another set of recent observations in which lupus was
found in both humans and dogs in two separate households and in several
of the personnel associated with one mouse colony raises the possibility
that one form of lupus might be transmitted from animals to man or vice
versa.

RHEUMATOID ARTHRITIS

The term *rheumatoid arthritis* applies to a syndrome of polyarthritis
which can, in most instances, be differentiated from acute rheumatic
fever, gout, degenerative joint disease, and pyogenic arthritis. Rheumatoid
arthritis is a systemic disease. No age is exempt, but the maximum incidence is the fifth and sixth decades in adult females. Women are far more
frequently affected than males in the ratio of approximately 4 to 1.

Juvenile rheumatoid arthritis is considered by most workers to be the
childhood equivalent of the adult syndrome, but in several clinical ro
spects it is different and in its several forms may represent separate diseases. Ankylosing spondylitis (Marie-Strümpell) and psoriatic arthritis
in their typical expressions are clinically distinct from peripheral joint
rheumatoid arthritis and are not included in this discussion.

It is highly probable that in many etiologically distinct conditions a
polyarthritis can occur that more or less closely mimics rheumatoid arthritis, e.g., the joint diseases of systemic lupus, sarcoidosis, ulcerative colitis, and psoriasis. A more precise classification can be achieved by the
criteria laid down by the American Rheumatism Association that are now
quite generally accepted. Apart from classifying cases into classical, definite, probable, and possible categories based upon the number of diagnostic features presented, the Association drew up an important list of
criteria, any one of which made untenable a diagnosis of rheumatoid arthritis. The classification and exclusion list is shown in Table 24-1.

The synovial membrane of the affected joints is usually swollen, edematous, and hyperemic, but the most striking features are the dense infiltrations of plasma cells and aggregations of lymphocytes into follicular structures sometimes complete with germinal centers. The subcutaneous nodules, which develop at points of pressure or friction, are a characteristic
feature with a histology that, apart from some confusion with granuloma
annulare, is pathognomonic. Involvement of the serous membranes is
common, and lesions in the heart and peripheral blood vessels are by no

Table 24-1. Revised Criteria of the American Rheumatism Association

---

Classical Rheumatoid Arthritis

This diagnosis requires seven of the following criteria. In Criteria 1 to 5 the joint signs or symptoms must be continuous for at least 6 weeks. (Any one of the features listed under "Exclusions" will exclude a patient from this category.)

1. Morning stiffness.
2. Pain on motion or tenderness in at least one joint (observed by a physician).
3. Swelling (soft tissue thickening or fluid—not bony overgrowth alone) in at least one joint (observed by a physician).
4. Swelling (observed by a physician) of at least one other joint (any interval free of joint symptoms between the two joint involvements may not be more than 3 months).
5. Symmetrical joint swelling (observed by a physician) with simultaneous involvement of the same joint on both sides of the body (bilateral involvement of midphalangeal, metacarpophalangeal, or metatarsophalangeal joints is acceptable without absolute symmetry). Terminal phalangeal joint involvement will not satisfy this criterion.
6. Subcutaneous nodules (observed by a physician) over bony prominences, on extensor surfaces, or in juxta-articular regions.
7. X-ray changes typical of rheumatoid arthritis (which must include at least bony decalcification localized to or greatest around the involved joints and not just degenerative changes). Degenerative changes do not exclude patients from any group classified as rheumatoid arthritis.
8. Positive agglutination test—demonstration of the "rheumatoid factor" by any method that, in two laboratories, has been positive in not more 5 percent of normal controls; or positive streptococcal agglutination test.
9. Poor mucin precipitate from synovial fluid (with shreds and cloudy solution).
10. Characteristic histologic changes in synovial membrane with three or more of the following: marked villous hypertrophy; proliferation of superficial synovial cells often with palisading; marked infiltration of chronic inflammatory cells (lymphocytes or plasma cells predominating) with tendency to form "lymphoid nodules"; deposition of compact fibrin, either on surface or interstitially; foci of cell necrosis.
11. Characteristic histologic changes in nodules showing granulomatous foci with central zones of cell necrosis, surrounded by proliferated fixed cells, peripheral fibrosis, and chronic inflammatory cell infiltration, predominantly perivascular.

Definite Rheumatoid Arthritis

This diagnosis requires five of the above criteria. In Criteria 1 to 5 the joint signs or symptoms must be continuous for at least 6 weeks. (Any one of the features listed under "Exclusions" will exclude a patient from this category).

Probable Rheumatoid Arthritis

This diagnosis requires three of the above criteria. In at least one of the Criteria 1 to 5 the joint signs or symptoms must be continuous for at least 6 weeks. (Any one of the features listed under "Exclusions" will exclude a patient from this category.)

Possible Rheumatoid Arthritis

This diagnosis requires two of the following criteria, and the total duration of joint symptoms must be at least 3 weeks. (Any one of the features listed under "Exclusions" will exclude a patient from this category.)

1. Morning stiffness.
2. Tenderness or pain on motion (observed by a physician) with history of recurrence or persistence for 3 weeks.

Table 24-1. (continued)

3. History of observation of joint swelling.
4. Subcutaneous nodules (observed by a physician).
5. Raised erythrocyte sedimentation rate or C-reactive protein.
6. Iritis.

Exclusions

1. The typical rash of *disseminated lupus erythematosus,* with butterfly distribution, follicle plugging, and areas of atrophy.
2. High concentration of *lupus erythematosus cells* (4 or more in two smears prepared from heparinized blood incubated for not more than 2 hours).
3. Histologic evidence of *periarteritis nodosa,* with segmental necrosis of arteries associated with nodular leukocytic infiltration extending perivascularly and tending to include many eosinophils.
4. Weakness of neck, trunk, and pharyngeal muscles, or persistent muscle swelling of *dermatomyositis.*
5. Definite *scleroderma* (not limited to the fingers).
6. A clinical picture characteristic of rheumatic fever, with migratory joint involvement and evidence of endocarditis, especially if accompanied by subcutaneous nodules of erythema marginatum or chorea. (A raised anti-streptolysin titer will not rule out the diagnosis of rheumatoid arthritis.)
7. A clinical picture characteristic of *gouty arthritis,* with acute attacks of swelling, redness, and pain in one or more joints, especially if relieved by colchicine.
8. Tophi.
9. A clinical picture characteristic of *acute infectious arthritis* of bacterial or viral origin with an acute focus of infection or in close association with a disease of known infectious origin; chills; fever; an acute joint involvement, usually migratory initially (especially if there are organisms in the joint fluid or response to antibiotic therapy).
10. *Tubercle bacilli* in joints or histologic evidence of joint tuberculosis.
11. A clinical picture characteristic of *Reiter's syndrome,* with urethritis and conjunctivitis associated with acute joint involvement, usually migratory initially.
12. A clinical picture characteristic of the *shoulder-hand syndrome,* with unilateral involvement of shoulder and hand, with diffuse swelling of the hand followed by atrophy and contractures.
13. A clinical picture characteristic of *hypertrophic pulmonary osteoarthropathy,* with clubbing of fingers and/or hypertrophic periostitis along the shafts of the long bones, especially if an intrapulmonary lesion is present.
14. A clinical picture characteristic of *neuroarthropathy,* with condensation and destruction of bones of involved joints and with associated neurologic findings.
15. *Homogentisic acid* in the urine detectable grossly with alkalinization.
16. Histologic evidence of *sarcoid* or a positive Kveim test.
17. *Multiple myeloma* as evidenced by marked increase in plasma cells in the bone marrow or by Bence Jones protein in the urine.
18. Characteristic skin lesions of *erythema nodosum.*
19. *Leukemia* or *lymphoma,* with characteristic cells in peripheral blood, bone marrow, or tissues.
20. *Agammaglobulinemia.*

Adapted from a committee of the American Rheumatism Association (1959): Diagnostic criteria for rheumatoid arthritis. In *Annals of the Rheumatic Diseases.* Copeman, W. S. C. (ed.) London, British Medical Association, pp. 50-51.

means rare. Splenomegaly and a generalized hyperplasia of lymphoid tissue may occur at all ages but is more frequent in Still's disease, i.e., a form of rheumatoid arthritis in children. Weight loss, anemia, lymphadenopathy, and a raised erythrocyte sedimentation rate are further evidence of the generalized nature of the condition. Although in many patients, especially those seen within 1 year of onset, the disease may soon become arrested, one of the main pathologic problems the disease presents is its extraordinary chronicity with evidence of active inflammation persisting for 30 years or more.

A variant of the disease in which the enlargement of the lymph nodes and spleen is a major clinical feature, usually accompanied by such signs of hypersplenism as anemia, leukopenia, and thrombocytopenia, has long been recognized as Felty's syndrome. Recently a classic case of Felty's type of rheumatoid arthritis was studied by Kunkel and his associates in a patient suffering from severe immunodeficiency with agammaglobulinemia.

With the continuing failure to implicate living organisms in the genesis of rheumatoid arthritis, and the absence of any consistent nutritional deficiency or of any metabolic disturbance such as characterizes gout, it is not surprising that many students of the disease continue to give serious consideration to the possible role of autoimmunity in its pathogenesis. The widespread study of the rheumatoid factor reaction has clearly established that it is due to an immune reaction by the host to one or more specific determinants present in his own γ-globulin. As this conclusion is of far-reaching significance for immunology in general, and for the nature of rheumatoid disease in particular, the steps leading to this conclusion will be followed in some detail.

Over the past 20 years evidence has accumulated that several abnormal proteins that are autoantibodies against γ-globulin circulate in the blood of patients with rheumatoid arthritis. The observation was made 40 years ago that the presence of some human sera enhances the agglutination of sheep red cells treated with rabbit anti-sheep cell serum. This property of some sera was not connected with rheumatoid arthritis until Waaler showed that the blood of a significant proportion of rheumatoid arthritis patients contained such a factor. The factor became generally known as *rheumatoid factor* (RA factor).

A clue to the nature of the rheumatoid factor was provided by the observation that a human serum fraction containing mostly γ-globulin would inhibit the reaction of the sensitized cell with rheumatoid arthritis serum. Subsequently, many experiments have established that RA factor can combine with normal human immunoglobulin, and this has formed the basis of several subsequent tests, all of which depend on the ability of rheumatoid sera to agglutinate particles that have a layer of normal or partially denatured immunoglobulin at their surface, e.g., sheep red cells

treated with tannic acid and exposed to human IgG or particles of polystyrene latex or the volcanic clay bentonite which had adsorbed IgG or
heated IgG. Basically, all of the different reactions are regarded as testing for the presence of antibody to immunoglobulin. But they are not
identical, for sometimes human immunoglobulin and sometimes animal
immunoglobulin are used as the coating for the particles. Moreover, although there is good concurrence in most instances, it is clear that in certain circumstances the different tests give different results; consequently
it is necessary to postulate that a number of rheumatoid factors with
different specificities are involved.

Recently the recovery of purified RA factor has been accomplished
from complexes with sensitized sheep red cells or with mildly aggregated
human IgG. This has led to its characterization as a macroglobulin, or
group of macroglobulins, with a sedimentation constant of 19S. Their
chemical, physical, and antigenic properties are identical to the proteins of the normal IgM class, which is known to contain a variety of antibodies. However, not all RA factor is in the form of macroglobulin; in
some patients it is of the 7S IgG class, and in a few, IgA rheumatoid factors have been demonstrated.

These findings support the assumption that the RA factor is an antibody. What, then, is the antigen that induces its formation? The specific
reaction in all the various tests with human or animal immunoglobulin
implies that the RA factors are antibodies to immunoglobulin G or anti-
antibodies. The occurrence of such antibody, an autoantibody, would
presumably lead to reactions with the antigen in the circulation. Indeed,
as might be expected, rheumatoid factors often circulate in the blood as a
complex readily detected in ultracentrifuge, with a sedimentation coefficient of approximately 22S. This complex becomes dissociated with a
change at acid pH to 19S IgM rheumatoid factor and to 7S normal immunoglobulin, IgG.

In numerous instances human RA factors have been found to react
specifically with the H chains of immunoglobulin G and may even be
specific for H chains of a particular subclass or allotype of human IgG.
In some instances detailed dissection of rheumatoid factors has revealed
immunologic specificity for specific hidden determinants on the IgG
molecule that are revealed only when the molecule functions as an antibody or when the molecule is chemically fractionated. RA factors generally interact more readily with immunoglobulin bound at a surface or
aggregated by gentle heating than with native IgG in free solution. Furthermore, materials with the properties of RA factors can be evoked in
rabbits by prolonged immunization with bacteria, and their level can subsequently be increased by injection of autologous immunoglobulin denatured by gentle heating. In addition, rheumatoid factors appear in high
frequency in the sera of persons having subacute bacterial endocarditis.

Considerations of this kind have led to the hypothesis that RA factors are antibodies against immunoglobulin molecules distorted in some way (e.g., by combination with antigen) so as to reveal determinants that would not normally be exposed on the native IgG molecules in solution. This hypothesis may be correct, but the genetic data and the association of RA with other autoimmune diseases indicate that some abnormal immunologic propensity must play a role.

Human IgG can be used to detect the RA factor in sections of tissue by first labeling it with fluorescein and then by gently heating to cause molecular aggregation. In sections of the lymph nodes, subcutaneous nodules, and synovial fringes from cases of rheumatoid arthritis such fluorescein-labeled heat-aggregated IgG is localized to plasma cells, to the Russell bodies within the latter, and to cells of the germinal centers of the lymph nodes.

The most striking histologic feature of the lymph nodes in rheumatoid arthritis is the follicular hyperplasia with prominent germinal centers. Plasma cells are also numerous in the medullary cords. Indeed, these histologic changes are similar to those produced in experimental animals that are repeatedly stimulated by antigenic materials, and the finding of RA factor in plasma cells provides additional evidence for the antibody-like nature of this entity. The presence of RA factor in the plasma cells of subcutaneous nodules and synovial fringes presumably implies that it is being formed there as a consequence of a local antigenic stimulus. The reason for the localization at these sites poses an intriguing but unsolved problem.

Even if the autoantibody nature of RA factor is accepted, it does not follow that any of the disease manifestations result from this autoimmune process. It is now clear that more persons have rheumatoid factor in their circulation without showing symptoms of rheumatoid arthritis than have rheumatoid factor in their serum together with rheumatoid arthritis (Table 24-2). An analogy could be drawn with syphilis, in which circulating 19S antibodies against an intracellular constituent, e.g., heart, may occur and give rise to the Wassermann reaction. These may be produced in response to the tissue destruction consequent to the treponemal infection. In this analogy the RA factors could be the consequence of infection with an unrecognized agent and without major pathogenic significance on their own. Also, the RA factors were originally described in diseases such as liver cirrhosis before they were even associated with rheumatoid arthritis, and patients with various conditions that are associated with hyperglobulinemia, such as sarcoidosis, also may show high titers. The latter may be present for prolonged periods in such patients without the appearance of arthritis. Finally, rheumatoid arthritis may occur in the subjects of hypo-γ-globulinemia. This, however, is a complex issue, since rheumatoid disease occurring in agammaglobulinemic patients may be

Table 24-2.   Diseases Associated with Rheumatoid Factor Activity

Frequent Association
  Rheumatoid arthritis (90%)
  Sjögren's syndrome (75%)
  Systemic lupus erythematosus (30%)
  Juvenile rheumatoid arthritis (25%)

Occasional Association
  Polyarteritis nodosa
  Systemic sclerosis
  Hypergammaglobulinemia due to any cause
  Leprosy
  Fibrosing alveolitis
  Chronic bronchitis
  Myocardial infarction
  Paroxysmal nocturnal hemoglobinuria
  Renal allografts
  Skin allografts
  Infectious mononucleosis
  Cryoglobulinemia
  Syphilis
  Multiple transfusions
  Multiple vaccinations
  Endogenous depression
  Leukemia
  Normal individuals, particularly in the older age groups

From Freedman, S. O. (ed.) (1971): *Clinical Immunology,* New York, Harper & Row Publishers, Inc. p. 223.

associated with small or even large amounts of rheumatoid factor. In the most extreme forms of X-linked agammaglobulinemia, however, rheumatoid arthritis has been seen without rheumatoid factors demonstrable by even the most sensitive techniques.

The RA factor has been shown to be present in symptom-free relatives of patients with rheumatoid arthritis. If such familial clustering is genetically determined, then, in view of the preponderance of the disease in females, it would be tempting to assume that a somewhat sex-limited form of inheritance is involved, such as a dominant gene on the X chromosome or a somatic chromosomal involvement. Thus far the evidence for clear genetic involvement is far from satisfactory, and it is best to think of this disease as often being familial, but not necessarily genetic, with hormonal influence being required for full expression.

Many patients with rheumatoid arthritis (40 percent in some surveys) possess antinuclear factors in their serum as shown by the fluorescent antibody technique. Conversely, rheumatoid factors occur with high frequency in relatives of patients with lupus erythematosus. The clinical association of rheumatoid arthritis and lupus erythematosus has long been recognized. These facts, taken together with the genetic data and the findings that several other diseases thought to be due to an autoimmune process (hemolytic anemia, ulcerative colitis, lymph-adenoid goiter, Sjögren's disease) are often associated, have led to the view that a genetically predetermined group of persons can lose their tolerance to antigenic components of their own tissues and develop an immunologic response at these sites. This basically is a statement of the forbidden clone concept of autoimmunity. The alternative view is that for reasons as yet unknown patients who develop rheumatoid arthritis or rheumatoid factors are infected chronically with exogenous agent/agents that perturb the immunologic system and that the altered immune response leads in some way to the tissue damage. This is the concept of the forbidden antigen.

There is substantial evidence from recent studies that special forms of 7S IgG rheumatoid factor complexing with IgG may be present in synovial fluid. Unlike other rheumatoid factors these can activate the complement cascade. Such factors could surely participate in the inflammatory events of rheumatoid arthritis. In addition, evidence that the complement system has been activated in the joint spaces has been presented. Finally, it is also clear that although some rheumatoid factors do not activate the complement system and cannot produce inflammation by this mechanism, they may activate other biologic amplification systems, and these engage effector mechanisms via another pathway.

Rheumatoid arthritis occurring during childhood takes three distinctly separate clinical forms; Still's disease, adult type of rheumatoid arthritis, and the pauciarticular form often associated with iridocyclitis.

The Still's form often presents as a septic-like disease with high spiking fever, extreme leukocytosis, lymphadenopathy, and significant splenomegaly. Later joint disease develops which can involve any joints and is quite symmetrical. Children with the Still's form often have a diagnostic skin rash that is an evanescent salmon pink and usually has small clear centers. Although usually not, the rash occasionally is urticarial and pruritic. This disease is almost never associated with a significant titer of rheumatoid factor. The synovitis, however, may produce serious secondary consequences including growth retardation, shortening of specific long bones, the jaw, or the fingers. The median duration is about 3½ to 4 years, but we have studied cases in which activity lasted for more than 25 years and produced awful crippling in spite of the most skillful therapy. This disease may first express itself on the day after birth, and frank Still's disease has occurred in children with agammaglobulinemia of the most extreme form. Although rare among the rheumatoid diseases of adults, this Still's type of rheumatoid arthritis occasionally is encountered in adults.

The second form of rheumatoid arthritis, which may occur at any age of childhood, is identical to the common rheumatoid arthritis of adult life. Rheumatoid factor occurs in high frequency. Joint involvement is symmetrical and all the features of the adult disease, including subcutaneous nodules and the presence of rheumatoid factor, are the rule.

The third form of rheumatoid arthritis occurring in children is the pauciarticular form. Often a misleadingly mild disease presenting, for example, with monarticular arthritis and only a slightly elevated sedimentation rate, this disease is of greatest importance because it is in such children that the destructive iridocyclitis occurs so frequently. The latter is often overlooked until irreversible damage to the eyes has occurred, and these patients are often treated primarily by ophthalmologists who do not recognize that the children have rheumatoid disease. Rheumatoid factor is almost always lacking in these patients.

Treatment of all forms of rheumatoid arthritis in adults and children requires frequent interaction between patient, family, and physician. These diseases are at once among the most frustrating and rewarding illnesses to treat. Basic to all treatment is gently persistent physical therapy. Therapy is, in good part, constructed around the thesis that a spontaneous remission may occur at any time. It is of utmost importance not to do harm with the therapy. Over 25 years of treating rheumatoid arthritis in some 500 to 600 children, the only deaths we have observed have been 5 iatrogenic deaths. Of the numerous drugs administered, none is generally accepted as being capable of inducing remissions. The goals of present day therapy are (1) to control pain as effectively as possible with agents that do as little harm as possible and (2) to prevent, minimize, or reverse deformities of joints while awaiting the hoped-for remission.

Salicylates in doses of 60 mg/lb, up to 3.0 gm or more per day in children have the greatest effectiveness coupled with the lowest incidence of serious toxicity. Their anti inflammatory effect, previously undisputed in acute rheumatic fever, has also been demonstrated in studies of rheumatoid subjects.

Indomethacin has proved to be relatively free from serious toxicity except in young children with severe and overwhelming infections that preclude its use. The clinical experience with indomethacin in rheumatoid arthritis has not been consistent. Most physicians use it as a trial, second to salicylate, before proceeding to treatment with more toxic drugs.

Phenylbutazone and its analogues are potent anti-inflammatory agents; they are not very effective in the average case of rheumatoid arthritis. Potential toxicity (myeloid depression and peptic ulceration) limits their usefulness.

Adrenocorticosteroids are the most effective agents available for suppressing inflammation and controlling pain in this disease. They, however, have a number of limitations. (1) Although pain may be dramatically suppressed by a given dose of corticosteroid, the disease (including progression of deformities) is not always controlled, and if the disease is sustained, the dose of drug may have to be progressively increased, and

serious, unwanted side reactions are the consequence. (2) It is very difficult, if not impossible, to discontinue corticosteroid therapy when the disease remains active, because of severe exacerbations which follow reduction of dosage. (3) Patients on long-term corticosteroid therapy may develop serious life-threatening complications in frequency and to degrees
that make rheumatoid arthritis seem almost inconsequential. A proposal
that corticosteroids be administered in a single dose every 48 hours (in
an effort to prevent complications of steroid therapy) has not been tested
systematically in rheumatoid patients. It has been our experience that
regimens using prednisone every other day are not as effective as very
small doses administered more frequently.

AMYLOIDOSIS

Amyloid is a hyaline hydrophilic substance, predominantly protein in
nature, which may accumulate in a variety of locations. It exhibits certain characteristic staining reactions, and when examined with the elec-
tion microscope is seen to contain numerous fibrils whose properties appear to be unique for this substance.

It is no longer practical to utilize the term amyloidosis to refer to the
condition of all patients in whom traces of amyloid can be detected histologically. Instead, amyloidosis should probably be defined as a cluster
of conditions, the chief manifestations of which are due to compression
of, or interference with, the function of vital tissues by the accumulation
of amyloid.

In recent studies it has been established that one form of amyloid
is made up entirely or largely of polymerized light chains of immunoglobulin molecules. Another form of amyloid, originally associated with
secondary amyloidosis, has been identified. The purified protein forms
fibrils. The cellular site of production of this amyloid protein has not
been definitely located, but the best evidence is that it may be produced
by reticular cells under appropriate stimulation. Are there really two
distinct forms of amyloidosis? It is our view that in most, if not all, instances amyloid comprises two major protein components, each of which
may be present in different concentrations in the amyloid complex and
capable of forming fibrils. One of these components is comprised of light
chains of immunoglobulins that are produced by plasma cells. The other
is a fibrillar protein produced in all likelihood by the reticulum cells. Both
components are present in most amyloids of the so-called primary and
secondary amyloidosis. Perhaps occasionally a so-called amyloid protein
can be made up of only one or the other of these components. Perhaps
the fibrillar non-light chain component has a special affinity for the light
chain component.

In so-called secondary amyloidosis most accumulations occur in the
kidney, spleen, and, usually to a lesser extent, liver, and proteinuria is the

most frequent and conspicuous initial manifestation. Traces or moderate accumulations of amyloid may also be noted in many different organs, including skin, adrenals and other endocrine glands, prostate, pancreas, stomach, small bowel, and aorta. The incidence of amyloidosis in rheumatoid arthritis may be as high as 6 percent. On the other hand, in one study secondary amyloidosis was noted in only 1 of 48 cases of long-standing rheumatoid arthritis. Congo red staining with polarization microscopy appears to provide, if properly used, an extremely sensitive and specific indication of the presence of amyloid.

The pathogenesis of amyloidosis has been the subject of numerous speculations and experimental studies extending over many decades. One of the most persistent concepts is that its genesis is related in some way to prolonged immunologic stimulus accompanied by prolonged hypergammaglobulinemia. In 1897 Krakow first demonstrated that amyloidosis can be induced in experimental animals by serial injections of live or dead bacteria. Subsequent studies by many workers have shown that amyloidosis can be induced in animals by serial injections of sodium caseinate, Freund's adjuvants, sodium ribonuclease, pentose nucleotides, and other antigens, and also following transfer of a transplantable tumor, a reticulum cell sarcoma, in mice.

It has been postulated that the relationship between the pathogenesis of amyloidosis and immunologic mechanisms may relate to a subtle imbalance between the prolonged immunologic stimulus and a defect in the response of the host. Examples include radiation chimeras and thymectomized rabbits. Amyloidosis is not infrequently observed in a disorder resembling wasting disease developed by NZB mice. Teilum has shown that a very high percentage of patients with primary immunodeficiency diseases, e.g., the common variable forms of immunodeficiency, develops amyloidosis. These many lines of evidence suggest that it is a disbalance of the immunologic mechanism leading to excessive stimulation of the overworked remaining immunologic system that favors amyloidosis. Neonatally thymectomized mice and aging mice of strains prone to develop autoimmunity and early defects of the T-cell system regularly develop amyloidosis, whereas aging mice whose immunologic systems remain in good balance for much longer periods develop little if any amyloidosis.

SARCOIDOSIS

Sarcoidosis was first described by Hutchinson and Boeck. Since the definitive histologic picture of cutaneous sarcoidosis was presented by Boeck, it is called Boeck's sarcoid.

Sarcoidosis is a systemic granulomatous disease of undetermined etiology and pathogenesis. Mediastinal and peripheral lymph nodes, lungs, liver, spleen, skin, eyes, phalangeal bones, and parotid glands are most often involved, but other organs or tissues may be affected. The Kveim reaction is frequently positive, and cell-mediated hypersensitivities to a wide variety of antigens are frequently depressed or absent. Other important laboratory findings include hypercalciuria and increased serum globulins. The characteristic histologic appearance of epithelioid tubercles with little or no necrosis is, of course, not pathognomonic, but a regular concomitant. The diagnosis is established, for clinical purposes, on the bases of consistent clinical features and biopsy evidence of epithelioid tubercles with a positive Kveim test.

The granuloma in sarcoidosis consists mainly of mononuclear cells associated with the presence of occasional giant cells. Typically the giant cell granulomas of sarcoidosis do not caseate or break down as do those in chronic tuberculosis. Sarcoid granulomas are found typically in the lungs, skin, lymph nodes, and spleen. However, in many cases it may present in the eye as a uveitis. As many as 50 percent of cases start as erythema nodosum in the skin.

About two thirds of patients with sarcoidosis have a marked deficiency of cell-mediated immunity, although no abnormality of humoral antibody formation is seen. A marked reduction in delayed hypersensitivity to tuberculin, histoplasmin, oidiomycin, trichophytin, or mumps antigen injected intradermally is encountered, and patients fail to convert to tuberculin positivity when immunized with BCG. Similarly they cannot be sensitized as readily as can normals to develop contact sensitivity to chemical sensitizing agents such as 2,4-dinitrochlorobenzene. Surprisingly, they appear to be able to reject skin allografts normally. These patients also show a defect in the reactivity of their circulating lymphocytes to be transformed by antigens *in vitro*. By contrast, lymphocytes of the lymphoid tissues are transformed by antigens to immunoglobulin-producing and secreting cells by antigenic stimulator *in vivo*.

Lymphocytes from sensitive donors and even transfer factor from sensitive donors can confer on patients with sarcoidosis cell-mediated immunity localized to the site of injection. Systemic cellular immunity can be established with either transfer factor or intradermal injections of intact lymphocytes. The basic deficit responsible for the immunologic perturbation in sarcoidosis is not yet clear.

The *Kveim test* resembles closely the "late" or Mitsuda reaction to lepromin in cases of tuberculoid leprosy. The granulomatous reaction may depend on the same mechanism as that which determines the accelerated formation of tubercles when tubercle bacilli are injected into a tuberculous guinea pig. However, until the nature of the antigenic component of the Kveim test is elucidated, it would be difficult to conclude that the reaction is certainly an immunologic one. The test consists of the intradermal injection of a heated (pasteurized) saline suspension of sarcoid tissue obtained from a sarcoid spleen or lymph node. In patients with active sarcoidosis a dusky red nodule develops slowly over a few weeks at the injection site. Histologic examination, which forms an essential part of the complete test, reveals sarcoid tissue (scattered miliary nodules of epithelioid cells and giant cells, with close resemblance to miliary tubercles, but lacking central caseation).

One common hypothesis of sarcoidosis attributes this disorder to many and varied antigenic stimuli. However, it seems unlikely that there are several different unrelated stimuli, since the same Kveim test suspension can give similar responses in cases of sarcoidosis all over the world. Also sarcoidosis has a sharply defined geographic localization in North America and Northern Europe.

To date little is known about the nature of sarcoidosis, although it is suspected that the reactions in these patients are variations of or deviations from the normal cell-mediated immunologic response. Fractionation of extracts from the spleen of sarcoidosis patients has shown that the active principle producing the Kveim reactions is probably present in the subcellular organelles associated with the liposomes of phagocytes. This suggests that the agent causing the reaction could be an infective organism. However, the antigen or agent is highly resistant to powerful chemical and physical agents, and in this way is unlike most infective agents. Much will be learned about the nature of this disease, once this agent is actually identified. Recent studies claiming to have demonstrated an infective agent from both sarcoidosis and granulomatous colitis have not yet been confirmed.

So far it has been shown that sarcoidosis responds to treatment with steroids (20 mg prednisone daily) which will inhibit the development of the Kveim reaction, although it will not block a reaction if therapy is started 4 to 6 weeks after injection of the Kveim antigen. Other immunosuppressive agents have not yet been found to be useful in this disease. Fortunately the disease in most patients is quite benign. However, iridocyclitis, uveitis, and central nervous system involvement can damage vital or crucial organs, and death or great disability may be the consequence. Atypical forms of the disease are sometimes encountered in children.

POLYARTERITIS NODOSA

"Periarteritis" was originally described by Kussmaul and Maier in 1866 as a fatal disease characterized by the presence of numerous macroscopic nodules along the course of arteries throughout the body. The term *polyarteritis* was later suggested as more appropriate, since there is involvement of arterial walls as well as periarterial tissue (Table 24-3). On microscopic examination the involved arteries, which are of the caliber of the primary branches of the coronary arteries or the hepatic arteries, show inflammation and necrosis of the vessel wall and thrombosis and perivascular exudate of polymorphs and eosinophils, with macrophages

Table 24-3. A Classification of Necrotizing Angiitis

1. Polyarteritis (polyarteritis nodosa, periarteritis nodosa)
2. Hypersensitivity or allergic arteritis or angiitis
3. Arteritis of serum sickness
4. Rheumatic arteritis
5. Allergic granulomatous arteritis or angiitis
6. Wegener's granulomatosis
7. Giant cell arteritis (cranial arteritis, temporal arteritis)
8. Takayasu's arteritis (aortic arch syndrome, young female arteritis)
9. Arterial lesions of hypertension
10. Arteritis following resection of coarctation of the aorta
11. Arteritis or vasculitis associated with
    a. Rheumatoid arthritis
    b. Sjögren's syndrome
    c. Systemic lupus erythematosus
    d. Systemic sclerosis (scleroderma)
    e. Dermatomyositis (polymyositis)
12. Drug-induced (nonallergic) arteritis
13. The isolated arteritic lesion
14. Secondary arteritis

From Shulman, L. E. (1971): Polyarteritis nodosa. In *Immunological Diseases*, Samter, M. (ed.). Boston, Little, Brown and Company, p. 1229.

and lymphocytes. Frequently the disease occurs in persons with an atopic background, asthma, and eosinophilia. Death usually is consequent to coronary thrombosis, cerebral hemorrhage, or gastrointestinal bleeding. The characteristic clinical tetrad seen in this disease includes abdominal pain, hypertension, peripheral nerve symptoms, and renal malfunction. The characteristic nodules can often be located in skin or occasionally in the blood vessels of the contents of the scrotal sac or may sometimes be seen in the eyegrounds on ophthalmologic examination. Males have the disease far more frequently than do females.

From 1940, what has been called polyarteritis nodosa has been repeatedly noted in serum sickness and in patients who have received sulfonamides, thiourea, diphenylhydantoin (Dilantin), iodides, penicillin, and other drugs. Following the description of similar vascular lesions in rabbits treated with large doses of serum proteins, the drug-induced human cases of polyarteritis nodosa were thought to be related to the Arthus-type hypersensitivity reactions to unspecified antigen. However, we think it wise to make a distinction between periarteritis nodosa and the diffuse nodular vasculitis of serum sickness.

The necrosis and fibrinoid changes in the media of small arterioles in polyarteritis nodosa in man are similar to the change in blood vessels in the Arthus reaction produced in experimental animals. Similar lesions have also been found in experimental and clinical serum sickness and after repeated streptococcal infections in experimental animals. In man polyarteritis nodosa has been associated with chronic bacterial infections, but there is also a marked association with drug therapy. In some cases the lesions have actually developed during a serum sickness type of disease known to be caused by a particular drug. In other cases an attack of polyarteritis nodosa has been precipitated in the same patient on different occasions by the use of a drug. The drugs that have been incriminated in this way are thiourea, thiouracil, and neoarsphenamine.

The actual nature of the lesion will depend on the level at which the antigen-antibody reaction occurs in the peripheral circulation and whether the lesion is due to the deposit of immune complexes in the vessel wall or whether there is antigen-antibody interaction across the vessel wall as in the Arthus phenomenon. Lesions may be hemorrhagic infarcts or nodular granulomata. Vascular lesions in the skin in various types of allergic vasculitis have been examined by immunohistochemical methods using the fluorescent antibody technique. In a number of cases deposits of immunoglobulin and complement have been demonstrated in the inflamed vessel wall with the same distribution as that found in the Arthus reaction in experimental animals. Deposits of bacterial antigens in the walls of inflamed vessels that have also been demonstrated in cases of nodular vasculitis in the skin developed in one case after streptococcal throat infections and in other cases with tuberculous lymphadenopathy. In both the idiopathic form of periarteritis nodosa and in the nodular diffuse allergic vasculitis associated with serum sickness or drug reactions, the lesions in the vessel show depoits of IgG, complement, and fibrin. Serum complement levels, however, are normal or high, except in the early phases when there is glomerulonephritis together with diffuse vasculitis associated with serum sickness.

Polyarteritis is a striking feature of Aleutian mink disease, which manifests interesting immunopathic properties and is of viral etiology. Viral illnesses in man (e.g., influenza) may induce a vasculitis but usually not an arteritis. This does not rule out, however, the possibility that the idiopathic form of periarteritis in man is due to a virus. In a number of recent studies periarteritis was associated with persisting infections with the virus associated with the so-called Australia antigens. Indeed, additional studies seem to associate much less inflammatory lesions of blood vessels of all sorts with antigen-antibody complement complex deposits in which Australia antigen and antibody to Australia antigen are offenders. These lesions, sometimes indistinguishable from the vascular lesions regularly attributed to degenerative vascular disease, may be of greatest significance. If it could be shown that this kind of apparently degenerative vascular disease is caused by a virus antigen-antibody complex, the consequences could be far-reaching. Prognosis for all forms of polyarteritis is serious; however, the idiopathic form is much more frequently fatal and less successfully treated than the form associated with the diffuse vasculitis of serum sickness in which an exogenous antigen can be identified. Adrenocortical steroids are quite effective in treating the latter disease.

Arteritis occurs spontaneously in various animal species, including an outbred albino strain (PN) of New Zealand mice, elderly Sprague-Dawley rats, and cats. In several other animal models, arteritis is evoked by various means, such as creating hypertension or giving carcinogens.

The immediate response to corticosteroids in adequate dosage is usually dramatic, with prompt relief from the symptoms and signs of illness. New arteritic lesions may be prevented. However, the long-term results are often disappointing, especially in the idiopathic form of the disease. The toxicity of large doses of adrenal steroids given over long periods frequently requires reduction of dosage to inadequate levels. Adequate data are not available as to whether life is prolonged by corticosteroid therapy. In a report from the Mayo Clinic, the 5-year survival after diagnosis for 110 patients with polyarteritis was 48 percent. Data on the response of polyarteritis to immunosuppressive agents are few; however, on several occasions we have seen dramatic responses with the azathioprine (Imuran)-steroid combination in patients who had the idiopathic form of the disease. Nitroblue-tetrazolium reduction, regularly negative in the form of periarteritis associated with diffuse vasculitis and serum sickness, has sometimes been strongly positive in the idiopathic cases we have studied. This finding is unexplained but could reflect a role played by bacterial infection, mycoplasma, large virus, or rickettsial agents in the pathogenesis. Australia antigen has been found to be positive in a substantial portion of cases and Australia antigen gamma globulin and complement, probably as complexes, have been demonstrated in the vascular lesions.

SERUM SICKNESS

Serum sickness is defined as a clinical symptom complex due to adverse immune reaction to heterologous serum administered for passive immunization. Although the classic clinical features and the immunologic nature of the pathogenesis were described in 1905 by von Pirquet and Schick, it is only in recent years that the immunopathology of serum sickness has been thoroughly investigated. It has striking pathologic and immunologic similarities to systemic lupus erythematosus and erythema nodosum.

Primary serum sickness occurs 7 to 12 days after injection of foreign serum and is characterized by fever, urticaria, lymphadenopathy, myalgia, and arthralgia or arthritis. The site of injection becomes erythematous and swollen 24 to 72 hours before the onset of systemic manifestations. Neuritis, vasculitis, and glomerulonephritis are the major complicating symptoms.

Injection of 100 ml of "native" horse serum has been estimated to induce serum sickness in more than 90 percent of recipients, and 10 ml, in approximately 10 percent. With the purified so-called despeciated horse serum globulin, for example, 0.5 ml of horse globulin containing 15,000 units of tetanus antitoxin, the incidence of primary serum sickness is much less.

The symptoms of accelerated serum sickness are essentially those of primary serum sickness but occur 1 to 3 days after injection. Reactions of an anaphylactic type occur within minutes after injection of serum and are accompanied by shock, hypotension, urticaria, dyspnea, wheezing, nausea, emesis, laryngeal edema, diarrhea, and occasionally death.

Primary serum sickness is managed by the administration of epinephrine, antihistamines, analgesics, and local application of antipruritics. Corticosteroid is reserved for the complications such as glomerulonephritis, persistent neuritis, or other manifestation of destructive vasculitis.

Serum sickness is a classic example of disease caused by antigen-antibody complexes. The immunologic mechanisms of the pathogenesis of serum sickness are discussed in Chapters 11 and 13.

Skin testing before the administration of foreign serum protein may detect the sensitized person. It is said that desensitization can be accomplished by administration of small, gradually increasing doses of the foreign protein one desires to use, but it is our opinion that when such evidence of prior sensitization to a foreign protein is demonstrated it is best to avoid the foreign protein if at all possible.

SJÖGREN'S SYNDROME

A triad of keratoconjunctivitis sicca, dryness of mouth with or without salivary gland enlargement, and rheumatoid arthritis constitutes Sjögren's disease. This syndrome occurs together with scleroderma, polymyositis, polyarteritis nodosa, or systemic lupus erythematosus (SLE). It is a benign, though distressing, chronic disease of unknown etiology occurring predominantly in women in the fourth to sixth decades; it may begin in childhood or advanced age.

Dryness of the mouth, inability to moisten food with saliva, and the need for frequent ingestion of water, both with and between meals, are the commonest symptoms. Excessive dental caries often result from the lack of saliva. Xerostomia may be associated with historical or clinical evidence of salivary gland enlargement in about one half of patients. The most common pattern is one of discrete episodes of swelling, usually of the parotid gland, superimposed on less marked, persistent bilateral enlargement.

Nearly all patients, especially those with the sicca complex not accompanied by a connective tissue disease, have hypergammaglobulinemia. On immunoelectrophoresis and by quantitative assay, hypergammaglobulinemia may be shown to be due to a diffuse increase in concentration of all three major classes of immunoglobulins, IgG, IgA, and IgM.

Almost all patients with Sjögren's syndrome, whether or not they have rheumatoid arthritis, have rheumatoid factor in their serum. Approximately 70 percent have antinuclear antibodies, identified by the immunofluorescent technique, and some have anti-DNA antibodies.

Although the incidence of lymphoid malignancies cannot be stated precisely, malignancy appears to occur more often in Sjögren's syndrome than in uncomplicated rheumatoid arthritis or other connective tissue diseases. It is postulated that the chronic state of immunologic and lymphoid hyperactivity in Sjögren's syndrome predisposes to the development of malignant lymphoma or pseudolymphoma. Alternatively it may be that immunologic impairment predisposes to both Sjögren's syndrome and lymphatic malignancy or that the Sjögren's syndrome is secondary to a slowly developing malignancy featured by immunodepression and immunoperturbation. Treatment with cyclophosphamide has been reported to bring histologic improvement in some cases.

MIXED CONNECTIVE TISSUE DISEASE

Recently a fascinating form of mesenchymal disease has been separated from the others in which the pathogenetic mechanism seems to have been quite clearly established. This is the so-called mixed connective tissue disease in which the pathogenesis has been shown to be due to antibody formation against an extractable nuclear component. The antinuclear antibody that is formed in this disease gives a speckled fluorescent pattern with peripheral blood or calf thymus cells. The antigen-antibody complex in turn activates the complement system and other biologic amplification systems associated with inflammation. The disease may present as a disseminated systemic scleroderma or as a lupus syndrome, sometimes with renal disease. Fortunately this form of mixed connective tissue disease tends to respond well to adrenal-steroid therapy.

WEGENER'S GRANULOMATOSIS

Wegener's granulomatosis is characterized pathologically by (1) necrotizing granulomas in the upper or lower respiratory tract, or both, (2) disseminated focal necrotizing vasculitis, involving both arteries and veins in lungs and other sites, and (3) glomerulitis or glomerulonephritis. Young or middle-aged adults of either sex are affected. The disease begins clinically as sinusitis in two thirds of the cases and as persistent pneumonitis in the other third. The disease really must be separated into two distinct components, the granulomatous component, which may last for weeks or occasionally for as long as 2 years, and the disseminated vascular component, which often destroys vital organs such as the kidneys. Systemic features either follow or coincide with the respiratory disease and include fever, rash, joint and muscle pains, peripheral neuritis, and nephritis. The latter aspects are secondary to the vasculitis. Anemia (97 percent) and blood eosinophilia (46 percent) occur as in polyarteritis and indeed may be more frequent than in the latter disease. Most patients ultimately develop renal failure, with about one fourth having severe hypertension. This disease expressed in full form is highly lethal, the average duration of life being 5 months after diagnosis. However, Carrington and Liebow have described 16 patients with a more "limited" form of this disease and a better prognosis. Nine had pulmonary lesions only, and 7 also had extrapulmonary lesions but did not have nephritis. Treatment of the disease with adrenal steroids or immunosuppressive regimens in the early phases prior to development of the disseminated vascular component may prevent extension of dissemination of the disease and permit gradual resolution of the initial phase.

For reasons not understood, corticosteroid therapy is even less effective in Wegener's granulomatosis once dissemination has occurred than in polyarteritis. Initial results of therapeutic trials with various immunosuppressive agents, including chlorambucil, azathioprine, and mechlorethamine hydrochloride, however, are encouraging. Once the disseminated vascular disease has developed, even immunosuppressive regimens frequently are without avail. The histopathology of renal lesions reveals little evidence of immunologic assault but greater evidence of fibrin deposition in the glomeruli. Mesangial deposits of immunoglobulins and complement have been described, as have small foci of the latter, at the sites of fibrin deposition. Further critical studies, especially of the vascular lesions of the skin, may as in anaphylactic purpura help disclose the pathogenetic processes in the disseminated vascular phase. A likely explanation for the characteristic granulomatous disease is that the first phase of this disease represents an infection, perhaps a chronic virus infection, to which a cell-mediated immune response is directed and that the second phase is an antigen-antibody complex injury with intravascular coagulation and focal vasculitis a consequence.

TAKAYASU'S ARTERITIS

Takayasu's arteritis is also known as aortic arch arteritis, aortic arch syndrome, pulseless disease, brachial arteritis, and young female arteritis. Originally the disease was thought to be confined to Oriental populations, but in recent years many cases from Europe and America, including some in Negroes, have been recorded. Most patients are young females, aged 9 to 45 years. Recent reports emphasize systemic manifestations similar to those of the collagen diseases and some interesting immunologic abnormalities.

The essential pathologic change is segmental arteritis of the aorta and its branches, with granulomas or diffuse inflammation (mainly lymphocytes and plasma cells) in the media and adventitia. Necrosis is most pronounced in the media. Thrombosis is common.

The levels of all of three main classes of serum immunoglobulins may be elevated. In one study, the levels of IgG, IgA, and IgM were raised by 26, 43, and 43 percent, respectively. Complement-fixing antibodies against aorta and hemagglutinating antiaortic antibodies have been found in patients. Whether these autoimmune phenomena are primary or secondary is not yet clear, but the likelihood that they play a pathogenetic role seems real. However, the crucial question in this disease, as in many other so-called autoimmune diseases, is why the lesions are localized to the characteristic sites. The possibility that infection again with an agent or agents capable of altering or revealing hidden host constituents would make the autoimmune phenomena secondary rather than primary in pathogenesis.

The prognosis of this disease is very poor; most patients die as young adults or in middle age. The most frequent causes of death are cerebral and cardiac insufficiency. The efficacy of treatment with corticosteroids and anticoagulants is not clearly established. Theoretically, corticosteroids would be most useful in the early phases when systemic features first appear. Selective arterial surgery for such lesions as thrombi and renal artery stenosis has been effective.

SELECTED REFERENCES

Systemic Lupus Erythematosus

Beernink, D. H., and Miller, J. J. (1973): J. Pediat. 82:113.
Dubois, E. L. (1966): Lupus Erythematosus. New York, McGraw-Hill, Inc.
Grausz, H., et al. (1970): New Eng. J. Med. 283:506.
Györkey, F., et al. (1969): New Eng. J. Med. 280:333.
Györkey, F., et al. (1972): Amer. J. Med. 53:148.
Perry, H. M. (1973): Amer. J. Med. 54:58.
Ritchie, R. F. (1970): New Eng. J. Med. 282:1174.
Rothfield, N., et al. (1972): New Eng. J. Med. 287:681.
Sharon, E., Kaplan, D., and Diamond, H. S. (1973): New Eng. J. Med. 288:122.

Rheumatoid Arthritis

Baumal, R., and Broder, I. (1968): Clin. Exp. Immun. 3:555.
Bland, J. H. (ed.) (1968): Rheumatoid arthritis. Med. Clin. N. Amer. 52:477.
Calabro, J. J. (1970): J. Pediat. 77:355.
Editorial (1972): JAMA 222:1555.
Franklin, E. C., et al. (1957): J. Exp. Med. 105:425.
Fremont-Smith, K., and Bayles, T. B. (1965): JAMA 192:1133.
Hannestad, K., and Mellbye, O. J. (1967): Clin. Exp. Immun. 2:501.
Harter, J. G., Reddy, W. J., and Thorn, G. W. (1963): New Eng. J. Med. 269:591.
Hollander, J. L., et al. (1966): Arthritis Rheum. 9:675.
Ropes, M. W., et al. (1959): Ann. Rheum. Dis. 18:49.
Rose, H. M., et al. (1948): Proc. Soc. Exp. Biol. (N.Y.) 68:1.
Schaller, J., and Wedgwood, R. J. (1972): Pediatrics 50:940.
Schroehenloher, R. E. (1966): J. Clin. Invest. 45:501.
Waaler, E. (1940): Acta Path. Microbiol. Scand. 17:172.

Amyloidosis

Aach, R., and Kissane, J. (eds.) (1972): Amer. J. Med. 53:495.
Barth, W. F., et al. (1969): Amer. J. Med. 47:259.
Binette, J. P., and Calkins, E. (1967): Arthritis Rheum. 10:107.
Cathcart, E. S., Mullarkey, M., and Cohen, A. S. (1970): Lancet 2:639.
Cohen, A. S. (1967): New Eng. J. Med. 277:522.
Glenner, G. G., et al. (1971): Science 172:1150.
Glenner, G. G., Ein, D., and Terry, W. D. (1972): Amer. J. Med. 52:141.
Krakow, N. P. (1897): Arch. Exp. Path. Pharmak. 40:195.
Milgrom, F., Kasukawa, R., and Calkins, E. (1966): J. Immun. 96:245.
Shirahama, T., and Cohen, A. S. (1967): J. Cell. Biol. 33:679.
Sutherland, D. E. R., et al. (1965): Lancet 1:130.
Teilum, G. J. (1964): J. Path. Bact. 88:317.

Sarcoidosis

Boeck, C. (1899): Norsk. Mag. Laeg. 14:1321.
Editorial (1971): Lancet 2:750.
Hutchinson, J. (1877): *Illustrations of Clinical Surgery.* London, Churchill.
Israel, H. L., and Goldstein, R. A. (1971): New Eng. J. Med. 284:345.
Refvem, O. (1954). Acta Med. Scand. 149 (Suppl. 294):1.
Second International Conference on Sarcoidosis (1961): Amer. Rev. Resp. Dis. 84(2):171.
Siltzbach, L. E. (1964): Acta Med. Scand. 176(Suppl. 425):74.
Siltzbach, L. E. (1969): Practitioner 202:613.

Polyarteritis Nodosa

Asherson, R. A., Asherson, G. L., and Schrire, V. (1968): Brit. Med. J. 3:589.
Kussmaul, A., and Maier, R. (1866): Deutsch. Arch. Klin. Med. 1:484.
Wagner, B. M. (1963): Arthritis Rheum. 6:386.
Wigley, R. D., and Couchman, K. G. (1966): Nature 211:319.

Serum Sickness

Proceedings of a symposium on immune complexes and disease. (1971): J. Exp. Med. 134:1.
von Pirquet, C. F., and Schick, B. (1905): *Die Serum Krankheit.* Leipzig, Wier, trans. by Schick, B. (1951): *Serum Sickness.* Baltimore, Williams & Wilkins.

Sjögren's Syndrome

Anderson, L. G., et al. (1972): Amer. J. Med. 53:456.
Bloch, K. J., et al. (1965): Medicine 44:187.
Hood, J., Burns, C. A., and Hodges, R. E. (1970): New Eng. J. Med. 282:1120.
Leventhal, B. G., Waldorf, D. S., and Talal, N. (1967): J. Clin. Invest. 46:1338.
Shioji, R., et al. (1970): Amer. J. Med. 48:456.
Sjögren, H. (1943): *A New Conception of Keratoconjunctivitis Sicca,* trans. by Hamilton, J. B. Sydney, Australian Medical Publishing Company.

Mixed Connective Tissue Disease

Holman, H. R. (1965): Ann. N. Y. Acad. Sci. 124:800.
Sharp, G. C., et al. (1969): Clin. Res. 17:359.
Sharp, G. C., et al. (1970): Clin. Res. 18:617.
Sharp, G. C., et al. (1972): Amer. J. Med. 52:148.

Wegener's Granulomatosis

Aach, R., and Kissane, J. (eds.) (1970): Amer. J. Med. 48:496.
Carrington, C. B., and Liebow, A. A. (1966): Amer. J. Med. 41:497.
Fauci, A. S., Wolff, S. M., and Johnson, J. S. (1971): New Eng. J. Med. 285:1493.

Godman, G. C., and Churg, J. (1954): Arch. Path. (Chicago) 58:533.
McIlvanie, S. K. (1966): JAMA 197:130.
Novack, S. N., and Pearson, C. M. (1971): New Eng. J. Med. 284:938.
Paronetto, F. (1969): In Textbook of Immunopathology, Miescher, P., and Muller-
    Eberhard, J. J. (eds.). New York, Grune & Stratton.
Roback, S. A., et al. (1969): Amer. J. Dis. Child. 118:608.

Takayasu's Arteritis

Asherson, R. A., Asherson, G. L., and Schrire, V. (1968): Brit. Med. J. 3:589.
Nakao, K., et al. (1967): Circulation 35:1141.
Strachan, R. W., Wigzell, F. W., and Anderson, J. R. (1966): Amer. J. Med. 40:560.

25

Immunologic Disorders of the Respiratory Tract

The respiratory tract, particularly the lungs, provides a unique relationship between man's internal and external environments. This relationship has long been recognized as being of importance in disease. Discovery of anaphylaxis and allergy around the turn of this century soon led to recognition that immunologic events are involved in the pulmonary manifestations of anaphylactic shock, asthma, and serum sickness. Hypersensitivity mechanisms were then suspected in a number of other pulmonary disorders. In the past four years many new studies of these diseases have been recorded, and it is now possible to organize the growing body of information more precisely according to all four types of allergic reactions and to have a beginning understanding of pathogenic mechanisms involved in the large group of pulmonary diseases in which immunologic reactions play an important part.

The four types of allergic reactions responsible for hypersensitivity diseases of the lungs are Type I (IgE dependent); Type II (cytotoxic, tissue specific antibody); Type III (immune complex disease); and Type IV (cell-mediated delayed hypersensitivity). Each of these immune reactions induces characteristic pathologic changes in the lungs caused by the release of chemical mediators, and each is associated with distinctive immunologic reactions that may be elicited by appropriate testing, so that diagnosis can now be reasonably accurate. The initial portion of this review is concerned with immunopathologic mechanisms, particularly as they occur in the lungs, and with the immunologic tests that aid in their recognition.

EXTRINSIC ALLERGIC PNEUMONIAS

The term *extrinsic allergic alveolitis* denotes cases of Type III (immune complex) allergic disease of the lungs that result from inhalation of antigens that are often thermophilic actinomycetes or fungal spores present in organic dusts derived from moldy material, although antigens derived from insects, animals, or birds may be present in dusts and may induce these allergic reactions. A number of diseases in this category have been

Table 25-1.   Causes of Extrinsic Allergic Pneumonitis

Disease	Source	Allergens
Farmer's lung	Moldy hay	Micropolyspora faeni
Mushroom worker's lung	Mushroom compost	Thermoactinomyces vulgaris
Bagassosis	Moldy sugar cane	Thermoactinomyces vulgaris
Malt worker's lung	Germinating barley	Aspergillus clavatus
Maple bark disease	Dry, moldy bark	Cryptosporium corticale
Suberosis	Moldy cork dust	?
Sequoiosis	Moldy sawdust	Graphium, Pullularia
Mill worker's lung	Mill dust	Sitophilus granarius
Coffee worker's lung	Coffee-bean dust	?
. . .	Vegetable dusts	Fungal & other flora
Byssinosis	Cotton	Cotton antigens
Bird breeder's lung	Feathers, droppings	Derived from species (parakeets, pigeons, chickens, etc.)
Pituitary snuff taker's lung	Powdered pituitary extracts	Bovine & porcine serum & pituitary tissue
Hypersensitivity pneumonitis	Contamination of air-conditioning or heating systems	Thermophilic actinomycetes

McCombs, R. P. (1972): Diseases due to immunologic reactions in the lungs. New Eng. J. Med. *286*:1245.

described; they are listed in Table 25-1 together with the antigens believed to be responsible.

It is readily apparent that the 30 m² or more of alveolar surface area are at considerable risk from inhaled allergens, and, of course, asthma is a well-recognized consequence. Less well known is the response in the non-atopic person to a variety of inhaled antigens, now generally recognized as extrinsic allergic alveolitis, as being more in keeping with the actual pathology.

An excess of antigen may be present in the region of the immune reaction, creating a situation in which toxic immune complexes can be formed. Spore counts in the air after shaking moldy hay peaked at nearly 1,600,000,000 spores per cubic meter, with more than 90 percent being actinomycetes 0.5 to 1.3 μ in diameter—small enough to reach the alveoli. It has been estimated that in a farmer working in an atmosphere of moldy hay as many as 750,000 spores per minute would be deposited in lung spaces where they might activate immunologic reactions if prior sensitization had occurred.

Attempts have been made to identify immune complexes in the lesions of extrinsic alveolitis. Electron microscopy showed that a protein was deposited in an irregular (lumpy-bumpy) fashion along alveolar capillary basement membranes in a patient with this disease. This finding is compatible with the presence of immune complexes. Wenzel et al. used immunologic techniques to study lung tissue from 4 patients with farmer's lung. In 2 patients acutely ill with farmer's lung, the walls of the bronchioles contained high concentrations of antibody to Micropolyspora faeni, whereas similar studies in 2 other patients with more chronic disease were negative. Immunoglobulins IgG, IgA, and IgM were found in plasma cells and lymphocytes scattered throughout the diseased lungs. All patients showed great numbers of histiocyte-like cells that contained the third component of complement, an indication that antigen-antibody complexes that had fixed complement in these lungs had been phagocytized. However, since neither necrotizing vascular lesions nor polymorphonuclear cells in numbers seen in Arthus reactions were observed, these authors suggested that this may be a Type II cytotoxic reaction in which the polysaccharide antigen of the mycobacterium is fixed passively onto cells that are then destroyed by the antibody. They also suggested that the histologic picture suggested that a Type IV immune reaction, cell-mediated immunity, might be involved.

The diagnosis of extrinsic allergic alveolitis may usually be made by clinical observations, the chief of which is the history of exposure to appropriate antigens. Confirmation of diagnosis may be possible by serologic and inhalation tests. Precipitins to the specific antigens causing the disease are present in the serums of most patients with extrinsic allergic alveolitis. Skin tests are not of much value because most of the antigens are locally irritating. An acute phase of the disease was reproduced in 12 of 15 previously sensitized farmers by having them inhale aerosols of water-soluble, Seitz-filtered extracts of moldy hay. The reaction was delayed for several hours and was characterized by a marked fall of static lung compliance, a lesser decrease in ventilatory function, but no indications of bronchial obstruction.

We have repeatedly seen this disease, not as a consequence of the classic exposure to molds or mycobacteria in the hay on the farm but in city dwellers from exposure to mycobacteria or fungi that grow luxuriantly in humidifiers or air conditioners that are not properly cleaned and decontaminated. The clinical picture is that these patients have pulmonary disease because they are allergic to the very air in their own homes. When they are hospitalized, often very sick with acute or chronic lung disease, they gradually recover, only to experience the disease again and again on returning home.

BRONCHIAL ASTHMA

Bronchial asthma is a major cause of respiratory difficulty. Clinically it consists of paroxysms of dyspnea associated with wheezing due to mechanical obstruction of the air flow in the lesser airways. It was already recognized in ancient times. Although in the uncomplicated form it is easy to manage, the advanced stage, particularly as exemplified by so-called status asthmaticus, is a difficult therapeutic challenge. As with many conditions in which the pathogenesis is not clear, opinions are divided, and divergent camps exist. Most internists and pediatricians (especially those dealing with respiratory illnesses), occupy one camp, the allergist another, and the pathologist is somewhat in the middle. This is a reflection of the uncertainty as to whether allergy is really the essential component of the acute attack from which most patients recover. Yet substantial evidence favors a decisive role for immunologic reactions in the pathogenesis of the disease. Most attacks of bronchial asthma occur in atopic patients, and there is evidence that the propensity to develop hay fever and asthma occur together in certain families and that genetic factors play a significant role in both diseases. It is reasonable to assume that the changes in bronchial tissue are similar to the changes in the skin and are induced by the transitory effect of the combination of an allergen with reagin or IgE type antibodies. Wheal and flare in the skin have been studied extensively. Edema develops, and various cell populations are attracted to the area; in the beginning, polymorphonuclears predominate, followed by eosinophils and frequently by basophils over a 24 to 48 hour period. The biochemical events in the skin and in the lung are probably the same, but the clinical expression differs. Vasodilatation, edema, and accumulation of cells occur, but the signs and symptoms of bronchial asthma reflect the action of the same or related mediators on smooth muscle and mucus-secreting glands that are not present in the skin.

Biopsy of the lungs of such patients may show typical eosinophilic infiltration and changes in basement membrane. Neither biopsy nor specimens obtained at autopsy contribute much information about the pathogenesis. For example, the lung of an individual with "pure" allergic asthma and that of the patient whose symptoms occur only during bouts of infection in either the upper or lower respiratory tract may not differ significantly when examined by conventional light microscopy, although there may be evidence of chronic bronchitis or pneumonitis in the latter.

Ever-increasing evidence supports the view that the final events that culminate in the clinical attack are similar in the various forms of asthma, regardless of etiology. The similarity of histologic findings has already been cited as an example. In addition, the responses of such patients to the administration of mediators such as histamine and the findings on studies of pulmonary function or pulmonary circulation support the view. Even if immunologic mechanisms in the form of complexes of IgE antibodies with appropriate antigens are a major cause, nonimmunologic factors such as the biologic amplification and effector processes can be influenced by hormonal regulation, and emotional or climatic changes may, for example, contribute to expansion of the pathophysiology in the asthmatic patient. In the past, two major types of asthma were described, the so-called extrinsic and intrinsic forms. These classifications undoubtedly served a useful purpose, but these terms are now mainly of historical interest. Hypersensitivity based on antibody-antigen reaction can produce pulmonary lesions and changes in function other than asthma. For example, allergic alveolitis, usually attributable to IgG rather than IgE antigen-antibody complex, seems clearly related to the inhalation of organic material which, when combined or complexed with IgG antibody, gives rise to a different syndrome and in a different anatomic location.

Of all of the organs of the body influenced by environment, next to the skin, the lung stands paramount in that it is constantly exposed to the air and its contents. Among its many functions are purification and temperature and humidity regulation. The general anatomy of the lung is important with reference to the ease with which particles may gain access. Most pollens which vary in size from 10 to 100 μ do not penetrate beyond the terminal bronchioles. Smaller particles such as the spores implicated in farmer's lung or allergic alveolitis measure 2 μ or less and penetrate into the air sacs and alveoli.

At least two types of antigen-antibody complex systems are closely related to induction of the asthmatic attack. The first is the combination of allergen with reagin. The conditions which encourage the production of reagin or skin-sensitizing antibody are not well understood but seem to be genetically determined. It might require either altered permeability of the nasal or bronchial mucous membrane or perhaps the presence of a particular variant of the antigen reactive cell system in so-called atopic individuals. Perhaps an immunodeficiency not yet recognized is responsible for the apparent excessive response in the IgE system. As an example, one can cite the high frequency of respiratory disease compatible with allergic rhinitis when patients who lack normal reaction of the IgA system do not also lack the IgE system. Thus far, however, no clear evidence indicating immunodeficiency has been defined in most atopic or asthmatic persons. Recent evidence suggests that excessive stimulation of the IgE antibody system may sometimes be attributable to a slowly developing IgA antibody system. Such a relationship could be genetically determined and might account for the so-called atopic individual.

The significance of elevated levels of IgE in the sera of atopic patients is not clear. One could assume this to be similar to the original description of elevated γ-globulin levels in the sera of immunized animals. However, significant elevations of IgE were found by Heiner and Rose in patients with cirrhosis and no evidence of allergy. The mere presence of reagin in the serum of an individual does not indicate clinical sensitivity. Skin test responses to pollen extracts may be positive without evidence of clinical sensitivity. Of perhaps greater significance is the response of the individual who on skin testing has large reactions to ragweed and grass, and hay fever and asthma due only to ragweed. A possible explanation may be found in the site of fixation of the reagin or the balance of the immune responses to the two separate allergens. Much more study is needed on these points. It is already clear that even within one class of immune responses different qualities and thus different functional characteristics of antibodies exist. Quality, as well as quantity, of antibody may count very much.

Present evidence, especially that brought forward by Ishizaka et al. indicates that IgE skin-sensitizing antibodies find a selective receptor on mast cells or basophils in lung and other tissues. This selective fixation leads to release of specific mediators, e.g., histamine, when antibody and antigen combine at the cell surface in the respiratory tract.

There is much evidence to support the contention that Arthus type reactions may also induce asthma, and this phenomenon clearly implicates a different type of antibody. The classic example is asthma occurring in allergic bronchopulmonary aspergillosis. Studies show clearly that mast cells may be tripped to release histamine and SRS-A by IgG antigen-antibody complexes, as well as by IgE antibody complexes.

Finally, there is the question of secretory immunoglobulin, predominantly IgA with its so-called transport piece. It is known that secretory IgA is rich in antibacterial and antiviral antibody systems. It once was thought that IgA contained small quantities of a reagin-like substance, but this no longer can be accepted. Little is known of any qualitative or quantitative changes in secretory IgA with reference to asthma, but, as mentioned above, deficiencies of IgA may lead to recurrent chronic rhinitis or sinopulmonary disease when the IgE system is intact. The effector mechanisms set in motion by the reaction of antigen and IgE antibody on the surfaces of cells in the lung can be modified dramatically by treatments directed toward interfering with the release of mediators from mast cells or with the influence of these mediators on secondary target cells once they have been released. Thus interference with the intracellular balance between cyclic AMP and cyclic GMP in mast cells can be achieved with the theophylline derivatives that inhibit degradation of cyclic AMP via the phosphodiesterase pathway. For example, aminophylline can have striking benefits controlling expression of asthma as can antihistamines and substances that inhibit action of SRS-A. Epinephrine and its physiologic congeners seem to act both on the target cells of the antigen-antibody reaction and on the secondary target cells, e.g., smooth muscle cells, to modulate the consequences of the antigen-antibody reactions. Indeed, refractoriness to treatment of asthmatics can often now be attributable to changes in the state of responsiveness of the cells to the modulators of the secondary events in patients with asthma, for example, to the so-called Beta blockade.

Adrenocorticosteroid therapy, also capable of modulating responses of the effector cells, can be a most useful drug for treatment and prevention of severe asthma. Care must of course be taken so that toxic unwanted side reactions are not produced, especially when chronic therapy is being employed. In severe asthma the persistent use of relatively small doses of prednisone, for example, can be most helpful. The most effective treatment is achieved, of course, by careful attention to the environmental exposure that initiates the attacks to avoid the offending allergens.

ALLERGIC RHINITIS (HAY FEVER)

Allergic rhinitis is a condition caused by exposure of the mucous membrane to inhaled allergenic materials and is mediated by specific immunologic mechanisms. The characteristic symptom complex includes sneezing, nasal congestion, and watery discharge, as well as conjunctival itching and often cough and mild bronchoconstriction. That nasal reactions may occur to allergens introduced orally or parenterally or be mediated by other immunologic mechanisms is distinctly possible, but proof of such mechanisms is still lacking.

Biopsy specimens of the nasal mucosa obtained during allergic reactions show principally a profound edema of the submucosal tissue. Some infiltration by eosinophils and a lesser number of granulocytes is seen, but even in a long-standing condition the mucosa is intact, and there is no evidence of tissue destruction. Further changes occur only when there is secondary infection that is not part of the allergic lesion.

Although the immunologic pathophysiology of simple allergic rhinitis explains many of the manifestations of the condition, mucosal hyperemia, swelling, and hypersecretion can be induced by a number of noxious stimuli that have nothing to do with allergy. It is to be expected, therefore, that additional processes, both physical and emotional, contribute to the picture of allergic rhinitis. Noxious physical stimuli such as heat or cold or irritating reactions that influence these responses may be more subtle.

In seasonal allergic rhinitis the relationship between allergic exposure, reaginic antibodies, cellular reactions, and eventual symptoms, as well as complications from concomitant reactions to physical stimuli, emotions, and infections, can often be recognized and defined. Year-round symptoms occur in patients allergic to and exposed to dusts, mold spores, mite components, and the like that may be perennially present in the environment. Nevertheless, a considerable number of patients suffer from a chronic, perennial, poorly remitting disease of the nasal mucous membranes in which the appearance of the nose suggests allergic sensitization, but no clear relationship between allergic exposure and symptoms can be established.

The nature of the defect, presumably hereditary, which confers the ability to develop allergic rhinitis is not known. It is often suggested that the capacity to develop reagins exists in unusual degree in individuals with hay fever or other allergic diseases. The serum level of IgE is, on the average, six times greater, for example, in atopic individuals than in normals. Furthermore, immunization to diphtheria toxoid more commonly produced wheal and erythema reactions in allergic than in nonallergic individuals. Nevertheless, nearly everyone can develop skin-sensitizing antibodies if injections of antigens of Ascaris, Trichinella, or horse serum are used as a stimulus. Moreover, polysaccharide antigens produce similar immunologic responses in normal and atopic individuals. The highest levels of IgE noted have been found in children not expressing atrophy who have intestinal parasites.

Another unexplained aspect of allergic rhinitis is the difference in susceptibility among allergic individuals to specific allergens. It is evident that allergic sensitivity is rarely due to a single antigen and that the typical allergic person commonly reacts to a number of allergens. In addition, he may demonstrate positive reactions on skin tests with allergens that do not seem to cause symptoms upon natural mucosal exposure. Why two allergic individuals living in the same locality and hence subject to the same type of exposure to allergens should develop clinical reactions toward different allergens is unknown, but such reactions would appear to have a genetic basis that may relate to the Ir gene determinants. Levine and others have linked certain of the atopic diseases to particular HL-A antigens, a finding that would be consistent with this relationship.

In seasonal rhinitis the severity of symptoms is clearly related to exposure to allergens. In the laboratory, exposure by inhalation of known concentrations of pollen produces a nasal response in proportion to the amount of pollen trapped on the mucous membranes. A similar quantitative relationship between exposure and severity of symptoms may be demonstrated during natural exposure to pollens.

Relatively little information exists concerning the evolution in individuals of the immunologically mediated reactivities over years of annual reexposure to allergens in the absence of specific immunologic treatment. From this fact derives some of the difficulty of evaluating prophylactic and treatment regimens. Carefully controlled clinical trials are needed to establish the usefulness of a new therapy. Clinical experience indicates that the symptoms of atopy gradually become less severe with aging, but whether this is due to a lessening of immunologic reactivity or to other factors has not been studied. Many persons, however, are still suffering from symptoms of hay fever at advanced ages.

Spontaneous remissions of seasonal and nonseasonal atopy are uncommon but well-documented. A small number of young and middle-aged adults spontaneously lose clinical sensitivity to ragweed pollen and also histamine-releasing activity of their leukocytes and skin test reactivity. The remissions may occur despite continuing seasonal exposure to ragweed, though the patient has been treated only with antihistamines. The occasional occurrence of spontaneous loss of clinical sensitivity and immunologic reactivity complicates the evaluation of any therapy and emphasizes the need for untreated control patients for purposes of comparison. Such loss of reaginic sensitivity could be attributable to development of competing antibodies, e.g., IgG antibodies, or could relate to the achievement of a new balance in the immunologic systems.

The drugs employed in treatment of allergic diseases like hay fever may, as with treatment of asthma, interfere with the release of histamine by mast cell granules or with the action of SRS-A or may counteract the influence of the effectors, e.g., histamine or SRS-A, at secondary target cells.

Immunologic treatment for hay fever and allergic rhinitis was introduced by Noon and by Freeman in 1911, although the immunologic nature of the condition was not recognized until a few years later. They thought that hay fever was due to an idiosyncratic reaction to a soluble toxin in pollen and suggested that a series of inoculations of pollen extracts might build up antitoxin. Noon performed eye tests by placing dilutions of pollen extract directly into the conjunctival sac and, after a series of inoculations, showed that higher concentrations of extract were required to produce a reaction in the eye. Freeman noted that patients so treated seemed to be relieved of their symptoms during the pollen season and that injections at intervals of two or three days were more apt to give rise to "toxic" reactions than those spaced at a week or more.

When the immunologic nature of diseases such as hay fever was recognized, this form of treatment came to be known as *desensitization,* a term selected to describe the protection provided to anaphylactically sensitized animals by sublethal inoculations of the antigen to which they are sensitive. This term and a substitute sometimes employed, *hyposensitization,* seem to us misnomers with respect to prophylactic inoculations for allergic rhinitis, asthma, and hay fever. Desensitization, as used in animal experiments, refers to the transient depletion of reagin-type antibodies and/or mediators of the anaphylactic reaction by the administration of sublethal doses of antigens. Sensitivity returns within hours to days when injections are stopped. True desensitization has been attempted in man, as for example when the need for penicillin or horse serum seems urgent and the patient is sensitive to this allergen. The desensitization regimen calls for administration of gradually increasing doses of antigen every 20 to 60 minutes until the patient can tolerate therapeutic levels. Levine and Redmond have shown that skin test reactivity to penicillin disappears during desensitization and reappears shortly after therapy is stopped. This technique has not been applied frequently enough to assess how often it is efficacious in atopic diseases. Inoculations of allergens in man, however, produce more prolonged but less complete protection. The basis for the protection achieved by administration of allergen parenterally probably resides in achievement of immunity utilizing a different class of antibodies, e.g., IgG antibodies, that can then compete with the cell-fixed IgE antibodies for available allergens. We believe, then, that *immunotherapy* or *immunodeviation* are more appropriate terms for such treatment.

A variety of regimens of immunotherapy for allergic diseases in man have been described. They generally involve a series of inoculations with extracts of the specific allergens that cause symptoms in the patient, starting with minute doses in weekly or biweekly injections followed by gradually increasing doses as are tolerated by the patient. The endpoint in dosage has usually been determined either by the occurrence of local or systemic allergic reactions to the injections or by the patient's satisfaction with relief of symptoms. Reduction of mucous membrane or skin sensitivity has not been used sufficiently to control adequacy of dosage.

It seems strange that the immunochemists have so far been unable to find any distinguishing features common to allergens in general that distinguishes them from other antigens. Immunologically pure allergens have not, in the past, been used to study the various properties of allergens and antibodies in allergic patients. With methods now available, chemically pure substances can be prepared and used for clinical studies. Attempts have been made to standardize pollen extracts using a precipitating system. Immunoelectrophoresis and isoelectric focusing have been used to study pollen extracts. It is now clear that pollen antigens exhibit a wide range of electrophoretic mobilities and comprise many distinct antigenic components. Eight, 10, or more antigens present in extracts of ragweed pollen can be distinguished in this way. But are these antigens allergens? We now have much evidence that these antigens precipitated by antisera may not represent the allergens responsible for sensitivity. However, one highly purified antigen from ragweed pollen does seem to be involved in production of ragweed sensitivity and manifestations of hay fever and asthma—the so-called antigen E. This well-defined allergen deserves much more study. If a single antigen or even a few antigens responsible for ragweed pollen sensitization can be isolated, purified, sequenced for amino acid composition, and synthesized, powerful new approaches for the management of allergic diseases may be at hand. The latter approach has been used to prevent and treat experimental allergic encephalitis of monkeys. A form of immunologic engineering could thus be introduced that could be of great benefit to man.

The ideal method of hyposensitizing hay fever and asthmatic patients has yet to be found. Multiple injections with aqueous extracts have been the method of choice for over 50 years. The hope that water-in-oil emulsions would be a safe and effective method of hyposensitization in one or a few injections has not yet been realized.

In vitro methods for measuring the beneficial responses in allergy have been the goal of many investigators. Anti-ragweed antibodies were measured in pre- and post-treatment sera by hemagglutination procedures. Both the bis-diazotized benzidine method and the tannic acid method with rabbit erythrocytes coated with ragweed extract have been used. No correlation of serum antibody titers, however, has been obtained with any of the hemagglutination procedures, clinical effects, or injection dosages used. In tests evaluating *in vitro* release of histamine by leukocytes, declining susceptibility to antigen-mediated histamine release has been observed, especially in children undergoing immunotherapy; however, the basis of this finding has not yet been clarified. Since we do not know yet what we must know, e.g., the sites of formation of IgE antibodies, the best methods of stimulating or avoiding stimulation of atopic antibody, the basis or best means of inducing immunodeviation, if that is what is desired, efforts at immunotherapy are at present crude and empirical.

PULMONARY HEMOSIDEROSIS

Heiner et al. (1962) described 4 patients who fulfilled the criteria for primary pulmonary hemosiderosis in that each had recurrent pulmonary disease, hemoptysis, iron deficiency anemia, and iron-laden macrophages in gastric or bronchial washings or at lung biopsy. Additional distinctive features included unusually high titers of serum precipitins to multiple constituents of cows' milk, positive intradermal skin tests to various cows' milk proteins, chronic rhinitis, recurrent otitis media, and growth retardation. The symptoms of each patient improved when cows' milk was removed from the diet and returned with reintroduction of milk. An almost immediate clearing of chronic rhinitis and cough in several subjects who were placed on a milk-free diet seems to have provided an early clue that a lasting improvement would result in the pulmonary status. Most of the subjects having an important element of sensitivity to cows' milk were small infants, although one was 15 years of age. Milk aspiration has been suggested as possibly having a role in some subjects with pulmonary disease related to milk ingestion, but this has not been proved to the satisfaction of all.

It should be emphasized that not all subjects with primary pulmonary hemosiderosis have unusual precipitins to cows' milk, and without this finding some do not change dramatically when placed on a milk-free diet. Further, high titers of anti-milk antibodies, including precipitating antibodies, have been observed in children who do not develop pulmonary disease on ingestion of milk. Thus, it has been extremely difficult to establish that pulmonary hemosiderosis is due to hypersensitivity to milk constituents. The quality, as well as quantity, of antibody associated with milk allergy and pulmonary hemosiderosis should be studied further. Heiner's studies suggesting that milk allergy can be associated with primary pulmonary hemosiderosis must rest more on the clinical response to removal of the allergen and re-exposure to the allergen than on the demonstrated association with circulating antibodies.

Several similarities between subjects having pulmonary hemosiderosis with sensitivity to cows' milk and infants who have milk-induced gastrointestinal bleeding and iron deficiency anemia have been recognized. Both are likely to have multiple precipitins to cows' milk proteins in high titer in their serums, and both are usually recognized between the ages of 6 months and 2 years. Symptoms and abnormal bleeding can be repeatedly induced in each by the ingestion of cows' milk, and symptom-free intervals without bleeding occur on a milk-free diet. There seems to be a direct relation between the amount of milk ingested and the severity of symptoms and bleeding in both groups. The exact pathogenetic basis for both diseases requires further elucidation.

We have seen infants in whom arthritis, typical skin lesions of anaphylactoid purpura, and pulmonary hemosiderosis are associated. In some, but certainly not all cases, cows' milk proteins may be implicated. In several such children renal lesions characterized by focal and local glomerulonephritis have been present. Treatment with adrenal steroids or adrenal steroids together with alkylating agents or azathioprine sometimes, but not always, yields clinical improvement. The renal lesions include rather extensive mesangial deposits of complement and immunoglobulins and progressively increasing irregular "lumpy-bumpy" deposits of complement and host immunoglobulins along the epithelial side of the glomerular basement membrane.

GOODPASTURE'S SYNDROME

The association of diffuse pulmonary hemorrhage with glomerulonephritis was first described by Goodpasture in 1919. Since then there have been a number of reports of this disease. In the later stages of the disease there may be diffuse mottling of the lungs due to deposition of hemosiderin. As mentioned in Chapter 31 there is evidence that the renal lesions are caused by an immune process which is autoimmune in that the antibody responsible for the damage to lung and kidney has been shown to react specifically with the basement membranes of these organs (Fig. 25-1). Further, the antibody can be eluted from the lesions of either organ and can be shown to be specific for the basement membrane components and used to produce disease in experimental animals. On immunohistologic examination of the kidney, immunoglobulin and complement can be demonstrated to be deposited in a smooth, fine, linear pattern along the basement membrane of the glomerulus. The deposition is thus of a very different character from that found in other forms of glomerulonephritis, serum sickness, and systemic lupus erythematosus, where it has a discontinuous, granular or "lumpy-bumpy" distribution, associated with the deposition of immune complexes as aggregates occurring on the glomerular basement membrane. Similar deposits of immunoglobulin or complement can be detected in the lung along the alveolar basement membrane.

The immunopathology in the kidney is identical to the pathology produced in the autoimmune glomerulonephritis in sheep by immunizing them with glomerular basement membranes obtained from either humans or monkeys. The specificity of the antibody responsible for this disease and for pulmonary and renal membranes is most fascinating, since glomerular capillary membranes and pulmonary membranes react specifically, but basement membranes of neither tubules nor gastrointestinal tract possess the responsible determinant. By contrast, patients with certain forms of intestinal malabsorption have circulating antibodies specific for basement membranes of the gastrointestinal tract and renal tubules, and patients with bullous pemphigoid have antibodies specific for basement membrane of the skin. If a virus plays a role, it is most likely one played by altering the membranes of the lung or kidney to reveal hidden determinants or to permit a breaking of tolerance and allow the development of the autoimmune disease. Antibody eluted from the glomeruli or lungs is specific for glomerular and pulmonary basement membrane antigens. The pathogenesis of the disease appears to involve a directed immuno-

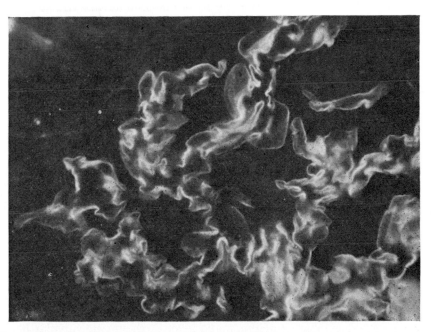

Fig. 25-1. Antibasement membrane antibody demonstrated by immunofluorescent microscopy in the glomeruli of a patient with Goodpasture's syndrome. A similar deposit of IgG antibody can be seen in the lungs.

logic assault against both glomerular and pulmonary basement membranes. The initiation of the disease could be the consequence of a pulmonary infection, e.g., with a virus.

In most instances, Goodpasture's syndrome is a very severe life threatening or lethal disease. Recently, however, intensive immunosuppressive therapy has led to apparent arrest and even reversal of the renal pathology in a few instances.

TONSILLECTOMY

The lymphoid tissue of Waldeyer's ring undergoes physiologic hypertrophy and hyperplasia, usually greatest between 2 and 5 years of age, in response to infections and antigenic exposure in this region. It is now known that tonsils contain both B- and T-cells with immunologic competence and that fantastic germinal center development occurs following antigenic stimulation at these sites. Further, it seems clear that many IgA- and IgE-producing plasma cells are spawned at these sites. Attempts to link the tonsils to bursal-equivalent functions by neonatal extirpation in mice, rabbits, and monkeys have thus far failed. Infections stimulating massive hyperplasia of the tonsils and adenoids are most prevalent during the early years, and as increasing resistance to infection develops, the frequency and severity of respiratory infections and tonsillar hypertrophy diminish rapidly. Under the stress of acute infection, tonsils and adenoids may undergo rapid enlargement, but as infection subsides, they generally return to their former state. One should not judge the tonsil by viewing it only under the conditions of its response to acute infection.

The surgical procedure known as adenotonsillectomy was attempted as early as 3000 years B.C. and has become one of the most, if not the most, frequent operations performed in the United States. Although a conservative attitude has developed toward adenotonsillectomy, the operation is still extremely common and probably is performed far too frequently. It is not without danger, 200 to 300 deaths from the elective procedure being reported each year.

Great variations in the indications for the operation emphasize the lack of understanding of the basic function of this lymphoid tissue and the consequences of its early removal. Because of the wide variety of indications, the lack of long-term follow-up, and performance of the surgical procedure usually at an age when spontaneous improvement in response to exposure to infection is to be expected, assessment of the results of adenotonsillectomy is extremely difficult. Tonsillectomized persons are neither more nor less susceptible to streptococcal infections, nor is the clinical course of streptococcal disease modified. There is also no effect on the development of rheumatic fever or rheumatic valvular heart disease. Streptococcal infections are less readily recognized in tonsillectomized children, who may thereby escape adequate treatment.

Some evidence indicates that the degree of antibody response in the nasopharynx to orally administered polio vaccine appears to be significantly higher when the vaccine is administered to children with intact tonsils. Also, pre-existing levels of local antibody may fall sharply after tonsillectomy and may persist at these levels for several months. These observations may provide an explanation for the observed epidemiologic relationship between tonsillectomy and bulbar and paralytic poliomyelitis and would suggest that the recently tonsillectomized child may still be more susceptible to natural infection with poliovirus and perhaps other viruses. Tonsillectomy predisposes to bulbar poliomyelitis, a finding not nearly so important now that effective immunization and even herd immunity to this disease have been accomplished in the United States. This relationship, however, should at least give the surgeon pause when a tonsillectomy is considered.

We are extremely conservative in recommending tonsillectomy or adenoidectomy. We have reserved this procedure for those rare circumstances when obstruction to the airway or drainage of the middle ear seems to be associated with persistent or recurrent infections of the middle ear. Even here we have so often been disappointed with the beneficial effects of tonsillectomy and/or adenoidectomy that we have considered recommending them only in the case of cancer of the tonsils or adenoids.

"COT DEATH"—SUDDEN DEATH IN INFANCY

Allergy to cows' milk proteins not only is considered to be a significant cause of gastrointestinal upsets associated with diarrhea in infancy, but can also be the cause of acute respiratory distress and under certain circumstances has been postulated to be the cause of sudden death in infancy between the ages of 1 and 6 months. Under experimental conditions it has been possible to produce sudden death from anaphylaxis in experimental animals by introducing a small quantity of cows' milk into lightly anesthetized animals that had been previously sensitized to cows' milk. Histologically, desquamation of the columnar or cuboidal epithelial cells of the bronchioles occurs so that these sloughed cells are deposited in large numbers in the lumen as single intact cells, many of which show no degenerative change. This picture is similar to that observed in the bronchioles of some human infants dying suddenly of unknown cause, where the lumen of the bronchioles is sometimes filled with many dispersed epithelial cells. It is of interest that death from anaphylaxis in the lightly anesthetized animal, equivalent to deep sleep in the human infant, was silent, sudden, and without violence, as might be expected if it was analogous to cot death and if the latter was due to inhalation of gastric contents by a sleeping infant highly sensitive to cows' milk. Although the degree of anaphylactic sensitivity to cows' milk in infancy is not known, conventional antibodies against cows' milk can be found in the serum of infants as early as 6 weeks of life. Significantly higher levels were found in the serum of bottle-fed than in breast-fed babies at 6 weeks of age.

Studies of sudden deaths in infancy disclosed that the serum of these children did not contain unusual quantities or qualities of anti-milk antibody. Further, cot deaths have occurred in many infants where no exposure to cows' milk could be implicated. If anaphylaxis to cows' milk is to be implicated in this treacherous disorder, it must be only one of several possible causes. Indeed, cot death in infancy—one of the most frequent causes of deaths of infants—remains an enigma that requires an answer. Attempts to link cot death to immune deficiency have failed. Although these findings are consistent with the hypothesis that has been current for some time that some cases of "cot death" may be caused by an anaphylactic reaction following the inhalation of cows' milk proteins, under these conditions it is most likely that sensitization occurs by the alimentary route. We are certainly not convinced that more than a few of many cases of cot death can be explained by anaphylactic reaction to cows' milk proteins. We believe it necessary to keep an open mind concerning the pathogenesis of this disorder that may kill more than 10,000 babies in the United States each year. This most perplexing disease of infancy still seems to us a wide open challenge to modern biomedical science.

SELECTED REFERENCES

Extrinsic Allergic Pneumonia

Emanuel, D. A., et al. (1964): Amer. J. Med. 37:392.
McCombs, R. P., (1972): New Eng. J. Med. 286:1186.
McMillan, R., et al. (1972): New Eng. J. Med. 286:681.
Nicholson, D. P. (1972): Amer. J. Med. 53:131.
Patterson, R., et al. (1973): Amer. J. Med. 54:16.
Wenzel, F. J., Gray, R. L., and Emanuel, D. A. (1970): J. Occup. Med. 12:493.

Bronchial Asthma

Callerame, M. L., et al. (1971): New Eng. J. Med. 284:459.
Cardell, B. S., and Pearson, R. S. B. (1959): Thorax 14:341.
Eidinger, D., Raff, M., and Rose, B. (1962): Nature (London) 196:683.
Heiner, D. C., and Rose, B. (1969): J. Allerg. 43:183.
Ishizaka, T., et al. (1969): J. Allerg. 43:168.
Kline, B. S., Cohen, M. D., and Rudolph, J. A. (1932): J. Allerg. 3:531.
Porter, R., and Birch, J. (eds.) (1971): Identification of Asthma. Edinburgh, Churchill Livingstone.
Siegel, S. C. (1965): J. Pediat. 66:927.
Stenius, B., and Wide, L. (1969): Lancet 2:455.
Taylor, B., et al. (1973): Lancet 2:111.
Tullis, D. C. (1970): New Eng. J. Med. 282:370.

Allergic Rhinitis (Hay Fever)

Bohrod, M. G. (1955): Progr. Allerg. 4:31.
Brostoff, J., and Roitt, I. M. (1969): Lancet 2:1269.
Freeman, J. (1911): Lancet 2:814.
Johansson, S. G. O., Mellbin, T., and Vahlquist, B. (1968): Lancet 1:1118.

Levine, B. B., and Redmond, A. P. (1968): J. Clin. Invest. 47:556.
Levine, B. B., Stenber, R. H., and Fortino, L. (1972): Science 178:1201.
Lichtenstein, L. M., and De Bernardo, R. (1971): Int. Arch. Allerg. Appl. Immun. 41:56.
Noon, L. (1911): Lancet 1:1572.
Piper, C. T. (1955): Med. J. Aust. 1:303.
Sadan, N., et al. (1969): New Eng. J. Med. 280:623.
Young, S. H., Zimmerman, R. E. P., and Smithwick, E. M. (1968): Pediatrics 42:976.

Pulmonary Hemosiderosis

Heiner, D. C., Sears, J. W., and Kniker, W. T. (1962): Amer. J. Dis. Child. 103:634.

Goodpasture's Syndrome

Beirne, G. J., et al. (1968): Ann. Intern. Med. 69:1207.
Everett, E. D., et al. (1970): JAMA 213:1849.
Markowitz, A. B., et al. (1968): Clin. Exp. Immun. 3:585.
Poskitt, T. R. (1970): Amer. J. Med. 49:250.
Proskey, A. J., et al. (1970): Amer. J. Med. 48:162.
Vazqucz, J. J. (1970): Arch. Intern. Med. 126:471.

Tonsillectomy

Editorial (1965): JAMA 194:234.
Evans, H. E. (1968): Clin. Pediat. 7:71.
Kaiser, A. D. (1932): Children's Tonsils In or Out: A Critical Study of the End Results of Tonsillectomy. Philadelphia, J. B. Lippincott Company.
Ogra, P. L. (1971): New Eng. J. Med. 284:59.

"Cot Death"—Sudden Death of Infancy

Committee on Infant and Preschool Child (1972): Pediatrics 50:964.
Ray, C. G. and Hebestreit, N. M. (1971): Pediatrics 48:79.
Shaw, E. B. (1970): Amer. J. Dis. Child. 119:416.
Stowens, D., Callahan, E. L., and Clay, J. (1966): Clin. Pediat. (Phila.) 5:243.

26

Immunopathology of the Gastrointestinal Tract

GASTROINTESTINAL ALLERGY

The term *gastrointestinal allergy*, as commonly used, refers to sensitization of the gastrointestinal tract. *Alimentary allergy*, on the other hand, refers to a hypersensitivity response triggered in other organs by food allergens. "Gastrointestinal allergy" is a diagnosis frequently entertained, occasionally evaluated, but rarely established.

Although there is little doubt that ingested foods may precipitate acute attacks of asthma, rhinitis, or urticaria or atopic eczema on a hypersensitivity basis, the occurrence of reagin-mediated hypersensitivity reactions confined solely to the gastrointestinal tract is much more difficult to document. When gastrointestinal manifestations of allergy have been documented, abdominal pain, vomiting, and bloody diarrhea have been the most frequent manifestation. Enzymatic abnormalities that may be present during the acute or chronic episode are transient and completely reversed when the offending antigen is avoided.

Unfortunately, gastrointestinal allergy is diagnosed more frequently on the basis of clinical impressions instead of properly controlled clinical studies. Because no suitable diagnostic tests exist at present, the diagnosis of gastrointestinal allergy still rests on the clinical documentation of symptoms after repeated challenges with the suspected food following periods when that food is completely removed from the patient's diet.

Rising titers of hemagglutinating antibodies and even precipitating antibodies to whole milk or milk proteins have been described in some infants with lactase deficiency and milk intolerance, but milk antibodies are apparently absent in the sera of most adults with the lactose intolerance syndrome. This peculiar tendency of children under the age of 3 years to develop circulating antibodies to food antigens has been observed in a wide variety of intestinal disorders and is not specific for the lactose intolerance syndrome. The most likely explanation is that absorption of whole milk proteins increases due to diminished proteolysis or to damage to the intestinal mucosa. Patients lacking IgA in their serums have a very high frequency of precipitating antibodies to milk proteins.

Although they sometimes develop a sprue-like syndrome, this does not correlate well with the presence or absence of high antibody titers to milk. However, when the local antibody system is defective, increased absorption of whole protein from the bowel is to be expected.

A type of protein-losing enteropathy thought to be due to gastrointestinal allergy has been described in six children, ages 3 to 10 years. These patients had diarrhea, vomiting, hypoalbuminemia, hypogammaglobulinemia, periorbital edema, iron deficiency anemia, and peripheral blood eosinophilia associated with other atopic manifestations such as atopic dermatitis, bronchial asthma, and rhinitis. In some of these patients it was demonstrated that the feeding of milk increased both the clinical symptoms and the enteric loss of protein, whereas the removal of milk from the diet appeared to reverse the entire process.

A somewhat similar syndrome of infancy has been described in which circulating antibodies to cow's milk were associated with gastrointestinal blood loss of up to 21 ml/day, iron-deficiency anemia, hypoproteinemia, and peripheral edema. Removal of milk from the diet apparently resulted in the reversal of the blood loss. In neither of these two syndromes is there any direct evidence that the underlying defect in the gastrointestinal mucosa is the result of antibody-mediated damage to tissue. Indeed, the exact immunopathologic basis has not been worked out for any form of gastrointestinal allergy.

Patients with several forms of primary immunodeficiency syndrome may develop a celiac disease picture or sprue-like syndrome. In some studies more than 50 percent of patients with primary immunodeficiency disease have shown evidence of protein-losing enteropathy. Similarly patients having an isolated absence of IgA have frequently developed a sprue-like syndrome. In the latter patients antibodies directed specifically toward basement membrane of the gastrointestinal tract and renal tubules have been found by Ammann, Roth, and Hong. However, the exact pathogenic basis of these forms of enteropathy have not been worked out.

ULCERATIVE COLITIS

Ulcerative colitis is an acute and chronic inflammatory disease of the colon and rectum characterized clinically by rectal bleeding, diarrhea, abdominal discomfort, and by numerous colonic and systemic complications. Ulcerative colitis was reported more than 100 years ago but remains a perplexing disease of unknown etiology, diagnosed by the exclusion of colonic disorders of known cause and by a characteristic gross appearance, radiologic picture and histopathology.

Since ulcerative colitis tends to be a chronic, recurrent disease with many complications, the outlook for return to complete health is uncertain, although many patients are able to live normal lives. Fatalities are most common during the initial one or two years of illness. Important causes of death are bowel perforation, peritonitis, carcinoma of the colon, massive hemorrhage, thromboembolism, and the problems associated with surgery, often undertaken in critical circumstances. Clinically a very difficult concomitant of ulcerative colitis is chronic active hepatitis. A form of rheumatoid arthritis may also accompany ulcerative colitis. Most evidence seems to indicate that this form of rheumatoid arthritis is quite different from the classic rheumatoid arthritis, and this form has thus been considered a variant of rheumatoid arthritis to be kept separate from the classic disease. We studied a patient whose disease began as myasthenia gravis that was successfully treated by thymectomy. Later this patient developed ulcerative colitis, progressive chronic active hepatitis, and a classic lupus syndrome with severe arthritis. Such conjunctions have argued strongly for an immunologic or infectious basis for ulcerative colitis.

The gastrointestinal tract is well endowed biologically to participate in and to generate immunologic reactions. The small intestine and colon are rich in lymphoid tissue, lymphocytes, and plasma cells and appear to be major sources of lymphoid cells containing and producing IgA. IgA, the predominant immunoglobulin in gastrointestinal and other external secretions, normally is combined with a secretory piece, a nonimmunoglobulin glycoprotein product of epithelial cells that may function to stabilize the secretory IgA molecule and enhance its protective role at mucous surfaces. The relationship of the IgA system to locally produced antibodies, or coproantibodies, is under investigation in several laboratories.

Abundant sources of antigen are present in the digestive tract, and immunologic responses follow the ingestion of or gastrointestinal instillation of a wide variety of chemical haptens, microbial antigens, plant substances, and dietary proteins, and are both cell-mediated and humoral. Immunologic responses have been described in rats and guinea pigs following direct stimulation of Peyer's patches with particulate antigens. Indeed, Muller in our laboratories has obtained evidence that extends the most important observations of Hess and co-workers in Bern. These findings confirm our observations several years ago that the epithelium overlying the Peyer's patches is a very special epithelium permitting particulate antigens to gain access to the Peyer's patches and to provide stimulation at that site. In this way the Peyer's patches like the bursa of Fabricius are stimulated in a most direct way by bacterial antigens in the gut. Muller has found that the gut lymphoid tissue stimulated in this way participates in an enteroenteric immunologic system that accounts for a major regional defense of the body. Thus particulate antigens can stimulate both cellular and humoral immune responses. The cellular immune responses spill over only very little to the systemic system. The humoral immune responses include IgA, of course, and the lamina propria plasma cell responses associated with it, but also apparently involve other secretory B-cell responses, including IgM and IgG responses. Cooper and co-workers have obtained morphologic and ultrastructural evidence for this special nature of the epithelium over both Peyer's patches and bursa.

Clear distinction must be made, in general, between the initiation of antibody synthesis by gut-associated lymphoid tissue and systemic im-munologic responses as a result of the passage of antigens into the blood stream. The systemic responses may reflect large antigen loads, physio-logic or organic changes in the integrity of the gastrointestinal mucosa, or differences in the rate and completeness of proteolysis of ingested anti-gens. Little is known of the effectiveness of the gastrointestinal barrier to oral antigens in infancy or adult life, in health or in diseases of the gas-trointestinal tract. Not only may antigen absorption occur, but intrave-nously administered antibody may be recovered in the enteric contents and feces of normal experimental animals. Specific antibodies have been identified in lymphoid tissues of the digestive tract, although usually without definitive evidence of the local production of the antibody. How-ever, local antibody synthesis in response especially to bacterial antigens when presented as whole organisms has been demonstrated. Although the role of the digestive tract in the immunologic unresponsiveness to a delayed contact sensitizer such as 2,4-dinitrochlorobenzene after feeding the hapten remains uncertain, there is clear evidence that cells in Peyer's patches and lymphoid tissue draining the gastrointestinal tract develop immunity and that IgA-producing plasma cells occupying the submucosa of the gastrointestinal tract derive selectively from precursors in Peyer's patches. Thus both a local antibody system for humoral immunity and a local immunologic system for cellular immunity may operate in the gas-trointestinal tract, but these two systems may remain relatively aloof from the rest of the peripheral lymphoid tissue and as cells exhibit an enteroenteric cycle. A local cellular immunity system originating in Pey-er's patches and functioning along the gastrointestinal tract in parallel with a local antibody system of similar origin is an exciting concept.

Autoantibodies that react with a polysaccharide antigen extracted from sterile fetal human colon can be found in the sera of some patients with ulcerative colitis. This antigen was also found in sterile fetal rat colon and could also be extracted from Escherichia coli 014. The incidence of this autoantibody is low, however, since it occurs in about 15 percent of patients with ulcerative colitis and no obvious relationship exists between its presence and the duration or severity of the disease. A similar anti-body to that described in human ulcerative colitis has been produced in experimental animals. Rabbits immunized with Escherichia coli 014 will produce antibodies that react with an antigen present in rat colon with the same distribution in the colon as for the antigens against which the autoantibodies from patients with ulcerative colitis react. However, there

has been a very strong suggestion that the primary factor in the pathogenesis of ulcerative colitis is some kind of allergic response to antigens
present in the diet or sometimes in bacteria of the gastrointestinal flora,
but clear evidence of either in the pathogenesis of the disease is lacking.

The autoantibodies against human colonic mucosa found in patients
with ulcerative colitis cannot be shown to be in any way cytotoxic for
the colon cells *in vitro*. However, evidence exists that autoimmune cell-
mediated immunologic mechanisms could be involved in the disease.
Since peripheral blood leukocytes from the patients with ulcerative colitis can be shown to be cytotoxic to human fetal colon cells in tissue culture, a colon-specific hypersensitivity reaction could be important in the
formation of tissue lesions in ulcerative colitis.

Both allergy to some factor in the diet and an autoimmune cell-mediated immune reaction possibly could participate in development of the
disease entity, ulcerative colitis. However, another immunologic process
that could also be involved is an immune reaction of the body against
the bacteria or other organisms invading the lower colon. The flora of
the colon in ulcerative colitis is different from that of the normal colon.
In ulcerative colitis there is a predominance of Streptococcus faecalis,
and Escherichia coli is often absent. Recent results in experimental animals have shown that if a strain of Escherichia coli specific for the particular animal is eliminated from the colon, either by immunization with
this organism or by treatment with antisera against the specific organisms, lesions develop in the colon similar to those of ulcerative colitis.
The disease, however, can be stopped if the specific strain of organism
is given by mouth and recurs if the treatment is stopped.

The significance of other "autoimmune processes" such as hemolytic
anemia, rheumatoid arthritis, and lupus erythematosus cells in patients
with ulcerative colitis is not understood. It has been suggested that the
phenomenon could develop either as an association of a severe chronic
inflammatory process or as a result of prolonged therapy with drugs such
as sulfonamides. These reactions could be consequent, of course, to increased absorbance of proteins from diet or to intestinal flora that cross
react with the normal constituents of the body.

Current methods of treating ulcerative colitis are not very satisfactory.
Local or systemic therapy with adrenocorticosteroid hormones helps in
many cases, but great care must be exercised so that toxic reactions do
not outweigh the advantages. Some have advocated immunosuppressive
therapy in which adrenocorticosteroids are coupled with immunosuppressive or anti-inflammatory drugs. The danger from both large doses
of steroids and steroid-immunosuppressive drug regimens is perforation
and septicemia. Recently antilymphocyte serum has been tried, and some
apparent influence reported, but again the results have not always been
impressive. Psychotherapy in general in our experience has added little

to management; however, good supportive mental hygiene by a strong and friendly physician may be salutary, since it minimizes fear and over-reaction of both parent and patient to this sometimes awful disease. Although it seems drastic, often the most conservative treatment of severe progressive disease or long-standing disease is surgical extirpation of the large bowel conserving the rectum and rectal sphincter. Dramatic reversal of all the toxic and of most, if not all, of the psychologic manifestations has regularly occurred following removal of the diseased bowel. True ulcerative colitis does not extend to the remainder of the bowel after surgical extirpation of the colon.

GRANULOMATOUS (ILEO) COLITIS—CROHN'S DISEASE

The acceptance of granulomatous colitis as a distinct clinical and pathologic entity has had an interesting course. In spite of reports of cases as far back as 1806, its full importance was not recognized until the 1932 publication by Crohn, Ginzburg, and Oppenheimer, which described the granulomatous involvement as limited to the ileum. In the very birthplace of our understanding of regional enteritis at the Mount Sinai Hospital in New York, where the early work on nonspecific granulomas of the intestine preceded the clinical presentation by Crohn and his colleagues, several authorities were most resistant to the concept of granulomatous colitis. It represents one of the very few occasions when an eponym, Crohn's disease of the colon, suggested by the English, was for a long time rejected by the very person so honored. Recently, Crohn has recognized the legitimate claims concerning the disease named for him and has permitted this entity to take its rightful place beside its older sibling, regional enteritis.

Of 100 patients with granulomatous disease of the bowel the process will be limited to the small intestine in about 50, to the colon in 10, and will include both small intestine and colon in 40. When a patient having what is thought to be ulcerative colitis has also disease of the small bowel, the correct diagnosis almost always is chronic granulomatous colitis.

Several recent studies on granulomatous colitis in children emphasize certain features that are distinctive for this group, as compared with ulcerative colitis or with older patients whose granulomatous disease is limited to the large intestine. In one report children with the onset of this disease before the age of 16 constituted about one fourth of all cases of granulomatous colitis, in contrast to only one seventh of the cases of ulcerative colitis. In another study of granulomatous colitis, the disease was first apparent in more than half of patients before the age of 21 and in only 1 patient after the age of 40. Such findings have led to the conclusion that more cases of granulomatous colitis than of ulcerative colitis begin in childhood.

The differentiation between ulcerative colitis and granulomatous colitis or Crohn's disease of the colon has received much recent emphasis, and many of the earlier immunologic studies of ulcerative colitis may have included patients with Crohn's disease. The morphologic features of sarcoid-like granulomas in the bowel, although virtually pathognomonic of Crohn's disease when present, suggest the occurrence of cell-mediated immunity against some antigen. This granulomatous reaction led to speculation about the possible role of immunologic mechanisms in this type of inflammatory bowel disease.

Despite data to the contrary, the frequent absence of both tuberculin sensitivity and reactivity to dinitrochlorobenzene in patients with Crohn's disease has raised the question of a depressed cellular immune responsiveness in such individuals in parallel with sarcoidosis. Divergent results perhaps reflect an incomplete knowledge of the heterogeneity of this disease. For example, the incidence of Mantoux-negative reactions was greatest in the subgroup of Crohn's disease with focal intestinal granulomas. In addition, clear statements often are lacking as to the site, activity, and duration of the disease.

Lymphocytes isolated from the peripheral blood of patients with Crohn's disease of the colon also may exert an *in vitro* cytotoxic effect on human colonic epithelial cells. Circulating anti-intestinal epithelium antibodies especially focused toward colonic cells have been demonstrated in patients with Crohn's disease. Serum hemagglutinating antibodies to Escherichia coli 014 have been observed in ulcerative colitis and Crohn's disease, regardless of the site of involvement. Healthy subjects, however, appear to have circulating antibodies to thyroid, gastric parietal cells, and nuclei as frequently as do patients with Crohn's disease. It seems likely that the autoantibodies in this disease reflect the tissue damage and are not etiologically significant.

Sera from patients with Crohn's disease have been reported to have a much lower incidence of hemagglutinating antibodies against casein and beta-lactoglobulin than do sera from patients with ulcerative colitis. This finding probably reflects the obvious differences in the amount of colonic surface mucosa lost in the two diseases. In all immunologic states involving the serum, antibodies are necessary but not alone sufficient to be the basis of symptoms. They may represent a secondary immunologic response to existing nonimmunologic colonic injury and play a protective role or aid in healing. On the other hand, an immune process developing secondarily may contribute to the tissue reaction in colitis and to chronicity. Finally, the possible involvement of an immune process mediated by lymphocytes merits further study in Crohn's disease as in ulcerative colitis. Especially it seems important to assess the reactivity of lymphocytes isolated from intestinal tissues in health and disease.

Recently Mitchell has claimed to have obtained from the lesions of Crohn's disease a virus that produces a transferable granulomatous disease in mice. Attempts to confirm his findings have been unsuccessful. It may be that the formation of granuloma in the mouse is brought about by the activation of a latent mouse virus due to the reaction to the foreign tissue derived from his patient. Search for a viral agent of slow virus type should, however, be continued in both sarcoidosis and the seemingly closely related granulomatous ileitis and colitis. Kveim tests have been reported to be positive more frequently in Crohn's disease than in the general population but less frequently than in sarcoidosis. This is also a most controversial point and at present writing confusion reigns in the medical literature about the relationship of Crohn's disease in its broadest definition and sarcoidosis.

The diagnosis of early granulomatous gastrointestinal disease often is missed because the disease presents as persistent or remitting fever of undetermined origin. In our experience fever of undetermined origin, systemic malaise, and failure to thrive associated with elevated erythrocyte sedimentation rate and abdominal discomfort, especially immediately after eating, are the most frequent early manifestations of the disease. The abdominal discomfort after a meal is often relieved by passage of gas. Appropriate roentgenologic studies including the follow-through gastrointestinal series and barium enema are regularly diagnostic if interpreted by an experienced roentgenologist. We have often diagnosed the disease roentgenologically in children whose roentgenograms were interpreted as ruling out this disease.

A most fascinating feature of this illness is its familial nature, multiple cases among siblings having been repeatedly described. However, no clear evidence of genetic origin has been presented. We have encountered what appears to be a small epidemic of Crohn's disease in a rural Minnesota community. One patient had an extreme form of antibody deficiency syndrome and yet had fulminant Crohn's disease. It was dramatic to study the histopathology of the Crohn's ileitis and colitis in this child whose lesions contained absolutely no plasma cells and to contrast these lesions with those seen in the immunologically vigorous person whose regional ileitis or granulomatous colitis lesions team with plasma cells. We have also reported studies of classic Crohn's disease in a patient with the extreme form of X-linked infantile agammaglobulinemia. This finding argues that autoantibodies sometimes seen in the disease are camp followers rather than pathogenetic agents and can be taken as indirect evidence that T-cell immunity or T-cell autoimmunity is a more important component than B-cell immunity or B-cell autoimmunity in the pathogenesis.

Treatment of Crohn's disease in both children and adults has been most unsatisfactory to date. Surgical removal of lesions may relieve symptoms, but recurrence is experienced in more than 50 percent of cases. Steroid treatment also may relieve symptoms, but control with dosages that can be given over a long period is not regular. The steroid-azathioprine immunosuppressive regimen and cyclophosphamide have both been said to be beneficial, but, again, results have not been consistent. Recently antilymphocyte serum has been tried, but the variable course of the disease and the minimal experience precludes drawing conclusions about this approach.

PERNICIOUS ANEMIA

The failure of absorption of vitamin B12 giving rise to typical megaloblastic anemia has also been known to be associated with a marked disturbance of gastric function. This has been classically demonstrated by a lack of hydrochloric acid in the gastric secretions. Atrophy of the gastric mucosa is associated with both a loss of the chief cells and a reduction in the number of gastric parietal cells. The association of atrophy of the mucosal cells of the stomach with marked infiltration with lymphoid tissue containing germinal centers has suggested that the deficiency in gastric intrinsic factor might be caused by an immunologic mechanism.

Two phases occur in the absorption of vitamin B12. The first is the coupling of vitamin B12 to intrinsic factor, and the second is the uptake of the Vitamin B12-intrinsic factor complex by the intestinal mucosa. Antibodies that can inhibit either of these phases have been detected in the sera of patients with pernicious anemia. In fact, two types of antibody have been detected in the serum. The first combines with the gastric intrinsic factor and can block the attachment of vitamin B12 to intrinsic factor (type 1: blocking antibody). The second type of antibody, which is less common, binds the vitamin B12-intrinsic factor complex (type 2: binding-site antibody) and can prevent the uptake of the complex by the intestinal mucosa.

Although these antibodies are present in the sera of a high proportion of patients with pernicious anemia and are found in the IgG fractions of the sera, it is recognized that their mere presence in the serum does not explain the mechanism of the disease. Finding antibodies against intrinsic factor in the gastric juice would be more important in explaining the mechanism of the failure of absorption of vitamin B12 than the mere presence of these antibodies in the serum.

Antibodies against the gastric parietal cells can be detected in a higher proportion of patients with pernicious anemia than can antibodies against intrinsic factor. However, the role of both antibodies against intrinsic factor and antibodies against the parietal cells in the pathogenesis of the disease is still obscure, especially since these antibodies are detected predominantly in the serum and not in intestinal or gastric secretions. It may be that the primary lesion is atrophy of the gastric mucosa as a result of cell-mediated or humoral antibody mechanisms and that the amount of intrinsic factor secreted into the gastric juices is reduced. The presence of antibodies in the serum may be a parallel phenomenon and not the direct cause of the malabsorption of vitamin B12 and the resulting mega-loblastic anemia. Antibodies against gastric parietal cells can occur in hypothyroid states without any evidence of pernicious anemia, although this antibody is rarely found in patients with a histologically normal gastric mucosa. Intrinsic factor antibodies have not been found in the absence of pernicious anemia.

Some idea of the mechanism of pernicious anemia can be obtained from studies of the response of these patients to treatment with predniso-lone (40 mg/day). This treatment enhanced vitamin B12 absorption and improved the histologic appearance of the gastric mucosa. The parietal cells began to appear in gastric biopsies. Both intrinsic factor and hydro-chloric acid reappeared in the gastric juice. Serum antibody levels against intrinsic factor and gastric parietal cells were reduced in only a proportion of the patients treated. In these studies it was suggested that antibody against gastric parietal cells was stimulated by the release of antigen from damaged gastric mucosa and that their presence was secondary to the actual disease process. It was apparently not the cause of the changes in gastric secretion and vitamin B12 absorption, as might have been suggested by earlier studies. The critical analysis by Twomey et al. of the occurrence of pernicious anemia in patients with primary immuno-deficiency disease seems most important. Pernicious anemia, absence of parietal cells, and gastric hypofunction are all seen with extraordinary frequency in such patients. These phenomena all occur at a much earlier age in this patient population than in apparently immunologically normal persons. In association with primary immunodeficiency diseases, perni-cious anemia occurs without demonstrable levels of antibody in the serum. These findings suggested to us that if an immunologic mecha-nism is responsible as the primary gastrogenetic mechanism in pernicious anemia it must be a cellular immune response.

SUGGESTED REFERENCES

Gastrointestinal Allergy

Ammann, A. J., Roth, J., and Hong, R. (1970): J. Pediat. 77:802.
Bayless, T. M., Partin, J. S., and Rosensweig, N. S. (1967): JAMA 201:128.
Buckley, R. H., and Dees, S. C. (1969): New Eng. J. Med. 281:465.
Good, R. A., and Rodey, G. E. (1970): Cell. Immun. 1:147.
Ingelfinger, F. J., Lowell, F. C., and Franklin, W. (1949): New Eng. J. Med. 241:303.
Matthews, T. S., and Soothill, J. F. (1970): Lancet 2:893.
Silver, H., and Douglas, D. M. (1968): Arch. Dis. Child. 43:17.
Waldmann, T. A. et al. (1967): New Eng. J. Med. 276:761.
Wilson, J. F., Heiner, D. C., and Lahey, M. E. (1964): JAMA 189:568.

Ulcerative Colitis

Aiuta, F., and Garofalo, J. A. (1972): New Eng. J. Med. 287:1151.
Barta, K., and Benysek, L. (1968): Digestion 1:107.
Broberger, O. (1964): Gastroenterology 47:229.
Burrows, W., and Havens, I. (1948): J. Infect. Dis. 82:231.
Cebra, J. J. (1969): Bacteriol. Rev. 33:159.

Chase, M. W. (1946): Proc. Soc. Exp. Biol. Med. *61*:257.
Cooper, G. N., and Turner, K. (1967): Aust. J. Exp. Biol. Med. Sci. *45*:363.
Cooper, G. N., and Turner, K. (1968): Aust. J. Exp. Biol. Med. Sci. *46*:415.
Craig, S. W., and Cebra, J. J. (1971): J. Exp. Med. *134*:188.
Goldstein, M. J., et al. (1969): Ann. Intern. Med. *70*:1067.
Gorbach, S. L., et al. (1968): Gastroenterology *54*:575.
Lowney, E. D. (1968): J. Invest. Derm. *51*:411.
Mitchison, N. A. (1953): Quart. J. Exp. Physiol. *38*:139.
Perlmann, P., and Broberger, O. (1963): J. Exp. Med. *117*:717.
Shorter, R. G., et al. (1968): Gastroenterology *54*:227.
South, M. A., et al. (1967): J. Pediat. *71*:645.
Springer, G. F., Williamson, P., and Brandes, W. C. (1961): J. Exp. Med. *113*:1077.
Taylor, K. B., and Truelove, S. C. (1961): Brit. Med. J. *2*:924.
Thomson, D., Thomson, R., and Morrison, J. T. (1948): *Oral Vaccines and Immunization by Other Unusual Routes.* Edinburgh, Livingstone.
Tomasi, T. B. Jr., et al. (1965): J. Exp. Med. *121*:101.
Watson, D. W., and Bolt, R. J. (1968): In *Progress in Gastroenterology,* vol. 1, Glass, G. B. J., (ed.). New York, Grune & Stratton, p. 391.

Granulomatous (Ileo) Colitis—Crohn's Disease

Appleman, H. D. (1970): New Eng. J. Med. *282*:1273.
Crohn, B. B., Ginzburg, L., and Oppenheimer, G. D. (1932): JAMA *99*:1323.
Crohn, B. B., and Yarnis, H. (1966): J. Mount Sinai Hosp. N. Y. *33*:503.
Eggert, R. C., Wilson, I. D., and Good, R. A. (1969): Ann. Intern. Med. *71*:581.
Farmer, R. G., Deodhar, S. D., and Michener, W. M. (1968): Ann. Intern. Med. *68*:1147.
Glotzer, D. J., et al. (1970): New Eng. J. Med. *282*:582.
Jalan, K. N., et al. (1970): New Eng. J. Med. *282*:588.
Jones, J. V., et al. (1969): Gut *10*:52.
Jones, W. W. (1965): Gut *6*:503.
Kirsner, J. B., and Goldgraber, M. B. (1960): Gastroenterology *38*:536.
Korelitz, B. I. (1968): J. Mount Sinai Hosp. N. Y. *35*:1.
Kraft, S. C., and Kirsner, J. B. (1966): Gastroenterology *51*:788.
Kraft, S. C., et al. (1966): Arch. Path. (Chicago) *82*:369.
Kraft, S. C., et al. (1967): Clin. Exp. Immun. *2*:321.
Lagercrantz, R., et al. (1966): Clin. Exp. Immun. *1*:263.
Lennard-Jones, J. E., Lockhart-Mummery, H. E., and Morson, B. C. (1968): Gastroenterology *54*:1162.
Lockhart-Mummery, H. E., and Morson, B. C. (1964): Gut *5*:493.
Marshak, R. H., Wolf, B. S., and Eliasoph, J. (1959): Radiology *73*:707.
Mitchell, D. N., et al. (1970): Lancet *2*:496.
Mitchell, D. N., and Rees, R. J. W. (1970): Lancet *2*:168.
Shorter, R. G., et al. (1969): Gastroenterology *56*:304.
Slaney, G. (1962): Ann. Roy. Coll. Surg. Eng. *31*:249.
Taylor, K. B., Truelove, S. C., and Wright, R. (1964): Gastroenterology *46*:99.

Pernicious Anemia

Castle, W. B. (1953): New Eng. J. Med. *249*:603.
Editorial (1970): Lancet *1*:458.
Fenwick, S. (1870): Lancet *2*:78.
Glass, G. B. J. (1963): Physiol. Rev. *43*:529.
Goldberg, L. S., and Fudenberg, H. H. (1969): Amer. J. Med. *46*:489.
Lillibridge, C. B., Brandborg, L. L., and Rubin, C. E. (1967): Gastroenterology *52*:792.
McIntyre, O. R., et al. (1965): New Eng. J. Med. *272*:981.
Taylor, K. B., et al. (1962): Brit. Med. J. *2*:1347.
Twomey, J. J., et al. (1970): Ann. Intern. Med. *72*:499.

27

Immunopathology
of Liver Diseases

CHRONIC ACTIVE HEPATITIS

In 1951, Kunkel et al. described a striking subgroup of patients with chronic hepatitis. These patients were usually young females with extreme hypergammaglobulinemia, massive plasma cell infiltrations in the liver, frequent arthritis, and a progressive downhill course, ultimately terminating with coarse nodular cirrhosis. No etiology was apparent in the patients. In 1953, Saint and his colleagues described two groups of patients with nonalcoholic chronic hepatitis on the basis of liver biopsy. Patients in the larger group had "active" disease marked by inflammatory cell infiltration and hepatocellular necrosis, and the other had inactive disease and scarring; the former were considered to have active chronic hepatitis and the latter inactive chronic hepatitis, probably equivalent to what is now called cryptogenic cirrhosis.

In 1955, Joske and King demonstrated the LE cell phenomenon in 2 patients with so-called active chronic viral hepatitis. In 1956, Mackay et al. described 5 further cases, mostly in young females with hypergammaglobulinemia; the syndrome was called lupoid hepatitis because there were some features (e.g., arthralgia) suggestive of systemic lupus erythematosus (SLE) and because the two diseases were considered to be caused by the same basic process—autoimmunization. In 1956, Bearn et al. suggested that although the hepatitis is frequently accompanied by manifestations of connective tissue disease, a wide range of clinical manifestations and a wide range of chronic active hepatitis can be associated. The features which distinguished this broad group of patients were the chronic, progressive hepatitis accompanied by significant increases in circulating gamma globulins. Lupus erythematosus may itself be accompanied on occasion by liver disease but here the pathogenesis is quite different and is associated with vascular inflammatory disease of the liver. In 1957, it was shown that the serum of patients with either lupoid hepatitis or systemic lupus erythematosus reacted by complement fixation with saline extracts of human tissues, particularly liver and kidney. This response became known as the autoimmune complement fixation (AICF) reaction. This reaction was also positive in another disease, primary biliary cirrhosis. Antibodies characteristic of chronic active hepatitis which are associated with the so-called atypical lupus erythematosus cells react with the antigens in smooth muscle. True anti-DNA antibodies and in our experience true lupus syndrome, are at best an infrequent associate of chronic active hepatitis.

The term *chronic active hepatitis* is currently used to describe a form of chronic liver disease which precedes, coexists with, and finally terminates in a coarsely nodular cirrhosis. Chronic active hepatitis is a clinical syndrome that develops in some patients who have icteric or anicteric subacute hepatic necrosis during viral hepatitis infection. Other causes for this clinical syndrome and the accompanying histologic features of necrosis, inflammation, and bridging fibrosis have not been excluded. The disease may begin abruptly and exhibit a severe and unusual course for viral hepatitis. However, in a majority of patients the course cf the disease is insidious and begins with weakness, fatigue, vague abdominal complaints, and liver function abnormalities.

Chronic active hepatitis can be defined by the following criteria: (1) persistent activity for at least 6 months, usually with relapsing or continuing jaundice and/or elevated levels of the serum transaminases, for example, 200 to 1000 units of glutamic-oxalacetic transaminase (GOT), (2) serum gamma globulin levels ranging from 2.0 to 10.0 gm/100 ml, (3) histologic features including patchy perilobular "piecemeal necrosis," hepatocellular regeneration, lymphoid-plasma cell infiltration, fibrosis, and progression to cirrhosis, (4) presence of autoantibodies, particularly to antigens of cell nuclei and smooth muscle, and (5) improvement with immunosuppressive drugs including corticosteroids and azathioprine or combinations of the two.

The increasing recognition of this syndrome in recent years emphasizes the importance of close clinical observation of all patients with viral hepatitis and early liver biopsy in patients who manifest an unusual course. The biopsy is required for correct classification in most patients suspected of having chronic active hepatitis. The earliest histologic lesions may simulate those of acute hepatitis, although plasma cells are regularly prominent. Plasma cell hepatitis or chronic active hepatitis may gradually slip into a very chronic cirrhotic condition with much lower levels of gamma globulin and much less plasma cell infiltration in the liver. This transition occurs over a variable time, often 2 to 4 years or longer. Thus patients with active chronic hepatitis usually have at the same time an incipient or established cirrhosis of the liver, and biochemical and histologic indices of active hepatitis and cirrhosis coexist throughout most of the course of the disease.

Histologically, masses of plasma cells and lymphocytes can be seen surrounding and infiltrating nodules of liver tissue (Fig. 27-1). The

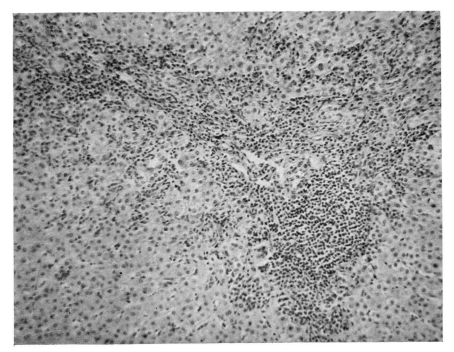

Fig. 27-1. Liver section of a patient with chronic active hepatitis. A characteristic feature is a massive infiltration of liver tissue by lymphocytes and plasma cells.

plasma cells can be shown to be making immunoglobulin, mostly of the IgG class, and more than two thirds of the cases have a high level of IgG in the serum. We have called the extreme form of the disease *plasma cell hepatitis* to emphasize the striking histologic characteristics of the disease, especially early in the course. Forty percent of patients have antibodies to nuclear constituents in their sera and 16 percent are said to have lupus erythematosus cells in the blood. Thyroid autoantibodies are also found in the sera of patients with this disease. As a result of the high incidence of antinuclear antibodies and lupus erythematosus cells, this disease has been thought by many to be a variant of systemic lupus erythematosus and has been called *lupoid hepatitis*. However, the incidence of the involvement of other organs, such as the kidney and brain, is much lower than in systemic lupus erythematosus, and the cause of the disease is not the same. Thus, it is important to keep these diseases separated. The most common systemic complication is arthritis. Occasional cases of renal involvement and arteritis in the skin have been described. Ulcerative colitis has also been described in association with this condition. We have studied dramatic cases in which other evidences of autoimmune phenomena and autoimmune disease have been accompaniments. For example, the onset of the disease in one of our patients was accom-

panied by recurrent parotitis, followed in turn by auotimmune thyroiditis and consequent hypothyroidism. She subsequently had an insidious
onset of liver disease and was found to have more than 8 gm/100 ml of
gamma globulin in her blood. Signs and symptoms of liver disease and
autoimmunity disappeared upon treatment with azathioprine alone. Two
years after discontinuing the anti-inflammatory immunosuppressive treatment the liver disease recurred, and the patient developed nonfamilial
diabetes mellitus. Thus, apparently autoimmune disease of the salivary
glands, thyroid, liver, and pancreas were all associated in this patient.

Chronic active hepatitis is characterized by a progressive relentless destruction of liver tissue with eventual complete failure of function, probably as a result of an immunologic interaction. The destruction of the
liver cells is thought to be an autoimmune process that may be triggered
by a virus infection, since in 25 percent of cases there is a suggestion of
a history of viral hepatitis. We have seen many cases in an area experiencing a high frequency of infectious hepatitis. Cases are clearly divided between those that are Australia antigen positive and Australia
antigen negative. This division does not distinguish any peculiar clinical
picture. Evidence has been presented that immune complexes in the liver
are associated with lesions of piecemeal necrosis; however, we have observed chronic active and progressive hepatitis in patients with the most
extreme form of congenital X-linked agammaglobulinemia. All the histologic characteristics of the disease, including coarse nodular cirrhosis and
piecemeal necrosis, have occurred in patients who apparently cannot form
gamma globulins or antibodies. Consequently, we believe that tissue
damage by a cell-mediated autoimmune mechanism associated with the
chronic virus infection may be more important than is currently realized
in considering pathogenetic mechanisms operating in these patients.

The influence of medical treatment on the course of chronic hepatitis
is important not only practically because the disease constitutes a significant health problem and greatly curtails life expectancy but also
theoretically because the effect of therapeutic agents can provide important clues to the pathogenesis of the disease. Current information suggests that prolonged treatment with a corticosteroid and azathioprine
improves both the clinical status and the liver function.

The effectiveness of aggressive treatment with corticosteroids was demonstrated in the mid-1950s and that of the immunosuppressive thiopur-
ines, 6-mercaptopurine, and azathioprine several years later. Adrenocorticosteroids cause a pronounced improvement, but large doses have to be
used, which in themselves cause toxic symptoms. Better results have been
obtained with prolonged courses of 6-mercaptopurine (5 to 100 mg daily)
or azathioprine (100 to 200 mg daily) for several years. Indeed, we have
treated some patients for as long as 10 or 12 years. During this time liver
function returned to near normal level. Whether these drugs act in their

anti-inflammatory capacity or as true immunosuppressive agents is not known.

Although the effect of chemotherapy on the eventual outcome of active hepatitis has been debated, corticosteroids and azathioprine certainly have a pronounced short-term action of suppressing all manifestations of the disease, as judged by the principal indices, the release of transaminase enzymes, hypergammaglobulinemic liver infiltration, and piecemeal necrosis. Data are insufficient on long-term prognosis with the treatment, but studies using both double blind control techniques and life-table evaluations indicate that in spite of the toxicity consequent to aggressive immunosuppressive and anti-inflammatory treatment, these measures are beneficial to the individual patient and to populations of patients.

SERUM HEPATITIS AND HEPATITIS-ASSOCIATED ANTIGEN (HAA)

Hepatitis has been a mysterious and sometimes intractable malady. Physicians have long recognized that its symptoms—inflammation of the liver accompanied by fever, weakness, loss of appetite, malaise, headache, and muscle pains and sometimes joint pain and mild arthritis—arise from two distinct types of infection. Hepatitis A, also called infectious hepatitis, is generally transmitted by fecal contamination of food and water and is responsible for some 90 percent of the more than 74,000 cases reported in the United States every year. Hepatitis B, also called serum hepatitis, is most frequently transmitted by infusions of blood from infected individuals. Although hepatitis B is responsible for less than 10 percent of the reported cases, it is considered the more dangerous form because those exposed to it are generally already ill. Furthermore the incidence of hepatitis B has been rising as a result of its spread by drug addicts and by increased use of paid donors by blood banks.

Until recently, little else was known about hepatitis, and even now there is neither a specific clinical test for either form of hepatitis nor a specific treatment other than rest and a nutritious diet. A major breakthrough occurred in 1964, however, when Blumberg et al. observed a foreign substance, initially called Australia antigen, in the blood of an Australian aborigine. No clinical significance of this discovery was immediately apparent until 1968 when Prince observed a similar substance in the blood of patients with hepatitis B. The two substances were quickly shown to be identical and to be specifically linked to hepatitis B.

Various terms and abbreviations which are synonymous with Australia antigen (Au) or antibody (anti-Au) have been used: hepatitis B antigen (HB Ag), hepatitis B antibody (HB Ab), Au/SH antigen, SH antigen, hepatitis antigen (HA), hepatitis-associated antigen (HAA), and hepatitis-associated antibody (anti-HAA).

Recent studies revealed that the particle is the DNA- or RNA-containing viral core that replicates in the hepatocyte nucleus and there presumably causes the tissue damage associated with hepatitis B. Through unknown mechanisms, the viral core, the presumed transmissible form of the virus, migrates to the cell cytoplasm where it is sheathed in the hepatitis B antigen coat. This mode of replication is similar to that of mouse leukemia (RNA) and herpes viruses (DNA), whose protein coats are also synthesized in the cytoplasm. Still more recent studies have established two subclasses of Australia antigen: Au a+ and Au b+.

The development of various tests for the detection of antigen and antibody has provided the methodology for studies of the immunology of viral hepatitis type B. The following tests have been used to detect the antigen with variable sensitivities: immunodiffusion, immunoelectrophoresis, complement fixation, passive hemagglutination, immune adherence hemagglutination, immune electron microscopy, radioimmunoassay, and new counter immunoelectrophoresis. Complement fixation, passive hemagglutination, immune adherence hemagglutination and new counter immunoelectrophoresis appear to be the most sensitive tests currently in use for detection of antigen. Radioimmunoassay and passive hemagglutination tests are the most sensitive for the detection of antibody.

Seroepidemiologic studies with the sensitive radioimmunoassay have shown an increasing frequency of anti-HAA with age; approximately 15 to 40 percent of adults have detectable antibody. Sera from young children are usually negative for anti-HAA. In certain institutions, however, a very high percentage of children have a high incidence of HAA. Further, in certain urban areas children may have a higher incidence of HAA than do children in the general population.

Infectious hepatitis is contagious under close and intimate contact which promotes the fecal-oral spread of virus. Therefore, immune serum globulin is indicated for family contacts and for persons in institutions where the disease is highly endemic; it is not indicated for the usual contact in office or school. Children, as well as adults, should receive immune serum globulin when exposed, even though such treatment does not prevent infection but only modifies the expression of the infection.

An active immunizing agent for the prevention of viral hepatitis type A is not available at the present. This development must wait until the agent has been successfully adapted to tissue culture. Patients having primary immunodeficiency diseases, especially those associated with agammaglobulinemia, are especially susceptible to infection with either infectious or serum hepatitis viruses. Fatal infections manifesting as acute fulminating hepatitis, acute yellow atrophy syndrome, progressive hepatitis, and chronic active hepatitis have all been observed. Since most cases of hepatitis occurring in agammaglobulinemic children have been fatal, patients with primary immunodeficiency disease should never be treated with plasma from a pool of donors.

The efficacy of immune serum globulin for the prevention of viral hepatitis, type B, has been a controversial subject for many years. Reports of its value have been mixed, ranging from evidence of some protection to none at all. Effective prophylaxis against this disease is a particular concern in great medical centers because of the high frequency of hepatitis associated with renal dialysis and transplantation surgery. This disease is a recognized occupational hazard of transplant surgeons and auxiliary personnel. In addition, of course, it presents real problems as a possible complication of transplantation surgery.

Active immunization against viral hepatitis, type B, has been reported. Inoculation of a boiled preparation of 1:10 dilution of MS-2 serum in distilled water has been shown to be immunogenic and not infectious. Two inoculations at four-month intervals appear to be more effective than one. However, one inoculation gives enough protection to prevent some cases of hepatitis and to modify others. These studies are being expanded at the present time.

Popper and Mackay postulated that the Australia-antigen particle of hepatitis type B represents an infectious agent different from viruses described so far. It is assumed that it consists of a very small amount of RNA-enzyme complex (virion) with an amount of host protein far in excess of the protein coat of most other viruses. These host proteins include various pre-existing structures of the liver cell. Acute type B viral hepatitis is regarded as a restricted immunologic response to the proteins in the complete B-antigen particle. It is presumed that if there is a hepatic antecedent of chronic liver disease , it will be B-antigen-positive hepatitis. Such chronic liver disease may be the result of one of two processes: (1) continued restricted immune reactions to the virion or, more probably, to the protein of the whole B-antigen particle, with infectivity persisting because of the presence of the virion and with a characteristic distribution of antigen in other organs (polyarthritis and polyarteritis); (2) florid and persisting autoimmune reaction to specific host components of broken-down B-antigen particles, occurring predominantly on females, persisting in the absence of the virion and of infectivity, and with great variation in the clinical manifestations, depending on the character of the antigenic components of the particle fragment and the organ localization of immune complexes. The nature of the autoimmunogen in the particle may determine whether a chronic aggressive hepatitis, primary biliary cirrhosis, or an overlapping syndrome develops. In our view, if this pathogenic scheme is to be taken seriously, it would have to be expanded to include cell-mediated immune mechanisms as well as immune complex injury and to permit expression by infectious hepatitis virus as well as by the HAA viruses, since many of our cases and those of others are both HAA antigen negative and anti-HAA negative and come from epidemics of infectious hepatitis.

Recently, Dudley et al., suggested that the competence of the cell-mediated (T-lymphocyte dependent) immune system would decide whether the infection is self-limited or persists with varying degrees of liver damage. They presented evidence that the persistence of HAA is associated with impaired T-lymphocyte function which itself may be a reflection of the continuing virus infection as, for example, occurs during acute or chronic infections with other viruses, e.g., measles, rubella, mumps, influenza, and oncogenic animal viruses.

PRIMARY BILIARY CIRRHOSIS

The cholangitic and cholestatic types of chronic liver disease include obstructive biliary cirrhosis, primary biliary cirrhosis, fibrosing cholangitis, and drug-induced "allergic" cholestasis, all of which show features of cholestasis including bile retention, pruritus, intestinal malabsorption, retention of alkaline phosphatase, and hypercholesteremia. Primary biliary cirrhosis (Hanot's cirrhosis, xanthomatous biliary cirrhosis) is the disease in this group which has been linked with autoimmunity.

The characteristic serologic reaction is with an antigen of mitochondria, first detected by complement fixation and responsible for the high incidence of positive reaction to the autoimmune complement fixation test (AICF). This antimitochondrial reaction is now detected by immunofluorescence, and frozen sections of rat kidney are a convenient source of antigen. The incidence of positive antimitochondrial reactions in primary biliary cirrhosis has been reported to be 80 to 100 percent.

In regard to antinuclear reactions, a positive LE cell test has not been described in this disease, but there is a moderate incidence, 30 to 40 percent, of positive tests for antinuclear factor to tissue nuclei and 75 percent for granulocyte nuclei.

SELECTED REFERENCES

Chronic Active Hepatitis

Bearn, A. G., Kunkel, H. G., and Slater, R. J. (1956): Amer. J. Med. 21:3.
Gajdusek, D. C. (1958): Arch. Intern. Med. (Chicago) 101:9.
Joske, R. A., and King, W. E. (1955): Lancet 2:477.
Kunkel, H. G. et al. (1951): J. Clin. Invest. 30:654.
Mackay, I. R., and Gajdusek, D. C. (1958): Arch. Intern. Med. (Chicago) 101:30.
Mackay, I. R., Taft, L. I., and Cowling, D. C. (1959): Lancet 1:65.
Miller, J., et al. (1972): Lancet 2:196.
Mistilis, S. P., and Blackburn, C. R. B. (1970): Amer. J. Med. 48:484.
O'Brien, E. N., et al. (1960): Aust. Ann. Med. 9:295.
Page, A. R., Condie, R. M., and Good, R. A. (1964): Amer. J. Med. 36:200.
Page, A. R., Good, R. A., and Pollara, B. (1969): Amer. J. Med. 47:765.
Saint, E. G., et al. (1953): Aust. Ann. Med. 2:113.
Sherlock, S. (1970): Amer. J. Med. 49:693.

Serum Hepatitis and Hepatitis-associated Antigen (HAA)

Blumberg, B. S., Alter, H. J., and Visnich, S. (1965): JAMA 191:541.
Dudley, F. J., Fox, R. A., and Sherlock, S. (1972): Lancet 1:723.
Editorial (1973): Lancet 1:85.
Giustino, V., Dudley, F. J., and Sherlock, S. (1972): Lancet 2:850.
Krugman, S., Giles, J. P., and Hammond, J. (1971): JAMA 217:41.
Lander, J. J., et al. (1972): JAMA 220:1079.
Popper, H., and Mackay, I. R. (1972): Lancet 1:1161.
Prince, A. M. (1968): Proc. Nat. Acad. Sci. 60:814.
Seminars on Viral Hepatitis (1972): Amer. J. Dis. Child. 123:275.
Soulier, J. P., et al. (1972): 123:429.

Primary Biliary Cirrhosis

Baggenstoss, A. H., et al. (1964): Amer. J. Clin. Path. 42:259.
Doniach, D., et al. (1966): Clin. Exp. Immun. 1:237.
Paronetto, F., Schaffner, F., and Popper, H. (1966): New Eng. J. Med. 271:1123.

28

Immunopathology
of the Neuromuscular Diseases

The nervous system occupies a unique position in the history of immunology. "Neuroparalytic accidents" were described as early as 1888, only three years after Pasteur introduced the rabies vaccine grown in rabbit spinal cord as an effective prophylaxis against rabies. These sometimes catastrophic reactions were probably the first indication that immunization might have deleterious effects. Although safer vaccines have been devised, the problem remains with any vaccine that contains constituents of central nervous tissue. Moreover, it was the subsequent analysis of these reactions to rabies vaccine that led to the discovery of experimental allergic encephalomyelitis (EAE), a prototype of autoimmune diseases. More recently, and in an apparently unrelated field, neurologic diseases were the first chronic systemic disorders of man that were shown to be caused by persistent infection with virus. These two themes, autoimmunity and persistent viral infection, now come together in the present analysis because of the possibility that persistent viral infection may alter either the antigenic composition or the reactivity of the host. Techniques are now available to evaluate the possibility that these factors may be important in the pathogenesis of several important diseases currently regarded as being due to unknown causes.

In experimental animals repeated injections of vaccines containing central nervous system (CNS) constituents as in immunization against rabies will occasionally produce demyelinating encephalomyelitis, i.e., post-rabies vaccination encephalomyelitis. This reaction occurs in some patients receiving the classic Pasteur form of immunization (Chapter 33). The pathogenesis of the human disease has not been analyzed nearly so well as have the experimental models, but it would seem that cell-mediated immunity toward a basic protein antigen of myelin is crucial. This serious consequence of rabies immunization is difficult to treat and can be devastating. It can be avoided by use of modern vaccines prepared from purified rabies virus grown in duck eggs instead of the virus preparation that also contains animal spinal cord or brain tissue.

In one of the most exciting chapters of modern immunobiology as it

448

relates to human disease, Eylar has discovered that deep in the molecule of the basic protein of myelin is a sequence of 7 amino acids that are responsible for its antigenicity and for its capacity to produce autoimmune allergic encephalomyelitis. By analyzing the molecule and synthesizing the antigenic component, Eylar has developed preparations capable of being used to produce tolerance rather than immunity. He has been able to prevent and to treat EAE by using defined antigens that favor development of tolerance over development of immunity. This type of molecular analysis of antigens promises to be of immense value in the study of autoimmune, isoimmune, and allergic disease.

MULTIPLE SCLEROSIS

The hypothesis that multiple sclerosis is the result of a sensitization to some component of the central nervous system derives in part from certain clinical features of the disease but rests primarily on pathologic similarities between multiple sclerosis in human and experimental acute demyelinating diseases. At best, this evidence is circumstantial. The evidence that immunologic phenomena are operating in multiple sclerosis is at the moment rather meager. Attempts to demonstrate that lymphocytes of patients with multiple sclerosis undergo blast transformation upon exposure to basic proteins or emulsions of normal or diseased whole CNS tissue have in general been negative. Although lymphocytes of animals developing experimental allergic encephalomyelitis after injection of central nervous tissue adjuvants or basic proteins and adjuvants from myelin readily transform and produce macrophage migration inhibition factor after exposure to either crude CNS emulsions or the purified basic protein antigen, lymphocytes from patients with multiple sclerosis quite regularly failed to exhibit this reaction. Similarly the search for humoral evidence of immunity to central nervous tissue constituents in multiple sclerosis has been quite disappointing. However, a gliotoxic effect of lymphocytes that recently has been described in patients with multiple sclerosis deserves further study. Although these negative results lend no support to the view that autoimmune phenomena cause multiple sclerosis, they do not rule out the possibility.

A more attractive concept of multiple sclerosis is that this disease is caused by a slow virus agent similar to that responsible for other demyelinating diseases of man, e.g., Jakob-Creutzfeldt disease. If this is the case, the agent may be a most bizarre virus-like agent highly resistant to usual disinfecting procedures. Scrapie, a chronic progressive demyelinating disease of sheep, has been shown to be caused by one of these peculiar slow virus agents (Chapter 33). If slow viruses play a role in the pathogenesis of multiple sclerosis, an important immunologic focus becomes the nature of the host-parasite relation to this peculiar class of agents.

This issue has not been effectively resolved at present. In recent years perhaps the most important discovery concerning multiple sclerosis is the evidence that multiple sclerosis is intimately linked to a particular region on a somatic chromosome that controls the mixed leukocyte culture reaction. This evidence, together with evidence that links certain other diseases intimately to the HL-A system, argues strongly that the Ir (immune response) region of the chromosome exists in man as well as in the mouse. Further, in man, as in the mouse, this genetic control is located either at the same site or at a site intimately linked to that which controls the mixed lymphocyte culture responses. Thus capacity to respond to certain antigens of microorganisms or even in host constituents and as a result capacity to develop and express certain diseases may be consequent to the host capacities expressed in the MLC or Ir locus that lies just distal to the 4 component of the HL-A system in man.

IDIOPATHIC POLYNEURITIS AND EXPERIMENTAL ALLERGIC NEURITIS

Idiopathic polyneuritis was described first by Landry in 1859, but little attention was paid to it until 1917 when Guillain, Barré, and Strohl published a particularly lucid description of two cases. In recognition of these pioneer contributions, idiopathic polyneuritis is frequently designated the Landry-Guillain-Barré-Strohl syndrome, although many other synonyms are also used. Usually we speak of the Guillain-Barré syndrome.

Idiopathic polyneuritis is a disease of unknown etiology. In recent years, the suggestion that an immune response against peripheral nerve may be implicated in its pathogenesis has gained support largely from studies that have mimicked the disease in animals by using as the sensitizing agent preparations of peripheral nerve or purified antigens obtained from peripheral nerve along with Freund adjuvant.

An uncommon disease but by no means rare, idiopathic polyneuritis in its usual form evolves subacutely over a period of several days to a few weeks. Evolution is complete within 10 to 11 days in more than half the cases, and within 3 weeks in more than 80 percent. A stable period of variable but usually brief duration leads into the recovery phase which proceeds to completion within a period of weeks to months. Satisfactory recovery has occurred in 85 percent of the cases by the end of 4 to 6 months, although some patients show permanent deficits of varying severity.

The pathologic lesions seen in idiopathic polyneuritis have been the subject of numerous reports. Most studies in recent years have emphasized mononuclear inflammatory infiltration of the peripheral nervous system as a major finding. Such infiltrates, when acute, consist primarily of lymphocytes. In more mature lesions, larger cells, probably a mixture of transformed lymphocytes and macrophages, predominate. Infiltrates generally surround small endoneurial and epineurial venules that are scattered randomly throughout the entire peripheral nervous system from the point where proximal motor and sensory roots give way in the central nervous system to the farthest distal myelinated nerve twigs. Cranial nerves, dorsal root ganglia, sympathetic chains, and sympathetic ganglia all show inflammatory lesions. In a recent pathologic study of 19 cases of idiopathic polyneuritis, inflammatory cellular infiltrates were found in the nerves of all 19. Increased spinal fluid protein in the absence of significant pleocytosis is a characteristic finding, but studies of this protein have revealed evidence of an immunologic reaction in these fluids. Thus the accumulation sometimes of very large amounts of protein in the spinal fluid must be accounted for on other grounds. Some evidence suggests that the protein accumulation is consequent to abnormality of circulation of the cerebrospinal fluid secondary to the swelling of the spinal cord nerve rootlets occluding the outlet pathway at the site of emergence of the spinal nerves from the spinal canal.

Almost all authors agree that segmental demyelination occurring in foci represents the predominant form of nerve fiber damage. Generally, the zones of segmental demyelination correspond geographically to the areas of inflammatory infiltration. Axonal interruption and consequent wallerian degeneration have been observed frequently, most often in association with inflammatory changes of particular severity. Electron microscopic studies of demyelination in idiopathic polyneuritis have revealed segmental myelin disruption in intimate association with macrophages or large mononuclear cells. The processes of these large mononuclears were shown to penetrate through Schwann cell basement membranes to reach the axonal surface.

Experimental allergic neuritis can be produced by immunization with peripheral nerve of most mammalian species. The antigen responsible for the disease has only been partly characterized and is not nearly so well defined as the basic protein from myelin, which has been not only fully sequenced but also synthesized for some species. It is usually thought of as being a constituent of peripheral nerve myelin, but this has not been established for certain. Experimental allergic neuritis, like experimental allergic encephalomyelitis, has been transferred passively by lymphoid cells, but not by serum. This evidence, taken together with the lymphocytic nature of the histologic lesions, has led to the view that the disease is consequent to a delayed type of hypersensitivity.

Evidence that man can develop peripheral neuritis derives from observations that some patients developing post-rabies vaccination encephalomyelitis also show evidence of peripheral neuritis. The desiccated spinal cord used for the offending vaccine undoubtedly contained spinal nerve rootlets as well as spinal cord. The pathogenesis of the Guillain-Barré syndrome in cell-mediated immunity to antigens from peripheral nerve by using blast transformation of T-cells and of the induction of the release of macrophage migration inhibition factor and other T-cell mediators by these antigens awaits further study.

An immunologically mediated neuritic syndrome that should be clearly separated from idiopathic polyneuritis is the brachial neuritis that occurs infrequently as a complication of serum sickness. In general, in this disease other signs of serum sickness are readily demonstrable but need not always be present. The pathologic lesion in this syndrome does not seem to differ in its essentials from lesions of serum sickness elsewhere in the body. The basic lesion is vascular and depends on an antigen-antibody complex injury. In other sites during serum sickness, antigen-antibody complexes deposit on endothelial surfaces and damage them, thereby leading to perivascular edema. Involvement of the upper cords of the brachial plexus is common in serum sickness neuritis. This is usually attributed to the especially large size of these roots in relation to the size of the exit foramina. Consequently, they would be expected to be particularly vulnerable to damage caused by impingement of the bony structures on the swollen nerves. In this syndrome lesions occur in other nerves, and occasionally a polyneuritic syndrome will complicate serum sickness. Thus it may very well be that different forms of allergic polyneuritis occur in man—one based on cell-mediated immunity in a directed immunologic assault and another based on the innocent bystander type of assault due to antigen-antibody complexes.

Experimental allergic neuritis can be prevented by immunosuppressive treatment. The argument that this disease may represent a reasonable model for idiopathic polyneuritis has provided a rationale for the widespread use of steroid immunosuppressive therapy in idiopathic polyneuritis. In chronic neuritis the efficacy is disputed. Measles is a naturally occurring immunosuppressive event. During measles, as is well known, there is profound anergy. It is of interest to note, therefore, that spontaneous remissions of chronic neuritis sometimes follow measles.

SUBACUTE SCLEROSING PANENCEPHALITIS (SSPE)

Subacute sclerosing panencephalitis (SSPE) is a distinct clinical and pathologic entity of children, adolescents, and young adults that may follow measles (rubeola) by a few months to several years. The patient usually passes through four stages characterized by lethargy, regressive speech, myoclonus, and incoordination. Rigidity, mutism, and loss of cerebral function, coma, and death ensue. The electroencephalogram shows characteristic abnormalities, and γ-globulin is increased in cerebrospinal fluid. Infection with a virus has been suspected because of the presence of inclusions in certain cells of the central nervous system.

Specific measles antibody levels are unusually high in both the serum and the cerebrospinal fluid. It has been established that the antibodies against measles are produced within the central nervous system and are not merely passing from serum into the spinal fluid. The characteristic inclusion bodies of both cytoplasmic and intranuclear types are found in the brains of these patients, and these are composed of myxovirus-like particles. Antigen that reacts with antisera specific for measles virus has been demonstrated in brain tissue of these patients by fluorescent microscopy.

Burnet has suggested that SSPE occurs in patients who either lose or lack to some degree the delayed hypersensitivity response to measles. Alternatively the possibility exists that these patients have a more generalized nonresponsiveness of the thymus dependent system. It is known that the measles virus can suppress cell-mediated immunity, and this influence might pave the way for this unusual complication of measles infection. However, studies of *in vitro* cellular immune reaction both to measles virus antigens and to other antigens in patients with established SSPE fail to produce any clue.

Discovery that subacute sclerosing panencephalitis (SSPE) is a chronic infection of the brain by a measles-like virus may represent the solution of an etiologic problem that had been unresolved for many years. On the basis of inclusion body findings it has been proposed that some forms of demyelinating disease in children are due to infection with virus similar to the chronic demyelinating virus infection of the CNS that often complicates distemper in dogs. An immunologic relationship has been established between distemper virus and measles virus, and immunologic and virologic studies have demonstrated that the central nervous system of patients with SSPE contains antigens present in measles virus.

Reviews of the behavior of various isolates of SSPE virus in tissue culture have shown that, unlike conventional strains of measles virus, the agent is tightly bound to cells; infectious virus can only be detected with difficulty, and the pattern of intracellular appearance and growth of its various components is different from that observed with classic measles virus. The pathogenetic significance of these findings remains uncertain. Equally confusing have been the few results published so far about the immunologic responses of patients with SSPE. By definition these patients have high titers of measles antibodies in their serum and cerebrospinal fluid. The status of cell-mediated immune reaction is much more variable, since there have been reports both of accelerated "sensitized" responses to measles antigens and of varying degrees of hyposensitivity or even anergy to different test antigens. In SSPE it has been demonstrated that immune complexes of viral antigen combined with antibody are circulating. This finding has led to a hypothesis involving genetically determined qualitative variation in the patient's response to measles infection in the pathogenesis of the disease, depending perhaps on mechanisms linked to histocompatibility genes, rather than on a unique virus or an abnormal result of simultaneous infection by two viruses. The families of patients with SSPE do not, however, show inherited quantitative defects in their antibody response to measles, but this does not completely exclude effects that seem to be important in some slow virus or temperate virus infections in animals. The concept that SSPE represents a slow virus phase of measles virus infection is most attractive and may have great implications with respect to the pathogenesis of many human diseases ranging from multiple sclerosis to chronic active hepatitis. The possibility also seems most attractive that this disease representing a very special immunologic relationship to the measles virus could reflect in part the function of the Ir genetic locus.

The unusually early age at which many patients with SSPE have their first conventional attack of measles suggests that an innate abnormality or propensity to develop the disease exists in patients who have a special immunologic relation to the virus. Infants may have a considerable amount of circulating maternal antibody and may also be somewhat less responsive immunologically than older children. Perhaps infection at just the right time in relationship to this developing immunologic maturation may be crucial in predisposing to this disease.

A study of the natural history and epidemiology of subacute sclerosing panencephalitis diagnosed in 219 patients in the United States between 1960 and 1970 revealed an apparent preponderance of cases in the southeastern part of the United States, with a frequency of up to 4 per million children, as opposed to a national average of 1 per million, a mean age of onset of 7.2 years, a sex ratio of 3.3 males for each female patient, and a history of clinical measles under 2 years of age in just over half the cases. The basis for these interesting epidemiologic facts is yet to be clarified. It does not seem to be explained by race alone.

SYMPATHETIC OPHTHALMIA

Sympathetic ophthalmia (uveitis) occurs in the normal eye, as a complication, following traumatic endophthalmitis of the other eye. Uveitis may occur in the second eye 10 to 21 days after the initial injury. The figures usually cited for this complication range from 1 in 20 to 1 in 200 cases of traumatic endophthalmitis. Sympathetic ophthalmia can sometimes be produced in the guinea pig, rabbit, and monkey by immunizing with uveal or retinal tissue in Freund's adjuvant. Passive transfer of the disease can be effected with spleen or lymph node cells but not with serum or antibodies in any of the experimental models. When a severe immunogenic uveitis is produced in one eye, a certain number of animals develop a low-grade uveitis in the second eye. These animals also demonstrate circulating antiuveal autoantibody.

Treatment of sympathetic ophthalmia generally employs topical and systemic adrenocorticosteroids, and there seems little doubt that these measures have a beneficial effect, especially when the disease is not particularly severe. However, often in severe cases treatment seems to be insufficient, and blindness can ensue. Prophylaxis with corticosteroids may be more effective in this disease than it is in experimental allergic encephalomyelitis, but the difficulty is determining which patients should be given a prophylactic regimen. Those cases of complicated injury where prophylaxis might be most helpful are also cases where the hazard of enhancing infection by adrenal steroid treatment is also the greatest. Topical steroid treatment is widely used in the normal eye following surgery or trauma to a diseased or damaged eye. At the earliest signs of uveitis or inflammation of the normal eye, systemic steroid treatment must be employed. This is often effective. Reports of the use of antilymphocyte serum are few, but from analysis to date it might be expected that this approach would offer the most effective treatment once the disease has been established.

When uveitis has been developed in experimental animals immunized with a homogenized suspension of homologous uvea in Freund's adjuvant, the disease is transient, starting with vitreous opacities followed by appearance of cells in the aqueous humor. Deposits are seen on the anterior lens capsule and the posterior surface of the cornea. In addition, plasma cells, lymphocytes and histiocytes infiltrate the ciliary body and extend into the adjacent vitreous, iris, and choroid. The external layers of the retina may also be secondarily involved. Precipitating antibody against uveal tissue antigens can be demonstrated in the serum. The animals also show delayed hypersensitivity reactions with soluble extracts of the uvea. Since the uvea contains antigens common to other tissues, delayed hypersensitivity reactions can also be evoked by skin testing, for example, with extracts of spleen. The disease in experimental animals appears to be analogous to human uveitis, which starts as a cyclitis and spreads to the entire uvea, and seems a good experimental model of sympathetic ophthalmia. We cannot predict, at present, who is destined to develop this kind of autoallergic disease. Extensive studies are needed to determine whether this disease is linked to histocompatibility and thus to Ir determinants. Such data may provide a clue as to who is more likely to develop this disease.

MYASTHENIA GRAVIS

Thomas Willis first described the clinical condition now known as myasthenia gravis in 1672. This disease, based on malfunction of the myoneural junction, is one of the most fascinating of the diseases having immunologic concomitants. A pathologic condition of the thymus has been associated with this disease for 60 years. The possible relationship of myasthenia gravis to altered immunologic parameters was first suggested in 1960. Myasthenia gravis has been described in association with virtually every disease having immunologic features, and a variety of tissue specific autoantibodies have been detected in the serum of patients with myasthenia gravis.

Strauss and his associates discovered that patients with myasthenia gravis frequently have autoantibodies against muscle demonstrable by complement fixation. They also found these autoantibodies to be directed against the Z bands of skeletal muscle. In other studies two types of reactivity have been recognized between serum and muscle tissue. The first, designated S, was with skeletal muscles and was capable of fixing complement; the second, a noncomplement-fixing reactivity designated SH, reacted with components of both skeletal and cardiac muscle.

Antimuscle antibody was found in serum obtained at one point in time from approximately 30 percent of patients with myasthenia gravis and from 95 percent of patients with myasthenia gravis and a documented thymoma. Approximately 20 percent of patients also had antinuclear antibodies, which can occur in one, two, or even all three major classes of immunoglobulins in a given patient. Approximately 30 percent show at least one form of antithyroid antibody. Paradoxically, however, no autoantibodies directed to the site of major pathologic physiology—the motor end plate of the myoneural junction—have been found. The autoantibodies frequently found in the circulation of such patients react as well with certain large clear cells present within the thymus itself. These cells, on careful microscopic study and electron microscopic analysis, can be shown to contain muscle fibers and are the so-called myoid cells.

Goldstein and Whittingham reported that they could produce an experimental model of myasthenia gravis by immunizing guinea pigs against either thymus or skeletal muscle with Freund's adjuvant. They related the pathogenesis of the muscular malfunction in this model to the release of a factor from thymus that is toxic to the myoneural junction. On the basis of these findings and some evidence that a similar factor may circulate early in the course of human myasthenia gravis, these authors postulated that the pathogenesis of this disease involves a vicious cycle which includes production of autoantibodies against muscle that react with the myoid cells (clear cells) in the thymus to cause inflammatory damage in the thymus. The latter process is thought to lead to release of a toxic peptide by the thymus that in turn interferes with function of the myoneural junction. If this toxic peptide acts on the myoneural junction in sufficient concentration over a long period, permanent damage to this organ can be the consequence. This rather extended speculative interpretation, several aspects of which have been questioned by other investigations, might not be so attractive if it did not explain so well many otherwise inexplicable aspects of this disease. For example, removal of the thymus early in the course of myasthenia gravis, especially in young females, frequently results in complete arrest of the disease and return to normal. Removal of the thymus three years or more after onset when the myoneural junction can be presumed to have been irreversibly damaged in many patients has much less of a beneficial influence on the course of the disease. In patients who develop myasthenia in association with a form of clear-cell tumor (myoid cell) of the thymus, removal of the tumor, together with removal of the normal thymus, will often correct the myasthenia. Further, the symptoms do not return, even though the tumor returns and extends widely, and antimuscle antibodies reach very high levels when the nontumorous portion of thymus is removed in such patients. Unfortunately, to date the toxic factor presumably produced by the thymus that has been diseased by the autoimmune assault has not been isolated and defined. The experiment of Nature, however, provided by a myasthenic mother who passively transmits a transient myasthenia to her fetus and newborn argues strongly for the role of a serum factor that can be transmitted across the placental barrier in the pathogenesis of this disease. Whatever the circulating factor responsible for malfunction and damage to the myoneural junction may be, its influence on the newborn persists only for a few weeks after birth.

The thymic factor with pathogenetic potential in myasthenia gravis is a most interesting compound. Recently, Goldstein and his co-workers in New York have been isolating this material and have defined a neutral peptide of some 7000 MW, which has a consistent influence on the myoneural junction. This material, which they have sequenced for amino-acid structure, also acts to influence differentiation of stem cells in the mouse and to conver Th 1 (or θ) surface isoantigenicity.

About 80 percent of patients with myasthenia gravis have thymic hyperplasia characterized by the presence of germinal centers within the medulla of the gland. Approximately 15 percent of myasthenic patients have a true tumor of the thymus. The thymoma associated with myasthenia gravis is usually well encapsulated and is quite regularly comprised of the clear cells (myoid cells).

Cholinesterase inhibitors—neostigmine, pyridostigmine, and ambenonium (Mysuran)—are widely used for symptomatic relief in patients with myasthenia. Since patients differ considerably in the degree of response to and the side effects from each of these agents, the dose and time schedule for the administration of anticholinesterase medication must be adjusted to the individual patient. In 1939 Blalock and co-workers reported dramatic improvement following thymectomy in their patient with myasthenia and provided hope for a surgical treatment which has been widely substantiated since their study. The indications for thymectomy generally are (1) an operable mediastinal mass (presumably a thymoma), (2) poor medical control of the disease in patients with no contraindication to surgery, and (3) generalized myasthenia gravis in patients under 40 and over 12 years of age of either sex who have had the

disease less than five years. The latter group can be expected to experience the greatest benefit. This influence is probably due to removal of
the source of the toxic peptide that is released by the inflamed or injured
thymus in this disease.

Thymoma, Myositis, and Candidiasis Syndrome. Montes et al. have
recently emphasized what they believe to be a new syndrome in which
candidiasis, myositis, and thymoma go together. In this syndrome tumors
of the clear cells of the thymus, which are probably myoid cells, are associated with what very likely is cell-mediated autoimmunity directed
against the muscles. As so often is seen with autoimmunity when immunodeficiency also exists, the myositis is presumably produced by this autoimmune assault. In this case the immunodeficiency is of the cell-mediated
immunologic system, and thus mucocutaneous candidiasis is seen. As
these authors suggest, it could well be that the tumor of the thymus producing the abundant and extensive population of clear cells is the primary event. This in turn might be expected to perturb the normal development of thymus dependent T cells and permit the chronic mucocutaneous candidiasis. The myositis, on the other hand, could reflect the
cell-mediated autoimmunity produced by reaction of the persisting peripheral T-cell system against the antigens on the clear cells or myoid cells
that are closely related but not identical to antigens present on normal
muscle cells.

The relationship between this disease and the autoimmunity against
muscle and clear cells of the thymus in myasthenia gravis is provocative.
Indeed the frequent muscle infiltration in myasthenia, the so-called
lymphorrhages, may reflect its existence. Surely what is needed in both
diseases is a professional analysis of evidence for cellular immunity to
components of muscle and clear cells of the thymus as well as better
definition of the nature of the clear cells in the thymoma, candidiasis, and
myositis syndrome. The paradox in myasthenia remains, however, since
neither the cellular autoimmunity nor the humoral autoimmunity in this
disease is directed toward the myoneural junction where the fundamental
pathologic physiology resides. Surely cellular autoimmunity cannot account for the major manifestations of myasthenia, since pregnant mothers
with myasthenia gravis transfer a transient myasthenia to their offspring
but could not possibly transfer lymphocytes in large numbers without producing extensive graft-versus-host disease.

SELECTED REFERENCES

Multiple Sclerosis

Adams, R. D. (1959): In *"Allergic" Encephalomyelitis,* Kies, M. W., and Alvord,
    E. C. Jr. (eds.). Springfield, Illinois, Charles C Thomas, p. 183.
Dowling, P., and Cook, S. (1968): Neurology *18*:295.
Mills, J. A. (1966): J. Immun. 97:239.

Oppenheim, J. J. (1968): Fed. Proc. 27:21.
Shiraki, H., and Otani, S. (1959): In *"Allergic" Encephalomyelitis*, Kies, M. W., and Alvord, E. C. Jr. (eds.). Springfield, Illinois, Charles C Thomas, p. 58.
Wolfgram, F., et al. (eds.) (1972): *Multiple Sclerosis: Immunology, Virology, and Ultrastructure.* New York, Academic Press.

Idiopathic Polyneuritis and Experimental Allergic Neuritis

Asbury, A. K., Arnason, B. G., and Adams, R. D. (1969): Medicine 48:173.
Austin, J. H. (1958): Brain 81:157.
Costaigne, P., Brunet, P., and Nouailhat, F. (1966): Rev. Neurol. 115:849.
Guillain, G., Barré, J. A., and Strohl, A. (1916): Bull. Soc. Med. Hop. Paris 40:1462.
Jackson, R. H., Miller, H., and Schapira, K. (1957): Brit. Med. J. 1:480.
Landry, O. (1859): Gaz. Hebd. Med. Chirurg. 6:472.
Markland, L. D., and Riley, H. D. Jr. (1967): Clin. Pediat. 6:162.

Subacute Sclerosing Panencephalitis (SSPE)

Bodmer, W. F. (1972): Nature (London) 127:139.
Bonteille, M., et al. (1965): Rev. Neurol. 113:454.
Brody, J. A., and Detels, R. (1970): Lancet 2:500.
Brody, J. A., Detels, R., and Sever, J. L. (1972): Lancet 1:177.
Burnet, F. M. (1968): Lancet 2:610.
Dayan, A. D., and Stokes, M. I. (1972): Brit. Med. J. 2:374.
Gerson, K. L., and Haslam, R. H. A. (1971): New Eng. J. Med. 285:78.
Horta-Barbosa, L., et al. (1971): Science 173:840.
Jabbour, J. T., et al. (1972): JAMA 220:959.
Link, H., Panelius, M., and Salmi, A. A. (1973): Arch. Neurol. 28:23.
MacCallum, F. O. (1972). Brit. Med. Bull. 28:105.
McDevitt, H. O., and Bodmer, W. F. (1972): Amer. J. Med. 52:1.
Sell, K. W., et al. (1973): New Eng. J. Med. 288:215.
Soothill, J. F., and Steward, M. W. (1971): Clin. Exp. Immun. 9:193.
ter Meulen, V., Katz, M., and Müller, D. (1972): Curr. Top. Microbiol. Immun. 57:1.

Sympathetic Ophthalmia

Epstein, W. V., Tan, H., and Easterbrook, H. (1971): New Eng. J. Med. 285:1502.
Graefe, A. von (1957): Graefe Arch. Klin. Exp. Opthal. 3:442.
Joy, H. H. (1935): Arch. Ophthal. (Chicago) 14:733.
Theobald, G. D. (1930): Amer. J. Ophthal. 13:597.

Myasthenia Gravis

Blalock, A., et al. (1939): Ann. Surg. 110:544.
Castleman, B., and Norris, E. H. (1949): Medicine 28:27.
Goldstein, G. (1968): Lancet 2:119.
Goldstein, G., and Whittingham, S. (1966): Lancet 2:315.
Montes, L. F., et al. (1972): JAMA 222:1619.
Osserman, K. E. (1958): *Myasthenia Gravis.* New York, Grune & Stratton.
Osserman, K. E. (1968): Ann. Intern. Med. 69:398.
Simpson, J. A. (1960): Scot. Med. J. 5:419.
Strauss, A. J. L., et al. (1960): Proc. Soc. Exp. Biol. Med. 105:184.
Strauss, A. J. L., and van der Geld, H. W. R. (1966): In *The Thymus: Experimental and Clinical Studies*, Wolstenholme, G. E. W., and Porter, R. (eds.). Boston, Little, Brown and Company, p. 416.
Strickroot, F. L., Schaeffer, R. L., and Bergo, H. L. (1942): JAMA 120:1207.
Willis, T. (1683): *Two Discourses Concerning the Soul of Brutes*, trans. by S. Pordage. London.

29

Immunologic Aspects
of Hematologic Diseases

A major finding which sharpened the differentiation between acquired and congenital hemolytic disorders was the discovery of the antiglobulin test by Coombs et al. and the application of this test to red cells of patients with acquired types of hemolytic anemia by Boorman et al. The red cells of many patients with acquired hemolytic disease exhibit positive antiglobulin reactions, but only rarely is a positive reaction reported in cases of congenital hemolytic disorders. The introduction of the antiglobulin test clearly focused attention upon the possibility that immune mechanisms are involved in the pathogenesis of these disorders.

IDIOPATHIC ACQUIRED HEMOLYTIC DISEASE

Idiopathic acquired immune hemolytic disease (AIHD) may not be associated with any demonstrable underlying disease process in one half to two thirds of the cases reported. In the remaining cases, the acquired hemolytic disorder appears to be secondary to some underlying diseases,

Table 29-1. Auotimmune Hemolytic Anemias

	Warm antibodies	Cold antibodies
Idiopathic	+	+
Collagen-vascular disease	+	
Infectious diseases (mostly viral)	+	+
Liver disease	+	+
Lymphoreticular malignancies	+	+
Solid neoplasms	+	
Idiopathic thrombocytopenic purpura	+	
Drugs (α-methyldopa)	+	
Primary agammaglobulinemia	+	
Infectious mononucleosis		+
Ulcerative colitis	+	
Thyroid disease	+	
Cardiac prosthetic valves	+	

From Freedman, S. O. (ed.) (1971): *Clinical Immunology*, New York, Harper & Row, p. 284.

e.g., malignant proliferative disorders of the lymphatic and reticuloendothelial tissues; connective tissue disorders; systemic lupus erythematosus (SLE); and, rarely, nonlymphoid tumors, viral infections, or inflammatory diseases of a chronic nature such as ulcerative colitis and sarcoidosis. In more than three quarters of cases of secondary AIHD the underlying disorder is clearly evident at the time the hemolytic process is recognized. The underlying disorder generally becomes evident within one year in almost all remaining cases. However, a small proportion of patients, perhaps 5 percent, experience hemolytic disease long before an underlying disorder is recognized.

When the autoantibody is optimally active at body temperature, it is termed a *warm antibody*. The autoantibody optimally active at lower temperature, i.e., 2° to 10°C is termed the *cold antibody*. Idiopathic and secondary cases of the AIHD are recognized in both cold and warm autoantibody categories (Table 29-1). Certain clinical and pathophysiologic differences are associated with the serologic distinction in the thermal optimum of the autoantibody (Table 29-2).

The blood in cases of idiopathic AIHD may sometimes show minimal or no anemia and only moderate but persistently elevated reticulocyte counts. In cases with more active hemolysis, however, anemia ranges from moderate to severe, and the reticulocyte count may be markedly elevated to 50 percent or more.

Table 29-2. Relationship of Antibody Characteristics to Coombs' Test Pattern in Acquired Immune Hemolytic Disorders

Pattern of Direct Antiglobulin Tests*	Characteristics of Antibody	Antibody Specificity
1. IgG alone	Warm antibody; nonagglutinating; presumably inefficient in CF	a. Often Rh-related b. Non-Rh c. Mixed
2. IgG + C	Warm antibody; nonagglutinating; effective in CF	Usually non-Rh
3. C alone (subthreshold IgG)	Same as (2)	Usually non-Rh
4. C alone	a. Cold agglutinins b. Donath-Landsteiner c. Drug-antibody complexes d. ? Other mechanisms	a. Anti-I, i, etc. b. Anti-P c. E.g., antiquinidine
5. IgM (or IgA) + C	Apparently nonagglutinating warm antibodies	Nonspecific

* Abbreviations: C = complement. CF = complement fixation to red cells.

Adapted from Leddy, J. P., et al. (1970): J. Immun. *105*:677, The Williams & Wilkins Co.; and from Engelfriet C. P., et al. (1968): Clin. Exp. Immun. 3:605.

As was shown by Leddy et al., a patient's red cells may be autosensitized (1) with IgG alone, (2) with both IgG and C components (IgG + C pattern), or (3) with C in the absence of detectable immunoglobulins (C alone pattern). A large proportion of patients have in their autoantibody populations a predominance of κ or λ light chains, which depart markedly from the normal κ:λ ratios found in these patients' whole serum or serum IgG, although both K and L molecules are present. The IgG_1 subclass has strongly predominated in virtually all of the autoantibody populations associated with AIHD, although some exceptions have been found.

In cases with the IgG + C pattern, the cell-bound C is due to the C-fixing activity of IgG antibody. In patients with the "IgG alone" pattern, the autoantibodies appear to have a lesser capacity to fix C, although other factors could be involved. The C alone pattern of red cell autosensitization may be seen in patients with cold agglutinin disease or with certain types of drug-related hemolytic anemia. In this pattern it is presumed that C components are demonstrated on the cells and antibody is not because the antibody has been lost while the C remains attached. An alternative and more attractive view to us is that C is demonstrable and antibody is not because of the tremendous 300- to 400-fold molecule for molecule amplification which may be achieved during engagement of complement by the antigen-antibody reaction (Chapter 11). Another possibility for the C-alone pattern is that abnormal red cells, as is the case with abnormal PNH cells, may be able to activate the complement system directly, particularly via the so-called alternate pathway and the properdin system.

Although the factors causing formation of erythrocyte autoantibodies remain obscure, good evidence exists that these antibodies have true autospecificity. Reactions with native determinants of the human red cell membrane rather than to altered membrane constituents or to exogenous allergens are clearly demonstrable in most cases of idiopathic hemolytic disease. Immune hemolytic anemia, however, can also occur in association with sensitivity to drugs like penicillin, quinidine, stibophen, and other agents. In at least some of the latter the hemolytic process is due to the adherence of antigen, antibody, and complement on the red blood cell surface which then is injured as an innocent bystander. A crucial and pertinent question about any autoantibody, however, is whether it really has a pathogenic role in the disease with which it is associated. There can be no question that this is regularly the case with autoimmune hemolytic anemia.

Immunoglobulin deficiency, in the form of generalized hypogammaglobulinemia or selective deficiency of one immunoglobulin, has been observed in a minority of patients with AIHD, with or without associated lymphoproliferative disease. Indeed, the frequency of autoimmunity of this sort is very high in immunodeficiencies. The Coombs' test in these patients is usually positive, however, and the autoimmunity may be attributed to the immunodeficiency. For example, patients having selective absence of IgA have Coombs' positive AIHD in extremely high frequency. The basis of this association of such autoimmune disease with immunodeficiency has been discussed extensively especially by Fudenberg. For us, the most attractive hypothesis to explain this relation is that the immunodeficiency permits the remaining immunologic system to be stimulated excessively by antigens that cross react with host constituents.

Corticosteroid therapy may be dramatically effective in inducing cessation or marked slowing of red blood cell destruction in approximately two thirds of patients with AIHD. Five to 10 percent of patients show essentially no response to corticosteroid therapy, and the remainder, variable minor degrees of improvement. Doses equivalent to 40 to 60 mg/m^2 of prednisone daily may be needed for 10 to 14 days, with gradual decrease of this dosage to one quarter to one half of the starting dose after hemolysis has slowed. These dosages should then be administered for prolonged periods. Antimetabolites, such as 6-mercaptopurine (or azathioprine) and thioguanine, employed on the theory that they may interfere with the synthesis of autoantibody have also been effective in some recalcitrant cases.

It has long been recognized that transfusion of patients with AIHD presents a serious clinical and serologic problem. If autoantibody is free in the serum, it may be impossible to find compatible donor blood. Transfusion of patients with AIHD is usually followed by increasing signs of blood destruction with increase in jaundice, hemoglobinemia in some cases, and not infrequently renal damage and clinical deterioration.

PAROXYSMAL COLD HEMOGLOBINURIA

Acute intermittent massive hemolysis following exposure to cold and accompanied by hemoglobinuria, sometimes by acrocyanosis, and less commonly by cold urticaria represents the clinical syndrome of paroxysmal cold hemoglobinuria. This form of disease was recognized in the latter part of the last century, but its relationship to autoantibodies was not known. By 1884 a frequent association with advanced syphilis was noted, and in 1904 Donath and Landsteiner described the complement dependent autohemolytic serum antibody (D-L antibody) that is responsible for the hemolytic disease.

Patients of any age can be affected, but the association with congenital syphilis assured that many of the cases reported in the nineteenth and twentieth centuries would be children. Typically, attacks occur in cold seasons, but the degree of chilling required to induce hemolysis is variable from patient to patient. Constitutional symptoms begin minutes to hours after cold exposure, and the urine turns dark red. In the most acute cases, aching pain in the back and extremities is noted; acute abdominal cramps and fever as high as 40°C may be seen.

The hemoglobin level can drop as much as 5 or 6 gm/100 ml within a few hours during severe attacks. Direct Coombs' tests on the patient's red cells at this time may be positive and remain positive for a brief time after the attack. The positive Coombs' reaction is due primarily to coating of unhemolyzed red cells with C components (sublytic C fixation).

The disease has always been rare. An acute transient form of the disease has been recognized, in temporal association with measles, chickenpox, mumps, infectious mononucleosis, or "flu-like" illness.

The D-L antibody is typically demonstrated by a two-phase test in which the patient's fresh serum is mixed with his own or another person's erythrocytes at 4° C, and the mixture is then warmed to 37° C. Intense or complete hemolysis of the red cells occurs. It should be noted that the average temperature of the blood in the capillaries of the skin of the extremities is 28 to 31° C. During severe chilling, conditions are presumably achieved in these superficial vessels which satisfy the temperature dependence for combination with antigen on the red cells of the D-L antibody.

The D-L antibody itself is an IgG antibody. Positive indirect antiglobulin reactions with potent anti-IgG serum can be obtained with D-L antibodies if the incubation and washing of red cells are carried out in the cold.

Cases associated with virus infection tend to clear spontaneously. In cases due to syphilis, effective treatment of the syphilis has often resulted in cure of the hemolytic disease.

The molecular basis of the Donath-Landsteiner hemolytic phenomenon has not been established with certainty. However, since the antibody does not combine with the red cell in the warm but will do so in the cold, it has been presumed that a conformational change occurs in the antibody in the cold which makes the IgG antibody combine with an antigen on the red blood cells at low temperatures but not at higher temperatures. When the cell combined with antibody is warmed in the presence of serum, hemolysis occurs from action of the temperature dependent enzymes of the complement system. Alternatively, it is possible that the reaction is based on conformational changes occurring in antigens within the red cell membrane rather than in the antibody. Definitive studies that explain all these relationships in precise molecular terms are still needed.

COLD AGGLUTININ DISEASE

In 1925 Iwai and Mei-Sai showed that cold autohemagglutination could have clinical significance. When the conjunctivae or nailbeds of a patient with strong autohemagglutination were chilled, he responded with arrest or sluggishness of the blood flow and even vascular occlusion in small vessels. This phenomenon was first seen in a patient who had Raynaud's phenomenon but apparently no hemoglobinuria. Subsequently, cases with hemoglobinuria as well as Raynaud's phenomenon have been reported, and others have exhibited only hemoglobinuria.

Cold agglutinin disease occurs in an acute, transient form or as a chronic disorder (Table 29-3). The acute form affects both sexes, and adults more frequently than children. It may develop as an infrequent complication of the elevated cold agglutinin titer that commonly follows Mycoplasma infection. As a rule, hemolytic anemia occurs only in patients who manifest unusually high cold agglutinin titers. In these cases the onset of red cell destruction is usually sudden, and the patient develops pallor, jaundice, and weakness a week or two after having recovered from pneumonitis.

Chronic cold agglutinin disease is particularly seen in the elderly of both sexes. A correlation of severity of symptoms with cold weather is also observed. Chronic anemia, for example, is more severe in winter

Table 29-3. Autoimmune Hemolytic Disease Mediated by Cold Autoantibodies: Clinical Syndromes

---

I. Due to cold agglutinins (anti-I, anti-i, etc.)

    A. Transitory elevation of cold agglutinins associated with infections (Mycoplasma infection, infectious mononucleosis, etc.)

        1. Coombs' positive RBC, anemia ± hemoglobinuria

    B. Persistent elevation of cold agglutinins

        1. Cold agglutinins in very high titer and exhibiting high thermal range: chronic hemolytic anemia; acrocyanosis; C-coated RBC; low serum C; no hemoglobinuria; features of lymphoproliferative disease may evolve

        2. Cold agglutinins in lower titer and with lower thermal range ($<31°C$): mild or no hemolytic anemia; normal serum C; episodes of acrocyanosis and hemoglobinuria when chilled

        3. Cases with certain features of (1) and (2)

II. Due to D-L antibody (anti-P)

    Note: All forms have primarily chill-induced acute hemolysis with hemoglobinemia and hemoglobinuria (paroxysmal cold hemoglobinuria)

    A. Transient antibody formation associated with viral infections

    B. Persistent antibody formation causes susceptibility to recurrent attacks on chilling

        1. Idiopathic (no underlying disease recognized)

        2. Late syphilis, particularly congenital (now a very rare cause of paroxysmal cold hemoglobinuria)

Adapted from Leddy, J. P., and Swisher, S. N. (1970): Acquired immune hemolytic disorders. In *Immunological Diseases,* Samter, M. (ed.). Boston, Little, Brown and Company, p. 1097.

months. Raynaud's phenomenon frequently involves the fingers, toes, ears, or nose.

Chronic cold agglutinin disease may be idiopathic, or it may accompany underlying neoplastic disease of the lymphoid or reticuloendothelial system. Some idiopathic cases gradually evolve into a lymphoproliferative disease resembling Waldenström's macroglobulinemia. Indeed, some workers feel that chronic cold agglutinin disease in general should be considered a variant of Waldenström's macroglobulinemia.

Cold agglutinins are distinguished from other red cell antibodies by their capacity to bring about agglutination at low temperature (optimally at 0° to 5° C) while having very little or no capacity to agglutinate normal human red cells at temperatures above 30° C.

The majority of cold agglutinins causing hemolytic anemia have anti-I specificity. The I antigen is related to the ABH blood group system. It is strongly expressed on almost all erythrocytes but is weakly represented in neonatal (cord) red cells. It is genetically absent in the red cells of about 1 in every 4000 to 5000 adults (phenotype i). Conversely, the i antigen is strongly expressed on cord red cells but more weakly on normal adult cells. Typically, cold agglutinins are 19S IgM antibodies. Anti-I cold agglutinins react particularly well with rabbit red cells at higher temperatures (37° C) than with human red cells.

In vivo, even a transient interaction of cold agglutinins with red cells in the cooler superficial blood vessels appears to cause significant C fixation. As the blood returns to the central circulation (37° C), the cold agglutinins are undoubtedly dissociated completely from the red cells, but C components remain irreversibly bound to the cell membrane where they either complete the sequence of C lysis or "decay" to a hemolytically inactive (sublytic) state in which the red cells are destroyed more rapidly than normal by the spleen. Episodes of acute intravascular hemolysis with hemoglobinemia and hemoglobinuria are explained by the potential of many agglutinins to produce outright C lysis under favorable circumstances.

Patients with chronic cold agglutinin disease may survive many years, suffering minimal disability. Most patients tolerate their mild or moderate anemia quite well. In more severe cases, death may ensue, especially from infection probably associated with immune deficiency, from an underlying neoplastic process, and occasionally from severe anemia or its complications. Other patients experience complications of transfusion therapy. The latter may be lethal or highly destructive as, for example, with development of hepatitis or severe hemolytic transfusion reactions. Splenectomy and corticosteroid therapy have both been disappointing. Chlorambucil and cyclophosphamide are reported to have helped some patients, and treatment with these agents deserves consideration in difficult cases.

DRUG-INDUCED IMMUNE HEMOLYTIC DISORDERS

The association of positive direct antiglobulin tests and drug-induced immune hemolytic anemia represents several models of immune injury of red cells mediated by exogenous chemical agents. Four mechanisms of immune phenomena are known to be involved in drug-induced hemolytic anemia: (1) the hapten mechanism, exemplified by penicillin-induced hemolytic anemia in which the drug or a metabolite of the drug become attached to the cell membrane and act as a hapten in a directed immunologic assault on the membrane with its attached hapten; (2) the immune complex (or "innocent bystander") mechanism, exemplified by quinidine-, quinine-, and stibophen-related immune red cell injury in which antibody to drug combines with drug in circulation and adheres to the red blood cell surface to activate the complement system at the membrane; (3) true autoreactive anti-red blood cell antibodies that appear during therapy, for example, with α-methyldopa, mefenamic acid, or the hydantoins; (4) apparently nonimmune binding of plasma proteins, including immunoglobulins and complement components, to red cells as with cephalothin.

Among patients receiving very large doses of penicillin G (10 to 30 million units/day) or somewhat smaller doses in the presence of renal failure, Coombs' positive red blood cells and anemia may be observed. The incidence is low, but this is probably the commonest form of drug-induced immune hemolysis. It has been established that immune injury of red cells depends on (1) firm binding of penicillin to the patient's red cells, (2) subsequent binding of certain (mainly IgG) antipenicillin antibodies, and (3) shortened *in vivo* lifespan of these antibody-coated red blood cells in the patient's circulation. Positive direct antiglobulin reactions appear to be mainly due to coating of the patient's red blood cells with IgG antibodies. The antibodies eluted from his red blood cells or serum are not reactive with normal, untreated red blood cells but are reactive with penicillin-coated red blood cells. In all cases hemolysis has stopped on cessation of penicillin administration. Corticosteroids appear to be ineffective in the face of continuing penicillin therapy.

Several drugs, although chemically unrelated, bring about immune injury of red cells, platelets, or leukocytes by another mechanism—adsorption of drug-antidrug antibody complexes to the cell surface with activation of C at the cell membrane. The drugs best documented to mediate red cell injury by this mechanism are quinidine, quinine, and the antiparasitic drug stibophen (Fuadin). As shown by Shulman, thrombocytopenic purpura related to quinidine, quinine, or apronalide (Sedormid) and, probably, aminopyrine-related granulocytopenia also are mediated in this way. Some patients display combinations of such immune cytopenias, for example, quinidine-induced purpura plus hemolytic anemia. The antidrug antibodies mediating red cell injury by this mechanism have almost always proved to be 19S IgM. The antibodies mediating platelet injury have been 7S IgG. This rule has even been shown to hold in a patient who had both hemolytic anemia with IgM antibodies and thrombocytopenic purpura with IgG antibodies with specificity for the same drug.

Treatment of this form of hemolytic anemia consists of discontinuing the offending drug. The rapidity of recovery depends mainly on the rate of elimination of the drug in question.

The antihypertensive drug α-methyl-3,4-dihydroxy-L-phenylalanine (Aldomet) has been associated with a remarkably high incidence of positive direct antiglobulin reactions, varying from 10 to 20 percent of patients taking the drug for 6 months or more. The incidence is highest in those receiving the larger doses, as high as 36 percent in patients receiving more than 2.25 gm/day.

In virtually all cases the positive direct antiglobulin reaction is of the IgG variety. The IgG antibodies in the patients' sera or eluted from their red blood cells share many characteristics of the warm-reacting (IgG) autoantibodies occurring in idiopathic AIHD. Similar hemolytic anemias have been observed in children treated for convulsive disorders with hydantoin compounds.

A significant number of patients with drug-induced hemolytic anemia develop antinuclear antibodies. Withdrawal of the drug is usually followed by return of the hematocrit toward normal within a few weeks. A few patients have developed frank lupus erythematosus even with renal disease in addition to the autoimmune hemolytic anemia.

This drug-induced immune injury of red blood cells differs radically from the other types of drug-induced immune injury to red blood cells in which the antibodies are clearly directed against the drug and the binding of antibody to the target cell cannot take place in the absence of the drug.

Patients receiving cephalothin (Keflin) have also developed a high incidence of positive direct antiglobulin reactions in which neither antidrug antibodies nor autoantibodies to recognized red cell antigens have been defined. Patients with azotemia or hypoalbuminemia have been especially prone to develop this disease, presumably because in these circumstances high blood levels of unbound cephalothin are present in the circulation. Since cephalothin cross reacts with penicillin, some cases may reflect prior sensitization to penicillin together with fixation of cephalothin to the red cell under appropriate circumstances.

PAROXYSMAL NOCTURNAL HEMOGLOBINURIA

A rare form of hemolytic disease that has a fascinating immunologic mechanism is paroxysmal nocturnal hemoglobinuria (PNH). This disease is widely distributed around the world, occurs in both sexes, and is most commonly expressed during the third or fourth decades of life. It is manifested by persistent or intermittent anemia, hemoglobinemia, and hemoglobinuria that increase during sleep. Urine may be quite clear during the day but is brown or reddish brown on arising. Hemosiderinuria occurs frequently, and PNH may be complicated by neutropenia, thrombosis, and late development of acute myelogenous leukemia. A considerable proportion of patients with PNH have had transient episodes of aregenerative anemia or aregenerative pancytopenia prior to the onset of the PNH. The connection of this strange disease to immunity is that PNH cells are capable of activating the complement system by combining with properdin which functions as one means of access to the third component of complement. Activation of the alternate pathway can lead to lysis or destruction of red blood cells that have abnormal surfaces. The observations that red blood cells in this disease are unusually susceptible to spontaneous lysis by the complement system stimulated continued investigation of the properdin system and led to the modern definition of this component of the alternate pathway of complement.

SICKLE CELL ANEMIA

In sickle cell anemia, another form of chronic hemolytic anemia, it has been shown that the increased susceptibility to infections, especially by pneumococcus organisms, is associated with a profound perturbation of the alternate complement pathway. This abnormality reduces capacity of the serum of patients with sickle cell anemia to opsonize pneumococci and accounts for their predisposition to infection. Perhaps in sickle cell anemia and in other diseases where hemolytic anemia is associated with abnormalities of the alternate pathway of the complement system, we are seeing in bold relief one of the most important functions of the complement system, namely, to eliminate cells with abnormal surfaces.

IDIOPATHIC THROMBOCYTOPENIC PURPURA

Idiopathic thrombocytopenic purpura (ITP) is the term applied to the clinical picture of thrombocytopenia associated with mild to severe bleeding phenomena. The thrombocytopenia has been characterized by abnormal platelet morphology on the peripheral blood smear, decreased life span of the platelets, and hyperplasia of megakaryocytes in the marrow.

The term *acute ITP* applies to thrombocytopenia with hemorrhagic manifestations in children. It is generally transitory, rarely lasting longer than three months. Eighty-five percent of patients are below 8 years of age, and both sexes are affected equally. In the United States the majority of patients with acute thrombocytopenia are encountered from December to June, with a higher incidence in the spring when bacterial and

Table 29-4.   Causes of Immunologic Thrombocytopenic Purpura

Idiopathic (ITP)
Post-transfusion purpura
Neonatal thrombocytopenic purpura
Autoimmune hemolytic anemia (Evans' syndrome)
Systemic lupus erythematosus
Other collagen vascular diseases
Lymphoproliferative disorders
Drug-induced
Viral diseases
Septicemia

From Freedman, S. O. (ed.) (1971): *Clinical Immunology*. New York, Harper & Row, p. 304.

viral infections are most common. Eighty percent of the patients have had an acute febrile illness within three weeks prior to the onset of the purpura.

Most patients with acute ITP have a benign course and recover completely within six weeks. The 7 to 10 percent of patients in whom thrombocytopenia persists longer than six months have chronic ITP. The mechanism responsible for it is apparently an antiplatelet autoantibody (Table 29-4). The incidence of cerebral bleeding, although much emphasized, is less than 5 percent and usually occurs within the first few days following the appearance of purpura. Hence by the time a decision for therapy must be made, the physician may be wise merely to observe the patient. Although adrenal steroids may bring about symptomatic relief, they do not accelerate recovery in acute ITP, and the incidence of chronic ITP has not decreased with their use. If steroids are employed at all, prednisone is the drug of choice and should be used in a dose of 1 mg/kg body weight. After two weeks the dose should be cut in half, and it is best to stop treatment by the fourth week. If the thrombocytopenia persists for longer than three months, a second trial with corticosteroids may be considered. Persistence of thrombocytopenia for more than six months is an indication for splenectomy. Such patients should be carefully evaluated for systemic lupus erythematosus, leukemia, and lymphoma. The latter evaluation may be tricky, and correct diagnosis is sometimes made only at laparotomy.

The thrombocytopenia of adults is generally a chronic disorder that lasts for years unless drug therapy or surgery alters the course. A few patients with ITP may have episodic disease, followed by either a spontaneous remission or a remission induced by corticoid therapy. The disease, however, may reappear years later, and the recurrence is often preceded by infection. In adults the disease occurs more frequently in females than in males. The autoantibody against platelets in this disease is usually of IgG class and thus can be transmitted across the placental barrier to produce transient thrombocytopenic purpura in the neonate.

Adrenocorticosteroids have been used successfully to increase the platelet count, decrease bleeding, and prolong life in chronic ITP. Usually a maximal oral dose of 1 mg/kg of prednisone daily is sufficient. Splenectomy often dramatically relieves symptoms and signs. Splenectomy is of additional value because it permits additional diagnostic opportunity. More complete laboratory procedures have sometimes revealed that the thrombocytopenia reflects SLE and is not an isolated manifestation. The spleen in SLE, unlike the spleen in ITP, regularly has marked follicular hyperplasia, reticulum cell hyperplasia, and plasmacytosis.

Abrupt development of thrombocytopenia in man has been noted following ingestion of certain drugs. Of the drugs in current use, sulfonamides, chlorothiazide derivatives, chlorpropamide, meprobamate, phenylbutazone, and quinidine are particularly implicated; quinidine has been implicated most frequently. These instances are due to drug sensitivity, and almost always the destruction of platelets is of the innocent bystander type of immune assault.

A rare form of purpura occurs following blood transfusions. This disorder is basically similar to drug-induced purpura but involves a platelet antigen (Pl) instead of drug. About one week after transfusion a sudden onset of severe thrombocytopenia has been described in certain patients. This may persist and may be accentuated by platelet transfusions. In this purpura the recipient (Pl negative) is immunized by a platelet antigen (Pl positive) in the transfused blood. The platelet antibody that develops binds to both autologous and homologous platelets. The mechanism for the thrombocytopenia is not completely understood.

When repeated platelet infusions are necessary, as in leukemia or idiopathic pancytopenias, immunization to histocompatibility antigens on the platelets may occur. The rapid destruction of the platelets under these conditions limits usefulness of the platelet therapy. This form of immunologic destruction of platelets can be avoided if HL-A matched donors are used for the infusions.

IMMUNE THROMBOCYTOPENIA AND IMMUNE NEUTROPENIA

Thrombocytopenia and neutropenia have been reported in association with the isoantibodies and autoantibodies (leukolysins, leukotoxins, leukoagglutinins, or thromboagglutinins). Severe neutropenia and infection can be found in newborn infants in association with maternal isoantibodies directed against a baby's leukocytes.

SELECTED REFERENCES
Idiopathic Acquired Hemolytic Disease

Boorman, K. E., Dodd, B. E., and Loutit, J. F. (1946): Lancet 1:812.
Coombs, R. R. A., Mourant, A. E., and Race, R. R. (1945): Brit. J. Exp. Path. 20:255.

Dacie, J. V., and Worlledge, S. M. (1969): In *Progress in Hematology* 6, Brown, E. B., and Moore, C. V. (eds.). New York, Grune & Stratton, p. 82.
Engelfriet, C. P., et al. (1968): Clin. Exp. Immun. 3:605.
Fudenberg, H. H. (1966): Arthritis Rheum. 9:464.
Good, R. A., and Rodey, G. E. (1970): Cell. Immun. 1:147.
Leddy, J. P., et al. (1970): J. Immun. 105:677.
Zuelzer, W. W., et al. (1970): Amer. J. Med. 49:80.

Paroxysmal Cold Hemoglobinuria

Dacie, J. V., Crookston, J. H., and Christenson, W. N. (1957): Brit. J. Haemat. 3:77.
Donath, J., and Landsteiner, K. (1904): Munchen. Med. Wschr. 51:1590.
Hinz, C. F. Jr. (1963): Blood 22:600.

Cold Agglutinin Disease

Iwai, S., and Mei-Sai, N. (1925): Jap. Med. World 5:119.
Schubothe, H. (1966): Seminars Hemat. 3:27.
Tönder, O., and Harboe, M. (1966): Immunology 11:361.
Wiener, A. S., et al. (1956): Ann. Intern. Med. 44:221.

Drug-induced Immune Hemolytic Disorders

Dausset, J., and Contu, L. (1967): Ann. Rev. Med. 18:55.
Shulman, N. R. (1964): Ann. Intern. Med. 60:506.

Paroxysmal Nocturnal Hemoglobinuria

Carmel, R., et al. (1970): New Eng. J. Med. 283:1329.
Evans, D. I. (1969): Brit. Med. J. 4:300.
Götze, O., et al. (1972): New Eng. J. Med. 286:180.
Rosse, W. F. (1971): Blood 37:556.
Sirchia, G., et al. (1970): Blood 36:334.

Idiopathic Thrombocytopenic Purpura

Dameshek, W., et al. (1963): New Eng. J. Med. 269:647.
Erslev, A. J., and Wintrobe, M. M. (1962): JAMA 181:114.
Hirsch, E. O., and Dameshek, W. (1951): Arch. Intern. Med. (Chicago) 88:701.
Lusher, J. M., and Zuelzer, W. W. (1966): J. Pediat. 68:971.
Schulman, I. (1964): Pediatrics 33:979.
Shulman, N. R., et al. (1961): J. Clin. Invest. 40:1597.
Shulman, N. R., Marder, V. J., and Weinrach, R. S. (1965): Ann. N. Y. Acad. Sci. 124:499.
Weintraub, R. M., Pechet, L., and Alexander, B. (1962): JAMA 180:528.
Wilde, R. C., Ellis, L. D., and Cooper, W. M. (1967): Arch. Surg. (Chicago) 95:344.

Immune Thrombocytopenia and Immune Neutropenia

Boxer, L. A., Yokoyama, M., and Lalezari, P. (1972): J. Pediat. 80:783.
Colombani, J. (1966): Seminars Hemat. 3:74.
Eisner, E. V., and Kasper, K. (1972): Amer. J. Med. 53:790.
Lalezari, P. (1966): Seminars Hemat. 3:87.
Shulman, N. R., Marder, V. J., and Hiller, M. C. (1964): Progr. Hemat. 4:222.
Shulman, N. R., Marder, V. J., and Weinrach, R. S. (1965): Ann. N. Y. Acad. Sci. 124:499.

30

Immunologic Aspects
of Endocrine Disorders

HASHIMOTO'S DISEASE—CHRONIC LYMPHADENOID GOITER

Hashimoto's disease, which occurs more frequently in the female than in the male, is associated with an enlargement of the thyroid gland that occasionally may be so great that it obstructs the airway. The gland feels rubbery on palpation; histologically the typical glandular structure is replaced or extensively invaded by lymphoid tissue. Depending on the amount of normal thyroid tissue replaced, the patient may show symptoms of hypothyroidism or of myxedema. The disease may ultimately lead to a secondary disorder formerly referred to as primary hypothyroidism without goiter.

The lymphoid infiltration within the gland consists mainly of small lymphocytes, histiocytes, and plasma cells, but typical germinal centers are found frequently in more or less well-organized lymph follicles, and plasma cells can be observed among the lymphocytes, usually in maximal numbers near the germinal centers. The presence of lymph follicles and germinal centers in the thymus of such patients indicates that the mechanism behind the disease is surely not limited to the thyroid itself.

Humoral antibodies in the serum of patients with Hashimoto's disease have been extensively studied, especially by Roitt, Jones, and Doniach in England and by Rose and Witebsky in the United States of America. These antibodies are directed against the cellular elements of the thyroid gland, as well as against thyroglobulin. Anticytoplasmic antibodies are detected by the complement fixation technique, and their titer seems better correlated to the course and severity of the disease of the gland than that of antibodies directed against thyroglobulin. A complement fixation titer of 1:32 is considered compatible with a diagnosis of Hashimoto's disease. Thyroglobulin antibodies are, however, quite ubiquitous; a titer of 1:2500 or greater is usually necessary before a diagnosis can be made. When the titer of antithyroglobulin is this high, these antibodies can be detected by the relatively crude technique of precipitation of thyroglobulin on an agar plate. In spite of its regular association with antibodies against a variety of constituents of the thyroid, Hashimoto's disease should not be diagnosed without a needle biopsy of the thyroid gland and histologic confirmation.

The pathogenetic basis of chronic "auto-allergic" thyroiditis has been studied extensively in experimental animals. A disease similar to that in the human can be produced in experimental animals by the injection of homologous or heterologous thyroid tissue in an adjuvant mixture. The disease thus produced consists of a marked lymphocytic infiltration of the gland with small lymphocytes and histiocytes. However, the disease differs from the human disease histologically in that plasma cells are at times relatively scarce and true germinal centers are rarely found in the gland.

The disease in experimental animals has been thought by many to be completely cell-mediated, as it is associated with the development of a state of delayed hypersensitivity to the intradermal injection of an extract of thyroid tissue and cannot be transferred passively with serum containing high titers of autoantibodies to the glandular tissue. Similar skin reactivity can be found in patients with Hashimoto's disease. However, passive transfer of the disease with lymphocytes has not been consistently positive, although no difficulty exists in transferring skin reactivity from a sensitized to a normal animal. Currently it is considered that the disease is caused by a combination of humoral and cell-mediated immune mechanisms. The role of humoral mechanism in the causation of the disease in the human is evidenced by the frequency of plasma cells in the gland and germinal centers in both the target organ and in the closely adjacent thymus.

How the immune mechanisms are stimulated to react against thyroid tissue is not known, but this point has been studied extensively by Weigle. He has shown that a tolerant state to thyroglobulin is maintained by continuous presence of thyroglobulin in the circulation. This tolerant state can readily be abrogated, however, by injection of either chemically altered thyroglobulin or thyroglobulin from disparate but closely related species. The possibility exists that antigens in the thyroid are made more immunogenic as the result of the action of viruses or chemical agents.

There is no doubt that genetic factors can cause a predisposition to chronic thyroiditis. A markedly high incidence of thyroid disease, of both Hashimoto's type and thyrotoxicosis, is observed in members of families of patients with Hashimoto's disease. Moreover, Hashimoto's disease has been described in both members of two pairs of uniovular twins. Thyroid disease has also been described in a number of patients with congenital diseases associated with abnormalities of the X chromosome. Two patients who had Turner's syndrome, an XO chromosome pattern with an enlarged or drumstick X chromosome, were also found to have Hashimoto's disease, and two patients with Klinefelter's syndrome, a disease also associated with an abnormal XXY chromosome pattern, were discovered to have thyroid malfunction and disease related to the Hashimoto type of pathology.

Hashimoto's disease has been found to be associated with a number of other diseases. These include chronic active hepatitis, rheumatoid arthritis, Sjögren's disease, systemic lupus erythematosus, and Addison's disease. One of the more striking associations is between immunologic disease of the stomach and the thyroid. Pernicious anemia, for example, is found in about 6 percent of patients with Hashimoto's type of thyroid disease. About a third of patients with immunologic disease of the thyroid have in their sera antibodies to gastric parietal cells, and about half have antibodies to gastric intrinsic factor.

Low levels of thyroid autoantibodies, usually directed against thyroglobulin rather than against the cytoplasmic components of the thyroid, have been found in approximately 5 percent of normal subjects. In the absence of overt thyroid disease, higher levels of such autoantibodies have been found in such immunologic diseases as systemic lupus erythematosus and chronic hepatitis and in family members when the propositus presents with a common variable form of primary immunodeficiency. Raised levels of thyroid autoantibodies have also been found in leprosy, especially in the lepromatous form, and in other long-standing chronic infections. This would indicate that patients with chronic diseases, where there are continuous stimulation of the immunologic mechanisms and possibly immunologic perturbation, develop the property to react with higher levels of antibodies to antigens widely available than do normal people. This is probably a nonspecific event similar to that produced in experimental animals with Freund's adjuvant. Because antithyroid antibodies have been observed in patients with isolated absence of IgA, immunodeficiency itself may be associated with frequent production of antithyroid antibody.

Antibodies to cytoplasmic components of the thyroid may be as significant in apparently normal people as in patients with Hashimoto's disease. Since postmortem studies on such patients have revealed focal thyroiditis not detected during life, the significance of these antibodies in producing or indicating disease may be quantitative.

Hashimoto's disease may be treated by a ten-day course of 60 mg/day prednisone followed by thyrotoxine or desiccated thyroid usually given in a dose of 90 to 100 mg or levothyroxine, 0.2 mg daily. This treatment produces a dramatic reduction in the size of the thyroid gland. Treatment with thyrotoxine alone is used by some, but the response will be slower than when it is combined with adrenal steroids.

THYROTOXICOSIS AND LATS

The immunologic basis of thyrotoxicosis (Graves' disease) has only recently been clarified. It has been known for some time that about 40 percent of patients with thyrotoxicosis have antibodies to thyroglobulin in their serum; thus it was reasonable to suspect that some immunologic process might be participating in the pathogenesis of this disease. Further, it has long been recognized that the number of lymphocytes in the blood and the bone marrow may be very high in this disease. The lymph node is frequently enlarged, and splenomegaly is found in some 10 percent of cases. Thymic hyperplasia is said to be present in one half of the victims studied at autopsy.

It is here important to reflect on the influence of thyroid function on immunologic responses. Excessive stimulation of the thyroid not only increases antibody production but also increases the rate of degradation of antibody, and thus following primary stimulation antibody responses are not unusual. Similarly in the opposite perspective, hypothyroidism decreases the rate of antibody synthesis and also the rate of antibody degradation. Thus the levels of antibody after stimulation have not been unusual. No one has yet done serious studies of the influence of thyroid hormone on the cellular immunities or the distribution of B and T lymphocytes in the circulation. It has been shown, however, that thyroid hormone is essential for normal development of the immunologic system.

Further, it has long been known that patients with Graves' disease possess in their serum a substance which stimulates thyroid function in experimental animals. The substance responsible was defined by Adams and Purves. A bioassay known as the McKenzie test is still used for the detection and quantitation of this substance. Stimulation of thyroid function has been assayed by the release of radioactive iodine from the thyroid glands of mice whose thyroids had been labeled previously with radioactive iodine and in whom pituitary thyroid-stimulating hormone (TSH) had been suppressed by pretreatment with thyroxin. This stimulator took longer to act than did TSH and so was called *long-acting thyroid stimulator* (LATS). Recently it has been shown that LATS is an immunoglobulin of the IgG class. LATS can be found in the serum of about 45 percent of patients with thyrotoxicosis, and a strong correlation between the presence of LATS and antithyroglobulin antibodies has been found. The concentration of LATS is especially high in the sera of patients with exophthalmos.

The role of TSH in the pathogenesis of thyrotoxicosis has been reexamined in the light of more recent findings. In most patients with thyrotoxicosis, instead of being increased, the level of TSH in the blood is usually less than that in normal individuals and increases in thyrotoxic patients only following effective treatment. The secretion of TSH by the pituitary is inhibited by a normal feedback mechanism due to the excessive amounts of thyroxin in the blood. Thus it is accepted now that thyrotoxicosis is not due to an excessive stimulation of the thyroid by pituitary TSH. Moreover, an inverse ratio between LATS and TSH has been found.

The role of LATS in causing thyrotoxicosis has been emphasized by the finding of thyrotoxicosis in babies born of mothers with high levels of circulating LATS. These neonates have goiters, prominent eyes, and classic signs of thyrotoxicosis which progressively disappear as LATS is decomposed. This again is a nice experiment of Nature that helps clarify the pathogenesis of an important disease of man. The LATS antibody is thyroid specific and probably combines with an antigen on the thyroid membranes. Antigen-antibody interaction on the surface of the cell seems to stimulate thyroid cells to excessive function. Evidence of acceleration of cell metabolism can be obtained from electron microscopic examination, which shows morphologic concomitants of increased protein synthesis and increase in the size of the Golgi apparatus associated with the increased secretion of protein. In a wide range of experimental systems the metabolic activity of cells has increased as a result of antigen-antibody interaction at the cell surface. Another possible explanation for the action of LATS is that it could remove an inhibitor of enzyme activity in thyroid cells and in this way increase their metabolic activity.

LATS antibody is not demonstrable by present techniques in the sera of all patients with thyrotoxicosis, but the positive responses increase if IgG concentrates from serum are used in the assay. The insensitivity of the bioassay almost certainly is responsible for the relatively low frequency (45 percent) of LATS positivity in thyrotoxicosis patients. The absence of LATS in serum of some patients, however, suggests that other causes for stimulation of thyroid cells may be found. Studies with the drug carbimazole, for example, may present one alternative. Treatment with carbimazole has been found to suppress hyperthyroidism in a proportion of patients with this disease. Those that responded to carbimazole treatment were the ones who lacked LATS in their sera. Patients who did not respond to carbimazole had LATS antibody and also antithyroglobulin in their sera and were the ones who had a strong family history of thyroid disease.

The presence of antithyroid antibodies in the serum of patients with thyrotoxicosis has been assessed in relation to the form of therapy that patients with thyrotoxicosis have been receiving. A certain proportion of patients with thyrotoxicosis become hypothyroid after treatment with radioactive iodine or after partial thyroidectomy. Examination of thyroids of patients who developed hypothyroidism after surgery revealed marked lymphocytic infiltration of the thyroid, germinal centers in some, and extensive plasma cell infiltration. Moreover, a higher incidence of cytoplasmic complement fixing antibody in the serum of these patients indicates a coexisting Hashimoto's disease. As a result of this finding many surgeons have learned to remove less of the thyroid gland if they find macroscopic evidence of lymphoid infiltration of the thyroid gland in patients with thyrotoxicosis. Although it has been suggested that the development of hypothyroidism following treatment with radioactive iodine is the result of an immunologic reaction, no correlation between the level of antithyroglobulin antibodies and antithyroid cytoplasmic antibodies has been found with the development of the hypothyroid state after treatment with radioactive iodine. Thus at present the clinical evidence does not appear to support the concept that immunologic reaction is responsible for this form of hypothyroidism. Further, the level of antithyroid antibody in patients with Graves' disease has not been found to be helpful in predicting response to antithyroid medications.

A higher incidence of LATS antibody has been found in the serum of patients with thyrotoxicosis with exophthalmos than in the serum of those without. Although exophthalmos can occur in the absence of demonstrable circulating LATS, it has been suggested that this antibody may facilitate the development of exophthalmos. The association of LATS with pretibial edema in thyrotoxicosis is even stronger. The finding of an association between exophthalmos and LATS has led to the use of adrenal steroid therapy and immunosuppressive therapy to combat this malady. With such treatment exophthalmos has often improved, and LATS has disappeared from the serum. Antimetabolites, e.g., azathioprine and methotrexate, have also been recommended for treatment of this sometimes most threatening manifestation.

In Graves' disease the thyroid microscopically shows hypertrophy and hyperplasia. Epithelial cells are large and columnar with irregular apical borders lining a follicular lumen that contains less than the normal amount of colloid. The thyroid follicles often show papillary infoldings. More often than not prominent lymphocytic infiltration and germinal center formation are seen. The confusion with Hashimoto's disease indeed may be considerable. Sometimes both the clinical and the histopathologic observations fail to distinguish between the two diseases, and both may actually be present at once. Some have emphasized the value in pathologic diagnosis of Askanazy cells that are present in Hashimoto's disease and absent in Graves' disease. These cells, which have pleomorphic nuclei and are acidophilic, are found in the lymphoid follicles. To us they are typical of the early elements of the germinal center.

ADDISON'S DISEASE

The immunologic nature of one form of Addison's disease has been suggested by the finding of lymphocytic infiltration of the adrenal gland and antibody in the circulation directed mainly against the cells of the zona glomerulosa. Some cases of adrenal atrophy have been associated with insufficiency of the anterior pituitary gland, in which case this gland has also been infiltrated with lymphoid tissue containing germinal centers. Antibodies have been detected against the steroid-producing tissues such as placental trophoblast cells, ovarian corpus luteum cells, and the interstitial cells of the testis. It is interesting that the antigen which appears to induce the highest antibody responses in these patients has the same cytoplasmic localization as the antigen in the thyroid cells to which antibodies appear in the circulation of patients with Hashimoto's disease.

Similar lesions of the adrenal glands can be produced in experimental animals by injection of homologous or autologous adrenal tissue in an adjuvant mixture. The disease thus produced is associated with the presence of antibodies against adrenal tissue in the sera of affected animals. As in the human disease antibodies are directed against components of the cells of the cortex and not against those of the medulla. Immunoglobulins have been found to be fixed in the diseased cortex. However, the experimental disease cannot readily be transferred passively with either cells or serum alone. This finding suggests that as with a number of experimental organ specific immunologic diseases, the lesions result from an interaction of both humoral and cell-mediated immunologic pathogenetic mechanisms.

It has been suggested that immunologic injury in Addison's disease is not limited to the adrenal gland but is part of a more widespread "polyendocrinopathy." This is because of the high incidence of thyroid disease, hypoparathyroidism, diabetes mellitus, and atrophic gastritis with this disease. These other conditions are, of course, not associated with the Addison's disease which is caused by tuberculosis of the adrenals nor are they present in the Addison's disease attributable to destruction of the adrenal by malignant infiltration or surgical extirpation. It is of interest that patients with immunologically based Addison's disease have a high incidence of antibodies to gastric intrinsic factor and gastric parietal cells in their serum but a low incidence of pernicious anemia. This disease complex may also include steatorrhea.

Although immunologically Addison's disease has a high degree of association with immunologic disease of the thyroid gland, the thyroid gland disease itself has a low incidence of association with Addison's disease. Thus although a patient with thyroiditis has a good chance of having atrophic gastritis, the chance of his having adrenal disease is low. However, if he has adrenal disease, the chance of his having thyroid disease is high. The association of thyroid disease and gastric disease appears to be one immunologic disease entity, and the polyendocrinopathy associated with adrenal disease, which may include thyroid disease, would appear to be a different independent and rarer disease entity.

Frequently the polyendocrinopathy of apparent immunologic origin is associated with chronic mucocutaneous candidiasis. This persistent infection in turn seems to be consequent to a perturbed immunologic defense function that may have as its common denominator failure of the normal biologic amplification of cellular immunity. If this, upon more definitive study, is really the case, it represents another intimate association of autoimmune disease and immunodeficiency.

Thyroid disease, pernicious anemia, and diabetes mellitus of the insulin dependent type also seem to be frequently associated with idiopathic Addison's disease. The basis for this strange constellation needs further analysis. It appears that if an individual is making autoantibodies to adrenal cortex, he stands a high chance of making antibodies to thyroid, gastric parietal cells, intrinsic factor, parathyroid, and other steroid-producing cells.

Autoantibodies against adrenal cortex, being IgG, can pass the placental barrier and enter the fetal circulation, yet normal babies have been born of mothers who have idiopathic Addison's disease with high titers of these antibodies detectable in the mother's serum and in serum obtained from umbilical cord blood. No evidence of any impaired function of the babies' adrenal glands has been observed. Thus if immunologic mechanisms are of importance in the etiology of idiopathic Addison's disease and are not secondary phenomena to injury based on other mechanisms, they operate through cellular immunity, e.g., delayed allergy or a synergism between delayed hypersensitivity and circulating antibody. This probably also holds true for the related conditions of idiopathic hypoparathyroidism and the autoimmune forms of premature gonadal failure.

DIABETES MELLITUS

Soon after the discovery of insulin and the initiation of its routine administration to diabetic subjects, certain immune responses to this hormone became evident. Three separate manifestations of immune responses to this antigen have been recognized to date: (1) insulin allergy, (2) insulin resistance, and (3) histopathologic changes, possibly of an autoimmune nature, that may be related to the etiology and pathogenesis of some cases of diabetes mellitus.

Employing antisera directed against insulin of various species, Berson and Yalow demonstrated that although immunologic specificity exists among these insulins, considerable cross reactivity is regularly demonstrable between them. Likewise, proinsulin cross reacts with insulin from the same species.

Allergic manifestations to insulin may take one of many forms. By far the most frequent response is a local dermal reaction characterized by burning and pruritus that appear soon after injection and by a typical wheal with erythema that may be followed by induration after a few hours. The reported incidence of these dermal reactions varies from 10 to 55 percent in various series. The serum of some patients with dermal reactions to insulin contains IgE antibodies capable of sensitizing normal skin to this hormone. Skin-sensitizing antibodies are known to persist for as long as three years after the cessation of insulin therapy. In one series skin reactions were elicited in 18 percent of diabetic patients who had not received insulin for more than one year. Other types of allergic responses to insulin include urticaria, angioneurotic edema, and rarely anaphylactic shock.

The finding of antibodies to insulin in subjects given this hormone raised the important question of whether the etiology and pathogenesis of some cases of diabetes mellitus might be attributable to an autoimmune process. For diabetes mellitus to be considered to reflect autoimmune pathogenesis, it must be shown that subjects with this disease manifest an immune response to homologous and/or autologous insulin. Further, evidence should indicate that at least some of the histopathologic lesions in diabetes mellitus result from an immunologic mechanism.

It is conceivable that the insulin molecule in subjects with diabetes mellitus is altered to change not only its biologic activity but also its antigenicity and in the latter case to obscure the development of antibodies as measured by the usual techniques using normal insulin as antigen. In some juvenile diabetics who die within six months of the onset of their disease, a lymphocytic infiltration of the pancreatic islets or "insulitis" has been found. Experimental evidence is now abundant to indicate that histopathologic lesions in the islets can result from either active or passive immunization of several species of animals with insulin.

Elucidation of the molecular structure of insulin has led to a better definition of the immunologic characteristics of the hormone to a description of species specificity attributable to variability in the sequence of minor amino acids. After five to six weeks of insulin therapy, the production of circulating antibodies to insulin is almost universal. Some circulating antibodies bind insulin avidly and in some cases lead to the development of insulin resistance requiring enormous daily doses of insulin. Although there are histopathologic data to suggest that diabetes mellitus could be an autoimmune disease in certain individuals, there is no compelling evidence at the moment that an immune response can be implicated in either the etiology or the pathogenesis of most cases of this disease. If, however, some cases of resistance to insulin or diabetes are attributable to autoimmunity, antigenic analysis and manipulation that have been used with the basic protein of myelin hold great promise. It may even be possible to reinitiate a tolerant state as a therapeutic or prophylactic measure.

PITUITARY DWARFISM

Pituitary disease, like other endocrinopathies, may be based on apparent autoimmune mechanisms. Unfortunately, to date definitive studies of these relationships are lacking and all studies are meager.

In mice, study of several genetically determined dwarfisms has revealed a dramatic association of growth failure and immunologic deficiency.

These relationships were first described by Baroni, who found that Snell-Bagg dwarf mice are regularly immunodeficient. This abnormality has also been studied by Pierpaoli and his associates and by Duquesnoy and Good. Although some details are in conflict, there can be no question that pituitary dwarfism in mice is associated with failure of normal development of both thymus dependent and thymus independent immunologic functions. The work of Pierpaoli et al. suggests that therapy with somatotropin and thyrotropin will replace the missing pituitary function in development of the thymus dependent lymphoid system. Duquesnoy and Good, however, could not reconstitute the system with purified somatotropin but could do so with less well-defined preparations and have concluded that a thymotropic hormone distinct from somatotropin is involved in normal development of the lymphoid system. From studies of Ames dwarf mice has come evidence that the active factor may be secreted in the milk.

That patients with primordial dwarfism associated with deficiency of somatotrophic hormone do not experience increased susceptibility to infection argues that either man and mouse differ in the vital influence of growth hormone on the lymphoid system or the thymotropic and lymphotrophic substance essential for differentiation of both immunity systems is not lacking in such dwarfs. Definitive studies of immunologic development in patients with various forms of pituitary dwarfism seem much in order.

IMMUNOREPRODUCTION

Selective damage of the germinal epithelium of adult guinea pigs was obtained after autosensitization or allogeneic sensitization with a single dose of testicular homogenate plus complete Freund's adjuvant. The allergic response developed between two and eight weeks later and was characterized by (1) congestion and serous edema in most of the intertubular spaces of the gonad and foci of perivascular cellular infiltration, including mostly plasmocytes and lymphocytes; (2) vacuolization and sloughing of the germinal cells, beginning with spermatids, finally involving spermatocytes and spermatogonial cells, with Sertoli's cells showing only striking vacuolization, but with their nuclei remaining intact; (3) absence of damage to Leydig's cells or other connective tissue cells, such as fibroblasts and scattered mast cells; (4) appearance of circulating antispermatic and cell-bound antibodies concurrent with the testicular lesion; and (5) spermia due to germinal cell destruction which rendered the animal sterile for months.

Experimental allergic orchitis is a complicated disease. That cell-mediated immunity may be involved is indicated by these facts: (1) The use of complete adjuvant is essential to the development. (2) Certain of these testicular lesions are correlated with delayed skin reaction rather than circulating antibodies. (3) Histology of the testis shows not only typical aspermatogenesis but also mononuclear cell infiltration. (4) Mononuclear cells from lymph nodes of sensitized animals can passively induce delayed hypersensitivity in the skin and some of the testicular lesions when transferred to normal recipients. Recent evidence indicates that both humoral antibody and cell-mediated immunity participate in its pathogenesis.

The possible role of the human testis in the immunologic response to autosensitization or allosensitization was substantiated during attempts to induce allergic orchitis in human volunteers. Biopsies of the testis showed numerous foci of tubular lesions with sloughing and cytolysis of germinal cells. The possibility that some cases of male sterility of unknown etiology have an immunologic pathogenesis was raised when sperm agglutinins were found in blood and semen of some sterile patients. Immunofluorescent studies using the patient's own serum show antibodies that attach to the heads of spermatozoa and to the perinuclear region of spermatids. Specific fluoresence seems to be located in the head and occasionally in the midportion or the tail. During immunologic assault the germinal cell may break down in the testis or the sperm may stagnate in the efferent duct. Thus the simultaneous presence of an inflammatory process and the abnormal immune responses to sperm antigens may be necessary to initiate an autoimmune response to sperm. Passive immunization of female mice and guinea pigs with antispermatozoal antisera may impair or abolish fertility.

For many years attempts have been made to produce antispermatic antibodies in normal women and to evaluate the influence of such antibodies on fertility without producing organic changes in the genital tract. The results suggest that circulating antibodies against sperm can impair fertility. Analysis of the data from various authors supports the contention that a small but statistically significant antifertility effect may even be attributable to ABO incompatibility between the couple, since A and B antigens are expressed on sperm. In experimental animals repeated breeding may be associated with either immunity or tolerance of a histoincompatible partner's skin. The tolerance is particularly likely to be observed if the histocompatibility barrier is not too great. Evidence has been presented that prostitutes frequently have immunity to sperm which makes them less susceptible than normal women to impregnation. Further evidence has been presented that immunization against sperm can yield antibodies against HL-A antigens. Such antibodies have a remarkable tendency to be monospecific. It is of interest that individual spermatozoa express only one histocompatibility HL-A haplotype as would be expected.

It thus appears that immunologic factors may participate in abnormalities of male and female reproduction. The immunologic basis of male sterility can be related to alteration of spermatogenesis or impairment of seminal plasma formation, or both. Maturation of spermatozoa appears to account for differences in their antigenic potency. Antibodies against testis can be shown not to affect adnexal glands but to immobilize epididymal spermatozoa. By contrast antibodies to seminal plasma react only with adnexal glands and seminal spermatozoa but not with the cells of the testes proper. In addition, some intrinsic antigens, probably accumulated in the acrosome, are common for testicular, epididymal, and seminal spermatozoa.

By studies of the potential immunologic relations in the reproductive machinery, it should be possible both to facilitate fertility when this is desired and to produce a variety of effective contraceptive techniques. One approach would be a contraceptive based on locally administered and slowly released antibodies directed against sperm.

RADIOIMMUNOASSAY AND ENDOCRINE PHYSIOLOGY AND PATHOLOGY

The radioimmunoassay is, in our opinion, one of the most important contributions made by immunobiology to the analysis of endocrine disorders. The technique, which has revolutionized endocrinology, was discovered accidentally by Berson and Yalow who were trying to determine the effects of an enzyme, insulinase, on the degradation of insulin in patients who had been given insulin. They observed that intravenous injections of radioactively labeled insulin disappeared more slowly from the blood of insulin-treated patients with diabetes than of untreated patients. The insulin couples with antibodies in the blood that prevent it from escaping from the circulation. This observation helped ultimately to explain insulin resistance because patients with insulin resistance had high titers, whereas most treated patients had only low titers.

During the course of their investigation Berson and Yalow discovered that labeled and unlabeled insulin were competing for the antibody combining sites and that this competition could serve as a basis for an insulin assay that is more suitable than chemical methods for detecting and measuring individual peptide hormones in plasma. Immunochemical reagents produced biosynthetically work very well. In the classic test the test antigen, insulin, is labeled with a radioisotope. To a solution containing this labeled peptide are added first highly avid antibody and later unlabeled antigen (insulin) solutions of known standards and of unknown test samples. After equilibrium has been reached, the amount of labeled insulin in the antigen-antibody complex is measured.

Satisfactory highly sensitive and highly specific assays have since been developed for assaying almost all of the known peptide hormones, as well as many other hormones, including some of the steroid hormones that can act as haptens. The high degree of specificity and sensitivity give radioimmunoassay its great value in detecting many of the endogenous hormones like insulin, glucagon, growth hormone, parathyroid hormone, ACTH, follicle-stimulating hormone, and chorionic gonadotropin. This relatively simple immunologic method has generated much fundamental new information in endocrinology. It has brought progress toward understanding the control of insulin secretion in health and disease. It has helped establish that endocrine-secreting tumors like the islet cell tumors of the pancreas may be autonomous of the normal physiologic controls. It has helped immeasurably in improving the hormone analysis and control of certain breast tumors by endocrinologic means. It has contributed in a major way to the understanding of the role of growth hormone in normal physiologic processes, as well as in gigantism and certain forms of dwarfism. Immunologic assay for hormones has just begun to pay major dividends in understanding the function and control of function of the parathyroids, adrenals, thyroid, and even the placentas. In addition, the patterns of polypeptide hormone secretion and degradation have become amenable to isolation and analysis. With this synergistic approach to understanding the influences of and handling such molecules, the future of macromolecular engineering for the benefit of man indeed looks bright.

SELECTED REFERENCES

Hashimoto's Disease—Chronic Lymphadenoid Goiter

Ardeman, S., et al. (1966): Quart. J. Med. 35:421.
Hashimoto, H. (1912): Arch. Klin. Chir. 97:219.
Loeb, P. B., Drash, A. L., and Kenny, F. M. (1973): J. Pediat. 82:17.
Masi, A. T., Hartmann, W. H., and Shulman, L. E. (1965): J. Chron. Dis. 18:1.
Roitt, I. M., Jones, H. E. H., and Doniach, D. (1962): In *Mechanisms of Cell and Tissue Damage Produced by Immune Reactions*, Grabar, P., and Miescher, P. A. (eds.). Basel, Schwabe, p. 154.
Rose, N. R., and Witebsky, E. (1968): In *Textbook of Immunopathology*, Miescher, P. A., and Müller-Eberhardt, H. J. (eds.) New York, Grune & Stratton, 1:150.
Shulman, S. (1971): Advances Immun. 14:85.
Weigle, W. O. (1965): J. Exp. Med. 122:1049.

Thyrotoxicosis and LATS

Adams, D. D., and Purves, H. D. (1956): Proc. Univ. Otago Med. Sch. 34:11.
Anderson, J. W., et al. (1967): J. Clin. Endocr. 27:937.
Burke, C. (1968): Amer. J. Med. 45:435.
Field, E. J., et al. (1970): Lancet 1:1144.
Hershman, J. M., et al. (1966): J. Clin. Endocr. 26:803.
Kaneko, T., Zor, U., and Field, J. B. (1970): Metabolism 19:430.
Kendall-Taylor, P., and Munro, D. S. (1971): Biochem. Biophys. Acta 231:314.
Lipman, L. M., et al. (1967): Amer. J. Med. 43:486.
McKenzie, J. M. (1968): Physiol. Rev. 48:252.
Papapetrou, P. D., et al. (1968): Lancet 2:1045.
Werner, S. C., et al. (1972): New Eng. J. Med. 287:421.

Addison's Disease

Blizzard, R. M., Chee, D., and Davis, W. (1967): Clin. Exp. Immun. 2:19.
Colover, J., and Glynn, L. E. (1958): Immunology 1:172.

Nerup, J., Andersen, V., and Bendixen, G. (1969): Clin. Exp. Immun. 4:355.
Nerup, J., and Bendixen, G. (1969): Clin. Exp. Immun. 5:341.

Diabetes Mellitus

Arquilla, E. R., et ·l. (1967): Vox Sang. 13:32.
Berson, S. A., and Yalow, R. S. (1959): J. Clin. Invest. 38:2017.
Berson, S. A., and Yalow, R. S. (1963): Science 139:844.
Dixon, K., Exon, P. D., and Hughes, H. R. (1972): Lancet 1:343.
Faulk, W. P., Tomsovic, E. J., and Fudenberg, H. H. (1970): Amer. J. Med. 49:133.
Irvine, W. J., et al. (1970): Lancet 2:163.
LeCompte, P. (1958): Arch. Path. (Chicago) 66:450.
Paley, R. G., and Tunbridge, R. E. (1952): Diabetes 1:22.
Tuft, L. (1928): Amer. J. Med. Sci. 176:707.
Whittingham, S., et al. (1971): Lancet 1:763.
Yasuna, E. (1940-41): J. Allerg. 12:295.

Pituitary Dwarfism

Baroni, C. (1967): Experientia 23:282.
Baroni, C., Fabris, N., and Bertoli, G. (1967): Experientia 23:1059.
Duquesnoy, R. J. (1972): J. Immun. 108:1578.
Duquesnoy, R. J., and Good, R. A. (1970): J. Immun. 104:1553.
Fabris, N., Pierpaoli, W., and Sorkin, E. (1971): Clin. Exp. Immun. 9:227.
Pierpaoli, W., Fabris, N., and Sorkin, E. (1970): In *Developmental Hormones and Immunological Maturation,* Wolstenholme, G. E. W., and Knight, J. (eds.). Ciba Foundation Study Group No. 36, London, Churchill.

Immunoreproduction

Beer, A. E., and Billingham, R. E. (1971): Advances Immun. 14:1.
Boughton, B., and Schild, H. O. (1962): Immunology, 5:522.
Freund, J., Lipton, M. M., and Thompson, G. E. (1953): J. Exp. Med. 97:711.
Katsh, S., and Katsh, G. (1965): Pacific Med. Surg. 73:28.
Henle W., et al. (1940): J. Immun. 38:97.
Laurence, K. A., Carpuk, O., and Peribachs, M. (1965): Int. J. Fertil. 10:13.
Mancini, R. E., et al. (1965): J. Clin. Endocr. 25:859.
Rümke, P. (1958): Proc. Roy. Soc. Med. 61:275.
Tyler, A., Tyler, E. T., and Denny, P. C. (1967): Fertil. Steril. 18:153.

Radioimmunoassay and Endocrine Physiology and Pathology

Berson, S. A., et al. (1956): J. Clin. Invest. 35:170.
Berson, S. A. and Yalow, B. S. (1959): J. Clin. Invest. 38:1996.
Hunter, W. D. (1967): In *Handbook of Experimental Immunology,* Weir, D. M. (ed.). Philadelphia, F. A. Davis, p. 608.

31
Immunopathology of Renal Diseases

ACUTE POSTSTREPTOCOCCAL GLOMERULONEPHRITIS

Glomerulonephritis occurs typically one to two weeks following onset of pharyngitis. Glomerulonephritis has a variable attack rate and appears to result from infection by a limited number of the 50 or so M types of streptococcal nephritogenic strains. The major nephritogenic M types remain 12, 4, 25, and 49, but not all strains of these types are nephritogenic.

Since the clinical course of acute poststreptococcal glomerulonephritis is predictable, at least on a statistical basis, it is important for physicians to search diligently for historical, bacteriologic, and serologic evidence in support of recent streptococcal infection when apparent acute hemorrhagic glomerulonephritis occurs in a community. Antibody titers to the extracellular antigens, streptolysin O (ASO), hyaluronidase, and streptokinase, or combinations of these antibodies, are elevated in 85 to 95 percent of patients with acute poststreptococcal glomerulonephritis. Additional evidence of streptococcal infection may be sought by evaluation of antibody titers to nicotinamide adenine dinucleotidase and deoxyribonuclease B.

Serum complement levels are almost uniformly decreased in acute poststreptococcal glomerulonephritis, and assay of either total hemolytic titers or specific components of complement has become an important clinical diagnostic method in this disease. Early in the course of the disease some patients will show low levels of all the complement components. In most instances, however, the complement profile reveals sparing of C1, C2, and C4 components coupled with severe depression of C3 and terminal components. This type of profile of complement components in the blood is like the profile that can be produced *in vitro* by endotoxin or cobra venom factor which spares the earlier components but activates the complement system by the alternate pathway. Unfortunately a number of other renal syndromes are also regularly associated with depressed serum complement levels (including some differential problems such as the acute exacerbation of persistent hypocomplementemic glomerulonephritis and lupus nephritis). Complement profile studies, immunologic analysis for evidence of preceding strepococcal infection, and the clinical picture help sort out these difficult diseases.

Children and young adults are most commonly afflicted, but the disease may occur in infants and in the very elderly patient. The severity of acute poststreptococcal glomerulonephritis varies from that seen in the asymptomatic patient, discovered only because of disease in a sibling, to gross hematuria, oliguria, anuria, azotemia, and death in cardiorenal failure.

With the more careful documentation of etiology and the frequent utilization of percutaneous renal biopsy studies, in recent years it has been possible to show that nearly all children and most adults with acute poststreptococcal glomerulonephritis recover completely. Edelman et al. concluded that less than 1.0 percent of children with acute glomerulonephritis developed chronic renal disease. This does not mean that renal abnormalities do not persist for long periods in some instances. After an epidemic in Trinidad pathologic changes lasted more than a year in a significant proportion of the patients.

Renal biopsy specimens obtained within a few weeks of the onset of clinical nephritis usually demonstrate diffuse proliferative glomerulonephritis. The glomeruli are enlarged and inflamed, and the capillary lumens are obliterated by swelling and by an increase in the number of endothelial and mesangial cells. Diffuse exudation occurs, and for the most part the cells of the exudate comprise polymorphonuclear leukocytes. A few lymphocytes, and in very early cases occasional eosinophils, may be seen. Biopsy specimens obtained at later times after onset commonly reveal decreasing proliferation and a focal pattern of the glomerulonephritis during recovery.

Fine or coarse granular deposits of IgG globulin and β1C-globulin (β1C, the third component of complement) along the glomerular capillary walls are revealed by immunofluorescent microscopy of kidney tissue from most patients with acute poststreptococcal glomerulonephritis (Fig. 31-1). Morphologically these deposits often have characteristics of rather large humps similar to those sometimes seen late in the course of "one shot" serum sickness. Once these humps containing immunoglobulin and complement are recognized as part of the picture of the disease they can be identified by light microscopy, especially when a trichrome stain and very thin section are employed. In a smaller percentage of patients with otherwise typical but less severe disease, interrupted linear deposits of either IgG or β1C or of both may be noted along the glomerular capillary walls and within the mesangial cells. These, however, are not like the fine linear deposits of immunoglobulin and complement seen in Goodpasture's syndrome or the Masugi or Steblay models of renal disease based on directed immunologic assault but in our experience are simply part of the pattern of deposition of immunoglobulin and complement in an indirect immunologic assault.

Electron microscopy of glomeruli from patients with acute glomerular nephritis frequently demonstrates rounded dense masses extending from

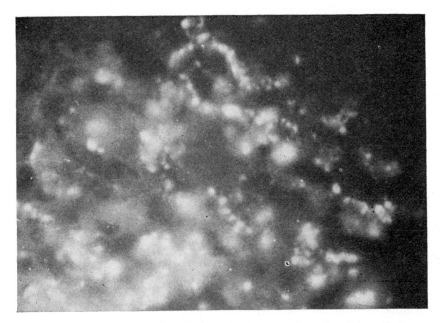

Fig. 31-1. Immunofluorescent studies of glomerulus in acute glomerulonephritis with hypocomplementemia. Isolated granular and nodular deposits of β1C are seen along the capillary loop (approximately × 800). For a more detailed description see Michael A.Γ., et al. (1971), J. Exp. Med. 134:208s.

the capillary basement membrane toward the epithelial cells. The densities, termed *humps*, are numerous in some patients and uncommon in others with clinically similar disease.

Sequential biopsy of renal specimens has revealed disappearance of both the immunoglobulins and the ultrastructural deposits as clinical recovery ensues.

Although recent studies have revealed evidence of cellular immunity in acute poststreptococcal glomerulonephritis, it seems unlikely that delayed hypersensitivity plays a significant role in this disease. An important point in the pathogenesis of poststreptococcal glomerulonephritis is the fact that patients often develop this disease as a consequence of skin infection with nephritogenic streptococci, even when the pharynx has apparently not been involved. By contrast, rheumatic fever does not seem to follow uncomplicated skin infections with group A β-hemolytic streptococci, but usually appears after streptococcal infection of the throat.

Treatment of children with acute glomerulonephritis involves primarily avoiding the dangers of hypertensive encephalopathy and cardiac failure. It has been shown conclusively that the hypertension in these patients can regularly be dramatically relieved with combinations of antihypertensive drugs, especially reserpine and hydralazine hydrochloride. If the renal damage is severe, low protein intake and even renal dialysis may be necessary to tide the patient over until the disease process begins to heal. Early studies indicated that ACTH or corticosteroids can sometimes induce rapid resolution of the inflammatory process. In our experience, however, such hazardous treatment is very rarely indicated in patients with this disease. Since few strains of streptococci are nephritogenic, antibacterial prophylaxis has not helped patients with this disease.

HYPOCOMPLEMENTEMIC GLOMERULONEPHRITIS

In 1965 West et al. described 7 children with persistent glomerulonephritis, low serum complement levels, and a lobular membranoproliferative glomerular histopathology which was thought to be particularly distinctive on silver methenamine staining. Herdman et al. identified 25 patients who had persistent hypocomplementemic glomerulonephritis. The average age at onset was 9.6 years (range 4 to 14.5 years), and slightly more girls than boys were represented. The clinical onset was characterized by gross hematuria in 9, asymptomatic proteinuria in 7, and insidious edema in 9. Seventeen of the 25 patients had a nephrotic syndrome at some time during their illness.

Serum complement titers (total hemolytic) may be remarkably low for many years, with fluctuations to normal on occasion and gradual return to normal in those who survived into adult life. The third component ($\beta 1C$) in the cases studied was usually distinctly low, with complete sparing of the earlier components of complement. The complement profile in these patients clearly reflects sparing of the C1, C4, and C2 and activation of the complement pathway at C3. Studies of the biologic half-life of C3 reveal a short half-life, an indication that this component is being activated and "used" more rapidly in this disease than in normal persons. Peripheral eosinophilia is common, and levels as high as 25 percent are sometimes observed. The clinical course of the disease is often slowly progressive; it is unusual for patients to develop renal failure in less than 5 years.

A lobular glomerulonephritis with striking hyperplasia and proliferation of the mesangium and duplication and splitting of the capillary basement membrane constitutes a prominent and accurate diagnostic histologic feature. Fluorescent microscopy demonstrates coarse granular deposits of IgG and $\beta 1C$-globulin along capillary membranes at the periphery of the lobules, a distinctive lobular pattern. Electron microscopy emphasizes the extent of the mesangial hyperplasia and the extreme degree of increase of the mesangial matrix. These features suggest that the splitting and the nonargyrophilic deposits seen by light microscopy reflect the mesangial abnormalities.

The etiology of this form of persistent glomerulonephritis is not known, but the prolonged reduction of complement levels, the distinctive histopathology, and the evidence of fluorescent microscopy suggest that this disease involves a distinctive form of glomerular assault and that an unusual immunologic mechanism may underlie the pathogenesis of the process. Some investigators have presented evidence that activation of the complement system is based on a circulating factor capable of attacking the third component of complement. In some patients with hypocomplementemic nephritis a serum factor would apparently activate the terminal complement sequence. Thus the pathogenesis of the disease seems to reside in a peculiar activation of complement.

Treatment of this disease is for the most part unsatisfactory. Although progression may be slow, in most instances it is progressive, with periods of apparent improvement. Some evidence suggests that this form of renal disease has identical morphology to a form of chronic progressive renal disease in adults, but rarely does clinically significant depression of serum complement levels occur. Treatment with a combination of heparin and adrenal steroids can bring about dramatic clinical and histologic reversal of the disease. Recently West et al. studied the effect of adrenocorticosteroid therapy on this disease. They found that although adrenal steroid treatment improved dramatically the C3 nephritic factor (C3NeF) ratio, this change was not accompanied by clinical improvement. These authors concluded that high levels of C3NeF are not associated with rapid renal deterioration in these patients and that lowering these levels was not of value. These relationships deserve additional study.

NEPHROTIC SYNDROME

The nephrotic syndrome is a clinical disorder characterized by marked proteinuria, hypoproteinemia, edema, and, usually, hypercholesterolemia. Common causes of nephrotic syndrome with known immunologic features are given in Table 31-1. About 75 percent of cases are due to primary renal disease, i.e., glomerulonephritis. Four pathologic categories are recognized: (1) "foot-process type" (lipoid nephrosis or minimal lesion nephrosis), (2) membranous, (3) proliferative, and (4) mixed.

In lipoid nephrosis, the renal lesion is noteworthy for its lack of inflammatory changes or basement membrane alteration. The glomerular basement membrane is usually completely normal or minimally altered focally. Deposits are most unusual, and the most striking change is fusion of the epithelial foot processes (podocytes). Deposits of immunologic reactants are not demonstrable in the glomerular capillary loop area by the fluorescent antibody technique. The etiology of this disorder remains a mystery. Recent claims that the disease is regularly associated with deposition of IgE in the glomeruli have not been confirmed after extensive and highly documented studies in a large series. Thus, either there may be a rare form of lipoid nephrosis associated with IgE deposition, which is not the general case in lipoid nephrosis, or directed immunologic assault is not the long-sought pathogenetic mechanism.

Table 31-1.   Causes of Nephrotic Syndrome with Known Immunologic
Implications

Primary Renal Diseases ("idiopathic")
  Membranous glomerulonephritis
  Proliferative glomerulonephritis (some cases)
  Idiopathic nephrotic syndrome of childhood
      ("lipoid" or minimal lesion nephrosis)
  Congenital familial nephrotic syndrome

Collagen-Vascular Diseases
  Systemic lupus erythematosus
  Sjögren's syndrome
  Polyarteritis nodosa
  Wegener's granulomatosis

Hypersensitivity Phenomena
  Insect stings
  Drugs
  Pollen injections
  Anaphylactoid purpura
  Cyclical nephrotic syndrome of pregnancy
  Associated with tumors

Serum Sickness

Infectious and Postinfectious Causes
  Subacute (proliferative) glomerulonephritis,
      poststreptococcal
  Infected ventriculoatrial shunt
  Quartan malaria
  Subacute bacterial endocarditis
  Syphilis (active)

Multiple Myeloma

Amyloidosis

Waldenström's macroglobulinemia

Adapted from Freedman, S. O. (ed.) (1971): *Clinical Immunology*. New York, Harper & Row, page 174.

In the membranous type of nephrosis, the glomerular lesion also seems, for the most part, to be noninflammatory. The thickening and irregularity of the capillary walls may be seen under ordinary light microscopy. Ultrastructural examination usually reveals electron dense deposits, most prominently located on the epithelial side of the basement membrane, although they may also occur in subendothelial and intramembranous locations. Immunofluorescent studies frequently reveal deposition of IgG and C3 in a discontinuous, closely packed, granular fashion along the glomerular basement membrane. This finding, coupled with the subepithelial deposits, suggests an "immune-complex type" of mechanism. The reason for the extremely tightly packed deposition of $\beta 1C$ and immunoglobulin, looking almost like a scalloping on the epithelial side of the glomerular basement membrane, is not clear. The morphologic similarity of these lesions to the lesions observed in a model of chronic glomerulonephritis produced by injection of renal tubular antigen led us to seek evidence that renal tubular antigen is involved in the human disease to no avail. Thus, the responsible antigen in the human disease remains obscure. It is of interest that complement components can often be demonstrated much more readily than can immunoglobulin components in the deposits. This finding again probably reflects the biologic amplification involved in the complement deposition.

In early studies of the metabolism of C3 in patients with chronic nephritis, low levels of this complement component were attributed, at least in part in some patients, to decreased synthesis and delivery of the component to the circulation. More recently, it has been shown that the characteristic complement profiles as in lupus may be a function of activation of both the primary and alternate complement pathways and in some patients having hypocomplementemic nephritis, by activation of the alternate pathway alone.

In the nephrosis associated with chronic proliferative glomerulonephritis, the pathologic lesions are characterized by a prominent proliferative, inflammatory component. A mixed lesion that has been described is likely a variant of proliferative glomerulonephritis with prominent membrane changes. Some patients with proliferative glomerulonephritis have various kinds of deposits in and around the glomerular basement membrane. The deposits are generally less dense and less discrete than those seen in classic membranous glomerulonephritis.

Serum complement levels are occasionally low in the nephrotic syndrome associated with childhood progressive glomerulonephritis, proliferative glomerulonephritis, and in some patients with membranous glomerulonephritis, but usually normal C levels are found. Complement levels, however, are consistently normal in lipoid nephrosis. The basic pathophysiologic abnormality in the nephrotic syndrome is, of course, an increase in glomerular permeability due to basement membrane damage.

The kidneys may excrete as much as 10 gm of protein in 24 hours. Patients with lipoid nephrosis are usually children and do not as a rule show hematuria or hypertension. They constitute the largest single group of childhood nephrotics and generally have a good prognosis. They respond well to treatment with adrenal steroids or with cyclophosphamide. In contrast, the membranous form of the nephrotic syndrome is generally seen in adults in whom the prognosis is poorer. Hematuria may occur, and hypertension is said to develop in about half the patients. The proliferative type of nephrotic syndrome which occurs in both adults and children may be clinically indistinguishable from other types of chronic progressive glomerulonephritis and is usually associated with a poor prognosis.

A special form of nephrotic syndrome is that occurring in infancy. In rare instances we have found this to be due to toxic chemicals, for example, $HgCl_2$, used as an antibacterial agent for soaking the infant's diapers. In most of these instances, however, the nephrosis is actually present at birth and is accompanied by very characteristic cystic changes in the renal cortex. This form of nephrosis has been quite common and very extensively studied in Finland. We have had extensive experience with the disease in Minnesota, which has a predominant Scandinavian population. Multiple cases have occurred in families. This disease has been attributed by some to isoimmunization, but our studies have failed to reveal any clear evidence of a primary immunologic assault on the kidney in these children. These included lack of evidence of isoimmunization to renal constituents in the mothers of such children. The disease is relentlessly progressive and most recalcitrant to therapy. The natural history is for these children to die from renal failure during the first three years of life. Recently, dramatic success in treatment of these infants has been experienced using renal transplantation, and the disease has thus far not reappeared in the transplanted kidneys.

Children with lipoid nephrosis respond dramatically to corticosteroid therapy. If they are steroid dependent, treatment with cyclophosphamide gives equally or more dramatic and surprisingly long-lasting remissions. Patients who do not respond to corticosteroids alone often benefit to some degree from the administration of immunosuppressive agents (cytotoxic drugs), either alone or in combination with corticosteroids. Satisfactory remissions have been obtained in more than 85 percent of nephrotic children with minimal renal lesions by the use of cyclophosphamide alone. The general use of cyclophosphamide, however, is discouraged to some degree by the report of the late appearance of a malignancy in one such case treated in Toronto.

CHRONIC GLOMERULONEPHRITIS

Chronic glomerulonephritis with or without the nephrotic syndrome represents a progressive renal disease of unknown etiology. In animals forms of naturally occurring chronic nephritis have been found in most species, sometimes in endemic forms. Deer, sheep, tigers, and mice frequently have chronic nephritis very similar to the disease of man. Usually immunopathologic dissection reveals a normal complement profile but varying evidence of immunoglobulin and complement deposition within the glomeruli. Sometimes both irregular "lumpy-bumpy" deposits of immunoglobulins of one class or another and complement components are found along the epithelial side of the glomerular membrane. Occasionally, as in Goodpasture's syndrome, evidence of directed immunologic assault is found, but in the absence of Goodpasture's syndrome this feature is rare in children and uncommon in adults. The only evidence of immunologic activity on immunofluorescent study may be extensive deposition in the mesangium of complement and immunoglobulin components. In experimental animals and in natural occurrence in animals, progressive glomerulonephritis is often attributable to persistent virus infections, and antigens of the virus, as well as immunoglobulins and complement, may be seen.

As in human chronic glomerulonephritis, the immunopathology includes both mesangial deposits of complement and immunoglobulin and irregular "lumpy-bumpy" deposits of these components and reflects the indirect form of immunologic assault. Experimentally chronic virus infections of great variety, including oncogenic viruses and viruses for which tolerance used to be claimed, e.g., lymphocytic choriomeningitis virus (LCM), produce this disease. To us it seems most likely that most cases of chronic progressive glomerulonephritis in man are due to the mechanism of persistent infection, antibody response to the infection, antigen-antibody complex formation, and destruction of the kidney secondary to these events. The mesangial deposits we take as a sign that this kind of disease process is going on and that these reflect normal functioning of the mesangium in handling antigen-antibody complexes as these circulate through the kidney. Occasionally the deposits in the mesangium and along the epithelial side of the membranes may be IgA rather than the more efficient complement fixing antibodies of IgG and IgM classes. Sometimes all major immunoglobulins are thus deposited.

Mixed Cryoglobulinemia and Renal Disease. In mixed cryoglobulinemia complexes of IgM and IgA and of IgG and IgM not only are responsible for renal damage but are evidence of the most extreme activation of the complement system. These disorders apparently represent autoimmunity to immunoglobulins involving antibodies that, unlike rheumatoid factor, fix complement with vigor. The pathology of the renal lesions in this disease is like that of chronic serum sickness or chronic glomerulonephritis. In these cases, however, the nephritis regularly is accompanied by arthritis, skin lesions reflecting a more generalized vasculitis, and often by pulmonary disease as well.

IDIOPATHIC RECURRENT HEMATURIA

Many patients experience recurrent episodes of hematuria in association with upper respiratory infections unrelated to the streptococcus. The pathogenesis of this provoking renal disease which sometimes progresses to chronic glomerulonephritis has remained obscure. However, recently Day has discovered that in one such patient recurrences of hematuria were associated with the presence in circulation of a factor capable of activating the complement system in the cold. This factor operating via the alternate pathway and utilizing the C3PA component of the serum appeared to be an unusual IgA molecule characteristic of the patient. The capacity to activate complement in the cold was removed by immunologic extraction of the patient's IgA from serum and restored with the patient's own IgA, but not with normal IgA. Perhaps IgA antibody selectively is involved in this form of nephritis.

RECURRENT URINARY TRACT INFECTION

Urinary tract infection is a frequent and sometimes severe acute disease, especially in children. Recurrent and recalcitrant urinary tract infections are often associated with congenital abnormalities of the urinary tract and are a sign of stasis in this system. They are valuable as a tip-off of serious and sometimes correctable congenital abnormality. It has not yet been possible to link them with immunologic deficiency of any type.

Recurrent and persistent urinary tract infections not associated with obvious congenital abnormality have been extensively studied in Sweden and the United States, but such studies of the systemic and local immunity systems have not yielded an explanation for the problem. Such studies have uncovered no abnormality of the local antibody system, but have presented some evidence that these patients excrete a more dilute urine than normal. It is our contention that further, more probing analysis of the relation of this condition to the vigor of the local antibody or local immunity systems in the kidney and bladder may yet be revealing.

Studies of the so-called "bladder sweat" of nephrectomized patients have shown that the local secretory antibody system may be of considerable vigor in this region. Other studies, however, have failed to demonstrate an abnormality in the function of this system in patients with recurrent urinary tract infection.

SELECTED REFERENCES

Acute Poststreptococcal Glomerulonephritis

Berger, J., Yaneva, H., and Hinglais, N. (1971): Advances Nephrol. 1:11.
Dillon, H. C. Jr., and Derrick, C. W. Jr., (1972): Hosp. Prac. 7:93.
Dodge, W. F., et al. (1972): New Eng. J. Med. 286:273.
Edelmann, C. M., Greifer, I., and Barnett, H. L. (1964): J. Pediat. 64:879.
Feldman, J. D., Mardiney, M. R., and Shuler, S. E. (1966): Lab. Invest. 15:283.
Fish, A. J., et al. (1970): Amer. J. Med. 48:28.
Macanovic, M., Evans, D. J., and Peters, D. K. (1972): Lancet 2:207.
Michael, A. F. Jr., et al. (1966): J. Clin. Invest. 45:237.
Perlman, L. V., et al. (1965): JAMA 194:63.
Rocklin, R. E., Lewis, E. J., and David, J. R. (1970): New Eng. J. Med. 283:497.
Schmidt, W. C., and Rammelkamp, C. H. Jr. (1958): Advances Intern. Med. 9:181.
Simon, N. S., et al. (1965): J. Lab. Clin. Med. 66:1022.

Hypocomplementemic Glomerulonephritis

Bardana, E. J. Jr., et al. (1970): Amer. J. Med. 49:789.
Chirawong, P., Nanra, R. S., and Kincaid-Smith P. (1971): Ann. Intern. Med. 74:853.
Day, N. K., et al. (1973): J. Clin. Invest. 52:1601.

Herdman, R. C., et al. (1970): Medicine 49:207.
McIntosh, R. M., et al. (1972): Lancet 1:1085.
Ogg, C. S., Cameron, J. S., and White, R. H. R. (1968): Lancet 2:78.
Vallota, E. H., et al. (1972): J. Pediat. 80:947.
West, C. D., et al. (1965): J. Pediat. 67:1089.

Nephrotic Syndrome

Barratt, T. M., and Soothill, J. F. (1970): Lancet 2:479.
Cornfeld, D., and Schwartz, M. W. (1966): J. Pediat. 68:507.
Drummond, K. N., et al. (1966): J. Clin. Invest. 45: 620.
Drummond, K. N., Michael, A. F., and Good, R. A. (1966): J. Canad. Med. Ass.
  94:834.
Farquhar, M. G., Vernier, R. L., and Good, R. A. (1957): J. Exp. Med. 106:649.
Gerber, M. A., and Paronetto, F. (1971): Lancet 1:1097.
Hoyer, J. R., et al. (1967): Pediatrics 40:233.
Hunsicker, L. G., et al. (1972): New Eng. J. Med. 287:835.
Lyons, H., et al. (1973): New Eng. J. Med. 288:124.
Mallick, N. P., et al. (1972): Lancet 1:507.
Ooi, B. S., et al. (1972): Arch. Intern. Med. 130:883.
Reeves, W. G., Cameron, J. S., and Ogg, C. S. (1971): Lancet 1:1299.
West, C. D., Hong, R., and Holland, N. H. (1966): J. Pediat. 68:516.
White, R. H. R., Glasgow, E. F., and Mills, R. J. (1970): Lancet 1:1353.

Chronic Glomerulonephritis

Bardana, E. J. Jr., et al. (1970): Amer. J. Med. 49:789.
Levitt, J. I. (1970): New Eng. J. Med. 282:1125.
McCluskey, R. T., and Baldwin, D. S. (1963): Amer. J. Med. 35:213.
Pickering, R. J., et al. (1971): J. Pediat. 78:30.
Relman, A. S. (1971): In Diseases of the Kidney, Strauss, W. B., and Welt, L. G.
  (eds.). Boston, Little, Brown and Company.

Idiopathic Recurrent Hematuria

Ayoub, E. M., and Vernier, R. L. (1965): Amer. J. Dis. Child. 109:217.
Brodwall, E. K., Oyri, A., and Oystese, B. (1971): Acta Med. Scand. 190:545.
Day, N. K., et al. (1973): J. Clin. Invest. 52:1698.

Recurrent Urinary Tract Infection

Bienenstock, J., and Perey, D. Y. (1972): Med. Clin. N. A. 56:391.
Feldman, B. H., Herdman, R., and Hong, R. (1971): Invest. Urol. 8:575.
Lincoln, K., Lidin-Janson, G., and Winberg, J. (1970): Brit. Med. J. 3:305.
Siegel, S. R., Sokoloff, B., and Siegel, B. (1973): Amer. J. Dis. Child. 125:45.
Tomasi, T. B. Jr., and Bienenstock J. (1968): Advances Immun. 9:1.
Uehling, D. T., and Steihm, E. R. (1971): Pediatrics 47:40.

32
Immunobiologic Aspects of Cardiac Diseases

Cardiac manifestations of immune injury are not uncommon in patients with clinical allergy and with serum sickness reactions following injection of foreign proteins or drugs. These manifestations range from mild transient effects, such as minor arrhythmias and electrocardiographic abnormalities, to such serious cardiac injury as coronary insufficiency, myocardial infarction, and pericarditis. Studies in experimental animals have amply documented the pathologic effects of antigen-antibody interaction on endocardium, myocardium, pericardium, and cardiac vessels.

Hypersensitivity to infectious agents has been postulated to play a role in the pathogenesis of infectious myocarditis due to viruses, bacteria, and protozoa, and such a mechanism could be responsible for the pathogenesis of certain cases of primary cardiomyopathy or idiopathic myocardial disease. Autoantibodies to heart have been demonstrated in many patients, especially those with rheumatic fever, postcardiotomy and postmyocardial infarction syndromes, endomyocardial fibrosis, and other cardiac disorders. For the most part these seem to be consequences rather than causes of cardiac pathology. Cardiac involvement occasionally occurs in rheumatoid arthritis, is frequent in systemic lupus erythematosus, scleroderma, some forms of polyarteritis nodosa, and amyloidosis.

RHEUMATIC CARDITIS

The carditis in rheumatic fever is an active inflammatory process associated with group A streptococcal infection. It affects heart valves, myocardium, and pericardium. The incidence of clinically recognizable carditis in initial rheumatic fever attacks in the United States is about 40 percent. Autopsies have revealed that most patients with rheumatic fever have inflammatory lesions of the heart even in cases of accidental death. Carditis is usually accompanied by other symptoms of rheumatic fever, such as fever, arthritis, and skin lesions, but may develop insidiously in association with vague constitutional symptoms or may appear in a fulminant form particularly in children.

Endocarditis, the most frequent manifestation of carditis, is characterized by murmurs reflecting involvement of the mitral, aortic, and rarely tricuspid valves. The onset of mitral and aortic valvular disease is signaled by the appearance of mid-diastolic murmurs at the left sternal border. Murmurs of mitral and aortic stenosis occur much later with progression or recurrence of carditis. The characteristic histopathologic lesion is the *Aschoff body*, a granulomatous lesion associated with foci of altered connective tissue in myocardium and endocardium, usually located in proximity to blood vessels.

Increased immunoglobulin levels, particularly of IgG and IgA, and elevated immune responses to streptococcal cellular and extracellular products support the concept that the hypersensitivity reaction might play a role in the pathogenesis of rheumatic fever. Further support of this concept is the 2 1/2 to 4 week interval between the initial streptococcal infection and development of rheumatic fever. In addition, the infrequent occurrence of rheumatic fever in infants infected with streptococci, together with the concentration of incidence in children between 4 and 16 years of age, has been taken as evidence of the importance of hypersensitivity in the pathogenesis of this disease. Patients who develop rheumatic fever following streptococcal infection also on the average develop higher titers of antistreptococcal antibodies than do comparable populations who do not develop rheumatic fever. The enhanced immune response in rheumatic fever is mostly related to streptococcal antigens; however, more vigorous than normal immunity mechanisms in these patients have not been substantiated.

Interest in the possible role of autoallergic mechanisms in the pathogenesis of rheumatic fever has been stimulated by several different lines of evidence, including (1) the high frequency of autoantibodies to heart that can be demonstrated by many techniques in sera of patients with rheumatic fever; (2) presence of bound gamma globulin deposits in myocardium and endocardium of rheumatic hearts; (3) demonstration of an immunologic cross reaction between components of group A streptococci and human heart tissue ; and (4) observation of autoantibodies reactive with particular heart constituents in sera of patients with rheumatic fever.

Postmortem immunopathologic studies of hearts from rheumatic fever patients and biopsy specimens of auricular appendages from patients with severe rheumatic heart disease have revealed deposits of bound immunoglobulins and complement, β1C- globulin, localized mainly in sarcolemmal-subsarcolemmal sites in cardiac myofibers and smooth muscle of vessel walls and of endocardium and in focal sites in collagenous tissue of interstitium. In cases of fatal rheumatic fever in children, massive immunoglobulin and complement deposits were observed throughout the myocardium of all four chambers of the heart. In the Aschoff nodule deposits of IgG and complement have also been demonstrated.

The frequency of autoimmune responses has been correlated with clinical activity of the rheumatic disease, with presence of carditis, and with the number of previous attacks of rheumatic fever.

The antibody response to streptococci varies with the site of infection. Antistreptolysin O, antistreptococcal deoxyribonuclease B (anti-DNase B), and antistreptococcal nicotinamide-adenine-dinucleotidase (anti-NADase) are all found to be elevated in patients with streptococcal pharyngitis, but in streptococcal impetigo only anti-DNase B is regularly elevated. Virulence among group A streptococci appears to be determined largely by the organism's ability to produce large amounts of M protein, and clinical immunity is determined by antibodies directed against this component.

Tagg and McGiven postulate that the heart-reactive antibodies in the sera of patients with rheumatic fever may reflect the autoimmune process in the pathogenesis of rheumatic fever. The nontoxicity of such sera for cultures of mammalian heart cells led these investigators to postulate that these antibodies do not have a primary pathogenetic role but are formed as part of an immunologic response to antigens in heart tissue that has been damaged by an unrelated cardiotoxic agent produced by streptococci.

Recently Wannamaker has reviewed the differences between Streptococcus pyogenes infections of the throat and skin and their sequelae, the most important of which is that rheumatic fever seems to follow only throat infections and that nephritis may complicate skin or throat infections. The nephritis seen in the summer and in hot countries is commonly a complication of skin infections; the nephritis and rheumatic fever seen in winter and spring, and in cooler countries, follows throat infections. The streptococci that cause skin infections commonly belong to a different set of serotypes from those isolated from the throat and were for a long time wrongly thought to lack M antigens; several have now been shown to be nephritogenic.

Studies have shown that Australian aboriginals have a high frequency of rheumatic heart disease but a low frequency of rheumatic fever that could be recognized by usual clinical criteria. They were found to have chronic protein deprivation as a rule and expressed certain cell-mediated antigens normally. This observation has been an important point of departure for extensive studies of the influence of the nutritional state on the immune responses and autoimmune diseases (Chapter 14).

Since persistence of streptococcal infection appears to be necessary for development of rheumatic fever, it is possible to prevent initial attacks and recurrences of rheumatic fever by recognition and treatment of the preceding streptococcal disease. In both military and civilian populations rheumatic fever occurred in a frequency of 2 to 3 percent following group A streptococcal infections. Evidence has been presented that this figure may be lower for children in civilian populations. By contrast, the frequency of recurrences of rheumatic fever once a person has had this malady has ranged from 25 to 70 percent in different series. This increased risk of rheumatic fever as a complication after streptococcal infection has been taken by some as strong evidence that hypersensitivity operates in the pathogenesis of this disease. Further, it is the basis for the strong recommendation that streptococcal reinfections must be prevented in patients who have had rheumatic fever by using appropriate prophylactic regimens based on penicillin or sulfadiazine.

Treatment of streptococcal infections of the pharynx or tonsils is directed toward eradication of group A streptococci and is essential for the prevention of rheumatic fever. Injection of long-acting benzathine penicillin or oral administration of penicillin for 10 days or more are recommended.

POSTCARDIOTOMY AND POSTMYOCARDIAL INFARCTION SYNDROMES

The trauma or damage to the heart or pericardium following surgical procedures, stab wounds, or pacemaker catheter placement, and acute myocardial infarction often results in a symptom complex variously termed the *postcardiotomy, postcommissurotomy, postpericardiotomy,* or *postinfarction* syndrome. It occurs from three days to several months after the initiating event and is characterized by fever and chest pain which may be mild or severe, crushing or dull, and may persist for hours or weeks. Frequently an associated pericarditis, most often with mild pericardial effusion, and a concomitant pleuritis with pleural effusion and, on occasion, pulmonary infiltrates are present. The effusions may be serous or hemorrhagic. Arthralgia may also occur. Other findings include leukocytosis, increased erythrocyte sedimentation rate, and positive test for C-reactive protein.

The syndrome is characterized by a high recurrence rate over a period of many months, lack of response to antibodies, and a favorable response to corticosteroid therapy. Participation of an immune mechanism in these syndromes is suggested by the occurrence of a latent period, clinical association with pericarditis, pleurisy, and arthralgia (manifestations often associated with immunologic diseases), and a prompt clinical response to corticosteroid treatment.

Autoantibodies to heart have been demonstrated by one or more techniques in almost all patients with postcardiotomy syndrome and in the majority of patients considered to have postmyocardial infarction syndrome. The relation of circulating autoantibodies to these clinical syndromes is still uncertain. Available evidence indicates that autoantibodies to heart in human sera are multiple and include reactivities for both particulate and soluble components of heart. These autoantibodies can be differentiated by absorption tests from the antibodies in rheumatic fever patients which exhibit cross reaction with Streptococcus and heart. Recently, however, the association of the postcardiotomy syndrome with infection from certain viruses contained in administered blood has been demonstrated; e.g., Au antigen, inclusion body virus, and other viruses have been implicated. Here the pathogenetic immunologic event may involve immune response to the virus rather than to the heart tissue. This explanation would not cover diseases of many patients, especially those with postinfarction syndrome.

VIRAL MYOCARDITIS

Viral myocarditis shows clinically a biphasic pattern. In children, the onset is characterized by malaise and general discomfort followed in 3 to 10 days by fever, tachycardia, arrhythmias, protodiastolic gallop, cardiac dilatation, and signs of congestive failure. In adults, the second phase may be manifested by fever, myalgia, weakness, and chest pain, with varible degrees of cardiomegaly or cardiac decompensation.

The failure to isolate virus from heart tissue, coupled with the clinically biphasic nature of viral myocarditis, has provoked the thought that a secondary immune process is involved in its pathogenesis and is directed against target antigens either endogenous or exogenous in pleura, pericardium, myocardium, and heart valves. Immunofluorescent studies of 55 hearts from routine autopsies have indicated that in 31 percent Coxsackie virus antigen in the myocardium was associated with focal damage to this layer. Since the usual viral infection is self-limited within the context of a normally developing immunity, the development of a chronic or progressive myocardial disease following viral infection would seem more probably related to a mechanism of autoallergic response to heart induced by viral infection, immunodeficiency, or immunodeviation produced perhaps by the virus itself.

CORONARY HEART DISEASE

Even coronary artery disease, the most common killer of Western man, cannot escape the consideration of the modern clinical immunobiologist. The possibility that immunologic mechanisms may play a role in coronary disease derives from several considerations which recently appeared. First of all, immunologic aging in which an immunologic disbalance occurs has been observed in certain inbred strains of animals. The vascular lesions that these animals develop include disease of large as well as small vessels, and coronary arteries are not immune. Secondly, studies of the influence of nutrition on immunity indicate that dietary manipulations of proteins, essential amino acids, calories, and fat can have profound influences on immunity and autoimmune reactions. These lines of reasoning are dreadfully indirect and would not be worthy of mention were it not for the fact that intimal disease, especially prominent in the coronary arteries, is a striking and regular concomitant of cardiac transplant rejection. This is especially the case when the cellular immune responses have been suppressed and a kind of immunoperturbation or immunodeviation has been produced and the chronic rejection reaction is largely or completely the consequence of circulating antibody. Such lesions occur whether the heart has been transplanted to replace a congenitally abnormal heart, a heart that has been irreparably damaged by old rheumatic disease, or it is the heart of a patient who himself had coronary disease. Similarly, intimal disease of larger vessels is often seen in kidneys of patients who have had chronic rejection reactions based largely on antibody rather than the better known acute rejections based largely on cellular immunity.

DEGENERATIVE VASCULAR DISEASE

Pathologists for many years have been concerned with degenerative changes in vessels of the heart, kidney, brain, and other vital organs. Hyalin fibrous alterations, especially in the intima of small vessels, have been thought to be one major concomitant of aging. Nowoslawski has recently obtained evidence (unpublished) that such hyalin-fibrous degenerative lesions are accompanied by deposition of antigen-antibody complexes and that these in turn might account for the vascular damage and be one basis of so-called arteriosclerotic heart and other organ disease. Much further study in this direction is surely needed.

SELECTED REFERENCES

Rheumatic Carditis

Dudding, B. A., and Ayoub, E. M. (1968): J. Exp. Med. 128:1081.
Hess, E. V., et al. (1964): J. Clin. Invest. 43:886.
Kaplan, M. H. (1969): Progr. Allerg. 13:408.
Kaplan, M. H., et al. (1964): New Eng. J. Med. 271:637.
Kaplan, M. H., and Dallenbach, F. D. (1961): J. Exp. Med. 113:1.
Tagg, J. R., and McGiven, A. R. (1972): Lancet 2:686.
Wannamaker, L. W. (1970): New Eng. J. Med. 282:23.
Wannamaker, L. W., and Ayoub, E. M. (1960): Circulation 21:598.
Zitnan, D., and Bosmansky, K. (1966): Acta Rheum. Scand. 12:267.

Postcardiotomy and Postmyocardial Infarction Syndromes

Kantor, G. L., and Johnson, B. L. (1970): Arch. Int. Med. 125:488.
Reyman, T. A. (1966): Amer. Heart J. 72:116.
Williams, J. F., Jr., Morrow, A. G., and Braunwald, E. (1965): Circulation 32:608.

Viral Myocarditis

Abelmann, W. H. (1973): Ann. Rev. Med. 24:145.
Sanders, V. (1963): Amer. Heart J. 65:707.

33

Immunologic Aspects
of Viral Infections

Long before the virus was clearly defined, an effective means of prevention of viral disease was developed by Jenner through the use of vaccination. Thus, the very beginning of modern immunobiology occurred in a pragmatic setting. The virus may now be defined as a peculiar piece of genetic material, either DNA or RNA but never both, which is ordinarily capable of committing a living cell to produce more viral nucleic acid and proteins, one or more of which is specifically associated with the new nucleic acid to form particles infective for other living cells.

The increased awareness of the prevalence of viruses and their frequency as etiologic agents of many human diseases, including cancer, led to the studies of their pathogenicity and immunity. For the time being, the relative paucity of effective chemotherapeutic agents active against viruses leaves vaccination as a major means of preventing some of the known viral diseases. The interaction of virus and host cells may lead to one of four consequences: (1) lysis of the host cell, (2) persistent infection and replication of virus, (3) integration of virus genome into the host cell, and (4) elimination of the virus, often together with the infected cells, from the host. As was discovered by Jenner and rediscovered by von Pirquet, the very difference between virus infection and the diseases of human cells infected by viruses is often the immune reaction to the viruses or to the bodily cells they infect (self + X). These relationships have recently been brought dramatically home to us when by cellular engineering we have introduced immunity into the equation for the virus (parasite) and host cell reaction, i.e., we have observed in many instances minimal or no manifestations associated with the virus infection in the immunologically unresponsive host transformed into violent disease as capacity for immune response is reconstituted.

Interestingly, viral infections may enhance or suppress immune responses of the host. The effect can be nonspecific or quite specific. The suppression can affect either humoral or cellular immunity or both. Further, immunosuppression of the host may activate silent infection or predispose to the opportunistic infection with other viruses, fungi, or bacteria. That antibodies play a major role in protection against bacterial diseases is undisputed and there is little to indicate that the viral diseases should escape from such a powerful defense mechanism. Viruses are neutralized by antisera unless they are already inside the cell. Studies on immunodeficiency diseases have elucidated further the mechanism of immunity to viral diseases. Patients with agammaglobulinemia suffer from bacterial infection with encapsulated pathogens, although they recover reasonably well from measles, varicella, mumps, and poliomyelitis. Further, their inability to form demonstrable amounts of antibody helps them to control and recover from most viral infections. These patients develop delayed hypersensitivity and immunity to infecting viruses. These findings support the contention that cell-mediated immunity plays a most important and perhaps crucial role in dealing with certain virus infections.

Virus infection may leave transient or "permanent" immunity in the host. A second attack of measles, smallpox, or yellow fever, for example, is rare, whereas multiple attacks of influenza and the common cold are well known. The latter may be due, in part, to the many different serotypes capable of causing the clinical disease.

The most devastating viral infections, e.g., smallpox, measles, yellow fever, poliomyelitis, and even rubella, have been or can be successfully controlled by means of vaccination. These approaches are now being extended to almost all reaches of the earth. For example, we can predict the elimination of smallpox from the globe during this decade through the anti-smallpox vaccination program being undertaken by WHO.

SLOW VIRUS INFECTION

Slow virus is a term used to indicate the slowness in the manifestation of disease caused by some viruses. Long incubation periods, rather than slowness of multiplication, are characteristic of the agents under appro-

Table 33-1. Examples of Slow Virus Infections

Man

    Kuru
    Jakob-Creutzfeldt
    Subacute sclerosing panencephalitis (SSPE)
    Progressive multifocal leukoencephalopathy (PML)*

Animals

    Scrapie (sheep and goats)
    Visna (sheep)
    Mink encephalitis (mink)
    Aleutian mink disease (mink)
    Lactic acid dehydrogenase (LDH) elevating disease (mice)*
    Lymphocytic choriomeningitis (LCM) (mice)*
    NZB mouse disease (New Zealand Black [NZB] mice)*

---

* Probable slow virus infection. Courtesy of Dr. Carlos Lopez.

priate conditions. In addition to long incubation periods ranging from a few months to a few years, progressive pathologic changes lead to the death of the host in slow virus diseases (Table 33-1). The reason for the long incubation periods of these diseases is not clear. Ineffective immune response of host may be the major factor, but further studies are required.

Recently the importance of these slow virus infections became more apparent, since studies of these viruses have shed new light on the possible identification of etiologic agents of human diseases of unknown cause which affect large segments of the population, i.e., multiple sclerosis, leukodystrophies, Parkinson's disease, cancer, collagen diseases, and many autoimmune diseases. During the past few years, four neurologic diseases of man have been shown to be caused by chronic persistent infections of virus: kuru, Jakob-Creutzfeldt disease, subacute sclerosing panencephalitis (SSPE), and progressive multifocal leukoencephalopathy. Epilepsia partialis continua, chronic viral encephalitis, and focal epilepsy with progressive brain lesions, including cytoplasmic viral inclusion bodies and rare cases of subacute herpes simplex encephalitis, can be added to the list.

RUBELLA AND CONGENITAL RUBELLA SYNDROME

In 1942 Gregg's pioneering observations on embryopathy stimulated intensive investigations of the relationship of maternal infections to congenital malformation. However, of all the congenital infections, none has had the dramatic impact or has caused more community concern than congenital rubella. Despite the widespread practice of therapeutic abortion for rubella in the first trimester of pregnancy, a conservatively estimated 30,000 children developed rubella-associated birth defects as a consequence of the epidemic of 1964 in the United States. Careful studies of children born of mothers who had rubella during the first trimester of pregnancy in the epidemic have revealed that none of these children escaped completely significantly lasting impact of the infection.

Recent scientific advances have provided techniques for documenting the magnitude of the tragedy in 1964 and interpreting the consequences of prior rubella epidemics. Fortunately, this stimulus has provided tools which soon should eradicate the rubella problem. The isolation of the rubella virus in tissue culture in 1962 made possible (1) the characterization of the natural history of postnatal and congenital rubella and (2) the development of rubella virus vaccines. The rapid progress in clarification of the rubella problem represents the combined efforts of investigative teams in a number of centers and reflects the power of modern biology.

Rubella virus is distinct from all other known viruses and is antigenically stable. There is no evidence to suggest the presence of different strains (e.g., influenza virus A, B, C) or different serotypes (e.g., poliovirus, types I, II, III). This presents an important advantage in development of an effective immunization program. The rubella virus has been tentatively placed in the paramyxovirus group; it contains RNA, is pleomorphic and ether sensitive, and has antigen that can be revealed by hemagglutination and complement fixation assays. Rubella virus is thermolabile; inactivation is rapid at 37° C and room temperature, but the virus can be stored for short periods at —20° C and for months at —60° C.

The rubella virus is shed in pharyngeal secretions and is spread directly by person-to-person exposure. Since persons with subclinical infections have both pharyngeal shedding and viremia, they may be contagious to others and may give birth to children with congenital rubella.

Rubella is a mild illness in children and young adults. In a classical case, occipital or postauricular lymphadenopathy, which may be tender and slightly painful, may precede the onset of the rash by several days. The onset of a rash two to three weeks after exposure may be accompanied by low-grade fever and malaise. The rubella exanthem is variable and has no diagnostic features. Especially in young children clinical rubella is also often manifested by extraordinary hematologic signs. Lymphocytosis with as many as 95 percent lymphocytes on differential count and striking apparently immature forms, basophilic forms, and even plasma cells may appear in the circulating blood.

Arthralgia and arthritis are so common in adults, especially women, that they must be considered typical manifestations of rubella. Fortunately, joint complaints are not so common in children. The arthralgia may be quite mild and limited to "morning stiffness," or full-blown arthritis with swelling, effusion, pain, and tenderness may simulate acute rheumatoid arthritis. Paresthesia, most typically "pins and needles" sensations, often accompanies the joint symptoms.

Rubella virus may be cultured from pharyngeal secretions and the serum as early as one week before onset of the rash. Detectable viremia ceases promptly after onset of the rash, usually in less than 48 hours, but pharyngeal shedding of virus may persist occasionally for up to two weeks. Urine and stool are unreliable sources of rubella virus.

Rubella antibody can be measured by neutralization, complement fixation (CF), immunofluorescence (FA), and hemagglutination inhibition (HI) antibody techniques. The rubella HI antibody test has the greatest general applicability, since it is a rapid, sensitive, and an economic procedure.

The absence of rubella HI or neutralizing antibody at the time of exposure indicates susceptibility. This is not necessarily true with CF antibody, since it usually does not persist very long after infection. The presence of any detectable rubella antibody at the time of exposure indicates past infection, and in pregnant woman freedom from the risk of rubella-induced congenital malformation.

In patients with clinical rubella, HI antibody is usually detectable within 24 to 48 hours after onset of the rash, and peak titers are reached within 6 to 12 days. The promptness of this response makes serodiagnosis of rubella difficult unless the first blood specimen is obtained before or within a few days after onset of the rash. Since the first antibody detectable in the primary response to rubella infection is specific IgM, demonstration that antibody found in the early days after a rash contains rubella IgM is diagnostic and rules out confusion with the booster responses occasionally observed following exposure of immune individuals to rubella. In the latter, IgG antibody is the kind observed.

Herd Immunity in Rubella Infection. Although herd immunity contributes significant protection of susceptibles in the case of poliomyelitis, smallpox, and probably measles, the situation is somewhat more complex in the case of rubella immunization with current strains of virus. Immunization with current rubella vaccines, although effective in protecting children from developing symptoms of rubella, is not so effective in protecting children from rubella infection. Under these circumstances herd immunity is practically inoperative. Indeed the only protection afforded nonimmunized persons by mass immunization is the degree to which the number of potentially infecting organisms available to the susceptible population is reduced. This means that with the available rubella vaccine susceptible girls must be immunized late in childhood and susceptible mothers right after delivery of a child.

Congenital Rubella. Many of the crucial steps of maternal-fetal rubella infection have now been documented. Maternal viremia may persist for approximately one week and may lead to placental infection, and fetal viremia. The viremia may produce disseminated fetal infection. Timing is of great importance. The major steps in organogenesis occur during the second through the eighth weeks after conception, when infection is of maximum hazard to the heart, eyes, and brain. By the fifth month of gestation, the fetus no longer seems susceptible to the chronic infection characteristic of rubella during the first 16 weeks. However, central nervous system damage apparently has occurred in children infected with rubella virus during the second trimester. During the second trimester, the fetus develops an increasing degree of immunologic competence, and perhaps the placenta becomes a more effective barrier to virus transmission. In contrast to thalidomide or radiation, where a single exposure during early pregnancy exerts its effect at that time only, the available evidence suggests that the chronic infection with rubella virus contributes to the acute illness seen during the newborn period in infants who have been infected earlier in development. These infants may show hepatitis, encephalitis, thrombopenic or vascular purpura, growth failure, bone lesions, progressive psychomotor retardation, and damage to hearing and sight. In one study the major manifestations of congenital rubella among 271 abnormal infants followed to the age of 18 months were congenital heart disease, hearing loss, cataract or glaucoma, psychomotor retardation, neonatal thrombocytopenic purpura, and death. The mortality rate of these congenitally infected infants exceeded 35 percent during the first year of life.

The long-term prognosis for children with severe multiple rubella defects, especially neurologic abnormalities, must be guarded. However, a recent 25 year follow-up of 50 patients who were among the original children described by Gregg and his colleagues has provided a note of optimism. Most of these survivors have made relatively good socioeconomic adjustments, despite hearing loss in 48 of the 50, cataracts or retinopathy in 26, cardiac defects in 11, and mental deficiency in 5.

Prevention of Rubella. The use of gamma globulin for prevention of rubella has been controversial for many years and has not yet been satisfactorily resolved. It is clear that administration of commercially available gamma globulin cannot be relied on to prevent rubella and that infection occurring despite attempted prophylaxis may be characterized by detectable viremia. However, better results may be obtained with specific hyperimmune or immediate postinfection gamma globulin.

In 1966, Meyer and his co-workers described completion of a small trial with rubella vaccine in which they used a strain of rubella virus (HPV-77) attenuated by 77 tissue culture passages in African green monkey kidney cells. Two other strains of attenuated rubella virus vaccine, the Cendehill strain and the RA27/3 strain, now have been tested in the United States and Europe.

The prime purpose of a vaccine against rubella is the prevention of the congenital rubella syndrome. This requires prevention of rubella during early pregnancy. Good correlation exists between provocation by the vaccine of hemagglutination-inhibiting (HI) antibodies and protection against clinical rubella. A relationship between the level of serum HI antibodies and subclinical infections has been found, and the incidence of subclinical reinfections is clearly lower among individuals who have high titers of antibody than among those with low HI antibody titers. Therefore, the level of serum antibodies induced by rubella vaccines and the persistence of these antibodies over the years may be important criteria. The induction and persistence of serum antibodies other than the HI and of the local secretory antibodies have not yet been definitively studied but may be even more important than HI antibodies in preventing the disease.

Infants with congenital rubella, as in other cases of persistent virus infection, were found to have high levels of 19S neutralizing antibody to the rubella virus, even at birth and in the immediate neonatal period.

Usually these children show a significant defect in their ability to develop IgG antibodies after loss of maternal antibodies and have lower than normal levels of IgG. Infants with the congenital rubella syndrome may occasionally exhibit failure of normal immunologic development expressed as a panhypogammaglobulinemia. Approximately 6 such cases have been described, and other variations of immunologic development have been encountered. Infants with congenital rubella were shown to be lacking anti-rubella antibody, and secretion of virus continues. The pathogenesis of persistent excretion of viruses in infants with the congenital rubella syndrome remains an immunologic paradox. The presence of circulating 19S rubella-virus-neutralizing antibody indicates that an immune response has been provoked by the virus and that tolerance in the usual sense is not operating. However, none of the circumstances of congenital viral infection that have been properly studied has revealed evidence of true immunologic tolerance, so in this regard rubella is not unusual.

CYTOMEGALOVIRUS INFECTIONS

Since Ribbert, in 1904, first reported the presence of inclusion bodies in the cells of the kidney and parotid gland of a stillborn infant and Jesionek and Kiolemenoglou similarly cited inclusions in the cells of the kidney, liver, and lungs of another stillborn infant, *cytomegalic inclusion disease* has been reported frequently as a disease of newborn infants, older infants, children, and adults.

Cytomegaloviruses are agents ubiquitous in nature. They produce protean clinical manifestations in man. Since the human cytomegaloviruses (CMV) were first isolated in 1956, it has been established that these agents may infect man by diverse natural or iatrogenic routes from the fetal to adult life. The cytomegaloviruses are members of the herpesvirus family. The criteria for the presumptive identification of this virus are (1) capacity to induce cytomegalia, (2) formation of intranuclear and often cytoplasmic inclusion bodies, and (3) a marked degree of host specificity. Immunologic approaches to identification of this virus are crucial, however, and the complement fixation test is widely used as the basic serodiagnostic procedure, as well as in epidemiologic surveys.

The CMV infections occurring after infancy are often asymptomatic. Intrauterine infection, however, can produce severe damage to the central nevous system, eyes, heart, and other organs. Infants infected *in utero* may excrete virus in the urine for months or years, despite the presence of high levels of circulating antibody. In patients with secondary immunodeficiency diseases, e.g., generalized neoplasia, and in renal allograft recipients, the latent virus may be activated to cause apparent diseases, or exogenous virus may establish new infection more readily than in normals. This virus, like other agents, may sometimes be introduced by blood transfusion. In recent studies at the University of Minnesota activation or expression of inclusion body virus infection was found to be linked to lethal pulmonary disease and even to serve as an apparent triggering agent in renal allograft rejection in patients on the transplantation service. Patients whose cell-mediated immunities are selectively depressed produce excessive amounts of antibody against CMV.

In so-called CMV mononucleosis a notable immunologic aberration has been reported. Antinuclear antibodies, rheumatoid factors, cold agglutinins, cryoglobulins, and hypersensitivity to penicillin may be expressed.

The mechanism and timing of fetal infection with cytomegalovirus remains somewhat obscure. Since congenitally infected infants are often, but not always, the firstborn of young women, it was thought that congenital transmission of virus may reflect maternal viremia-associated primary infection. Other evidence indicates that in some infants cytomegaloviruses may be acquired during the birth process via cervical secretions. Nonetheless, it seems clear that congenital infection damaging a variety of organs can be attributed to this disease.

In the United States minimal infection rates of cytomegalovirus at birth are approximately 1 percent as assayed by the presence of the virus in urine. Starr and his co-workers suggest that 10 percent of neonatal viral excretors will exhibit some degree of neurologic sequelae. This would indicate that at least 3700 infants of 3.7×10^6 born in 1970 will be affected. At present no therapy is available. Interferon, fluorodeoxyuridine, and iododeoxyuridine have been tried in some instances with apparent benefit.

INTERFERON, AND OTHER ANTIVIRAL AGENTS

The ability to treat and control a wide spectrum of viral diseases that affect man has long been the goal of medical research. At the present time this goal has been partially attained through (1) active immunization with live attenuated or killed virus vaccines, (2) passive immunization with gamma globulin, (3) improved sanitation and control of vectors of virus transmission, such as the mosquito, and, finally (4) the first limited steps toward chemotherapy with the use of iododeoxyuridine (IDU) in herpes simplex virus keratitis. Although each of these measures has been of benefit in specific infections, their application for the general control or treatment of viral infections has not been possible.

This situation was abruptly altered in 1957 when Isaacs and Lindenmann, while studying interference between influenza viruses, discovered that elimination of the viral particles from allantoic fluids of influenza-infected chick embryos did not eliminate the capacity to induce interference. They named the soluble mediator of the interference phenomenon "interferon." The question raised by their findings was whether this was just another interesting facet of viral interference or whether it represented a major breakthrough with far-reaching implications not only for the interference phenomenon but also for the elucidation of metabolic processes involved in viral replication, for our understanding of host defenses and the mechanisms by which we actually recover from some viral infections, and as a potential chemoprophylactic or chemotherapeutic tool.

The interferon system is a mechanism of cellular defense or a form of immunity that man shares with most animals, some as primitive as the teleost fishes. This natural defense system operates in numerous viral infections by means of interferons, which are proteins produced by appropriately stimulated vertebrate cells. An interferon is operationally defined by its ability to confer antiviral resistance upon normally susceptible animal cells, usually of the same species.

Interferon formation by cells or tissues is stimulated by a variety of agents: viruses, nucleic acids, synthetic polymers, tilorone (a low molecular weight aromatic amine), bacterial products, and other natural inducers. The induction of interferon is an event that proceeds from the exposure of cells to the stimulating agent; the normal cellular machinery is thereby engaged for the production of proteins. Agents that stimulate the production of interferon in cells exposed to them have been referred to as interferon *inducers. Induction* and *production* are terms used interchangeably in the interferon literature. The first process, however, precedes and probably should be kept separate from the second. A further distinction should be made between the stimulation of antiviral resistance in cells and the formation of interferon. Certain agents provoke antiviral resistance in the absence of detectable interferon.

In general, interferon is most active in the cells of the same species of animal that produces it. A clear exception to this general rule is the cross reactivity between interferons of man and rabbit. Viral-induced interferon from human skin fibroblasts, for example, showed 20 times more antiviral activity in rabbit kidney cells than in the human cell system.

At least two molecular species of interferon have been described. One has a molecular weight greater than 100,000, and the other is a smaller molecule with a molcular weight of about 20,000 to 40,000. Some evidence for subunit structure has been presented. Differences in molecular size may indicate different cell sources producing interferon and may suggest more than one gene that codes for these molecules.

A variety of techniques of modern protein chemistry have been applied to the concentration and purification of interferon. Although purifications of several thousand times have been reported and specific activities over 1000 units per microgram of protein recorded, the best estimate now is that the most highly purified preparations are still very impure.

The lack of standard methods and reagents, as well as the biologic variation of cells in culture, has made comparison and even repetition of results from different laboratories difficult.

Capacity to produce interferon resides in the host genome of vertebrate cells and is not a function of the virus genome. Depression of the interferon cistrons located in the cell's DNA apparently permits the formation of messenger RNA, which then carries to the ribosomes the coding for the production of interferon proteins. Interferon production can be inhibited or suppressed by actinomycin D at a dose that can prevent DNA-dependent RNA synthesis or by inhibitors of RNA or protein synthesis administered before or with the inducer. Interference with production of these compounds also may be achieved with chemical carcinogens, corticosteroids, cyclophosphamide, or X-irradiation.

In viral infections interferon acts intracellularly to limit viral synthesis. It has no effect on viral attachment or penetration of virus into the cell or its release from the cell. The true biologic function of interferon is not clear. It may be a major factor in the intact host in recovery from viral infections, for it is present early in infection, during viremia, and before pathologic change occurs.

For clinical use administration of exogenous interferon would have real advantages. Repeated doses clearly afford antiviral and antitumor effects in experimental systems. Fortunately interferon is only weakly antigenic, or in homologous species may not be antigenic at all. Toxic effects have not been observed in animals. Interferon injections given subcutaneously, intramuscularly, intravenously, or intraperitoneally can provide antiviral protection in experimental systems. However, major logistic problems exist in production of sufficient quantities for effective dosage of patients. Methods are currently under study to produce sufficient quantities of human interferon (by mass cultures of human leukocytes or cell lines from other tissues). Also much work is under way to stabilize and characterize the interferon produced. Although it has now been a long time since interferons were discovered and the bright future predicted for these agents has been tarnished by frustration and passage of time, hope still exists that ways will be found to use these substances in manners and forms that will be practical and beneficial to man.

Perhaps more promising even than interferon for the immediate future are chemical agents that take advantage of developing understanding of the crucial relationships of viruses to human cells and the molecular biology of the function and persistence of viruses as parasites. For example, antimetabolites like BUDR and FUDR already are exerting significant clinical benefit in both topical and systemic therapy of viruses of the pox and herpes classes. Further, the semicarbasones, which are inexpensive and relatively nontoxic, have shown promise in prophylaxis for smallpox infection. Recently derivatives of Rifampin, useful in antituberculosis therapy and in treatment of leprosy, have apparently been used *in vitro* to interfere with viral influences on cells, e.g., malignant transformation.

VIRUSES AND DELAYED HYPERSENSITIVITY

Viruses clearly can induce delayed hypersensitivity. The practice of immunization with attenuated smallpox virus is an example of the production of delayed allergy and immunity following viral infection.

The observations concerning the responses to viral infection of patients with a variety of clinical syndromes, all accompanied by immunologic defect, support the view that cellular immunity, probably a function of T-cells is of importance in resistance to, and even immunity to, some viruses. Among the most important viruses frequently encountered to which cell-mediated immunity can represent effective defense are vaccinia, varicella, and herpes simplex. Measles seems to represent a special situation.

Skin reactivity of the tuberculin type to viral antigens has been demonstrated in man and animals following infection with a number of viruses, including smallpox, influenza, mumps, and herpes simplex. A positive reaction seems to be indicative of immunity.

A model in which manifestation of disease is associated with the immune response is lymphocytic choriomeningitis (LCM) infection in mice. Mice infected *in utero* or shortly after birth with LCM virus develop persisting infection capable of initiating destructive humoral immunity, but the virus is not eliminated from the body. Virus persists in high titer in the blood and many organs. The animal is resistant to challenge with LCM, but specific antibodies are hard to detect by conventional means. This response to infection was once considered to result from acquired immunologic tolerance to the virus. Normal mature animals inoculated with the same agent become ill, react to the virus with both cellular and humoral immunity, and if they do not die, recover completely. If treated with irradiation or drugs to suppress the immune response, however, the mature animal may develop the same host-parasite relation that is observed in newborn animals. Evidence that such animals fail to eliminate the virus because they lack T-cells and T-cell immunity to the agent has been developed experimentally with the demonstration that reconstitution of the immune response by thymus or spleen cells markedly reduces the viremia and virosis.

As was discovered by von Pirquet and clarified by the recent *in vitro* studies of Smithwick and Berkovich, patients having positive skin reactions to tuberculin may temporarily lose this response during clinical measles or following the administration of attenuated measles vaccine. This anergic state may last for weeks. Lymphocytes from such known tuberculin-positive individuals obtained during measles infection fail to undergo blast transformation when exposed *in vitro* to tuberculin.

The American Academy of Pediatrics recommends that children with positive tuberculin reactions "should be placed on antituberculous therapy before being given live measles vaccine" because of the possibility that exacerbation of tuberculosis may occur on administration of measles vaccine as it has during natural measles infection. The temporary loss of skin reactivity and the diminished *in vitro* mitogenic response to tuberculin during measles infection is assumed to result from an interaction between virus and lymphocyte. A variety of other viral agents can profoundly affect cellular immunities, perhaps by means analogous to those used by the measles virus. We have recently been quantifying responses of lymphocytes in healthy laboratory personnel. Not infrequently the number of cells capable of responding to this mitogen are much reduced in the blood. Almost invariably change in responsive cells is associated with a prodrome of a virus respiratory disease.

IMMUNIZATION AGAINST VIRAL DISEASES

Smallpox

Smallpox vaccine is prepared from vaccinia virus that has been maintained alternately on the skin of a rabbit and the skin of a sheep or a calf. The virus is scarified into a wide area of cleaned and shaved skin. Material from the mature vesicular eruption is then collected by a sharp spoon and is ground and suspended in 1 percent phenol. Glycerol is added and the vaccine is stored at $-10°$ C. This form of vaccine is often known as glycerinated lymph.

Smallpox vaccine is also grown in embryonated eggs of chickens or ducks in tissue culture of suitable cells such as bovine amnion. The virus obtained this way is free of bacteria and is further purified, freeze-dried, and stored at a temperature below $10°$ C. This is the form most commonly used today, but in susceptible persons it may induce sensitivity to egg protein or reactions to protein.

Vaccination is carried out by first preparing a clean area of skin, placing vaccine on the skin, and inoculating into the epidermis by a single scratch about 1 cm long or by the multiple pressure method. In a primary reaction a red elevated papule is noted at the third or fourth day after vaccination, which is followed by vesiculation, intense inflammation, and pustulation by the ninth day. Some degree of pyrexia and tenderness of regional lymph nodes regularly occurs. The lesion then begins to subside, a scab forms, and the entire lesion heals by approximately the eighteenth day. Only vaccination which results in vesiculation should be accepted as being successful. *Vaccinoid* or accelerated response is seen in persons revaccinated within a few years after a successful primary vaccination. These reactions are characterized by the same events cited above except that the lesions evolve more quickly, are more intense very early, but do not become as extensive as in the primary response, and subside more promptly. After successful vaccination immunity to small-pox lasts about 3 years. Thereafter it wanes gradually until 20 years later no protective effect is seen.

In the highly immunized person an immediate reaction occurs. In this response almost immediately evidence of delayed hypersensitivity is ex-perienced, and usually neither vesicle nor pustule is experienced. Patients with the most extreme form of X-linked infantile agammaglobulinemia have repeatedly been infected with vaccinia virus. Although they may have a slightly prolonged primary reaction, they become immune with-out producing circulating antibodies in demonstrable amounts and can develop accelerated and even immediate immune reactions almost as readily as can persons with vigorous humoral immunity. Their clinical immunity must depend on the vigorous cell-mediated immunity which they can be shown to develop to the virus.

Apart from bacterial infection of the site of vaccination and occasional keloid formation, three major complications have been observed—gener-alized vaccinia, vaccinia gangrenosa, and postvaccinal encephalitis. The former two occur during the second week after vaccination and are pres-ent in children with defects of the T-cell immunity system. These pa-tients regularly die of either of these complications, although treatment using massive doses of immune serum and immune cells has sometimes been effective. Postvaccinal encephalitis is also a most serious and prob-ably the most frequent complication. The highest incidence has been noted between 6 and 12 years of age. Symptoms appear first during the second week after vaccination and are characterized by the features of disseminated encephalomyelitis. Since this complication occurs 10 to 30 times more often between 6 and 12 years of age than in infants under 1 year of age, if vaccinia is to be used, it is advantageous to vaccinate in-fants before they reach 2 years of age.

The second complication also occurs with high frequency in persons having eczema of any kind, but particularly in children with atopic ec-zema. Patients with Wiskott-Aldrich syndrome have been particularly vulnerable on three counts. They have well-established deficits of cellular immunity, eczema, and insufficient platelets. Thus they often develop disseminated hemorrhagic and gangrenous vaccinia (Fig. 33-1).

Recently, after agonizing discussion, routine vaccination of infants against smallpox has been removed from recommended routine immuni-zations in the United States. This is because the complications cited above now outweigh the risks of the smallpox itself. The reasoning be-hind this discontinuation is that in the United States (1) we now have strong herd immunity to smallpox, (2) only one virus, easily identifiable, in one vector, man, is responsible for the disease, (3) we have on reserve an immunizing agent that can be called upon should an epidemic break

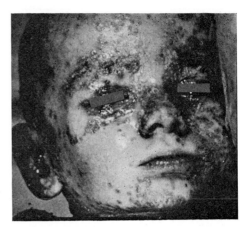

Fig. 33-1. Hemorrhagic and gangrenous vaccinia after smallpox vaccination in an infant with severe combined immunodeficiency disease. Such complication is usually fatal.

out, (4) chemical prophylaxis against this disease is effective and could be used in the United States if necessary, and (5) the development of a killed-virus-antigen vaccine or further attenuated virus vaccine seems close at hand.

Poliomyelitis

The Salk polio vaccine, a killed virus vaccine that was introduced in 1954, consisted of strains of virus derived from each of the three main antigenic groups which were grown in monkey kidney cells maintained in tissue culture and then inactivated with formalin. The trial results indicated that vaccination provided a marked, but not complete, protection against paralytic disease. Three injections of the vaccine were usually given, but later indications were that a fourth dose resulted in a higher and much better maintained antibody response.

This vaccination, which proved most effective in diminishing the incidence of central nervous system disease because of an essential viremia antecedent to the latter was for the most part abandoned in the United States in favor of a live virus vaccine. The primary base of this abandonment was the demonstration that immunization permitted virus infection of the gastrointestinal tract. It was presumed that such immunization, although most effective in preventing clinical paralysis from polio infection, could not eradicate the infecting viruses. To the surprise of many, the Swedes have been using an improved killed virus vaccine. With widespread use of this vaccine they have succeeded in eliminating not only clinical polio but also infection with this virus from their land.

Infection with poliovirus, even when subclinical, is followed by long-lasting immunity, and subclinical infection (if this could be guaranteed) would, therefore, appear to be an ideal form of prophylaxis. To achieve this end, Cox and then Sabin developed attenuated strains of poliomyelitis virus which can multiply in the cells of the human intestinal tract and stimulate immunity, but which have lost the ability to invade and attack the central nervous system. Sabin's strains of virus can be grown in monkey kidney tissue culture under conditions similar to those for growing virus for inactivated vaccine. Live vaccine composed of a mixture of attenuated strains of the three main types of poliomyelitis virus has been administered orally to many millions of children in several countries of the world. The virus has been found not only to grow in the intestinal tract of the children who were consciously infected but also to spread to other children or adults in contact with them. Intervals of 4 to 6 weeks should be allowed to elapse between successive feedings of the virus, the reason being that one type of poliovirus may be prevented from establishing itself in the intestines while one or both of the other types are multiplying, a process that may last 4 to 6 weeks after the initial infection.

Among the advantages of oral vaccines are that they are relatively cheap, since much smaller quantities of virus can be used to establish infection, they are easy to administer on a large scale, being simply placed on a lump of sugar or actually incorporated into sweets, and they presumably can better defend against infection and transmission of the mild viruses. Such vaccines can be preserved in a frozen state for long periods of time.

Oral poliovirus vaccine also has the advantage that it can be used in the face of an epidemic; large numbers of persons can be immunized by feeding the vaccine during a very short period. Field trials have shown that such procedures can effectively halt the course of an epidemic. On the other hand, injection of killed vaccine was thought not to prevent the vaccinated subject from being locally infected and shedding the virus. Thus the normal cycle of transmission of the virus in the community was expected not to be broken, and the vaccinated subject was thought to be a possible carrier.

The relative merits of inactivated and attenuated vaccines have led to much controversy that is not yet resolved. Occasional adults and very few children have developed poliomyelitis from a strain of the vaccine virus. In immunodeficient patients, both adults and children, exposure to live virus has produced continuing infection that may have serious consequences.

Rabies

In 1885 Pasteur vaccinated, apparently successfully, a boy who had been bitten by a rabid dog with a suspension of dried spinal cord from a rabbit which had been infected with virulent rabies virus. Drying the infected nervous tissue had successfully attenuated the virus in it. Rabies in man is a disease of a variable, but generally a long, incubation period, and Pasteur considered that sufficient time might be available to immunize the patient in the interval between the bite and the onset of the disease. The Pasteurian method, using dried infected rabbit spinal cord, is still used in some countries, but most health authorities now favor a vaccine (Semple type) prepared from the ground-up brains of infected sheep or rabbits in which the virus is killed with phenol or β-propiolactone. The presence of nervous tissue in the vaccine makes it potentially dangerous. It may cause demyelination in the patient by a process apparently analogous to the experimental allergic encephalomyelitis that can readily be produced in several different species of animals by injecting either homologous or heterologous brain tissue with adjuvants. The reported incidence of this complication following rabies vaccination varies from country to country but is probably 1:4,000 to 1:10,000 of patients treated with vaccines containing central nervous system tissue.

Bites and other wounds should be given local treatment by thorough washing with soap and water. Severe bite wounds on the face or finger call for immediate application of antirabies serum, some of which should be infiltrated beneath the wound if possible. The serum is prepared in horses and "refined" by pepsin digestion. The recommended dose of serum is 40 IU/kg body weight. At least 14 daily doses of vaccine should be given, and in high risk cases, in which serum is also given, further doses of vaccine should be given 10 and 20 days after the conclusion of this treatment. These later injections of vaccine are likely to produce extremely painful local lesions, especially when central nervous system tissue is present in the vaccine.

In recent years vaccine free from encephalitogenic nervous tissue has been prepared from a virus grown in duck embryos and inactivated with β-propiolactone. This is already extensively used for prophylactic vaccination of veterinary and other workers whose occupations involve contact with possibly rabid animals. A different approach to the preparation of safe rabies vaccine is to grow the virus in the brains of very young animals. Infected brains of rats and mice harvested before the start of myelination are a rich source of fixed rabies virus, yet are nonencephalitogenic when tested in guinea pigs. Human subjects injected with them have developed very satisfactory high concentrations of neutralizing antibody.

Yellow Fever

Yellow fever vaccine is another live vaccine. It was developed when it was found that a certain strain of yellow fever virus (17D) would multiply in chick embryo tissue cultures and retain its virulence for mice, but after 100 passages become attenuated and quite avirulent for man. It must be borne in mind that the vaccines contain a considerable amount of egg protein which can cause severe reactions in persons with atopic hypersensitivity to eggs. The vaccine is prepared in freeze-dried form and is reconstituted in saline solution immediately before use. It retains its potency, when dried, for at least a year at $0°$, but loses potency within a few days at room temperature. All vaccine not used within 30 minutes after reconstitution should be discarded because of the instability of the virus.

A single subcutaneous dose (usually 0.5 ml) establishes immunity within 10 to 12 days, which endures for at least 6 years. If both smallpox and yellow fever immunization are required, yellow fever inoculation should always precede smallpox vaccination by at least 4 days. If small-pox vaccination has been carried out first, there should be an interval of 21 days before yellow fever inoculation. This relationship of immuniza-tions is necessary to avoid interference of the one virus with the other. Recently a mouse brain 17D vaccine has been introduced. Two vaccina-tions by the scratch technique, using this preparation, separated by an interval of 14 days have been shown to give 98 percent protection against yellow fever.

Measles

In certain of the developing countries measles has a high mortality, and even in the United States the morbidity and mortality attributable di-rectly and indirectly to native measles infection is sufficient to make an effective prophylactic vaccine necessary. Unfortunately none of the live virus measles vaccines available at present is completely satisfactory. At-tenuated live measles virus vaccines have been developed by repeatedly passing measles virus through human, monkey, and chick embryo cells. The vaccines produce long-lasting immunity but have sometimes pro-voked severe pyrexial reactions and more rarely, central nervous system reactions, e.g., convulsions.

Inactivated virus vaccines have failed to provide long-lasting immu-nity and are therefore not of much value except perhaps for prophylaxis against severe reactions that might otherwise be encountered with live virus vaccines. Indeed, prior immunization with killed vaccine has set the stage for a most severe skin reactivity that reveals an underlying sensi-tivity while permitting infection with native virus or even vaccine virus. This hypersensitivity reaction, which can be lethal, controverts the use of the killed virus vaccine in any of its present forms. The measles vaccine currently in use in the United States, although producing some reactions, should be widely used because it is safe and effective. Moreover, it has the potentiality of achieving an effective herd immunity.

Influenza

Successful prophylactic vaccination against influenza is difficult to achieve. The humoral immunity produced is short-lived. Influenza viruses vary in their antigenic constitution from one epidemic to another. The first influenza A strain was isolated in 1933, and antigenic variation within this strain was recognized when viruses recovered from different epidemics were found to be antigenically different from one another. In 1946 an antigenic variant, A1, appeared in Australia and spread so that all epidemics for the next few years were caused by this virus. In 1956 another new A variant appeared, A2 or Asian virus, which was responsible for the pandemic of 1957. In 1940 in New York a virus markedly different in its antigenic make-up appeared and was called type B. Antigenic variants of this have also been found since 1940. Another variant, type C, is known but has not caused epidemics. Still more recently the Hong Kong variant has appeared, which is an additional variety of the A strain.

During the 1957 epidemic caused by the "Asian" variety of influenza A a vaccine containing the new strain of virus was prepared, and a controlled mass immunization effort was mobilized in time to test its efficacy. Clinically significant infection was cut to approximately one third in the group vaccinated with the new vaccine.

Influenza vaccine is prepared by growing strains of virus in the allantoic cavity of chick embryos, as currently recommended by the World Influenza Center of the World Health Organization. The allantoic fluids are inactivated with 0.01 percent formaldehyde in the cold, and the virus is purified (e.g., by centrifugation) and resuspended in buffered saline. Such treatment destroys infectivity but permits retention of hemagglutinating activity for fowl red cells and antigenicity. The vaccine is stable at 2° to 10° C for at least 18 months and for about one week at room temperature. Two adequately spaced doses of killed vaccine are recommended for primary immunization, although one dose may be given when an epidemic is imminent. Administration of the recommended influenza vaccine is especially important for the elderly and for patients having chronic lung, heart, and renal disease.

Given as a single deep subcutaneous injection, not less than 10 days before exposure to infection, it may be expected to confer protection for a few months. In some vaccines a mineral carrier or oily adjuvant is incorporated, and although higher antibody titers have been obtained, these types of vaccines have not been generally accepted. A living attenuated virus vaccine that is used as a nasal spray has been developed in Russia. Unlike the killed vaccine, this live prophylactic is said to be effective even when used in the face of an influenza epidemic. This vaccine has not yet been evaluated in the United States. We visited the laboratories in the Soviet Union where the vaccine was being evaluated, and the data supporting its effectiveness seemed quite impressive.

The great pandemics of influenza seem always to be attributed to appearance of a new immunogenetic variant of the virus. This phenomenon has been attributed by Beveridge and others to hybrid forms of virus developing when a human strain and a native animal strain of the virus infect the same host at the same time and hybridize within commonly infected cells.

Mumps

Mumps is a common childhood disease that may be severely and even permanently crippling when it involves the brain, testis, ovary, auditory nerves, or pancreas. Usually the meningoencephalitis is self-limited, and permanent damage either does not occur or is minimal and not easily measured. Adult males may be permanently sterilized by mumps. These serious complications seem to justify development and application of a safe and effective live virus vaccine. Buynak and Hilleman in 1966 developed a live, attenuated mumps virus vaccine referred to as the Jeryl Lynn strain, level B. Given subcutaneously, this vaccine produces a non-contagious infection causing only a mild reaction that results in a mumps antibody response in almost all recipients.

Recently Kupers et al. reported a significant depression of the tuberculin skin reaction following inoculation with the live, attenuated mumps vaccine. If this finding is confirmed and established, it may be advisable to do tuberculin skin tests before vaccination with live, attenuated mumps virus, just as with measles vaccination, and to watch carefully for untoward influences of the vaccine attributable to its capacity to induce an anergic state.

SELECTED REFERENCES

Slow Virus Infection

Day, S. B., and Good, R. A. (eds.) (1972): *Membranes and Viruses in Immunopathology.* New York, Academic Press, Inc.
Eklund, C. M., Kennedy, R. C., and Hadlow, W. J. (1967): J. Infect. Dis. *117*:15.
Gajdusek, D. C., Gibbs, C. J., and Alpers, M. (1966): Nature *209*:794.
Gajdusek, D. C., et al. (1968): Science *162*:693.
Gibbs, C. J., et al. (1968): Science *161*:388.
Johnson, R. T., and Mims, C. A. (1968): New Eng. J. Med. *278*:23.
Kenyon, A. J., et al. (1973): Science *179*:187.

Rubella and Congenital Rubella Syndrome

Dent, P. B., et al. (1968): Lancet *1*:291.
Gilmartin, R. C., Jabbour, J. T., and Duenas, D. A. (1972): J. Pediat. *80*:406.
Gregg, N. M. (1942): Trans. Ophthal. Soc. Aust. *3*:35.
Hancock, M. P., Huntley, C. C., and Sever, J. L. (1968): J. Pediat. *72*:636.
International Conference on Rubella Immunization (1969): Amer. J. Dis. Child. *118*:1.
Kilroy, A. W., et al. (1970): JAMA *214*:2287.
Klock, L. E., and Rachelefsky, G. S. (1973): New Eng. J. Med. *288*:69.
Menser, M. A., Dods, L., and Harley, J. D. (1967): Lancet *2*:1347.
Meyer, H. M., Parkman, P. D., and Panos, T. C. (1966): New Eng. J. Med. *275*:575.
Mims, C. A. (1968): Progr. Med. Virol. *10*:194.

Montgomery, J. R. et al. (1967): *157*:1068.
Olson, G. B., et al. (1968): J. Exp. Med. *128*:47.
Plotkin, S. A., Klaus, R. M., and Whitely, J. P. (1966): J. Pediat. *69*:1085.
Rawls, W. E. (1968): Progr. Med. Virol. *10*:238.
Rubella Symposium (1965): Amer. J. Dis. Child. *110*:345.
Schimke, R. N., Bolano, C., and Kirkpatrick, C. H. (1969): Amer. J. Dis. Child. *118*:626 .
Weinstein, L., and Chang, T. (1973): New Eng. J. Med. *288*:100.
White, L. R., et al. (1968): J. Pediat. *73*:229.

Cytomegalovirus Infections

Jesionek, and Kiolemenoglou (1904): Munch. Med. Wschr. *51*:1905.
Krech, U. H., Jung, M., and Jung, F. (1971): *Cytomegalovirus Infections of Man.* Basel, S. Karger.
Ribbert, H. (1904): Zbl. Allg. Path. *15*:945.
Starr, J. G., Bart, R. D., and Gold, E. (1970): New Eng. J. Med. *282*:1075.
Weller, T. H. (1971): New Eng. J. Med. *285*:203.

Interferon and Other Antiviral Agents

Glasgow, L. A. (1965): J. Pediat. *67*:104.
Grossberg, S. E. (1972): New Eng. J. Med. *287*:13.
Hossain, M. S., et al. (1972): Lancet *2*:1230.
Isaacs, A., and Lindenmann, J. (1957): Proc. Roy. Soc. London (Biol.) *147*:258.

Viruses and Delayed Hypersensitivity

Burnet, F. M. (1968): Lancet *2*:610.
Kupers, T. A., et al. (1970): J. Pediat. *76*:716.
Miller, L. H., and Brunell, P. A. (1970): Amer. J. Med. *49*:480.
Olson, G. B., et al. (1968): J. Exp. Med. *128*:47.
Smithwick, E. M., and Berkovich, S. (1966): Proc. Soc. Exp. Biol. Med. *123*:276.
Starr, S., and Berkovich, S. (1964): New Eng. J. Med. *270*:386.
Torphy, D. E., et al. (1970): J. Pediat. *76*:405.

Immunization against Viral Diseases

Arbeter, A. M., et al. (1972): J. Pediat. *81*:737.
Beveridge, W. I. B. (1972): *Frontiers in Comparative Medicine.* Minneapolis, Minnesota, University of Minnesota Press.
Buynak, E. B., and Hilleman, M. R. (1966): Proc. Soc. Exp. Biol. Med. *123*:768.
Editorial (1971): Lancet *2*:1127.
Feigin, R. D., Guggenheim, M. A., and Johnsen, S. D. (1961): J. Pediat. *79*:642.
Hilleman, M. R., et al. (1967): New Eng. J. Med. *276*:252.
Imagawa, D. T. (1968): Progr. Med. Virol. *10*:160.
International Conference on Rubella Immunization (1969): Amer. J. Dis. Child. *118*:1.
Karzon, D. T. (1972): J. Pediat. *81*:600.
Krugman, S. (1971): J. Pediat. *78*:1.
Krugman, S., et al. (1965): J. Pediat. *66*:471.
Kupers, T. A., et al. (1970): J. Pediat. *76*:716.
Kuwert, E., et al. (1972): Deutsch. Med. Wschr. *97*:1893.
Meyer, H. M. (1968): J. Pediat. *73*:653.
Miller, L. H., and Brunell, P. A. (1970): Amer. J. Med. *49*:480.
Riker, J. B., et al. (1971): Pediatrics *48*:923.
Warin, J. F., Harker, P., and Mayon-White, R. T. (1972): Lancet *2*:810.
Wilkins, J., Williams, F. F., and Wehrle, P. F. (1972): Amer. J. Dis. Child. *124*:66.

34

Bacterial, Fungal, and Parasitic Diseases

TUBERCULOSIS

Tuberculosis is a chronic infection causing overt signs and symptoms in only a fraction of infected individuals. Infection with Mycobacterium tuberculosis is indicated by positive tuberculin reaction, and at present less than 15 percent of the population in the United States show positive tuberculin tests. However, in the developing countries, the rate of M. tuberculosis infection is higher and ranks among the highest causes of mortality and morbidity. Similarly in times of malnutrition, even in otherwise highly developed nations, as existed in postwar Europe, tuberculosis jumps to the fore as one of the greatest threats to the existence of man.

In addition to infections with M. tuberculosis, infection with a group of acid-fast bacilli variously termed atypical, anomalous, anonymous, or unclassified mycobacteria occurs. The latter are antigenically related to M. tuberculosis and can be assigned to four categories on the basis of various cultural characteristics: (I) photochromogens, (II) scotochromogens, (III) nonchromogens, and (IV) rapidly growing pigmented organisms. Infections with these organisms can produce granulomatous disease that is localized to skin and lymph nodes or lungs or is even widely disseminated throughout the body. Another allergic disease recently attributed to the atypical acid-fast bacilli, as well as other organisms that can grow in humidifiers or air conditioners, is the farmers' lung illness attributable to allergy to organisms in the home. As Rich has clearly pointed out, in the hypersensitive animal a bland antigenic substance behaves as though it were an acute toxin, inducing reactions varying from mild inflammation to necrosis of tissue and even death when given systemically.

In delayed hypersensitivity, convincing evidence has never come forth that humoral antibody bears any causal relationship to the tissue reactivity or damage. Presumably the destructive activity of the antigen in delayed hypersensitivity results from a direct interaction with sensitized T-cells with which the antigen comes into contact. Further, factors produced by intermediary cells analogous to histamine release from mast cells and the pharmacologic agents that act in antibody-conditioned responses have been demonstrated in bacterial allergy. Nevertheless, materials—lymphokines—released by lymphocytes themselves on contact with antigen when injected into the skin can cause increased capillary permeability, inflammation, accumulation of mononuclear cells, and tissue destruction.

How far is tuberculin hypersensitivity responsible for the disease manifestations in man? This is a difficult and controversial problem. As in many other such complicated problems, analysis will depend upon accurate measurement of the many simultaneous and interacting phenomena. In tuberculous infection in man we are sadly deficient in methods for measurement of such factors, and the argument from artificial experiments, often employing relatively vast doses of bacillary products, is filled with pitfalls.

Tubercle bacilli of various kinds can cause severe toxic reactions if injected in sufficient quantity. However, there is no indication that, weight for weight, the bacterial bodies of virulent strains are any more toxic than are those of attenuated or avirulent strains of mycobacteria.

The idea that hypersensitivity accounts for the tissue damage in human tuberculous infection such as the caseation and cavitation, as well as the general toxemia, lassitude, and wasting, is based on analogies drawn from the experimental infections in guinea pigs.

The events of the Koch phenomenon are often compared with results of so-called primary and postprimary (or reactivation) types of disease in man. The primary complex consists of the usually small peripheral pulmonary granuloma (Ghon focus) with enlarged granulomatous draining lymph nodes. This may be compared to an early state of affairs in the guinea pig. However, whereas in the latter the progressive multiplication of tubercule bacilli and their spread by lymphatic channels eventually leads to generalized miliary tuberculosis and death, in man the primary complex usually regresses to a small fibrotic and sometimes calcified pulmonary focus which may include for prolonged periods living tubercle bacilli. Even though such an individual remains intimately exposed to persons with open tuberculosis, it is rare to find evidence at autopsy that a second primary complex has occurred. Reactivation disease takes the form of a gradually evolving caseous and fibrotic pulmonary focus without lymph node involvement. The inference is that this altered behavior in the reactivation stage depends upon the acquisition of hypersensitivity. An event such as sudden bronchopneumonic extension or cavitation is regarded as the more violent manifestation of such hypersensitivity.

The complexity of these relations, however, has become apparent in subsequent analysis. Although it seems quite certain that some manifestations of tuberculosis may be attributable to cell-mediated immunity, it has become even more apparent that resistance to the virulent forms of the tubercle bacillus also is attributable in large measure to delayed allergy and cell-mediated immunities. An experiment with a similar infection has shown that specific T lymphocyte-mediated immunity can, after engagement with antigen, stimulate proliferation and activation of the phagocytic population of cells and can enhance resistance to facultative intracellular bacterial pathogens like tubercle bacilli. Furthermore, BCG immunization is effective in proportion to the cell-mediated immunity produced, and patients with extreme forms of agammaglobulinemia who have intact cellular immunities can resist primary infection effectively with human tuberculosis bacilli and BCG. By contrast, immunodeficient patients who lack the cellular immune mechanism often develop fulminating and lethal tuberculosis, atypical acid-fast infections, and even disseminated BCG infections or BCGosis.

The classic Mantoux test employed for the detection of delayed hypersensitivity in tuberculosis is carried out by intradermal injection of Old Tuberculin (OT), or purified protein derivative (PPD). The OT is used on the basis of dilution: 0.10 ml of 1:10,000 dilution (equivalent of 0.00002 mg of PPD) is generally employed as an initial test dose and is referred to as "first strength" or "1 unit." The "second strength" dose is 0.00005 mg of PPD or 1:100 dilution of OT.

The skin test is read at 48 hours or 72 hours. The lower limit of a positive reaction is 5 mm of induration, but recently 8 to 10 mm have become a more generally accepted criterion of positive reaction. Reactivity to tuberculin in man may be depressed by some intercurrent events, measles (natural and vaccinated), poliomyelitis, mumps (natural and vaccinated), and other situations where cell-mediated immunity is impaired. It may indeed be that such intercurrent events temporarily lessen the vigor of cell-mediated immunity and account for reactivation of tuberculosis more than does the hypersensitivity to which reactivation of the disease was previously attributed.

The vaccine most widely used in man and experimental animals for induction of immunity against tuberculosis is composed of attenuated viable organisms called BCG (bacille Calmette Guérin). The vaccination provides protection in more than 80 percent of recipients. Development of antimicrobial drugs, isonicotinic acid hydrazide (INH), para-aminosalicylic acid (PAS), and streptomycin have, of course, enhanced the effective control and treatment of tuberculosis in man and the prevention of the devastating complications from dissemination of the organisms to children.

LEPROSY

At least 12 to 15 million persons are estimated to have leprosy in the world today. Mycobacterium leprae is accepted as the etiologic agent of human leprosy and was the first bacterium to be identified under the microscope as the cause of a disease in man.

Infection by M. leprae results in a chronic inflammatory response that varies greatly in its histologic and clinical features. Two polar forms of leprosy have been defined, i.e., tuberculoid and lepromatous leprosy.

Tuberculoid leprosy is so called because of its resemblance to cutaneous tuberculosis. This disease is a granulomatous inflammatory disease. The classic dermal lesion is a well-defined plaque that is erythematous or hypopigmented and has elevated margins. The histopathology resembles that of sarcoidosis with foci of well-developed epithelioid cells extending into the papillary stoma up to the basal cells of the epidermis. Giant cells of the Langhans type are frequent with this form of disease. Nerve destruction is a characteristic. Clinically the patient with this form of disease can be expected to do relatively well, except for the paresis or paralysis secondary to peripheral nerve damage.

Lepromatous leprosy represents the other polar form of the disease and is by far the more serious. Multiple macules with poorly defined borders or small nodules may be scattered symmetrically over the entire body. Involvement of nasal mucous membranes is almost universal, and large numbers of leprosy bacilli are shed from these lesions.

Between the two poles of pure tuberculoid and pure lepromatous leprosy may be found many other forms of the disease complex that share some, but not all, of the characteristics of the polar types. Some forms of leprosy, however, defy simple classification.

Mitsuda, in 1919, reported that intradermal injection of a boiled emulsion of bacteria (integral lepromin) obtained from lepromatous nodules caused no reaction in patients with lepromatous leprosy but a positive reaction in apparently normal patients and in those with tuberculoid leprosy. The reaction to this mixture of antigens is a biphasic phenomenon, i.e., a typical tuberculin type of reaction within 48 hours and a progressive local inflammation of the site producing a nodule that may undergo central necrosis at 3 to 4 weeks.

Dharmendra partially separated bacilli from tissues, prepared an extract, and resuspended the bacilli in a concentration of 1 mg of dry bacterial powder per 10 ml of carbol-saline. This type of lepromin induces positive reactions at 48 hours, probably a reflection of delayed allergy. The late reaction at 3 to 4 weeks is minimal.

The lepromin reaction is not specific for leprosy because most normal adults give positive results. Vaccination with BCG has been shown to induce a positive lepromin reaction in lepromatous leprosy in more than 50 percent of instances. Young children are generally lepromin negative and become lepromin positive as they grow older. Recently, Lim et al. have found lepromin reactions to be frequently negative in adults in Minnesota where exposure to tubercle bacilli is very low.

Growing evidence indicates that patients with leprosy may have some degree of generalized impairment of the delayed hypersensitivity responses; i.e., they have a depressed lymphocytes response to PHA stimulation, a depressed skin reaction of the delayed type, depleted thymus dependent areas of lymph node, and skin allograft rejections somewhat less vigorous than in normal persons. Patients with lepromatous disease frequently exhibit a marked elevation of the gamma globulins and hypoalbuminemia. Approximately 85 to 95 percent of sera from lepromatous patients contain demonstrable antibodies to M. leprae and other mycobacteria and frequently have a biologically false positive test for syphilis. The best evidence indicates that the cell-mediated immunities of these patients to lepra bacilli or their components are much more grossly defective than are the cell-mediated immunities to other organisms. Interestingly, we have recently found that the number of B lymphocytes in the circulation are both relatively and absolutely increased in patients with lepromatous leprosy.

The keystone to effective therapy in leprosy is diaminodiphenylsulfone (DDS) and its analogues which presumably act on M. leprae by competitive inhibition of para-aminobenzoic acid to form active analogues of dihydropteroic acid. The establishment of a model for experimental leprosy by Rees in neonatally thymectomized or athymic mice has provided a new way of studying the pathogenetic mechanism and chemotherapy of leprosy. In addition, it has recently been established that the 9-banded armadillo is extremely susceptible to infection with M. leprae without any manipulation. These two experimental models make it certain that rapid progress in control of infections by lepra bacilli will be made. Already it is apparent that improved antibiotics will be available. For example, rifampicin and its derivatives seem to be much more potent than is DDS. One of the major problems of effective treatment of lepra bacilli is the reaction that may be induced by this therapy. Erythema nodosum leprosa, a serious and frequent complication even of untreated lepromatous leprosy, is a common concomitant of effective therapy. The reaction can sometimes be controlled by treatment with adrenal corticosteroids. However, thalidomide treatment seems even more effective in controlling such reactions, but its mechanism of action remains obscure.

Transfer factor has been used in attempts to alter reactivity to Dharmendra lepromin of patients with lepromatous leprosy. This treatment not only converted some patients from negative to positive reactors but seemed to produce mild symptoms like those sometimes seen in so-called reversal reactions. These observations have raised hopes that more vigorous treatment with the dialyzable transfer factor of Lawrence may have promise in clinical treatment of this disease.

Another novel form of therapy has recently been proposed by Lim et al. In these studies most dramatic clinical, bacteriologic and histopathologic improvement has been attributable to cellular engineering achieved by weekly injections of allogeneic leukocytes from different donors. This method has resulted in extraordinarily rapid elimination of bacteria from the tissues and apparently has promise in both lepromatous and tuberculoid leprosy. Controlled studies of this approach are needed, and its mechanism of action must be precisely elucidated. At present the working hypothesis is that the mismatched leukocytes react with host antigens to produce lymphokines that activate and facilitate function of macrophages of the lepromatous patient. Objections to this approach have been raised on the basis of experiments in mice that show that graft-versus-host reactions can activate oncogenic RNA virus infections. However, rather extensive experience with graft-versus-host reactions in bone marrow transplantation programs has not revealed any evidence of activation of RNA viruses of any kind in man. Worries about the hazard from graft-versus-host reaction in this form of therapy have not been supported by experience to date and seem to us to be unfounded because patients with lepromatous leprosy regularly reject skin allografts. Perhaps the most important aspect of these studies is that they show the potential of cellular engineering in treating persistent infections. Whether cells themselves will be required or whether their products can substitute or be safely induced to take the place of the lymphoid cells themselves will only be established by further careful experimental and clinical studies. This approach using cellular engineering may be effective for chronic virus infections, malignant disease, other persistent bacterial infections, and even some parasitic diseases.

A specific staphylococcal lysate has been tested in the nonspecific therapy of leprosy. This product of staphylococci seems to be able nonspecifically to stimulate cell-mediated immunities. In controlled studies in patients with lepromatous leprosy this staphylococcal product was shown to have a beneficial influence in the treatment of lepromatous leprosy.

BRUCELLOSIS

Three species of Brucella are known to cause brucellosis in animals and man: Brucella abortus, Brucella melitensis, and Brucella suis. Human beings, especially veterinarians and farmers, can be accidentally infected from domestic cattle or other animals. The symptomatology is often related to the development of delayed hypersensitivity to the brucella organism.

Theobald Smith first recognized the remarkable intracellular proliferation of brucella organisms in bovine fetal membrane of aborted material. Why do the brucellosis organisms have such predilection to the reproductive organs for its multiplication? Recent studies indicate that the tissues of animal species highly susceptible to infection by brucellae con tain large amounts of erythritol, whereas tissues of highly resistant animal species contain little or none of this carbohydrate molecule, a chemical essential for growth of brucellae *in vitro.* This discovery may have wider implications for other kinds of infection, natural immunity, and host-parasite relationships.

In man, following invasion of the blood stream, the organisms quickly localize in reticuloendothelial tissues, e.g., liver, spleen, bone marrow, and lymph nodes. The key cells of host defense against brucellae appear to be macrophages. The evolution of the noncaseating granuloma is considered to be a reflection of cell-mediated immunity and host defense. The most common complication is spondylitis. Suppuration of the liver, spleen, and kidney is most often associated with Brucella suis infection, whereas meningitis can be due to any of the three species.

The most commonly recognized immune response is the appearance of agglutinins at the end of the first week of infection, and the highest titers occur between the second and fourth weeks. The 19S IgM agglutinins appear first; 7S IgG agglutinin is detected later. The persistence of 7S IgG agglutinins indicates continuing active disease. Since the 7S IgG antibodies can fix complement, the complement-fixation reaction is a sensitive test for the detection of active brucellosis.

The chronic stage of human brucellosis is reached usually in 3 to 6 months, and the blocking antibodies, IgG, may appear with a concomitant prozone phenomenon. Precipitins for the carbohydrate fraction of brucellae have been detected in the blood of patients with acute illness of experimental brucellosis. This carbohydrate fraction of the organisms can elicit an immediate skin reaction and Prausnitz-Küstner transfer, and the latter is almost certainly a reflection of an IgE antibody against brucella antigen. These 7S antibodies appear to be a valuable distinguishing feature in differentiating active from inactive disease in patients having ill-defined complaints, sterile blood cultures, and low titers of brucella agglutinins.

Brucellosis can be designated as a disease of intracellular parasitism. Intracellular brucellae are protected from the bactericidal action of human sera and from antibiotics.

Immunization with Brucella abortus strain 19 has been highly effective in cattle but a disappointment in sheep and goats. In Russia, strain 19 has been used as a live vaccine in man, but because of frequent complications it has not been recommended by the World Health Organization (WHO) for general use throughout the world. The most effective treatment of brucellosis is the use of tetracycline.

HEMOPHILUS INFLUENZAE

In 1933, Fothergill and Wright described the occurrence of Hemophilus influenzae type B meningitis to be inversely related to the presence of bactericidal activity of blood for this organism. They pointed out that while the incidence of influenzal meningitis was highest in children 2 to 36 months of age, unusual in neonates, and rare in older children and adults, blood bactericidal activity was usually present in neonates, declined in infants at about the age of 2 months, and remained absent until about the age of 3 years. An increasing proportion of children over 3 years of age acquired such activity so that by age 10 or above the blood of all tested individuals demonstrated bactericidal antibodies.

Hemophilus influenzae causes several human diseases; the most significant morbidity and mortality rates occur in infants and children. The exact incidence of disease caused by this organism has not been established.

The most serious disease caused by Hemophilus influenzae type B is bacterial meningitis in children under the age of 4 years in the United States and throughout the world. A recent increase in the absolute, as well as the proportional, frequency of meningitis due to this organism has been reported. In spite of antibiotic therapy, the mortality rate remains at about 10 percent, and neurologic sequelae persist in a substantial proportion of survivors.

Hemophilus influenzal meningitis occurs most frequently in children between the ages of 6 months and 3 years when antibody titers to these organisms are very low. Maternal antibodies transferred across the placenta are presumed to be effective in protection of neonates from this disease. Rather surprisingly, however, Norden et al. and Greenfield et al. observed that young children infected with Hemophilus influenzae type B often do not show an antibody response in the convalescent period following infections. The reason for the apparent inadequacies of the response of children to this organism at this age needs further study. Children 6 months to 2 years have a well-developed immunity system and show vigorous immune responses to many infections and antigens. Explanation could be achieved by considering the antigen of these pathogens to be one to which the responsiveness develops late in ontogeny. Alternatively, these findings could be explained by increased susceptibility of the host at this age to development of immunologic paralysis to the quantities of antigen delivered by the infecting organisms producing the disease. Fortunately existing immunologic methodology will permit definitive studies to distinguish between these hypotheses. The susceptibility of children to Hemophilus influenzae during the period of their lives when antibody responses to these organisms are low is consonant with the known susceptibility of agammaglobulinemic patients of all ages to Hemophilus infections.

HISTOPLASMOSIS AND COCCIDIOIDOMYCOSIS

Histoplasmosis and coccidioidomycosis can be classified in the group of fungal infections manifested by hypersensitivity mechanisms. The development of clinical disease is mainly related to the development of hypersensitivity, both cell mediated and humoral, to the organism. The hypersensitivity develops usually within 14 days after initial infection when the clinical symptoms become apparent. The acute disease is then localized to the sites in the lung in most cases and pursues a benign course.

In this disease, as in tuberculosis, the primary infection, although localized and successfully contained in most of the cases, may become reactivated later in life, especially if the immune function of the host is impaired. The antigens widely used for skin testing are the mycelial phase antigen called histoplasmin and coccidioidin, in parallel with the terminology for tuberculin. The intradermal test is read in the same manner as is the tuberculin test. Three types of serologic tests have been used in histoplasmosis: complement fixation, precipitation, and agglutination. Serologic tests do not correlate well with immunity, but appear to reflect the activity of infection. This is especially true when 19S IgM antibodies are present in the serum.

Histoplasma capsulatum, Blastomyces dermatitidis, and Coccidioides immitis may yield antigens that cross react with each other. It has been established that preexisting histoplasmosis may become disseminated when adrenal corticosteroids are used for the treatment of concomitant diseases, e.g., sarcoidosis and leukemia. For this reason corticosteroid therapy is contraindicated in the presence of a positive skin test or other evidence for histoplasmosis. Patients with extreme forms of humoral and B-cell immunodeficiency may resist and control histoplasma infections very well in spite of their inability to form detectable amounts of circulating antibody. This is presumably a function of the efficacy of cellular immunity and its biologic amplifications. By contrast, the disseminated forms of both histoplasmosis and coccidioidomycosis are associated with negative skin test reactions to these organisms and their products.

Treatment of histoplasmosis by intravenous administration of amphotericin B has met with encouraging results. Toxic effects on the kidney may require careful monitoring of dosage.

CRYPTOCOCCOSIS

Cryptococcosis is a chronic infectious disease caused by the fungus Cryptococcus neoformans, a common saprophyte in nature, acquired by the respiratory route, with a focus of infection, usually subclinical, in the lungs and occasionally with hematogenous dissemination characteristically to the meninges but also to the kidneys, skin, bone, and other organs. The most frequent form is a self-limited respiratory disease in which hypersensitivity to the organism is of high order. Here again, both cellular and humoral immunity may be involved in development of the symptoms and signs of this infection. Erythema nodosa is frequent and probably is based on antigen-antibody complex injury. With immunologic elimination of the organisms all manifestations cease, and the host is left immune to reinfection.

Numerous striking epidemiologic and clinical aspects of this disease, however, indicate forcefully the importance of predisposition and immunity. Cryptococcus neoformans is most ubiquitous in man's environment. But disease caused by it occurs mainly in patients with Hodgkin's disease, diabetes mellitus, immunosuppressive (azathioprine) therapy, acute and chronic (especially lymphatic) leukemia, hypogammaglobulinemia, and, to a lesser extent, corticoid therapy, sarcoidosis, tuberculosis, and other fungal diseases. Meningitis used to be universally fatal until the development of specific chemotherapy. In patients with disseminated active disease, it has often been difficult to demonstrate significant responses of circulating antibody or delayed cutaneous hypersensitivity. The histopathology of the disseminated disease is marked by a minimal inflammatory response in the brain and meninges and by only a minimal and, in a sense, inadequate cytologic and biochemical response in the cerebrospinal fluid.

Of historical interest is the fact that the first patient reported by Busse in 1895 had remarkable lymphadenopathy, and it had been appreciated almost as early that there is a marked association of cryptococcosis with Hodgkin's disease. This association has been so striking as to lead to the suggestion that this fungus may be etiologically related to Hodgkin's disease. Of 60 patients with cryptococcosis, reported by Zimmerman and Rappaport, 18 had Hodgkin's or related diseases.

Since the advent of organ transplantation and the necessity for artificial suppression of the immune response by specific drugs (e.g., azathioprine) a number of cases of severe disseminated and indeed fatal cryptococcosis have occurred in this population. Cryptococcosis infection, interestingly enough, has been handled well in patients with primary B-cell humoral immunity deficits, but as with Hodgkin's disease overwhelming infection has accompanied primary deficits of cell-mediated immunity.

CANDIDIASIS

Infection with Candida albicans ranges from the generally benign oral thrush of infancy to severe systemic involvement. Within this spectrum are a number of patients with chronic mucocutaneous candidiasis, characterized by persistent C. albicans infection of the skin, nails, scalp, buccal mucosa, and vaginal mucous membranes. Endocrinopathy sometimes is associated with the infection and usually consists of hypoparathyroidism, hypoadrenalism, or hypothyroidism. Although the mucocutaneous infection is very resistant to therapy, systemic candidiasis develops rarely, if at all.

Chronic mucocutaneous candidiasis can be associated with a form of cellular immune deficiency. Chilgren et al. have described 3 patients who

failed to manifest delayed hypersensitivity when challenged with a battery of intracutaneous skin tests. These patients also failed to respond to
active sensitization with 2,4-dinitrofluorobenzene. Similar generalized
cutaneous anergy has been described in 3 other patients.

Defective cellular immunity, both *in vivo* and *in vitro,* was shown in
one patient. There was complete anergy, with negative intradermal tests
for delayed hypersensitivity with eight antigens and a lack of response
to dinitrochlorobenzene after contact sensitization. A skin graft has not
been rejected after more than a year. The patient's lymphocytes responded by proliferation *in vitro* to stimulation with phytohemagglutinin,
but not with mumps or Monilia antigens. His cells neither responded nor
were stimulated in a one-way mixed lymphocyte culture. His serum inhibited the proliferative response of normal control lymphocytes stimulated with Candida and mumps' antigens, and allogeneic cells.

These abnormal responses seem to be the result of the serum factor inhibiting the proliferative response of the small lymphocytes. The defect
appears to be genetic, as there are other affected members in the family.

The chronic granulomatous form of mucocutaneous candidiasis has
been treated successfully on several occasions with transfer factor of
Lawrence. In these instances most devastating infection has been allevi-
ated. By contrast, transfer factor has regularly failed in the nongranulo-
matous form of chronic mucocutaneous candidiasis. After long-term intensive therapy with amphotericin B, a patient who had been entirely anergic
to a broad battery of antigens responded vigorously after chronic infection
had been eliminated. This experience provides evidence that the candida
organisms themselves have in some unknown manner capacity to suppress
the capacity of the host to develop delayed allergic reactions.

Candida organisms possess many antigens that can be demonstrated
when antisera from prolonged immunization of rabbits is reacted against
candida culture fluid using an immunoelectrophoresis technique. When
sera from normal persons are run against these antigen preparations,
many precipitating antibodies against candida products can be demonstrated. Sera of patients with chronic mucocutaneous candidiasis, by contrast, show high concentrations of antibody to a few antigens and seem to
be lacking antibodies that normal persons usually develop against many of
the antigens. Using these methods to study other persistent fungus or
bacterial infections is indicated. Systemic candida infections and candida
septicemia are sometimes associated with absence of the enzyme myeloperoxidase in the granulocytes. This abnormality is not seen in leukocytes
of patients with chronic mucocutaneous candidiasis.

PARASITIC INFESTATIONS

Parasitic infection can induce all or any of the known forms of hypersensitivity: anaphylaxis, serum sickness (including fever), atopic reac-

tion, and delayed hypersensitivity. Occasionally parasites cause unusual and intriguing immunologic reactions that cannot be correlated with the natural history of the disease. For instance, antigens have been discovered which are common to the schistosomes and the tissues of their mammalian hosts—mouse red blood cells or hamster liver. This raises an important question concerning enhancement of the pathogenicity of an infectious organism which may result from "biologic mimicry."

Worm infections have several unique immunologic characteristics. These organisms are potent inducers of eosinophilia and of the homocytotropic IgE antibody. Cell-mediated mechanisms appear to play important roles in both immunity and hypersensitivity to these parasitic organisms. It is the rule rather than the exception that the worms go through several developmental stages in the host, each of which may be related to different disease manifestations based on immune mechanisms. Finally, in contrast to the other infectious agents—viruses, bacteria, fungi—the various stages of the worms in the definitive hosts (those in which sexual reproduction occurs) do not themselves undergo multiplication, a phenomenon that has implications in respect to concepts of immunologic disease.

Worms have long been known for their unique ability to evoke eosinophilia. Very high levels of circulating eosinophils are seen in the diseases caused by worms which migrate through the tissues. These include ascariasis, strongyloidiasis, trichinosis, certain filarial infections, and the acute stages of schistosomiasis. The tissue lesions caused by many of these organisms are also characterized by large numbers of eosinophils and tremendously high levels of IgE. A type of eosinophilic pneumonia, Löffler's pneumonia, is found in ascaris infections. A tropical eosinophilia has been shown to be due to filarial infections. Eosinophilic meningitis of the South Pacific is apparently caused by Angiostrongylus cantonensis, a nematode with an interesting rat-slug life cycle.

Experimental studies have demonstrated recently that the eosinophilia induced by the injection of Trichinella larvae into rats is a T lymphocyte-mediated immunologic reaction. Many of the parasitic worms are powerful inducers of IgE. These antibodies are found in these diseases both in serum in high concentration and bound to tissues and are apparently responsible for anaphylactic and atopic reactions. Ogilvie first observed that a rat intestinal nematode, Nippostrongylus brasiliensis, induced formation of a very high concentration of IgE antibodies. Since then, homocytotropic antibody formation has been demonstrated in a variety of worm infections, including schistosomiasis, trichinosis, filariasis, and ascariasis. Recently it has been suggested that the cell-mediated reactions may be an important or even primary factor in the establishment of immunity to certain parasitic worms. Evidence has been presented indicating that immunity to Trichostrongylus colubriformis, a nematode para-

18

site of ruminants, can be transferred with cells but not with serum. Delayed skin reactions transferable with spleen cells occur in guinea pigs with trichinosis.

Swimmer's itch, a sensitization phenomenon, was shown by MacFarlane in New Zealand to be due to infection with Cercaria longicauda and by Olivier in the United States to be due to the cercariae of Trichobilharzia stagnicolae, Trichobilharzia ocellata, and Schistosomatium douthitti. This disease is common in swimmers using lakes in the midwestern United States. Primary exposure was followed by virtually no reaction in some subjects, but in most, immediate pruritus was noted, followed within 30 minutes by the development of a small macule that faded in approximately 10 hours. Small papules (2 mm in diameter) appeared 5 to 12 days later. On secondary or repeated exposures, a similar immediate reaction is seen, followed in 6 to 15 hours by the development of large papules (8 mm in diameter) accompanied by erythema, edema, and pruritus. The results of some further experiments by Olivier suggested that this secondary reaction was quite specific. A person sensitized to T. stagnicolae cercariae cross-reacted upon exposure to the closely related T. ocellata cercariae, both of avian origin, but developed only a primary reaction on exposure to S. douthitti cercariae, which are of mammalian origin. MacFarlane's studies included skin biopsies. In unsensitized subjects virtually no reaction occurred until 7 days, and even then it was relatively slight. Secondary reactions at the time of papule formation revealed edema and massive round cell invasion of the dermis and epidermis.

Katayama fever, most severe in infections with Schistosoma japonicum, occurs only in those patients experiencing very heavy initial infections with S. mansoni, and has not been reported in patients with schistosomiasis haematobium. The pathology of Katayama fever is virtually unknown. The few postmortem studies of acute schistosomiasis japonica show massive infection with huge numbers of eggs in the liver and intestines. The onset of Katayama fever occurs after several weeks of stimulation of antibody formation by the cercariae in the presence of the migrating schistosomules. Antibody levels are, however, relatively low at the time of its occurrence. The fever is associated with outpouring of antigens derived from the eggs of the pathogenic organism. Many of the antigens of the pathogens cross react with those of the other schistosomes, but some appear to be unique. It is possible that the conditions of antigen excess are conducive to the formation of soluble antigen-antibody complexes of a type leading to the development and fever or manifestations of serum sickness. The potential hazard of renal injury from such antigen-antibody complexes has not thus far been realized in these diseases, but it seems likely that careful searching might reveal such evidence. In some of the parasitoses as, for example, in trichinosis, adrenal steroid therapy will suppress dramatically the fever and apparent toxicity. Only specific antiparasite regimens together with time will eliminate these sometimes serious diseases.

Filariasis. The many different species of filariae that affect man produce a wide variety of clinical signs and symptoms, including localized skin swellings, recurrent febrile episodes, blindness, chronic upper respiratory disease, and marked increases in the size of the genitalia and limbs—elephantiasis. Many of these manifestations have been ascribed to hypersensitivity reactions. Tropical eosinophilia is apparently a response to the microfilariae, and elephantiasis is generally believed to be due primarily to the adult worms. Tropical eosinophilia resembles a chronic respiratory tract infection, but it is accompanied by pronounced eosinophilia. Microfilariae may circulate in the blood and tissues for days and even months. The exact immunopathology of these disorders remains to be elucidated, but both cellular immunities, IgE anaphylactic pathogenesis, and antigen-antibody complexes are probably involved in the several expressions of the disease. Intravenous administration of thiacetarsamide (Caparsolate sodium) in a dosage of 1.0 mg per kg daily is most effective against adult worms. Hetrazan (diethylcarbamazine) in an oral dosage of 2.0 mg per kg t.i.d. for 3 or 4 weeks is effective against microfilaria.

Malaria. Malaria infections are accompanied by hepatosplenomegaly, recurrent fever, and the anemia of obvious pathogenesis. Until recently little has been known of the immunopathology of this, perhaps the most frequent severe or fatal infectious disease of man. However, recent studies demonstrating that antigen-antibody complex type of assault is the basis of the nephrotic syndrome so frequently seen in the quartan type of malaria indicate that modern immunobiology can provide incisive analysis of the pathogenetic basis of components of this infection. That such analysis may be crucial also to the understanding of important diseases related to malaria is suggested by the epidemiologic association of malaria with EB virus (Herpes 3) infection in the pathogenesis of Burkitt's lymphoma.

Pneumocystis carinii Infection. Pneumocystis carinii is the pathogen that produced a highly lethal form of epidemic pneumonia among prematures and debilitated newborn infants in central Europe after World War II. This form of pneumonia, also called plasma cell pneumonia, is characterized by interstitial mononuclear inflammation coupled with a honey-combed, pink-staining exudate when studied by usual H and E sections. The pathogen, which has not yet been cultured, is readily demonstrated in the exudate in a cystic form exhibiting small nuclei. It may be located either intracellularly in phagocytes or more commonly free in the exudate by Giemsa stain (Fig. 34-1). The pathogen, either a yeast or protozoan, is also readily demonstrable when the tissues are stained

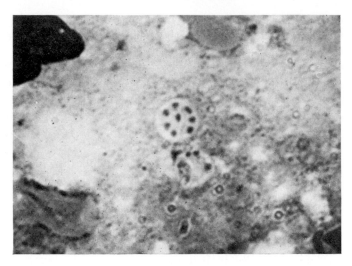

Fig. 34-1. A typical form of Pneumocystis carinii found in imprint preparation of lung biopsy. Giemsa stain [From Burke, B., and Good, R. A. (1973): Medicine 52:24. By permission of The Williams & Wilkins Co., Baltimore.]

with silver methenamine. With the return of the population of central Europe to good health and good nutrition plasma cell pneumonia caused by Pneumocystis carinii has almost completely disappeared. Infection with the same organism, however, has been encountered in Britain, Canada, and the United States and more recently again in Europe in patients suffering from either primary or secondary forms of immunodeficiency. This pathogen, ubiquitous in nature, is one of the most frequent causes of death in children with combined immunodeficiency disease. Infection with Pneumocystis carinii occurs as a frequent complication of immunodeficiency accompanying leukemias and lymphomas, combined immunodeficiencies, and iatrogenic immunodeficiencies as in transplanted patients or in patients under chemotherapy for cancer. Although in our experience both cell-mediated and humoral types of immunodeficiencies have been accompanied by this infection, severe defects of humoral immunity have been most frequent. In two families, for example, 5 male children with classical X-linked infantile agammaglobulinemia succumbed to Pneumocystis carinii pneumonia. These children had normal thymus as well as normal thymus dependent regions of their lymph nodes but lacked germinal centers and plasma cells in the classical expression of their disease. Less frequently, apparently isolated defects of cell-mediated immunity have also been associated with pulmonary infections with Pneumocystis.

Although these pathogens can occasionally be demonstrated in sputum or on bronchial swabs, the latter have generally failed as diagnostic measures. Consequently upon clinical suspicion based on even moderate pulmonary infiltration, especially when accompanied by cough or rapid respirations in a patient with immunodeficiency, an open pulmonary biopsy using minimal anesthesia, a small incision, and peripheral biopsy has been of low morbidity, no mortality and of high diagnostic value in our experience. Specific diagnosis is of paramount importance because most cases of this disease that are recognized early enough can now be treated effectively with pentamidine in a dosage of 4 mg/kg for 10 to 14 days. It has been reported that the diagnosis of this disease could be indicated by the presence of IgM antibodies in the blood of a healthy parent or a sibling of an immunodeficient patient. We prefer the more direct diagnostic method for this infection, since treatment is quite effective if initiated early.

SYPHILIS

Syphilis is caused by the highly parasitic Treponema pallidum, and man is the only known natural host. The first lesion, or chancre, appears about 3 weeks after the infection. At this time the reaction to serologic tests for syphilis (STS) may be negative, but within a week or so the STS become positive. In most instances the chancre heals spontaneously and is followed by secondary lesions of syphilis in 6 to 12 weeks. Sore throat, malaise, fever, lymphadenopathy, and a skin eruption are characteristic manifestations of secondary lesions. The STS are always positive in secondary syphilis. The secondary stage may heal spontaneously and becomes latent syphilis, which is characterized by persistent positive STS without any clinical manifestations. Latent syphilis may last many years. About 10 to 15 percent of untreated patients with syphilis develop latent syphilis.

Experimental studies in rabbits and man indicate that syphilis gives rise to partial immunity and that the degree of immunity appears to be directly related to the duration of infection. Although the discovery of the causative agent of syphilis and the ability to transmit it to laboratory animals provided useful means of studying immunity to syphilis, the inability to grow T. pallidum has been the major problem for further study.

The serologic tests currently used are (1) nontreponemal tests, e.g., Venereal Disease Research Laboratory (VDRL) tests, and (2) treponemal tests that employ T. pallidum, Nichols' strain as the antigen, e.g., T. pallidum immobilization (TPI) test and fluorescent treponemal antibody absorption (FTA-ABS) test. At the turn of the century Wassermann demonstrated that an antigen extracted from the liver of a syphilitic patient is reactive with antibodies in the sera of patients with syphilis. However, subsequent studies have shown that Wassermann antibody is not reactive with the spirochete itself, and the "Wassermann antigen" can be extracted not only from syphilitic livers, but also from normal livers, as well as from numerous other tissues. Cardiolipin, derived from the heart, is the familiar reagent now used in nontreponemal serologic tests. This Wassermann antibody, therefore, is an example of autoantibodies produced as a consequence of T. pallidum infection and undoubtedly may play a role in the production of the syphilitic lesions. It is well known that reactions to the standard STS do occur in many other diseases, such as lupus erythematosus, leprosy, and certain virus diseases, and are called biologic false positive reactions to STS. The meaning of these reactions is not clear, but the false positive tests are now more frequent than the STS reactions indicative of syphilis itself.

Total serum-globulin levels are abnormally high after infection with T. pallidum. In primary syphilis the level of IgM is increased, and both IgG and IgM levels are increased in secondary syphilis. Increased levels of IgM have been reported in congenital syphilis. Recommended regimens for treatment of early syphilis consist of (1) benzathine pencillin G, single injection 2.4 million units or equivalent dose of procaine or aqueous penicillin, (2) tetracycline (oral), total 30 gm, 3 gm/day for 10 days, or (3) erythromycin (oral), total 20 gm, 2 gm/day for 10 days.

IMMUNIZATION AGAINST BACTERIAL INFECTIONS

Passive Immunization

In active immunization the person or animal immunized produces his own antibody; this soon enters his circulation, and injections of his serum or plasma will then transfer the antibody to animals of his own or other species. By this means—passive immunization—antibody can be provided for inexperienced animals or man at a speed much greater than is practicable by active immunization. A number of antibodies may be produced in man by subclinical or clinical infection, e.g., measles antibody, or by deliberate active immunization, e.g., tetanus antitoxin, and used for passive immunization of other persons. These antibodies have the great advantage that they are homologous proteins; they are therefore destroyed at the usual rate for these proteins and do not excite the antibody response necessarily provoked by the corresponding foreign proteins. The main disadvantage is their low concentration in the plasma. By appropriate processes of concentration, measles antibody gamma globulin preparations, for example, can be effectively concentrated in serum. Many other antibodies exist in normal serum, but for only a few, like those directed against hepatitis A, can a sufficiently high concentration be obtained to be clinically useful.

However, with hyperimmune serum or human serum from a recent convalescent, immune antibodies most useful in passive transfer therapy or prophylaxis have been obtained. Such measures are effective against tetanus, pertussis, snake venoms, chickenpox, vaccinia, smallpox, and other infections or consequences of infection. Indeed because of the practicality today of plasma phoresis methodology, human hyperimmune gamma globulin preparations for passive immunization should become more readily available. In a most important study of the potentialities of this form of immunotherapy, it was shown that the antibody titers of policemen in Philadelphia who had been immunized with antigens such as pertussis can be maintained at very high levels for prolonged periods by regular weekly plasma phoresis. The latter apparently inhibits piling up of antibody to a crucial level and the engagement of a negative feedback mechanism.

The lack of high titer human serum has been overcome in the past by immunizing horses against the appropriate antigen—particularly against bacterial toxins—and using the serum of these animals for passive prophylaxis. A straightforward case occurs in prophylaxis against tetanus. When a nonimmunized person suffers a wound likely to give rise to tetanus, the common manner of minimizing the risk is to immunize him passively with tetanus antitoxin prepared in the horse, in which antitoxin levels of 300 units per ml or more are raised to 1500 units per ml or more by refining and concentration. If this serum is injected intramuscularly or subcutaneously, high concentrations of circulating antitoxin can be provided within less than 24 hours and considerable protection afforded.

In certain circumstances, when newborn infants are exposed to serious risk of infection, it may be of value to immunize them passively by actively immunizing their mothers. For example, in some parts of northern Africa it is customary to dress the umbilical cord with dung paste, and neonatal tetanus is common. Attempts to change long-established customs are unlikely to be effective, and immunization of the mothers against tetanus with toxoid, with consequent placental transfer of tetanus antitoxin to the fetus is far more likely to protect the newborn child. To provide high levels of passively acquired antitoxin at birth and for about 10 days afterwards, the second or third dose of toxoid should be injected 10 to 14 days before the expected date of birth. Subsequent active immunization will be necessary for the child.

A similar method is sometimes used for preventing lamb dysentery. Pregnant ewes are immunized with Clostridium welchii type B toxoid, so that the ewe reaches the maximum of her secondary response at the time of the birth of the lamb. High concentrations of antibody are secreted in the colostrum from which the lamb is able to absorb the antibody. As lamb dysentery is a disease of the first few days of life only, no subsequent active immunization of the lamb is necessary. This method has obvious advantages compared to another at one time in common use —the immunization of newborn lambs with Clostridium welchii type B horse antiserum. Since Clostridium welchii type B toxoids with increased

potency have been developed, the former technique has largely super-
seded the latter.

Active Immunization

Typhus. Vaccination against scrub typhus has not proved effective because of the large number of different strains of the causative agent,
Rickettsia nipponica. A more effective prophylactic vaccine can, however, be prepared against epidemic (louse borne and murine) typhus,
by growing the rickettsiae in the yolk sacs of embryonated eggs (or in
the lungs of small rodents or the peritoneal cavities of gerbils) and killing the microorganisms with formaldehyde. The killed rickettsiae are
concentrated and purified by shaking an aqueous suspension with ether
or fluorohydrocarbons.

The vaccine is administered by subcutaneous injections, repeated at
frequent intervals (e.g., every six months), while exposure to infection
continues. It does not prevent infection, but renders the illness milder
and very markedly reduces mortality. Treatment with suitable antibiotics is the method of choice.

Cholera and Plague. Cholera vaccines are prepared to contain equal
numbers of organisms from smooth strains of the two types of Vibrio
cholerae, Inaba and Ogawa, which are killed by heat or by a bactericidal agent. One ml contains at least 8000 million vibrios. The dosage
schedule is similar to that of enteric vaccines, and indeed the two are
sometimes combined. Experience in the Middle and Far East suggests
that cholera vaccines have some measure of success in prophylaxis,
though not in treatment, of cholera. It seems to us, however, that an inappropriate route of immunization with cholera vaccine has been used.
Studies of oral immunization with these agents surely are in order. Recent studies in our laboratories have established the existence of a local
cellular immunity system in the gastrointestinal tract which is quite
aloof from the systemic cellular immunity system. It seems important,
now, to begin to think of immunization purposes of domains—the respiratory domain, gastrointestinal domain, skin and peripheral domain, and
genitourinary domain. It may very well be that more effective active
immunization in the future can be accomplished if this concept is
utilized.

Plague vaccine is prepared from culture of the capsulated form of
Pasteurella pestis in such a manner that the final vaccine contains the
greatest possible amount of capsular material. The organisms are commonly killed with formaldehyde, and the vaccine made up to contain
3000 million bacteria per ml, in a medium containing 0.5 percent phenol
and not more than 0.025 percent formaldehyde. The dosage schedule is
similar to that of enteric vaccines. Plague vaccine is of value as a pro-

phylactic where plague is endemic or when it might occur in epidemic proportion.

Enteric Fever. A vaccine of killed typhoid bacilli was first employed by Almroth Wright in 1897. In animals it has been shown that vaccines containing the O somatic antigen can protect against intraperitoneal challenge or even against infection by mouth in epidemics caused by naturally occurring virulent strains. The H or flagellar antigens apparently give no protection. The usual vaccine has been prepared from smooth virulent organisms killed by heat and preserved with 0.5 percent phenol. Statistics derived from World War I and the African campaigns of 1940-43 indicate that such a vaccine was effective in reducing morbidity (of the order of tenfold) and mortality due to typhoid. Another antigen of Salmonella typhi, named Vi because it was characteristically associated with virulent strains, could also be important in protecting mice. The Vi antigen is preserved in antigenic form much more effectively when the vaccine is killed with 70 percent alcohol and the vaccine subsequently stored in 25 percent alcohol. Considerable question concerning the effectiveness of these vaccines, particularly in preventing gastrointestinal symptoms, has been raised in subsequent studies. Here again, advantage might be obtained by immunization via the gastrointestinal domain rather than just using the peripheral route.

Current vaccines against enteric organisms are prepared from a single strain or from several strains of S. typhi, S. paratyphi A, S. paratyphi B, an S. paratyphi C that are smooth and have the full complement of O somatic antigens and in the case of S. typhi and S. paratyphi C also contain the Vi antigen. They are killed by heat or by a bactericide chosen to retain maximum antigenicity. The number of organisms per ml is 1000 million S. typhi and 500 to 750 million S. paratyphi A, B, and C. The vaccine is given in two subcutaneous doses, usually with an interval of a month between them, and the second dose contains twice as many organisms as the first (recommended doses are 0.5 and 1.0 ml of phenolized vaccine or 0.25 and 0.5 ml of alcoholized vaccine). It is not uncommon for enteric vaccines to cause temporary general malaise, mild fever, and local tenderness. This is probably due to their content of endotoxin and is less with vaccines extracted with alcohol. In recent field trials carried out in Guiana both an acetone-killed and a phenolized typhoid vaccine were shown to confer a high degree of protection from systemic illness and death. These vaccines, however, all have been disappointing in the protection afforded against the gastrointestinal component of typhoid and paratyphoid infections. Here again, extension of the concept of immunization to using the local cellular and humoral immunity systems may be valuable.

Diphtheria. Purified toxin treated formalin (formol toxoid, FT) forms the basis of all preparations used to achieve antidiphtheria immunization today. Its antigenic effect is increased, and the number of injections necessary is cut down by adsorption onto aluminum hydroxide (to give APT, alum-precipitated toxoid) or onto hydrated aluminum phosphate (to give PTAP, purified toxoid aluminium phosphate). The latter is a less variable and slightly more powerful prophylactic. The virtual disappearance of diphtheria in Britain between 1941 and 1951 was largely due to almost universal immunization of children with two doses of diphtheria APT.

The earlier the immunization the better, even though in the first three months or so maternally transmitted antitoxin may interfere to some degree with the immune response to injected toxoid. This effect can be overcome by the use of a larger dose of toxoid. Routine immunization of infants starting at three months or earlier is advised. In practice, diphtheria prophylaxis is often started at two months, along with pertussis vaccine.

A single boosting dose (formol toxoid) is given at the time of entry to school, and another booster dose at the age of 9 to 11 years. The reason for using formol toxoid rather than APT or PTAP for the boosting doses is that statistical evidence shows that when alum-containing vaccines are given during epidemics of poliomyelitis, a small but significantly increased risk of paralysis affecting the injected limb may be encountered. Further, annoying local reactions are more frequent with secondary exposure to precipitated toxoid. Vaccines containing Hemophilus pertussis also appear to have a similar effect. The consensus among persons concerned with immunization programs is that it is necessary to use an adjuvant along with formol toxoid in order to ensure adequate immunization with the first two doses, and since these should be given at an early age when local reactions are less severe, APT or PTAP is recommended.

Older children or adults immunized with the usual diphtheria prophylactics sometimes exhibit delayed reactions of varying degrees of severity. This is particularly likely to occur after actual infection by the diphtheria bacillus has already occurred in earlier life. It has been found that such reactions are less common when toxoid-antitoxin floccules (TAF, toxoid combined with a quantity of antitoxin slightly less than the equivalence ratio) are used, and for this reason TAF is recommended by some authorities when the first immunization has been delayed. Before immunizing adults it is usual to use the Schick test to look for the presence of antitoxin, indicating previous prophylactic immunization or effectively immunizing clinical or subclinical diphtheria.

Whooping Cough (pertussis). Little doubt exists that when vaccines are used which are properly prepared from a mixture of freshly isolated, fully virulent phase I organisms which are carefully killed by formalin or merthiolate, immunity against whooping cough can be obtained. However, there is reason to believe that many of the vaccines used in the past have been ineffective. Studies, especially in Britain, have shown that vaccination reduces the incidence of pertussis by 80 percent and that the cases occurring in the vaccinated groups are on the average less severe and of shorter duration than in the control populations.

In view of the severity and the prevalance of whooping cough in infants, early protection is mandatory. Many authorities recommend that the first injection should be given at 2 or 3 months of age, followed by two further injections at monthly intervals. Some have even urged immunization beginning immediately after birth. Much debate concerns booster doses. One may be required at school entry age, but from the available figures, it is clear that pertussis is a killing disease only in the first year of life, and at 5 years the average child should be in a position to cope with an attack of pertussis without immunization. The danger of producing serious central nervous system disease with pertussis vaccine has made many pediatricians wary of giving these immunizations to children who have had brain injury at birth or who have abnormalities of development of the brain or propensity to seizures.

Alum-precipitated vaccines are sometimes used in America and seem quite effective. Diphtheria, pertussis, and tetanus combinations in this form are now standard immunizations for American children.

Tetanus. Formalized preparations of purified tetanus toxin are used This is a fairly potent antigen, and its administration is free from unpleasant reactions. Immunization may be begun at any age, but since the risk of tetanus is present at all ages, immunization is advised during infancy. Immunity depends on the presence of antitoxin in the blood and this does not occur naturally nor does it even follow recovery from tetanus. The dosage of the potent tetanus toxin producing devastating disease is below the amount required to immunize. The usual course consists of two injections separated by an interval of 1 month, followed by a third injection 6 to 18 months later. Booster doses used to be regularly given, but long-lasting immunity to the toxoid has made it clear that much of this ritual has been unnecessary. A booster dose given at the time of injury is all that is necessary after the usual childhood series.

When a person is not known to have been immunized or has been incompletely immunized, 3000 to 5000 units of tetanus antitoxin should be given intramuscularly upon exposure, e.g., a wound, to confer temporary passive immunity. The dose is not reduced for a child. The injection should be repeated at weekly intervals as long as the risk of tetanus persists. When homologous (human) tetanus antitoxin is available, it can be used for such prophylaxis, especially in cases in which hypersensitivity reactions to horse serum proteins are probable. In the same circumstances, and when human serum is not available, hypersensitivity reactions may be avoided by a switch to bovine tetanus antitoxin, which is reported to give reactions only rarely in those who have previously reacted to horse serum.

Patients receiving passive immunization should also be actively immunized with tetanus toxoid. Theoretically this is best done 6 to 8 weeks after passive immunization. Second or repeated prophylactic treatments with horse antitoxin should be avoided. The danger of anaphylaxis is great and serum sickness and immune complex injury should not be produced if they can be avoided. Further, if antibodies against the foreign protein exist in the circulation, the antitoxin will be simply lost by immune elimination. It is therefore dangerous to rely on passive immunization for protection.

Since the above recommendation that active immunization shall be given at some time after the use of passive protection may prove to be inconvenient or impracticable, the use of aluminum phosphate precipitated tetanus toxoid (PAPT) or aluminum hydroxide precipitated toxoid (APT) as a more powerful stimulus than soluble toxoid has been recommended for use at the same time as passive protection with antitoxin. Thus 3000 units of tetanus antitoxin may be injected into one arm intramuscularly and followed immediately by an injection into the other arm of 0.5 ml of PAPT. This procedure would normally be followed 4 to 6 weeks later by a booster dose of 0.5 ml of PAPT.

The combination of antibiotic protection with a long-acting penicillin preparation and active immunization with PAPT or APT at the time of injury may act in the previously nonimmune subject to prevent tetanus infection until adequate active immunity has developed.

Fatal cases of tetanus result from wounds in nonimmune persons which often are not regarded as being sufficiently serious for prophylactic antitoxin, e.g., thorn injuries, insect bites, slivers, and minor trauma. Passive immunization cannot protect against this hazard because it will not be used. Active immunization, especially in atopic persons, avoids the serious reactions of hypersensitivity to foreign serum proteins.

BCG Vaccination. Immunization against tuberculosis has employed a variety of strains of organisms presumably all derived from the original attenuated strain developed by Calmette and Guérin in France in the 1930's. Although it has been difficult to standardize these preparations, infection with BCG organisms has clearly been an effective immunization against tuberculosis in many countries of the Western world. The beneficial effect of this form of immunization was most clearly shown in controlling the tuberculosis epidemic that followed World War II. In some regions like Scandinavia, for example, BCG immunization has been a routine public health measure. Immunization using viable organisms capable of producing a mild infection may be accomplished in several ways. The gastrointestinal route, subcutaneous injection, and dermal scarification have been employed. The latter has been most widely used. Except in children deficient in cellular immunity where disseminated infection with BCG can be lethal, BCG infection rarely causes serious difficulty. The immunity produced by BCG infection usually is effective for at least 6 to 8 years.

In the United States utilization of BCG is generally confined to highly susceptible populations, e.g., nursing and medical staffs of large hospitals, contacts of known cases of tuberculosis, and American Indians. Currently enthusiasm for the possible use of BCG as an adjunct to immunotherapy in cancer is seeing widespread trial of a variety of regimens of BCG immunization in Europe and the United States (Chapter 15).

BCG immunization may also protect against related organisms such as atypical acid-fast organisms and to a degree against the lepra bacillus. The best form of BCG vaccine available today seems to be the freeze-dried preparation. This should be kept at very low temperatures for prolonged storage, but can be kept for shorter intervals at conditions more readily available, a week or so at room temperature and up to a year at ice box temperatures. The liquid forms of the vaccine are most unstable.

One major disadvantage of the use of BCG in widespread immunization against tuberculosis is that such immunization creates cell-mediated immunity to tuberculoprotein and thus the value of the Mantoux test for detection of active tuberculosis is lost. It is most unlikely, however, that effective immunization against tuberculosis without Mantoux conversion will be possible, since the major defense against facultative intracellular bacterial pathogens like the tubercle bacillus involves cell-mediated immunity.

The Mantoux Test. This test gives a measure of the degree of delayed hypersensitivity of an individual towards tuberculoprotein and is an indication that he or she has had a past or has a present infection with tubercle bacilli. The test is performed by injecting intracutaneously 0.1 ml of a standardized solution of tuberculoprotein prepared either from Old Tuberculin (OT, a concentrated filtrate from cultures of human or bovine strains) or from Tuberculin Purified Protein Derivative (PPD, a preparation of partially purified protein from the culture filtrate of human strains). The amount injected is defined in terms of tuberculin units that are related to the activities of the International Standard Preparations. One tuberculin unit is defined as the activity contained in 1/100,000 ml of the standard OT, or in 0.000028 mg of the Standard Tuberculin PPD. A feature of tuberculoprotein is that it adsorbs rather readily to glass, and consequently extra precautions need to be taken in cleaning glassware that has contained tuberculoprotein. Further, when dilutions are used containing less than 1000 units per ml these must be freshly prepared from a concentrated stock solution.

It is advisable to use a small dose, 10 tuberculin units or even less, for a first test, since tuberculin-sensitive patients may develop severe reactions with higher doses. A positive reaction consists in the development at the injection site (forearm) of induration and surrounding erythema which become apparent after 12 hours and reach the maximum size at 48 to 72 hours. The usually accepted criterion is that the area of induration should measure at least 6 mm in diameter when examined at 48 hours. If the subject does not react to so small a dose, further tests should be done with larger doses until no reaction is obtained to 100 units. Only then may an individual be regarded as being truly tuberculin negative.

In children's clinics it is sometimes more convenient to employ the "patch" test. The skin is carefully cleaned with acetone, and gauze impregnated with a solution of OT in a jelly is applied under plaster and left in contact with the skin for 48 hours. When the gauze is removed a tuberculin-sensitive child will show a red, slightly raised area at the site of contact with the gauze. A positive reaction is reliable, but negative reactors require confirmation by an intracutaneous test.

Occasionally in medical practice, but more commonly in veterinary practice, a question arises whether a positive tuberculin test indicates infection with a particular type of mycobacterium (e.g., M. tuberculosis of human, bovine, or avian strains, or M. balnei or ulcerans, or, in cattle, M. johnei). Tuberculin preparations have been made from each of these different organisms in the hope that the intensity of the skin response to the particular tuberculin from the infecting organism will be greater than those to other tuberculins. In practice it is found that extensive cross reactions between the different preparations exist. Until it proves possible to standardize one preparation in terms of another in animals which are infected with each separate organism, it will remain difficult to interpret such skin tests defining the particular strain of mycobacterium causing disease.

It has recently been called in question whether weak reactions to 100 TU indicate in all cases that the subject has been infected with human or bovine tubercle bacilli, or whether contact with saprophytic acid-fast bacilli could be responsible. Evidence indicates that, at least in this country, such weak positive reactions should still be regarded as evidence that infection with Mycobacterium tuberculosis has occurred unless clear evidence to the contrary has been developed. The best evidence indicates that the presence of a positive Mantoux test shows the presence of viable mycobacteria in the body. When organisms are completely eliminated as in childhood infections treated effectively with antibiotics and chemotherapeutics, the Mantoux test converts to negative. Thus this form of delayed T-cell allergy is probably not different from other forms of cellular immunity in which the duration of the hypersensitivity state, although prolonged, is finite.

SELECTED REFERENCES

Tuberculosis

Alarcón-Segovia, D., and Fishbein, E. (1971): Chest 60:133.
Barclay, W. R. (1973): JAMA 223:199.
Boyden, S. V. (1958): Progr. Allerg. 5:149.
Curry, F. J. (1967): New Eng. J. Med. 277:562.
Diagnostic Standards and Classification of Tuberculosis (1961): New York, National Tuberculosis Association.
East Africa/British Medical Research Councils (1972): Lancet 1:1079.
Editorial (1967): Lancet 2:1185.
Editorial (1969): Lancet 1:192.
Editorial (1972): Lancet 2:412.
Houck, V. N. (1972): JAMA 222:1421.
Minden, P., et al. (1972): Science 176:57.
Rich, A. R. (1951): *The Pathogenesis of Tuberculosis.* Springfield, Illinois, Charles C Thomas.
Rosenthal, S. R. (1966): *BCG Vaccination against Tuberculosis.* Boston, Little, Brown and Company.
Runyon, E. H. (1965): Advances Tuberc. Res. 14:235.
Schachter, E. N. (1973): JAMA 223:93.
Strieder, J. W., Laforet, E. G., and Lynch, J. P. (1967): New Eng. J. Med. 276:960.
Vall-Spinosa, A., et al. (1970): New Eng. J. Med. 283:616.

Leprosy

Bullock, W. E. Jr. (1968): New Eng. J. Med. 278:298.
Bullock, W. E. Jr., Fields, J. P., and Brandriss, M. W. (1972): New Eng. J. Med. 287:1053.
Bullock, W. E. Jr., Ho, M. F., and Chen, M. J. (1970): J. Lab. Clin. Med. 75:863.
Dharmendra (1942): Leprosy in India 14:122.
Lawrence, H. S. (1972): New Eng. J. Med. 287:1092.
Lim, S. D., Fusaro, R. M., and Good, R. A. (1972): Clin. Immun. Immunopath. 1:122.
Mitsuda, D. (1919): Hifuka Hinyoka Easshi 19:697.
Rees, R. J. W. (1966): Nature 211:657.
Turk, J. L., and Waters, M. F. R. (1969): Lancet 2:243.

Brucellosis

Braude, A. I. (1951): J. Infect. Dis. 89:87.
Reddin, J. L., et al. (1965): New Eng. J. Med. 272:1263.
Shaffer, J. M., Kucera, C. J., and Spink, W. W. (1953): J. Exp. Med. 97:77.
Spink, W. W. (1956): *The Nature of Brucellosis.* Minneapolis, The University of Minnesota Press.
Spink, W. W., et al. (1962): Bull. WHO 26:409.
Williams, A. E., Keppie, J., and Smith, H. (1962): Brit. J. Exp. Path. 43:530.

Hemophilus Influenza

Anderson, P., Johnston, R. B. Jr., and Smith, D. H. (1972): J. Clin. Invest. 51:31.
Anderson, P., et al. (1972): J. Clin. Invest. 51:39.
Fothergill, L. D., and Wright, J. (1933): J. Immun. 24:273.
Greenfield, S., et al. (1972): J. Pediat. 80:204.
Norden, C. W., et al. (1972): J. Pediat. 80:209.
Parke, J. C. Jr., Schneerson, R., and Robbins, J. B. (1972): N. Carolina J. Pediat. 81:765.
South, M. A. (1972): J. Pediat. 80:348.
Sproles, E. T., et al. (1969): J. Pediat. 75:782.

Histoplasmosis and Coccidioidomycosis

Biggar, W. D., Meuwissen, H. J., and Good, R. A. (1971): Arch, Int. Med. *128*:585.
Class, R. N., and Cascio, F. S. (1972): New Eng. J. Med. *287*:1133.
Clinicopathological Conference (1973): Amer. J. Med. *54*:73.
Diamond, R. D., and Bennett, J. E. (1973): New Eng. J. Med. *288*:186.
Froman, A., and Kaluzny, A. A. (1969): JAMA *210*:1737.
Furcolow, M. L. (1962): Lab. Invest. *11*:1134.
Furcolow, M. L. (1963): JAMA *183*:823.
Salvin, S. B. (1963): Prog. Allerg. 7:213.
Segal, C., Wheeler, G., and Tompsett, R. (1969): New Eng. J. Med. *280*:206.

Cryptococcosis

Busse, O. (1895): Virchow Arch. Path. Anat. *140*:23.
Diamond, R., and Benr.ett, J. E. (1973): New Eng. J. Med. *288*:186.
Zimmerman, L. E., and Rappaport, H. (1954): Amer. J. Clin. Path. *24*:1050.

Candidiasis

Canales, L., et al. (1969): Lancet 2:567.
Chilgren, R. A., et al. (1969): Lancet *1*:1286.
Folb, P. I., and Trounce, J. R. (1970): Lancet 2:1112.
Hermans, P. E., Ulrich, J. A., and Markowitz, H. (1969): Amer. J. Med. *47*:503.
Montes, L. F., et al. (1972): JAMA *222*:1619.
Roe, D. C., and Haynes, R. E. (1972): Amer. J. Dis. Child. *124*:926.
Valdimarsson, H., et al. (1972): Lancet *1*:469.

Parasitic Infections

Brown, I. N. (1969): Advances, Immun. *11*:267.
Burke, B. A., and Good, R. A. (1973): Medicine *52*:23.
Ching, W. (1958): Clin. Med. J. 76:1.
Damian, R. T. (1967): J. Parasit. *53*:60.
Daroff, R. B., et al. (1967): JAMA *202*:679.
DeVita, V. T., et al. (1969): New Eng. J. Med. *280*:287.
Dineen, J. K., and Wagland, B. M. (1966): Immunology *11*:47.
Donohugh, D. L. (1963): New Eng. J. Med. *269*:1357.
Editorial (1970): Lancet 2:1121.
Gelpi, A. P., and Mustafa, A. (1968): Amer. J. Med. *44*:377.
Kagan, I. G., et al. (1967): Clin. Pediat. 6:641.
Kim, C. W. (1966): J. Infect. Dis. *116*:208.
MacFarlane, W. V. (1949): Amer. J. Hyg. *50*:152.
Nelson, G. S. (1966): Helminth. Abst. *35*:311.
Ogilvie, B. M. (1964): Nature *204*:91.
Olivier, L. (1949): Amer. J. Hyg. *49*:290.
Repsher, L. H., Schröter, G., and Hammond, W. S. (1972): New Eng. J. Med. *287*:340.
Robbins, J. B. (1967): Pediat. Res. *1*:131.
Rosen, L., et al. (1962): JAMA *179*:620.
Rosen, P., Armstrong, D., and Ramos, C. (1972): Amer. J. Med. *53*:428.
Sadun, E. H., Schoenbechler, M. J., and Bentz, M. (1965): Amer. J. Trop. Med. *14*:977.
Seeler, R. A., et al. (1973): Amer. J. Dis. Child. *125*:132.
Sengers, R. C. A. (1971): Lancet *1*:594.
Strejan, G., and Campbell, D. H. (1968): J. Immun. *101*:628.
Symmers, W. St.C. (1904): J. Path. Bact. 9:237.
Warren, K. S., and Domingo, E. O. (1970): Amer. J. Trop. Med. *19*:292.
Zvaifler, N. J., et al. (1967): Exp. Parasit. *20*:278.

Syphilis

Braunstein, G. D., et al. (1970): Amer. J. Med. 48:643.
Delhanty, J. J., and Catterall, R. D. (1969): Lancet 2:1099.
Harner, R. E., Smith, J. L., and Israel, C. W. (1968): JAMA 203:545.
Neisser, A., and Bruck, C. (1911): Arb. Kais. Gesund. 37:203.
Schroeter, A. L., et al. (1972): JAMA 221:471.
Youmans, J. B. (ed.) (1964): Med. Clin. N. Amer. 48:571.

Immunization against Bacterial Infections

Ashcroft, M. T., et al. (1967): Lancet 2:1056.
Balagtas, R. C., et al. (1971): J. Pediat. 79:203.
Benenson, A. S. (1970): Control of Communicable Diseases in Man. New York, The American Public Health Association.
Editorial (1972): Lancet 2:168.
Editorial (1972): Lancet 1:625.
Gotschlich, E. C., et al. (1972): J. Clin. Invest. 51:89.
Hornick, R. B., et al. (1970): New Eng. J. Med. 283:686.
Horstmann, D. M. (1971): New Eng. J. Med. 285:1432.
Miller, L. W., et al. (1972): Amer. J. Dis. Child. 123:197.
Parish, H. J. (1968): Victory with Vaccines: The Story of Immunization. London, E. & S. Livingstone Ltd.
Red Book (1970): Report of the Committee on the Infectious Diseases, 16th ed., American Academy of Pediatrics, P.O. Box 1034, Evanston, Illinois.
Robbins, J. B., and Pearson, H. A. (1965): J. Pediat. 66:877.
Smith, D. T. (1970): Clin. Pediat. 9:632.
Status of Immunization in Tuberculosis in 1971 (1972): Washington, D. C., U. S. Government Printing Office.
Steigman, A. J. (1968): J. Pediat. 72:753.

35
Clinical Transplantation

KIDNEY TRANSPLANTATION

The transplantation of a functioning human kidney to a patient suffering from chronic renal failure has developed as the prototype for human organ transplantation. More renal allografts have been performed than the sum of all other human organ transplants combined. For this reason, more is known of the factors involved in renal allograft immunity and survival than is known about any other human organ. As of May, 1973, 13,361 renal transplantations in 12,113 recipients had been reported to the ACS/NIH Organ Transplant Registry. At least 5,500 recipients were alive as of May 31, 1973. The longest survival was 16.5 years for a renal transplant from an identical twin donor, 13.9 years for transplants from sibling donors, 10 years for those from parent donors, and 8.9 years for those from cadaver donors.

If a renal or other organ is to be transplanted, a syngeneic transplant is ideal. Thus, whenever possible, a monozygotic twin should be employed. In the majority of instances, however, a sibling matched with the potential recipient at the major histocompatibility determinants should be chosen as the organ donor. Next best are other first degree relatives of the best possible histocompatibility match. Other carefully typed, live volunteers have been used as donors quite successfully and have included (1) recipients' spouses, (2) unrelated volunteer subjects, and (3) patients undergoing nephrectomy of a normal kidney for reasons such as the presence of ureteral lesions or the use of a ureter for the drainage of spinal fluid in hydrocephalus.

Living donors should, of course, be carefully screened with regard to their own renal function. Normal anatomic configuration of the kidneys and the lower urinary tract must be assured by appropriate radiologic examinations, including aortograms, to assess the renal arterial supply. Since 20 percent of normal individuals have multiple renal arteries and since such arteries are end arteries, this common anomaly may lead to problems at surgery which will result in at least partial kidney necrosis. The risk in a young adult volunteer following nephrectomy is almost negligible.

In centers where there has been a reluctance to employ live donors, or in situations where no suitable living donor has been available, cadaver kidneys have been transplanted. The criteria for establishing death of the donor vary from group to group but usually include the absence of respiration and heart beat and a flat electrocardiogram and electroencephalogram. When the agonal period is prolonged, histocompatibility typing and an assessment of renal function may be performed prior to death. The best possible matching, of course, can be achieved if a large number of potential recipients are always available to take advantage of the kidneys that become available, for example, from accident victims.

The kidney should be removed and transplanted as soon after death as possible to avoid acute tubular necrosis. If transplantation must be delayed, the organ should be perfused and cooled. In general, better results have been obtained with cadaver kidneys taken from individuals under 65 years of age.

Elaborate schemes, e.g., Eurotransplant, where numerous centers collaborate over all of western Europe to make available the best matches of donor and recipient, have been developed. In spite of this, the nature of histocompatibility testing and the nature of genetic responsibility being what they are (Chapter 16) for allograft rejection, full house HL-A matches in the general population do not work nearly as well as they do when siblings are matched because the HL-A system, although closely linked to the control of major histocompatibility determinants genetically, does not itself contain the genetic determinants which it is being used to indicate. Perhaps as matching using the more relevant MLR determinants improves, the success expected from HL-A matched sibling donors can be extended to the non-sibling matches from the general population.

Renal Graft Rejections

In experimental animals renal grafts may be rejected in a number of different ways. If as in grafts of rabbit kidney to dog the experimental animal possesses circulating antibodies against the donor kidney at the time of transplant, a generalized vascular damage that is complement-dependent occurs within the grafted kidney. Complete necrosis and cessation of all renal function ensues often within 2 to 5 minutes. This immediate graft rejection is dependent on antibody and complement and involves damage to endothelium, platelet-dependent localized intravascular occlusion, and leukocytes of the peripheral blood. In these circumstances rapid ischemic necrosis causes too rapid a loss of function and death of the kidney.

In man the form of graft rejection most similar to this is that which occurs when antibodies are present in the circulation of the recipient to antigens present in the kidney or blood cells of the donor. This kind of rejection is sometimes seen when the donor and recipient are mismatched according to the major blood group antigens. Other specific antigenic bases have also been observed, and in these circumstances the immediate early failure of the graft signals the prior immunization of recipient to host constituents. This form of renal allograft rejection is called the *hyperacute rejection.* Both experimentally and clinically it has been impossible to manipulate to permit prolonged renal function.

The second form of rejection reaction is referred to as the *acute rejection reaction.* This is the sort of rejection which is seen in most experimental renal allografts across major histocompatibility barriers when the rejection occurs in experimental animals between closely related species, as, for example, between sheep and goats. The rejection reaction may have components of both humoral and cellular immunity, but the cellular component dependent on T-cell immunity is the predominant modality. Here rejection is accompanied by extensive infiltration of lymphocytes, histiocytes, and even plasma cells of host origin in the grafted organ. This form of rejection reaction can be almost completely prevented by neonatal thymectomy and depression of T-cell immunities. Even when the rejection reaction has come into play it can often be reversed by so-called immunosuppressive therapy with adrenal corticosteroids, antimetabolites, and antilymphocyte serum. Vascular damage and glomerular lesions are usually minimal in this form. However, depending on the duration of this form of rejection, antibody dependent components may come into play and be demonstrable by appropriate techniques. Indeed acute rejections in some species, particularly sheep, seem predominantly to be attributable to B-cell immunities.

Chronic rejection reaction, the third type of rejection, is seen experimentally, especially when grafting occurs between animals matched at the so-called major histocompatibility determinants—HL-A region in man, H-2 in mice, and AgB in rats—and mismatched at one or several minor histocompatibility determinants. Chronic rejections are also seen when antilymphocyte, antimetabolite, and adrenal steroid therapy has been effective in suppressing the acute rejection reaction. In the latter rejections clear evidence of IgG, IgM, or IgA antibody assault on the renal glomerules or blood vessels has been demonstrated. Low grade cellular T-cell immunities perhaps dependent on relatively small numbers of sensitized T-cells play a role in most cases.

Special forms of hyperacute rejection, the fourth type of rejection reaction, have also been observed in the human renal transplantation experience. A kidney undergoing rejection by either the cellular or humoral mechanism can be extensively vulnerable to influences of endotoxins and other substances capable of initiating intravascular coagulation. On several occasions clear evidence of the operation of this mechanism has been documented in man.

The fifth type of kidney graft rejection has emerged from our recent studies. In conducting a renal pathology conference together with one of the largest renal transplantation services over a 2 1/2 year period, we had an opportunity to see all deaths and all renal graft rejections. Evidence of classic renal allograft rejection was observed infrequently in patients who had been treated by modern immunosuppressive and anti-inflammatory measures. Chronic rejection patterns, rare hyperacute rejections, and a most interesting fifth type of rejection reaction were seen instead. With suppression of the host's immunity mechanism all sorts of strange bacterial, viral, and fungus infections were encountered and often caused death. One of the latter forms of chronic infection, that due to the cytomegalovirus, seemed to play a crucial role in the rejection reactions. Humoral immunity and other local or systemic reactions to the virus, we believe, play a significant role in rejection of a graft that would otherwise be well tolerated.

A sixth form of rejection reaction for kidney allografts does not relate to host response to the graft, but the graft's catching, if you will, the destructive influence responsible for the original destruction of the host's own kidney. On numerous occasions we and others have obtained evidence that the very pathologic process present in the recipient's kidneys at nephrectomy has either promptly or more gradually reappeared in the transplanted kidney and been responsible for its destruction.

BONE MARROW TRANSPLANTATION

Inadequate development of an organ due to congenital disease may result in death in early life. An example of this is the category of birth defects such as severe combined immunodeficiency disease, which is presumed to be caused by a failure to develop lymphoid stem cells. It is primarily because of these experiments of Nature that bone marrow transplantation represents an exciting chapter in the history of biomedical investigations of organ grafting for the treatment of pathologic processes. Injury to bone marrow by drugs, chemicals, or by radiation is a major clinical problem. The possibility of adverse reactions in which bone marrow is destroyed as a side effect is a frequent threat to the patient taking certain drugs.

Bone marrow and its ancillary lymphatic tissues are usually procured and transplanted in ways quite different from those used in organ transplants. Needles and syringes are used to aspirate the normal red bone marrow from the cavities inside bones. Suspensions of the living cells are then made in an appropriate vehicle, so that the cells can be injected directly into the blood stream or peritoneal cavity of the recipient. The stem cells of the marrow lodge in the recipient's bones in the spaces that normally contain red marrow; there they grow and repopulate the cavities. This procedure is not as artificial as it seems because the stem cells of bone marrow normally circulate in small numbers in the blood of mammals. They are present along with the other blood cells that were originally produced by division and differentiation of stem cells of the same type as those residing in the marrow.

A major achievement in bone marrow transplantation and related areas of research has been a new understanding of the complicated patterns of cell migration through the marrow, peripheral blood, lymphatic tissues, and thymus. This field of investigation, a form of experimental hematology, is now a major activity of many laboratories throughout the world.

Bone marrow transplants between identical twins have been successfully carried out on at least 13 occasions; one of the recipients was a worker who, in an accident, had been exposed to an apparently lethal dose of radiation from a particle accelerator. He survived with the aid of the transplant. A summary, with literature citations, of most of these transplants between identical twins appears in Bortin's compendium of 203 reported cases of human marrow transplants. Bortin cites recovery in 5 of 7 individuals who received marrow from an identical twin as treatment for aplastic anemia. With identical twins, proving that transplantation of marrow has actually been accomplished is a problem because there is no way of recognizing donor cells in the patient.

One other situation in which marrow transplant is beneficial or potentially so in experimental animals is seen in hereditary anemia in mice. If the genetic relationship of donor and recipient is very close, the anemia is curable. Hereditary anemia (for example, sickle cell anemia, or thalassemia) is a major disorder in some human populations, but attempts to transplant normal bone marrow have not yet succeeded in altering the course of the disease. The situation in this fascinating disease of mice touches upon another major generality. Both development of lymphoid and hematopoietic cells and freedom from damaging effects of graft-versus-host reaction are strongly favored by an ideal match according to major histocompatibility determinants.

Direct demonstration of the presence of donor cells in marrow is usually accomplished by examining the chromosome number or chromosome structure when the donor and recipient have different chromosomal karyotypes. Another technique is to react the cells with cytotoxic antibody directed against the antigenic differences between the donor and the host. Red blood cell types, histochemical differences, and differences in cell products between donor and host are also used as markers.

When the autologous donor cells or cell products come into contact with lymphatic tissues (lymph nodes, spleen, and so on) of the host, nothing happens because of the genetic identity. An immune response is not induced if the lymphatic tissues treat the donor material as "self," and there is no host-versus-graft reaction. Cell transplants between identical twins and within a highly inbred strain of animals are treated as if they were autologous.

With all other types of genetic relationships between donor and host, the outcome is different. When grafted cells and cell substances that are not genetically identical with host tissues come into contact with lymphatic tissues of the host, they activate these tissues because they are recognized by the tissues as "non-self," not having been there when the tissues first developed. The lymphatic tissue system proliferates to produce cells and substances that attack the graft and destroy it. This is the host-versus-graft reaction that causes the failure of allogeneic or homologous grafts and of xenogeneic or heterologous grafts.

Bone marrow from one strain of mouse placed in a normal adult mouse of a second strain is rejected; this is the host-versus-graft reaction in an allogeneic graft. Similarly, rat bone marrow given to a normal adult mouse undergoes the same fate as a skin transplant or organ graft.

If the lymphatic tissue system is severely injured or modified in any of a variety of ways, it loses its ability to recognize "non-self" substances and it may not reject the allograft. A common means of producing this effect, immunosuppression, is to treat the animal or patient with azathioprine, cyclophosphamide, antilymphocyte serum, or whole-body ionizing radiation.

Histocompatibility typing is a means of measuring the closeness of the genetic relationships between donor and host in the allograft experiment. In ordinary mongrel populations, such as man or domestic animals, outbreeding, not inbreeding, is the practice; hence rejection of an allograft is always anticipated. There are, however, degrees of allograft relationships, somewhat like the range of relationships seen in blood grouping, and if matching (determination of histocompatibility) of donor and host is undertaken, it may make the job of immunosuppression less difficult and the success of grafting more certain.

Tissue typing for determining the degree of compatibility is now an important area in transplantation research and practice, even when powerful immunosuppressive agents are available. It shows why, whenever practical, family donors are used after the degree of histocompatibility has been determined.

The idea that a graft of foreign cells can attack the host came to the attention of transplantation investigators in the early 1950s. This phenomenon, graft-versus-host reaction, is not seen with skin, kidney, heart, liver, and many other organ allografts, but it is a major, still unsolved, problem in the transplantation of foreign bone marrow, white blood cells, and lymphatic tissues. This special group of tissues is frequently referred to as "blood-forming tissues."

The major sites of injury in graft-versus-host reactions are the lymphatic tissues, hematopoietic tissues, the skin, the intestine, and the liver of the host. The failure of lymphatic tissues to regenerate as they do in syngeneic grafts means that the recipient animal or man cannot adequately control the microorganisms present in the flora of the skin, intestine, and other tissue.

The graft-versus-host reactions in bone marrow transplantation in humans have been of overwhelming importance and are the major problem in these experiments. Such reactions are also of great importance in monkey and dog marrow grafts between unmatched donor and recipient.

A long-range goal in marrow transplantation is to use marrow grafts as a means of promoting acceptance of other organs, such as liver, heart, and kidney. Investigations in the mouse have shown that, once the foreign marrow is established, skin taken from the same donor as the marrow can then sometimes be successfully transplanted without further immunosuppression. The transplantation of foreign bone marrow in laboratory animals constitutes the important feasibility experiment for many of the goals in organ transplantation, in particular that of achieving immunosuppression with only a single "pulsed injury" to the host.

Bone marrow transplantation experiments indicate the possibility of cure for at least two types of immune deficiency disorders in man. In the Swiss type of hypogammaglobulinemia, the patient is not able to reject foreign cells, thus showing an absence of the host-versus-graft reaction. In this disorder, numerous other measures of normal immune function also reflect the absence of effective lymphatic tissue and its ability to respond to antigenic stimuli. A bone marrow transplant can cure this situation, provided there is histocompatibility between the marrow donor and the recipient, so that a lethal graft-versus-host reaction does not develop. The longest observation, to date, of a child treated with a marrow transplant for this rare disease is 5 years. This successful marrow allograft, which has corrected an inborn error in the metabolism of the immunity function, has persisted to the present. Because the patient developed an iatrogenically induced, immunologically based pancytopenia, a second marrow transplant from the same donor was used to switch the recipient's blood type from A to O and correct his pancytopenia. He now lives completely well and has full immunologic vigor 5 years following the first transplant. Further, 5 years after the second transplant he still has his sister's blood type and marrow cells of female karyotype. This startling achievement signals the opening of an era which will use such cellular engineering as treatment for human disease. Numerous additional examples of marrow transplants to treat combined immunodeficiencies successfully are now available. In some instances, even when a full-house match of a sibling is available, engraftment is difficult. The latter may be related to the newly described autosomally inherited deficiency of adenosine deaminase, which could be interfering with development or differentiation of the grafted cells in much the same way it influenced development of the host's own cells. Not every patient so treated has survived the graft-versus-host reaction, but those who have appear to be cured. The Wiskott-Aldrich syndrome has also been partially reversed by marrow graft. The ability of marrow stem cells, when grafted, to generate a new lymphatic tissue system of donor-cell origin and a new thymus is one of the remarkable features of these cells.

It now appears that determinants at the MLR locus are more closely related to the graft-versus-host reaction than are those at the HL-A locus. For a bone marrow transplant Dupont et al. have used the mixed leukocyte culture technique to select a donor whose determinants at the HL-A locus were completely mismatched with those of the recipient but whose determinants at the MLR locus were matched. This transplant completely corrected the immunodeficiency in a patient with severe combined immunodeficiency.

The cure of thalassemia and of sickle-cell anemia in man has been another goal for marrow grafting, but successful results have not yet been attained. In the genetic anemias the host-versus-graft reaction must be avoided through histocompatibility matching of donor and host and through treatment of the host with immunosuppressants. The graft-versus-host reaction is still a major hazard, even when the take of the marrow graft is assured. One area where grafting with matched sibling donor marrow has already been effective in correcting human disease has been the aplastic anemias and pancytopenias. Combinations of lethal irradiation or massive doses of cyclophosphamide coupled with methotrexate to suppress the graft-versus-host reaction have been repeatedly successful in both animals and man when matched sibling donors of marrow have been used. At present it seems possible to correct approximately one half of such patients with aplastic anemia by bone marrow transplantation using a matched sibling donor. By contrast to severe combined immunodeficiency where a matched sibling donor marrow does not induce fatal graft-versus-host reactions, approximately one fourth to one third of marrow transplants using a matched sibling donor have led to fatal graft-versus-host reactions. The synergistic destructive effect of the cytotoxic chemicals used to suppress the host-versus-graft and the graft-versus-host reactions represents a major problem that has not yet been completely resolved. Studies in animals and man indicate that antilymphocyte globulin, especially that which has specificities directed toward T-lymphocytes, can be used to treat effectively the ongoing graft-versus-host reaction.

ENZYME ENGINEERING BY TRANSPLANTATION

The manifestations of some inborn errors of metabolism result from reduced or absent enzyme activity. For example, glucocerebrosides accumulate in reticuloendothelial cells of individuals with Gaucher's disease because their tissues possess subnormal activity of glucocerebrosidase, an enzyme which splits glucocerebroside to glucose and ceramide. Different degrees of severity of the disease may depend on the completeness of the enzyme deficiency. In Fabry's disease, deposition of a sphingolipid, trihexosyl ceramide, in tissues and blood vessels results from a deficiency of ceramide trihexosidase, a specific alpha-galactosidase that removes the terminal galactosyl groups from trihexosyl ceramide. Accumulation of this material in glomerular capillaries causes renal failure, usually in the third or fourth decade.

Replacement of missing enzymes by infusion in glycogenosis and in Fabry's disease has not been particularly rewarding, although it has altered the disease. The preparation and purification of enzymes is difficult, the half-life of the enzymes is short, and it is uncertain whether intravenous infusion delivers the enzyme to appropriate sites. Alternative approaches to treatment of genetically determined enzyme deficiencies have been suggested.

Renal transplantation has been performed on several patients with Fabry's disease with the dual purpose of relieving terminal renal failure and contributing the deficient enzyme, ceramide trihexosidase. Severe crises of pain were abolished in one patient, although mild attacks continued in another. In addition, the transplanted kidney seemed to contribute significant enzyme activity. In both patients transplanted at the University of Minnesota by Desnick et al. the plasma concentration of trihexosyl ceramide fell to normal, and the concentration of ceramide trihexosidase increased, although only to about 10 percent of the normal concentration. Whether these findings indicate that significant enzyme activity has been contributed by the graft will only be clear when the separate effects of restoration of effective glomerular filtration and administration of immunosuppressive drugs upon plasma-trihexosyl-ceramide have been established.

The kidneys of one of the patients of Desnick et al. were left in situ. After the transplantation of a renal allograft the activity of ceramide trihexosidase in her urine became normal and the urinary sediment lipid, thought largely to represent desquamated renal tubular cells, was reduced. The authors concluded that the lipid deposits in her own kidneys had diminished. Her kidneys were not biopsied. A double-dose pyelogram showed concentration of contrast material, whereas there had been none when she was uremic. The evidence that any lipid deposits have cleared is fragmentary and unconvincing, but the possibility is certainly worth further detailed study and manipulation.

Renal transplantation has also been undertaken for end-stage renal failure in cystinosis, a condition in which the enzyme deficiency has yet to be identified. Proximal tubular function was normal for up to 32 months, except during rejection crises. Biopsies of renal allografts up to

25 months after transplantation have shown interstitial accumulation of cystine but no deposits in glomeruli or tubular cells, although these may yet develop. Interstitial deposits have been found both in allografts from parent donors (who presumably were heterozygotes for the disease) and in an unrelated donor. In one case no cystine deposits were found in the renal allograft after 11 months. In none of these children did the deposits of cystine in cornea or bone marrow diminish after renal transplantation.

The enzymatic defect in Wilson's disease is also unknown. Speculation that the defect lies primarily in the liver and may therefore be corrected by orthotopic liver transplantation has been encouraged by the remarkable outcome of liver transplantation on a boy with cirrhosis, very probably (but not certainly) due to Wilson's disease. He had extensive deposits of copper in his liver, and for several months after transplantation he had a "massive cupruresis." No copper was found in biopsy specimens of the transplanted liver taken at 6 and 17 months after transplantation.

The evidence that sufficient enzyme activity can thus be contributed to arrest or reverse the deposition of metabolites in other tissues is incomplete and unconvincing, except perhaps in Wilson's disease. Another disease which may fall into this same category is congenital nephrosis. This disease is characterized by progressive renal destruction and presence of the nephrotic syndrome at birth. It has seemed to be especially frequent in Finland and Minnesota. In our studies the absence of evidence of immunologic assault coupled with evidence of progressive damage to the kidney tubules, as well as to the glomeruli, has suggested to us that this disease may have as its basis a toxic metabolite probably produced in the kidney. Renal transplantation at Minnesota in multiple cases has completely corrected the disease, and the new kidneys seem to be functioning normally and not showing any evidence of tubular or glomerular disease. Finally the renal disease associated with deficiency of the C1r component of complement has been corrected by renal transplantation, and total hemolytic complement and C1r levels have returned toward normal. This entire area is in a state of rapid flux and development and much new information can be expected within the next few years.

TRANSPLANTATION OF OTHER ORGANS

Heart Transplantation

The first human heart allograft was reported through the news media in December of 1967. Subsequent events generated an unprecedented degree of interest that served to focus public attention on the ethics of human organ transplantation in general, and of heart transplantation in particular. The human cardiac transplantation, dramatic as it was, had been, however, based on a solid substructure of experimentation in animals that was led by Shumway of Stanford University. As of May, 1973,

208 cardiac transplantations have been reported to the ACS/NIH Organ Transplant Registry. Of 32 recipients who were alive, 6 recipients have survived more than 4 years.

The medical problems encountered in heart transplantation are somewhat different from those associated with renal allografts. First, since the heart is an unpaired organ, only cadaver donors can be employed. Furthermore, unlike the situation in renal failure, where life can be maintained for an almost indefinite period by artificial means, the ability to prolong life in severe cardiac disease is often extremely limited. For both of these reasons prospective histocompatibility testing is more difficult in cardiografts, and greater reliance must often be placed on the use of immunosuppressive agents. It must also be remembered that even if heart transplantation were to become a feasible procedure without the necessity of typing for transplantation antigens, the number of prospective donors is extremely small with respect to the number of potential recipients.

The suggestion that a transplanted heart might react differently from other transplanted tissues is based on the fact that the heart is a simpler functional unit than organs such as the kidney or liver. Although muscle tissue may be somewhat less antigenic than blood leukocytes, no evidence supports the new concept that the heart is less vulnerable to rejection than are other human allografts. It is interesting that most of the successful heart allografts have been achieved by the surgeons who worked out the methodology first in experimental animals. It seems certain to us that with cardiac transplants, as with other organ transplants, methodologies will gradually be improved so that in spite of the difficulties attendant to the procurement of the graft and the technical components of the operation, allografts of the heart will be used in reconstructive surgery.

Lung Transplantation

As of May, 1973, at least 32 whole lung allografts obtained from cadavers or from living donors have been performed. Although the usual survival time following lung transplantation has been from a few days to a few months at best, the longest survivor lived for 11 months after the operation.

The most serious problems that must be solved to permit lung transplantation include: (1) the transplanted lung is particularly susceptible to infections, (2) the ability of the lung to clear secretions is dependent to some extent on an intact nerve supply which is lost during the transplantation procedure, (3) the lung has a double circulation which includes the necessity for the bronchial arteries to provide nutrition to parts of the pulmonary parenchyma, and (4) a latent period between the time of transplantation and the resumption of normal pulmonary function is difficult to overcome.

Liver Transplantation

The feasibility of hepatic allotransplantation has been established by experimental studies in which animals have been kept alive for prolonged periods after complete hepatectomy and liver replacement. The problems of liver allotransplantation in man are complicated by a number of specific problems peculiar to this organ. Orthotopic transplantation of the liver is difficult technically, and although heterotopic procedures have been described for the implantation of auxiliary livers, none is yet ideal.

The liver too is an unpaired organ, and therefore only cadaver donors can be employed. Because the human liver is extremely sensitive to ischemic damage, the major difficulty with human liver allotransplantation has been the preservation of adequate liver function between the time of donor death and the actual transplantation procedure. As of May, 1973, 190 liver transplantations in 186 patients had been reported to ACS/NIH Organ Transplant Registry. Eighteen were alive and one recipient had survived more than 4 years.

Very little information concerning the immunology of liver allograft rejection has been developed. However, it has been reported that the migration of peripheral leukocytes in a patient who had received a liver transplant could be inhibited by incubation with fetal liver homogenate at a time when there was biochemical evidence of rejection. A liver biopsy obtained at the same time showed liver cell necrosis and infiltration of lymphocytes and plasma cells in the portal areas. Successful treatment of the rejection crisis with prednisone returned the migration index to normal. These observations would support the contention that liver allograft rejection in man is mediated by cellular immune mechanisms.

No recipient of a heterotopic graft survived beyond one year. Despite the poor survival rate, the fact that recipients of human liver allografts could live for a year or more after operation is encouraging. Here again, improvements of technique and improvements in management of the allograft rejection are occurring, and liver allografts will ultimately become part of the therapeutic and reconstructive armamentarium.

Pancreatic Transplantation

For diseases of the pancreas, 32 transplants in 32 recipients had been reported by May, 1973. Of the 3 surviving recipients, one has survived more than 1 1/2 years. Most of the recipients were juveniles with severe diabetes with vascular complications, nephropathy, and chronic renal failure. Since these patients were poor risks for chronic hemodialysis or for renal allotransplantation alone, the objective was to transplant a kidney and a pancreas from the same cadaver donor. The principal technique used was the transplantation of the entire pancreas with the attached duodenum into the recipient's iliac fossa. In the immediate postoperative period, there was evidence of adequate pancreative function in some patients.

Corneal and Scleral Transplants

The human cornea holds a unique position in the history and biology of human transplantation. It enjoys a relatively privileged existence on the surface of the eye because, under normal circumstances, it is avascular. Preservation of corneal tissue, although often thought to be simple, is very difficult; viable corneas obtained several hours after death can sometimes be kept in transplantable form for only a few days. Corneas have been stored in tissue banks and shipped for long distances with some degree of preservation. Since immunosuppressive therapy is not always required in order to avoid rejection, corneal transplantation has been a well-established, even though difficult, clinical procedure for many years.

Surprisingly little is known about the immunology of corneal transplantation, but it has been established that the cornea contains tissue isoantigens as well as antigens of serum proteins. The most important isoantigens appear to be intracellular, concentrated in the epithelial layer, and closely related to erythrocyte antigens. High titers of circulating anticorneal antibodies have been detected 5 to 20 days after transplantation, but these appear to be more closely related to the development of iridocyclitis than to the failure of the graft. Rejection of corneal allografts, however, promptly occurs if for any reason the graft becomes vascularized.

Similarly, a high incidence of success has been achieved with scleral allografts without the use of immunosuppressive agents. The sclera, like the cornea, may therefore be considered as a somewhat privileged site, although little is known of the immune response following the allotransplantation of scleral tissue in humans.

It should be noted that in both corneal and scleral allografts, the transplanted tissue may serve both allostatic and allovital functions. Most of the available evidence indicates that successful corneal allografts are associated with the continued viability of the transplanted tissue. Nevertheless, it remains possible that, under certain circumstances, the donor tissue may function as an architecturally intact superstructure that is gradually replaced by normal recipient tissue.

As a result of recent studies at the University of Minnesota organ culture methods have been developed which seem to have great advantages in preservation of corneal tissues over techniques previously employed. Interestingly, after a critical period in culture the preserved cornea seems to resist allograft and xenograft rejection much better than do fresh corneas or corneas stored in the more conventional manner.

Bone and Cartilage Transplantation

It has been known for half a century that human bone can be transplanted successfully. Studies performed in both man and experimental animals have demonstrated that a bone allograft obeys the general rules governing transplantation of other allografted tissues. The transplanted cells are destroyed within 1 to 2 weeks by the various mechanisms of immune rejection. However, the dead skeleton of the transplanted bone still retains osteogenetic inductive capacity. Thus the dead allograft is slowly recognized by host blood vessels, and the transplanted bone is slowly removed and replaced by new bone of host origin. From these observations, it would appear that transplanted bone functions in an allostatic rather than in an allovital capacity.

Unlike bone transplants, transplanted cartilage functions as an allovital graft. It has long been known that cartilage can be transplanted successfully between individuals of different genetic backgrounds without suppressing immune function of the recipients. The first experimental study of cartilage transplantation was described by Bert in 1865. Chondrocytes are the only mammalian cells that can be transplanted into allogeneic recipients without provoking an immune response. For example, sex chromatin studies have revealed that donor cells remain in place for many years after grafting. Since cartilage allografts behave as autografts, no immunosuppression is required. At present cartilage allografts are used in clinical practice primarily for reconstructive surgery of nose, ears, and skull defects.

The use of osteochondral allografts to resurface joints has been an area of active investigation over a long period. Allografts of this type have been performed successfully in experimental animals, but only when the underlying metaphysis did not exceed 2 to 3 mm in thickness. When the supporting shell of underlying bone was thicker, the bony layer underwent absorption and collapse. Although similar transplants have not as yet been reported in man, it is possible that they may play an important part in providing functional, resurfaced joints in the future.

Spleen Transplantation

Recent interest in splenic allotransplantation has been generated by the suggestion that the spleen may be a source of antihemophilic globulin (AHG, factor VIII). The evidence for this hypothesis has come primarily from studies in dogs with hemophilia where splenic transplantation has occasionally returned AHG levels to normal, or close to normal. At the time of writing, a single heterotopic splenic transplant for hemophilia had been performed in man. The allograft was removed on the fourth postoperative day because of rupture of the transplanted spleen. However, the spleen does perform other functions far more important than its possible role as one contributory source of AHG, and future efforts to replace these functions may be needed.

Because it is uncertain whether the human spleen is the major site of AHG production, the risks of surgery and immunosuppression probably are not justified by the potential benefits. Moreover, AHG concentrates are more widely available and are more potent than they have been in the past.

Skin Transplantation

The history of the study of rejection of skin allografts is, in a sense, the history of transplantation itself. The intralymphatic situation of the skin allograft, the peculiarities of its vascular attachment to the host, and the highly antigenic properties of the epidermis have made skin allografts the most exacting test of human histocompatibility. For exactly the same reasons, attempts at the allogeneic transplantation of skin between humans have almost invariably failed. In fact, the failure to reject a skin allograft has become an important criterion for the assessment of immunologic deficiency states. It seems rather ironic that the organ which has been of such aid to the investigator in the field of transplantation could be the last tissue to be successfully allotransplanted.

At present, the function of the skin transplant appears to be limited to fulfilling an allostatic role in situations where large areas of skin have been denuded by extensive burns, ulcerated infections, or impaired vascular supply. Again studies at the University of Minnesota suggest that organ culture techniques may be used to render human and animal skin transplantable across major histocompatibility barriers. Already allogeneic transplants clearly identifiable as being of donor origin by the most critical criteria have remained in place for several years, and animal skin grafts have bridged both allogeneic and xenogeneic barriers for periods of greater than one year and are still in good condition. Cultured xenogeneic transplants have also been kept in place for many months. Whether this extraordinary achievement can be applied practically in cellular and enzymatic engineering is still to be determined.

SELECTED REFERENCES

Kidney Transplantation

Fine, R. N., et al. (1970): J. Pediat. 76:347.
Najarian, J. S., and Simmons, R. L. (1972): *Transplantation*. Philadelphia, Lea & Febiger.

Opelz, G., Mickey, M. R., and Terasaki, P. I. (1972): Science *178*:617.
Proceedings of the First International Symposium on Clinical Organ Transplantation (1972): Transplant. Proc. *4*:427.

Bone Marrow Transplantation

Bortin, M. M. (1970): Transplantation *9*:571.
Dupont, D., et al. (1973): Transpl. Proc. *5*:905.
Good, R. A. (1970): JAMA *214*:1289.
Thomas, E. D., et al. (1971): Blood *38*:267.
Thomas, E. D., et al. (1972): Lancet *1*:284.
van Bekkum, D. W., and deVries, M. J. (1967): *Radiation Chimaeras*. New York, Academic Press, Inc.

Enzyme Engineering by Transplantation

Clarke, J. T. R., et al. (1972): New Eng. J. Med. *287*:1215.
Desnick, R. J., et al. (1972): Surgery *72*:203.
DuBois, R. S., et al. (1971): Lancet *1*:505.
Fabry, J. (1898): Arch. Derm. Syph. *43*:187.
Groth, C. C., et al. (1971): Lancet *1*:1260.
Mahoney, C. P., et al. (1970): New Eng. J. Med. *283*:397.

Transplantation of Other Organs

ACS/NIH Organ Transplant Registry (1972): Second Scientific Report. JAMA *221*:1486.
Bert, P. (1865): C. R. Acad. Sci. (Paris) *61*:587.
Najarian, J. S., and Simmons, R. L. (1972): *Transplantation*. Philadelphia, Lea & Febiger.
Russell, P. S., and Winn, H. J. (1970): New Eng. J. Med. *282*:786.

36

Immunologic Perturbation
in Malignant Diseases

Lymphomas and leukemias are manifestations of lymphoproliferative neoplastic processes. In leukemias the malignant cells are widely disseminated from the earliest stages, whereas in lymphomas the disease often remains localized for prolonged periods and only becomes disseminated at a later stage. One form of lymphoma, so-called Hodgkin's disease, which has a variety of histologic variants, is often granulomatous in nature. Immunologic abnormalities have been associated with each of the basic forms and variants of lymphoma and leukemia. The most consistent and profound abnormalities, however, are seen in Hodgkin's disease and in chronic lymphatic leukemia. The immunologic perturbations occurring in these diseases often have provided new insights as to the basic pathogenetic mechanisms of diseases and basic insights concerning the organization and function of the lymphoid system.

HODGKIN'S DISEASE

Hodgkin's disease is an acquired disorder of the lymphoid system characterized by progressive glandular enlargement without appearance of characteristic cells in the blood. In most instances the condition begins as or progresses to a systemic illness with fever, chills, sweats, itching, weight loss, and anemia. The diagnosis is made by biopsy and is based on the histologic features which reveal loss of the usual architecture of the node, fibrosis, eosinophilia, and characteristic cellular elements— Reed-Sternberg cells, multinucleated giant cells with characteristic nucleoli. Several distinct pathologic forms can be identified. These include lymphocyte-predominant, nodular-sclerosing, mixed, and lymphocyte depleted forms.

In the absence of treatment or when treatment (radiotherapy) does not eradicate the process, the condition is fatal. Survival is occasionally less than a year but is quite variable, sometimes many years. In recent years evidence has accumulated that localized forms of the disease can be cured by intensive radiotherapy to the independent lymphoid chains of the involved nodes. A variety of chemotherapeutic compounds including the alkylating agent, vinblastine, and the methylhydrazine derivative, procarbazine, can induce useful remissions. Indeed, combinations of these agents, together with irradiation, have produced dramatic remissions even in the presence of widely disseminated Hodgkin's disease.

Patients with Hodgkin's disease have been known for many years to be inordinately susceptible to certain infections, particularly those attributed to tubercle bacilli, other acid-fast organisms, fungi (especially cryptococcus), and the herpes and pox viruses. By contrast they have little difficulty with infections produced by pneumococci, streptococci, Hemophilus influenzae bacilli, and Pseudomonas. This susceptibility to infection is due to cellular immunodeficiency present early in the course of Hodgkin's disease and increasing with progression of the disease. This defect is demonstrable before treatment is given and increases with pro gression of the disease regardless of treatment. The deficiency can be markedly enhanced by treatment with X-ray or cytotoxic agents.

The terminal patient with Hodgkin's disease can also lose ability to form antibody and even become hypogammaglobulinemic, but it is not clear that this late deficit is not a function of therapeutic efforts. Patients in good general condition with localized or moderately advanced disease retain the ability to form normal amounts of antibody to many antigenic stimuli and have normal or slightly elevated gamma globulin levels. However, Aisenberg has emphasized that a slight defect in antibody formation in such favorable Hodgkin's patients may be present. A depressed response to primary (as opposed to secondary) antigenic stimuli can be demonstrated to some antigens.

Phagocytic function appears to be intact in patients with Hodgkin's disease. Secondary infections with a variety of organisms are characteristic of the advanced stages of Hodgkin's disease. For example, fungi (Candida, Torula, Aspergillus, Actinomyces, and Histoplasma), viruses of the herpes group (herpes zoster and cytomegalovirus), and certain protozoa (Pneumocystis carinii and Toxoplasma) frequently cause infection. The frequency of infectious complications in Hodgkin's disease can be appreciated from the National Cancer Institute series of 51 cases reported by Casazza et al. Of all episodes of infections, 56 were bacterial, 17 viral, 10 fungal, and 3 protozoal.

The immunologic deficiency in Hodgkin's disease involves that function which in experimental animals has been shown to be thymus dependent, and many features of the Hodgkin's patient resemble the immunologically deficient thymectomized animal.

LYMPHOMAS AND LEUKEMIAS

Chronic Lymphatic Leukemia

Between one third and one half of patients with chronic lymphatic leukemia develop extreme hypogammaglobulinemia. Markedly increased susceptibility to infection with both high grade encapsulated pyogenic pathogens, e.g., pneumococci, as well as viruses, fungi, enteric and iso-teric bacteria, may be seen. As was shown first by Cone and Uhr, patients with chronic lymphatic leukemia have deficiencies of both cellular and humoral immunities. Failure to express delayed allergic reactions and to form antibodies has been demonstrated.

During the last two years studies quantifying both B-cell and T-cell populations have revealed deficiencies in the number of the normal B- and T-cells and evidence of monoclonal malignant expansion of the B-cell population in this disease. Usually this monoclonal expansion in-volves B-lymphocytes of the μ variety and thus far the majority of these cells containing μ "receptors" have been positive as well for κ light chains. A few instances of chronic lymphatic leukemia representing monoclonal malignant expansion of lymphocytes possessing IgG or IgA have been encountered.

At this writing the paradox of chronic lymphatic leukemia is the im-munodeficiency involving the T-cell line. Whether this depression is sec-ondary to the extension of the malignant B-cells into areas ordinarily oc-cupied by T-cells that provide the regions for normal expansion of T-cell populations upon antigenic stimulation or whether this deficiency re-flects an influence of an etiologic or pathogenic agent, e.g., virus, remains to be determined.

Lymphoma, Lymphosarcoma

Susceptibility to infections is much more variable in patients with lymphosarcomas or lymphomas than in patients with Hodgkin's disease. In some instances susceptibility to infection is a major problem in these diseases; in other instances vigorous immunologic mechanisms seem to sustain capacity for resistance to the microbial invader. Thus far analysis of the immunologic mechanisms in these patients, the perturbations of immunity present in these diseases, and relations to state of the evolu-tion of the disease have not been well studied.

It is already clear that the diseases referred to as lymphoma and lym-phosarcoma show great heterogeneity. For example, some are largely fol-licular in nature, some pleomorphic, and some monotonus in morphology. In some instances the lymphosarcomas represent monoclonal B-cell ma-lignant expansions; in other instances no evidence of this type of differ-entiation can be demonstrated. Autoimmunities and autoantibodies in the serum are encountered frequently in patients with lymphosarcoma. Sometimes these are monoclonal, but usually they are polyclonal auto-antibodies. The high frequency of such autoimmunities (Chapter 15) and the fragmented direct data thus far available indicate that immuno-deficiency is a common concomitant in lymphosarcomas of various types.

Once the lymphosarcoma has become widely disseminated, of course, increased susceptibility to infection and immunodeficiency are the rule. Much more study defining the immunologic status with a suitable spectrum of quantifiable analytic methods from the earliest stages to death in patients with lymphosarcoma is sorely needed.

Acute Lymphatic Leukemia of Childhood

Rather surprisingly, patients with so-called acute lymphatic leukemia of childhood usually show very little perturbation of immunologic parameters when studied early in the course of the disease. These patients usually have normal immunoglobulin levels, and both antibody production and development of cellular immunities are quite normal. However, very early in the disease they show rather extreme deficits of granulocytes, platelets, and red blood cells. The deficits of platelets, granulocytes, and possibly monocytes may render these patients more susceptible to bacterial infections than are normal persons. Just what cell type is being clonally expanded by malignant proliferation in acute lymphatic leukemia is not yet clear. On several occasions, however, we have seen acute lymphatic leukemia apparently appear first in the thymus as it does in mice. Such patients may present thymic mass and outflow obstruction before peripheral manifestations of leukemia occur. After a few days, however, they may then express typical acute lymphatic leukemia. This has also been encountered in patients with X-linked infantile agammaglobulinemia who have no B-cells. Further, recent studies using certain antisera apparently directed toward T-cell species determinants have recognized tentatively some of these cases as having a T-cell proliferation. For studying the influence of therapy on immunity in children with acute lymphatic leukemia Frommel et al. found that prolonged anticancer chemotherapeutic regimens with multiple drugs and sometimes coupled with radiation therapy can produce severe immunosuppression in these patients. Indeed, even severe hypogammaglobulinemia has occurred. After drug therapy has been discontinued, however, immunoglobulin and antibody production return promptly to normal. In a few instances during continuing infection extraordinary "dysgammaglobulinemia" (exceedingly high levels of IgM) has been encountered. Further careful quantitative studies of parameters of immunity are needed in this disease as well.

So-called acute myeloid leukemia of young adults is a disease in which ability to resist infection is often a paramount feature. Again definitive analysis of immunologic capacity has not been carried out in most cases, and such studies are much needed. However, the major defects of defense in these patients seem to be attributable to lack of mature, fully functional granulocytes and monocytes in the circulation. Table 36-1 summarizes the general picture of immunodeficiency associated with lymphoma and leukemia.

Table 36-1. Immunodeficiency Associated with Lymphoma and Leukemia before Treatment

	Inflammatory response	Humoral immunity	Cellular immunity
Acute leukemia	Decreased	Normal	Normal
Chronic lymphatic leukemia	Normal	Depressed	Depressed
Hodgkin's disease	Normal	Normal or slightly depressed	Depressed

MULTIPLE MYELOMA

Multiple myeloma belongs to so-called "plasma cell dyscrasia" which represents a group of conditions characterized by an unbalanced or disproportionate proliferation usually of a single number of clones of plasma cells resulting in an excessive production of a homogeneous protein, i.e., IgG, IgA, IgM, IgE, or IgD, with constituent heavy or light chain polypeptide components. In addition to multiple myeloma, Waldenström's macroglobulinemia, the heavy chain disease of IgG and of IgA, and the majority of cases of so-called primary amyloidosis are collectively grouped as plasma cell dyscrasia. Although the exact etiology of multiple myeloma and other plasma cell dyscrasias has not been fully elucidated, some evidence suggests that chronic stimulation of the lymphoreticular apparatus may play a predisposing role to development of this disease. In a few instances the myeloma proteins have been identified as the antibodies they all probably are. When this has been accomplished, the titers of antibodies have been fantastically high.

Dunn in 1957 described plasma cell tumors in the ileocecal region in association with local ulceration in C3H mice. Potter induced plasma cell tumors in BALB/c mice by the intraperitoneal injection of a variety of substances, including Freund's adjuvants, mineral oil, and plastics. In another interesting study New Zealand red rabbits immunized with group A-variant streptococcal vaccine produced very high concentrations of homogenous monoclonal gamma globulins with specific antibody activity directed to the immunizing antigen. Since the induction of this monoclonal hyperplasia is observed only in a small fraction of immunized animals, the influence of environmental or genetic factors or both may be important. Occasionally mink with Aleutian disease if kept alive long enough will develop monoclonal gamma globulin and apparently have a form of myeloma.

Analysis of multiple myeloma by Kunkel and his co-workers culminated in definition of the molecular nature of antibody and the structure and function of the immunoglobulins. Bence Jones protein, a key to the chemical analysis of immunoglobulin structure, is the light chain of the immunoglobulin molecule. Study of such patients has been most important in another perspective. The monoclonal proliferation of plasma cells is associated with significant deficiency of formation of all the normal immunoglobulins and antibodies. These patients consequently are extremely susceptible to infection with pneumococcus and other high grade encapsulated bacterial pathogens. By contrast, they resist infections with many viruses, fungi, and enteric pathogens very well. Cell-mediated immunities and allograft rejection in these patients are quite normal.

It is now possible to classify the M globulins and Bence Jones proteins in man into five major heavy chain classes, i.e., IgG, IgA, IgM, IgE, and IgD, and two light chain classes, i.e., α and κ. In clinical practice, M type globulins are first detected by electrophoretic analysis of the serum proteins, Bence Jones proteins by the demonstration of proteinuria by precipitation with 20 percent sulfosalicylic acid followed by electrophoresis. The distinguishing monoclonal features are evidenced by their electrophoretic homogeneity, the so-called M component.

Multiple myeloma characteristically displays features of plasma cell neoplasia manifested primarily by widespread skeletal destruction and is frequently associated with anemia, hypercalcemia, impairment of renal function, and increased susceptibility to infections. Amyloidosis, coagulation defects, and symptoms and signs related to the production of cryoglobulins or increased serum viscosity are also seen. The diagnosis of myeloma is generally made by (1) X-ray demonstration of bony destruction, (2) M-component in serum electrophoresis, or in urine, or both, and in increased number of plasma cells in bone marrow. The symptomatic stage of myeloma is usually preceded by an asymptomatic period, in which M-type serum or urinary proteins, or both, are demonstrable.

WALDENSTRÖM'S MACROGLOBULINEMIA

The syndrome of macroglobulinemia was first recognized by Waldenström in 1944. This is a form of a plasma cell dyscrasia involving the abnormal proliferation of IgM-producing cells. The excessive proliferation of these cells results in the production of monoclonal (M-type) IgM and associated clinical syndrome characterized by anemia, bleeding, and other manifestations connected with the increased serum macroglobulins. Both males and females are affected with equal frequency. The disease usually begins in the fifth and sixth decades but may be preceded by many presymptomatic years.

As the disease slowly evolves, lymphadenopathy, splenomegaly, and hepatomegaly develop into a clinical pattern resembling a malignant lymphoma or lymphatic leukemia. Skeletal lesions like those seen in myeloma are exceptionally rare in macroglobulinemia. Histologic studies of the bone marrow and lymph nodes in macroglobulinemia generally demonstrate a proliferation of lymphocytic and/or plasmacytic forms with intermediate and apparently transitional cell types. A variety of analyses confirm the synthesis of γ-globulin in these cells.

When macroglobulinemia becomes symptomatic, anemia is the most common presenting manifestation and is frequently profound. Hemoglobin levels as low as 4 to 6 gm/100 ml are the rule. Usually the anemia is due to a combination of factors, including accelerated red cell destruction, blood loss, and decreased erythropoiesis. Coating of erythrocytes with IgM is apparently responsible for the marked rouleau formation, autoagglutination, positive Coombs' reactions, and cross-matching difficulties encountered in many cases.

A large percentage of IgM globulins have specific physicochemical properties that are responsible for specific symptom patterns in certain cases. These properties include cold insolubility (cryoglobulins), high intrinsic viscosity, and the capacity to form complexes with coagulation factors and other plasma proteins. Cryoglobulin-related symptoms include Raynaud's phenomenon, cold sensitivity, cold urticaria, and vascular occlusion with gangrene following cold exposure. Viscosity-related manifestations are most evident in the retinal vasculature, where a pattern of patchy venous bulging and localized narrowing develops, frequently associated with hemorrhages, exudates, and visual impairment. Circulatory impairment in the central nervous system due to increased plasma viscosity produces changing patterns of neurologic signs and symptoms (e.g., transient paresis, reflex abnormalities, deafness, impairment of consciousness, or coma paraproteinemicus) frequently terminating with cerebral vascular hemorrhage. Cardiac decompensation and pulmonary symptoms may also develop secondary to increased viscosity in the systemic and pulmonary vascular beds. Protein-protein interaction with formation of complexes between IgM and coagulation factors (fibrinogen, prothrombin, factors V and VIII, etc.) is an important contributing factor to the bleeding diathesis (particularly epistaxis, oral mucosal bleeding, and purpura) exhibited in many cases. Interference with platelet function (platelet agglutination) and capillary damage secondary to increased serum viscosity are additional factors contributing to bleeding manifestations.

The presymptomatic cases are usually detected initially by the finding of an unexplained elevation of erythrocyte sedimentation rate on routine examination, followed by electrophoretic demonstration of an M-type serum protein and its characterization as IgM by ultracentrifugation or immunoelectrophoresis, or both. The majority of γ-M globulins are euglobulins and give a positive Sia water-dilution reaction, but this is not specific for macroglobulins, since certain IgG globulins are also Sia-positive euglobulins.

Hematologic abnormalities in addition to anemia include an absolute lymphocytosis with "atypical, immature, and plasmacytic" forms that occasionally reach leukemic proportions in macroglobulinemia. Neutropenia, thrombopenia, and eosinophilia are also observed. Bone marrow aspirations characteristically reveal an increase in lymphocytic-plasmacytic forms, accompanied by eosinophils and mast cells in many cases. Some of these patients also have high frequencies of infection and deficiencies of capacity for antibody and other immunoglobulin synthesis. Patients with macroglobulinemia do not in general have nearly as regular or severe an increased susceptibility to infection or immunologic deficit as is observed in patients with myeloma or Hodgkin's disease.

The principal indications for therapy are anemia, bleeding manifestations, and symptoms related to increased plasma viscosity. When the last are severe and threaten central nervous system function and vision, plasmaphoresis is indicated as a temporary measure. Sufficient plasma should be removed to lower viscosity, and the red cells returned. In certain cases, prompt and dramatic improvement in clinical status follows the removal of as little as 500 ml of plasma. Repeated plasmaphoresis for several weeks may be required until effective chemotherapy can be instituted.

Chlorambucil (Leukeran) is the chemotherapeutic agent of choice in macroglobulinemia. As with the chemotherapy of myeloma, continuous drug administration is necessary even during prolonged periods of apparently complete remission. More limited studies with melphalan and cyclophosphamide indicate these to be less effective agents in macroglobulinemia than chlorambucil. Prednisone may be of some value in the control of capillary bleeding.

HEAVY CHAIN DISEASES

IgG heavy chain (Fc fragment) disease is a rare form of plasma cell dyscrasia characterized by a lymphoma-like clinical pattern and the synthesis of excessive quantities of the Fc fragment of the heavy chains of IgG. Of reported cases, a strong male predominance is observed. Clinical features include lymphadenopathy, hepatosplenomegaly, an unusual erythema and edema of the soft palate, weakness, recurrent fevers, and marked susceptibility to bacterial infections. In the first case studied by Franklin and his co-workers a diffuse elevation of serum γ-globulins was documented in the prodromal period preceding the development of the monoclonal type serum pattern. These features, along with the electron microscopic finding of virus-like particles in some of the abnormal lymphocytic-plasmacytic cells in this case, suggest a possible viral etiology. As with other plasma cell dyscrasias, antecedent chronic RES stimulation can be inferred. Anemia, leukopenia, and thrombopenia presumably related to hypersplenism have been prominent features. Eosinophilia is a frequent concomitant. Bone marrow aspirations and lymph node biopsies demonstrate proliferation of plasma cells and lymphocytes. Further, eosinophils and large reticulum or reticuloendothelial cells are abundant.

The characteristic γ-globulin abnormality in IgG heavy chain (Fc fragment) disease is evidenced by the finding in both serum and urine of high concentrations of this specific immunoglobulin fragment. By conventional electrophoresis these proteins appear as homogeneous peaks usually in the fast gamma or beta mobility range. Specific identification is accomplished by immunoelectrophoretic analyses. It is of interest that four of seven of these proteins have been found to be structurally related to the IgG_1 subtype, and three to the IgG_3. The significance of this unexpectedly high frequency of IgG_3 is obscure.

Among 8 cases, considerable variability in the clinical course has occurred. Survival from the time of onset of symptoms ranged from four months to five years. Bacterial pneumonia and sepsis were the immediate cause of death in most cases. Irradiation of the spleen produced temporary remissions with hematologic improvement in 3 cases. Limited trials of cyclophosphamide, melphalan, and steroids yielded little or no benefit. The capacity of these patients to form normal antibodies and the normal immunoglobulins is defective. Appropriate studies of T-cell immunities are not yet available nor are quantitations of the number of normal T-cells and B-cells.

IgA heavy chain (α-chain) disease is the most recently identified plasma cell dyscrasia. This disease was defined by Seligmann and his associates. The clinical pattern in 4 cases was the syndrome previously described as the Mediterranean type of abdominal lymphoma. The predominant features were a diffuse lymphoma-like proliferation in the small intestine and mesentery, chronic diarrhea, and malabsorption unresponsive to gluten withdrawal. Although genetic factors were considered to be of major importance, the disease is not restricted to the Mediterranean population, and possible dietary and environmental factors must be considered.

Chronic diarrhea, malabsorption, and progressive wasting have been the major features of all cases. Biopsies of the small intestine have demonstrated a profound infiltration of the lamina propria by abnormal plasma cells. On electron microscopy these cells show an abundance of endoplasmic reticulum arranged in unusual whorl-like configurations. Intestinal absorption studies of the small intestine show thickened mucosal folds, segmentation, and dilated intestinal loops. Bone marrow aspirations show moderate increases in plasma cells, and skeletal X-ray studies reveal moderate diffuse osteoporosis but no destructive lesions.

The association of IgA heavy chain disease with the small intestine is of special interest, since IgA-producing plasma cells predominate in the lamina propria of the gastrointestinal tract. In a South American case the symptoms of sprue antedated the apparent neoplasia by several years.

However, Seligmann's cases showed an abrupt onset without preceding intestinal disease. Thus although suggested, the role of antecedent infection in the pathogenesis of IgA heavy chain disease cannot yet be defined.

IMMUNODEFICIENCIES IN OTHER CANCERS

In many forms of widely disseminated malignancy severe deficiency of cellular and humoral immunity has been reported. How many of those deficits already described are to be attributed to the malignancy, how many to the etiologic agent or factor, and how many to efforts of surgeons and physicians to treat the cancers still need to be analyzed and defined in precise quantitative terms. Further, as immunotherapy of both specific and nonspecific nature is developed, means for monitoring their influence will need to be available.

At present it is already clear from both clinical and laboratory analysis that immunotherapy will become a part of the method of treatment of some cancers. As a consequence, quantitative analyses of immunodeficiencies in cancer and those consequent to therapeutic efforts are sorely needed and must be developed and provided to guide the hand of the therapist.

SELECTED REFERENCES

Hodgkin's Disease

Aisenberg, A. C. (1964): New Eng. J. Med. 270:508.
Casazza, A. R., Duvall, C. P., and Carbone, P. P. (1966): Cancer Res. 26:1290.
Chawla, P. L., et al. (1970): Amer. J. Med. 48:85.
Cole, P. (1972): JAMA 222:1636.
Good, R. A., and Finstad, J. (1968): In Proceedings, International Conference on Leukemia-Lymphoma, Zarafonetis, C. J. D. (ed.). Philadelphia, Lea & Febiger.
Jackson, H. Jr., and Parker, F. Jr. (1947): Hodgkin's Disease and Allied Disorders. New York, Oxford University Press.
Kaplan, H. S. (1968-69): Harvey Lect. 64:215.
Kelly, W. D., et al. (1960): Ann. N. Y. Acad. Sci. 87:187.
Rubin, P. (1973): JAMA 223:164.

Lymphomas and Leukemias

Beilby, J. O., et al. (1960): Brit. Med. J. 1:96.
Frommel, D., Good, R. A., and Hong, R. (1969): Helv. Paediat. Acta 19:26.
Good, R. A., et al. (1962): Fed. Proc. 21:30.
Green, I., and Corso, P. F. (1959): Blood 14:235.
Gutterman, J. U., et al. (1973): New Eng. J. Med. 288:169.
Larson, D. L., and Tomlinson, L. J. (1953): J. Clin. Invest. 32:317.
Miller, D. G., Lizardo, J. G., and Snyderman, R. K. (1961): J. Nat. Cancer Inst. 26:569.
Opie, E. L. (1910): Arch. Intern. Med. (Chicago) 5:541.
Sbarra, A. J., et al. (1965): Cancer Res. 25:1199.
Sbarra, A. J., et al. (1964): Cancer Res. 24:1958.

Multiple Myeloma

Braun, D. G., and Krause, R. M. (1968): J. Exp. Med. 128:969.
Cone, L., and Uhr, J. W. (1964): J. Clin. Invest. 43:2241
Dunn, T. B. (1957): J. Nat. Cancer Inst. 19:371.
Fink, K., Adams, W. S., and Skoog, W. A. (1971): Amer. J. Med. 50:450.
Kunkel, H. G., Slater, R. J., and Good, R. A. (1951): Proc. Soc. Exp. Biol. Med. 76:190.
Leader, R. W., et al. (1963): Amer. J. Path. 43:33.
Mellors, R. C. (1965): J. Exp. Med. 122:25.
Osterland, C. K., et al. (1966): J. Exp. Med. 123:599.
Porter, D. D., Dixon, F. J., and Larsen, A. E. (1965): Blood 25:736.
Potter, M. (1962): J. Exp. Med. 115:339.
Turin, G. M. (ed). Combined Staff Clinic (1968): Amer. J. Med. 44:256.

Waldenström's Macroglobulinemia

Fessel, W. J. (1962): Acta Med. Scand. 173 (Supp. 391):1
Morel-Maroger, L., et al. (1970): New Eng. J. Med. 283:123.
Seligmann, M., et al. (1967): Amer. J. Med. 43:66.
Waldenström, J. (1970): Diagnosis and Treatment of Multiple Myeloma. New York, Grune & Stratton.
Waldenström, J. (1944): Acta Med. Scand. 117:216.

Heavy Chain Diseases

Franklin, E. C., et al. (1964): Amer. J. Med. 37:332.
Seligmann, M., et al. (1968): Science 162:1396.

Immunodeficiencies in Other Cancers

Augustin, R., and Chandradasa, K. D. (1973): Lancet 1:102.
Carey, R. M., et al. (1973): Amer. J. Med. 54:30.
Johnson, F. L., et al. (1972): Lancet 2:1273.
Meyer, R. D., et al. (1973): Amer. J. Med. 54:6.
Penn, I., and Starzl, E. (1973): JAMA 223:99.
Rosenthal, S. R., et al. (1972): JAMA 222:1543.

Appendix

I. PRACTICAL GUIDE FOR APPROACHING IMMUNOLOGIC PROBLEMS IN CLINICAL PRACTICE

A. Clinical situations in which immunologic studies are helpful and often necessary
   1. Recurrent or unusual infections
   2. Diseases that are related to autoantibodies
   3. Fever of unknown origin
   4. Collagen mesenchymal diseases
   5. Failure to thrive—persistent thrush, persistent diarrhea
   6. Cancer
   7. Organ transplantation
   8. Myeloma, macroglobulinemia, Hodgkin's disease, leukemias
   9. Infectious complication after surgery
   10. Unusual reactions to therapeutics
   11. Unusual reactions to common infection
   12. Neurologic diseases (ataxia, multiple sclerosis, etc.), eczema, purpura, sprue
   13. Diseases of unknown etiology
   14. Apparent allergic diathesis

B. Initial steps for immunologic workup
   1. History and physical examination
   2. Routine clinical laboratory tests that provide useful information:
      a. CBC—hemoglobin, total WBC count, differential count and absolute counts of neutrophils, lymphocytes, and eosinophils
      b. NBT test (See references)
      c. Erythrocyte sedimentation rate
      d. Urinalysis for formed element and protein
      e. Chest x-ray
      f. Isohemagglutinin and red cell type
      g. Bone marrow examination

C. Advanced steps for immunologic workup
   1. Serum electrophoresis and immunoelectrophoresis
   2. Quantitation of serum immunoglobulins: IgG, IgM, IgA, IgE, IgD
   3. Skin test: mumps, PPD, SKSD, Candida, Trychophyton, lepromin, Schick's test, Dick test, PHA, DNCB, and allergens
   4. Serum complement levels
      a. Total hemolytic titer
      b. Quantitation of each component
      c. Opsonization
      d. Quantitation of by-products of complement sytem (C3PA, properdin, inhibitors, and stabilizers)
      e. Consequences of complement action by chemotaxis, immune adherence

5. Evaluation of specific antibody response, e.g., pneumococcus polysaccharides, diphtheria and tetanus toxoids, isoantibodies (Anti-A, Anti-B, etc.), killed polio vaccine
6. Lymphocyte stimulation with PHA, specific antigens, e.g. staphylococcus Esch. coli, and candida and allogeneic cells (MLC test)
7. Macrophage migration inhibition (MIF) test
8. Identification of T- and B-lymphocytes (See Appendix III)
9. Phagocyte function tests
     a. Phagocytes bactericidal test—Maloe's technique
     b. Changes in metabolism of phagocytes during phagocytosis
     c. Rebuck skin window
     d. Chemotactic test of phagocytes
10. Tests for autoantibodies
     a. Coombs' test (direct and indirect)
     b. LE test, antimuscle, antithyroid, antibasement membrane antibodies
     c. Fluorescent antinuclear antibody (FANA) test
     d. Autoantibodies directed against specific tissues or organs or against lymphoid cells
11. Tests of lymphocyte cytotoxicity to cells, tissues, or organs
12. Lymphocyte proliferative responses to cellular, organ, or histocompatibility antigens
13. Lymph node biopsy following antigenic stimulation (use of World Health Organization recommendations for evaluation of lymph node morphology. Bull. WHO 47:375, 1972)

D. Additional procedures frequently used in clinical immunobiology
1. Methyl green pyronine (MGP) staining for plasma cells in tissue
2. Radio immunoassay for antigens, antibodies, and hormones
3. Passive hemagglutinin test
4. Hemadsorption test
5. Prausnitz-Küstner passive transfer
6. Immunofluorescent study of blood, cells, and tissues
7. Skin biopsy for detection of GVH reaction, autoantibodies

REFERENCES

NBT Test as a Diagnositc Aid

Feigin, R. D. (1971): New Eng. J. Med. 285:347.
Matula, G., and Paterson, P. Y. (1971): New Eng. J. Med. 285:311.
Park, B. H. (1971): J. Pediat. 78:376.
Park, B. H., et al. (1972): Lancet 1:1064.
Park, B. H., Fikrig, S. M., and Smithwick, E. M. (1968): Lancet 2:532.

Evaluation of Immune Function

Fudenberg, H., et al. (1971): Pediatrics 47:927.
Good, R. A., and Bergsma, D. (eds.) (1968): Immunodeficiency Diseases in Man. New York, National Foundation Press.

II. USE OF ACTIVE AND PASSIVE IMMUNIZATION

Table II-1. Revised Schedule for Active Immunization and Tuberculin Testing of Normal Infants and Children in the United States

2 months	DTP[1]	TOPV[2]
4 months	DTP	TOPV
6 months	DTP	TOPV
1 year	Measles[3]	Tuberculin test[4]
1–12 years	Rubella[3]	Mumps[3]
1 1/2 years	DTP	TOPV
4–6 years	DTP	TOPV
14–16 years	Td[5]	and thereafter every 10 years

Based on the approval by the Committee on Infectious Diseases, American Academy of Pediatrics, October 17, 1973.

[1]DTP—diphtheria and tetanus toxoid combined with pertussis vaccine.
[2]TOPV—trivalent oral poliovirus vaccine. The above recommendation is suitable for breast-fed as well as bottle-fed infants.
[3]May be given at 1 year as measles-rubella or measles-mumps-rubella combined vaccines.
[4]Frequency of repeated tuberculin tests depends on risk of exposure of the child and on the prevalence of tuberculosis in the population group.
[5]Td—combined tetanus and diphtheria toxoid (adult type) for those over 6 years of age in contrast to diphtheria and tetanus (DT) containing a larger amount of diphtheria antigen.

Tetanus Toxoid at Time of Injury

1. For clean, minor wounds, no booster dose is needed by a fully immunized child unless more than 10 years have elapsed since the last dose.
2. For contaminated wounds, a booster dose should be given if more than 5 years have elapsed since the last dose.

Indications for Rubella Vaccines

1. Unvaccinated school children, particularly girls approaching puberty.
2. Seronegative women of childbearing age who are not pregnant and who are on an acceptable regimen of pregnancy prevention for two months following vaccination. To extend vaccine use to this group, it will be essential to establish additional serologic testing programs.
3. Preschool children, especially those attending kindergarten, day care centers, and other similar groups.

Routine Smallpox Vaccination—No Longer Recommended

1. The risk of smallpox in the United States is now insufficient to justify continuing the routine primary vaccination of infants and children. Smallpox vaccination occasionally results in severe adverse reactions, some fatal.
2. Current state or local regulations and statutes may conflict with the immediate implementation of the new policy. Physicians and health officials should collaborate to facilitate this change.

3. Smallpox vaccination is still recommended for certain individuals:
  a. Medical and hospital personnel should be vaccinated regularly. They are principally at risk if a smallpox epidemic should occur.
  b. Travelers to those few areas where smallpox remains endemic or where vaccination is required must be immunized.
4. All vaccine recipients should be screened carefully for the known contraindications. These precautions can reduce complications to an absolute minimum.

Table II-2.   Clinical Use of Passive Immunization

Diseases	Type of Preparation	Doses	Comments
Measles	Hyperimmune globulin (Human)	0.1 ml/lb IM	As soon as possible after exposure
Infectious hepatitis	Hyperimmune globulin (Human)	Single or short term exposure—IM 0.01–0.02 ml/lb Prolonged or continuous exposure —0.03–0.06 ml/lb IM	As soon as possible after exposure
Rh hemolytic disease	Anti-Rho globulin (Human)	1.0 ml IM	Within 72 hours after delivery
Replacement therapy for congenital agammaglobulinemia	Gamma globulin (16.5%, Human)	1.5 ml/kg (loading dose) 0.6 ml/kg/25–30 days IM	
Pertussis	Hyperimmune globulin (Human)	1.25 ml IM	
Tetanus	Tetanus immune globulin (Human)	3000–6000 U for treatment 250–500 U for prevention IM	As soon as possible after injury
Rubella (1st trimester)	Gamma globulin (Human)	20 ml IM	
Varicella-Zoster in immunodeficiency diseases	Varicella-Zoster immune globulin (Human)	0.1–0.6 ml/lb IM	
Transfusion hepatitis	Gamma globulin (Human)	Up to 10 ml IM	
Mumps	Gamma globulin (Human)	2.5–7.5 ml IM	
Vaccinia	Vaccinia immune globulin (VIG) (Human)	0.3 ml/kg for prophylaxis 0.6 ml/kg for treatment IM	

Table II-3. The Concentrations of IgG, IgM, IgA, and Total Gamma Globulin in the Serum of Normal Persons (Mem ± 1 S. D.)

Age	No. of Subjects	Level of G		Level of M		Level of A		Level of Total Globulin	
		mg/100ml (Range)	% of Adult Level	mg/100ml (Range)	% of Adult Level	mg/100ml (Range)	% of Adult Level	mg/100ml (Range)	% of Adult Level
Newborn	22	1,031±200 (645-1,244)	89±17	11±5 (5-30)	11±5	2±3 (0-11)	1±2	1,044±201 (660-1,439)	67±13
1-3 mo	29	430±119 (272-762)	37±10	30±11 (16-67)	30±11	21±13 (6-56)	11±7	481±127 (324-699)	31±9
4-6 mo	33	427±186 (206-1,125)	37±16	43±17 (10-83)	43±17	28±18 (8-93)	14±9	498±204 (228-1,232)	32±13
7-12 mo	56	661±219 (279-1,533)	58±19	54±23 (22-147)	55±23	37±18 (16-98)	19±9	752±242 (327-1,687)	48±15
13-24 mo	59	762±209 (258-1,393)	66±18	58±23 (14-114)	59±23	50±24 (19-119)	25±12	870±258 (398-1,586)	56±16
25-36 mo	33	892±183 (419-1,274)	77±16	61±19 (28-113)	62±19	71±37 (19-235)	36±19	1,024±205 (499-1,418)	65±14
3-5 yr	28	929±228 (569-1,597)	80±20	56±18 (22-100)	57±18	93±27 (55-152)	47±14	1,078±245 (730-1,771)	69±17
6-8 yr	18	923±256 (599-1,492)	80±22	65±25 (27-118)	66±25	124±45 (54-221)	62±23	1,112±293 (640-1,725)	71±20
9-11 yr	9	1,124±235 (799-1,456)	97±20	79±33 (35-132)	80±33	131±60 (12-208)	66±30	1,334±254 (966-1,639)	85±17
12-16 yr	9	946±124 (726-1,035)	82±11	59±20 (35-72)	60±20	148±63 (70-229)	74±32	1,153±169 (833-1,284)	74±12
Adults	30	1,158±305 (569-1,919)	100±26	99±27 (47-147)	100±27	200±61 (61-330)	100±31	1,457±353 (730-2,365)	100±24

From Stiehm, E. R., and Fudenberg, H. H. (1966): Pediatrics 37:715.

Table II-4. Concentrations of IgE and IgD in the Serum of 132 Healthy Children

Age (Years)	IgE (ng/ml)		IgD (mg/100ml)	
	Arithmetic Mean±S.D. (Range)	Geometric Mean (95% confidence)	Arithmetic Mean±S.D. (Range)	Geometric Mean
2-2.5	137±47 (73-185)	129 (58-286)	—	—
3 (2.5-3.5)	140±58 (64-260)	129 (57-294)	0.95±0.63 (<1-1.93)	0.79
4 (3.5-4.5)	178±93 (62-308)	154 (48-494)	1.14±0.83 (<1-3.17)	0.91
5-6 (4.5-6.5)	209±119 (63-487)	183 (64-523)	1.11±0.67 (<1-2.55)	0.92
7-8 (6.5-8.5)	251±167 (65-535)	199 (46-861)	2.14±1.47 (<1-6.56)	1.71
9-10 (8.5-10.5)	256±158 (69-530)	209 (53-828)	2.78±2.42 (<1-9.11)	1.95
11-12 (10.5-12.5)	239±169 (69-715)	196 (55-703)	2.96±1.65 (<1-6.41)	2.68
13-15 (12.5-15.5)	330±212 (54-840)	268 (69-1040)	3.62±3.71 (<1-20.15)	2.45

From Berg, T., and Johansson, S. G. O. (1969): Acta Pediat. Scand. 58:513.

III. IDENTIFICATION OF T- AND B-LYMPHOCYTES

Extraordinary progress within the past two years has given reliable means of identifying the components of the two cellular immunity systems in man. The recognition and identifications of the cellular components have proceeded so rapidly that they seem certain to be modified considerably in years to come. Nonetheless, the basic approaches will doubtless be the ones to be used and further developed by physicians; thus a brief presentation of these methods of analysis seems appropriate in this volume.

T-Lymphocytes

Table III-1 sets down present concepts of the functions of T-cells and Table III-2 the means by which the functional adequacy of this cellular population can be assessed in man. Perhaps the three most useful means of quantifying the numbers of T-lymphocytes in the circulation include:
1. Capacity of T-lymphocytes to bind at 37° C to sheep red blood cells, thus forming rosettes. This spontaneous, nonimmune rosette formation must not be confused with the rosette formation that also can be produced with sheep red blood cells based on antibody at the surface of B-lymphocytes. The latter reaction occurs in the cold.
   The rosette technique is a method of visualizing receptors on cell surfaces and is based on the following principle: the suspected *receptor-bearing* lymphocytes are mixed with signal cells that carry the corresponding *receptor-binding* substance on the surface. The receptor-binding substance can be a natural substance on the signal cells or can be coupled artificially to signal cells. The re-

ceptor-bearing cells will then bind the signal cells around their surface and form "rosettes."

2. Several antisera specific for T-cells have been prepared. The methods used in their preparation include immunization of rabbits or goats with fetal thymus lymphocytes followed by exhaustive absorption with established human lymphoid cell lines (B-cell line). An alternative method is the immunization of rabbits or goats with peripheral lymphocytes or lymph node lymphocytes from patients with X-linked infantile agammaglobulinemia and later absorption of antisera with human lymphoid cells as above. Such specific anti-T-cell antisera are cytotoxic for T-cells in the presence of complement, thus permitting the identification of T-lymphocytes. The numbers of T-lymphocytes demonstrated in the circulation by these methods can be shown to be 60 to 80 percent in healthy persons. This method can also be adapted to fluorescent microscopic identification of T-lymphocytes.

3. The lymphocytes responding by blast transformation to certain mitogens, e.g., PHA and concanavallin A (Con-A) in solution are largely T-cells. To quantify this response, we have developed a technique that employs direct culture of 50 lambda of peripheral blood, short-term incubation, and relatively short periods of pulse labeling. It has been possible to relate the response obtained to the number of T-lymphocytes in the circulation under most conditions.

Table III-1. Functions and Properties of T-cells

1. Initiate delayed allergic reaction
2. Initiate graft-versus-host reaction
3. Respond with blast transformation to PHA or allogeneic cells in vitro
4. Participate in killer function against tumor cells
5. Participate in solid tissue allograft rejection
6. Contribute a major specific component in one of the bulwarks of bodily defense against certain viruses, fungi, and facultative intracellular bacterial pathogens
7. Participate in immunosurveillance against cancer

Table III-2. Tests for Adequacy of T-cell Function

1. Quantitative response of cells in whole blood to PHA—in vitro transformation
2. Dose response analysis of PHA responsiveness in vitro
3. In vitro response of lymphocytes to allogeneic lymphocytes
4. Development of delayed allergy to ubiquitous antigens: SK-SD, mumps, Candida, trichophyton, PPD
5. Development of contact allergy to 2-4 dinitrochlorobenzene
6. Count of small lymphocytes
7. Capacity to reject allograft of skin
8. Presence of an abundant cell population in deep cortical areas of lymph nodes following antigenic stimulation
9. Vigorous defense against fungi, virus, and facultative intracellular bacterial pathogens
10. Enumeration of nonimmune rosettes with sheep red blood cells

B-Lymphocytes

B-lymphocyte functions are recorded in Table III-3, and methods of quantifying B-cell functions in Table III-4. Three new methods for quantifying and identifying B-lymphocytes have been developed and are coming into general use.

1. Based on the surface immunoglobulins of lymphocytes, the first of these methods depends on fluorescent staining of surface immunoglobulin on B-lymphocytes by a technique developed by Pernis et al. Thus the percentage and absolute numbers of lymphocytes having IgM, IgG, IgA, IgD, and IgE immunoglobulins at their surface can be quantified.

2. With a second method based on Fc receptors on B-lymphocytes, specific binding of aggregated gamma globulins to B-lymphocytes was demonstrated by Dickler and Kunkel. The binding was shown to be irreversible and independent of complement, pH, and temperature. The protein content of the medium and the divalent cations and the site on the B-lymphocyte membrane responsible for binding aggregates might be distinct from those of surface immunoglobulins. The Fc receptor described by Basten and associates is probably responsible for the binding of the aggregated gamma globulins.

3. Applying a technique based on the receptor for antigen-antibody complement complexes, Nussenzweig and his colleagues demonstrated a population of lymphoid cells in many mammalian species, including man, which is capable of binding anti-antibody-complement (EAC) complexes. These lymphocytes can be readily identified and isolated by virtue of their ability to form rosettes with sheep erythrocytes (C) which have been sensitized with rabbit antibody (A) against the Forssman antigen and complement (C). These cells bind immune complexes through a membrane receptor for C3.

Each of these techniques permits identification and quantification of B-lymphocytes. In healthy persons the number of cells identified by each is in good agreement with the number obtained with each of the other techniques. Further, the median percentage of B-lymphocytes by each method is approximately 20 percent. This figure agrees with the 65 to 85 percent figure for T-lymphocytes obtained by the T-cell rosette techniques. In disease, however, the number of B-cells quantified by the several criteria may differ, and the number of T-cells and the number of B-cells may not add up to approximately 100 percent as is the case in health.

Each of these approaches, of course, provides new methodology that should make possible much clarification of primary and secondary immunodeficiencies and understanding of the development and involution of the lymphoid system.

T- and B-lymphocytes seem also to be distinguishable morphologically from one another using scanning electromicroscopy coupled with cutical point dying. The T-lymphocytes under these conditions are generally free of cytoplasmic surface projection while the B-lymphocytes possess an extensively filamented surface.

Table III-3.　Major Function of B-cells

1. Produce surface immunoglobulin made up of specific antibodies in receptor distribution
2. Secrete immunoglobulins and antibodies
3. Provide primary defense against high grade encapsulated bacterial pathogens and certain virus infections
4. Detoxify proteins, polysaccharides, and other toxins
5. Prevent recurrence of virus and certain bacterial infections

Table III-4.   Tests to Evaluate B-cell Function

1. Quantification of levels of all major classes of immunoglobulins by radial immunodiffusion or radioimmunoassay
2. Evaluation of fractional catabolic rate and/or synthesis rates for individual immunoglobulins
3. Concentration of antibody to antigens widely distributed in nature, e.g., isoagglutinins, antistreptolysin-O, Schick test, antiviral antibody
4. Quantification of antibody response to killed polio virus vaccine
5. Quantification of antibody response to diphtheria and tetanus toxoids
6. Antibody responses to polysaccharide antigens from pneumococcal, meningococcal, and Hemophilus
7. Concentrations of IgA and analysis of amount and form of IgA in saliva
8. Quantification of immunoglobulin subclasses
9. Specific identification of bacteria causing frequent pneumonia, sepsis, conjunctivitis and meningitis (The organisms that particularly plague patients with B-cell defects include pneumococci, streptococci, Hemophilus influenzae, meningococci, and Pseudomonas aeruginosa.)
10. Quantification of numbers of B-lymphocytes in blood by immunofluorescent detection of surface immunoglobulins, Fc receptors for IgG, or C3 receptor rosettes
11. Quantification of number of immunoglobulin-synthesizing cells by immunofluorescent staining of cytoplasmic immunoglobulin

REFERENCES

T-Cells

Bach, J. F., et al. (1969): Transplantation 8:265.
Brain, P., Gordon, J., and Willetts, W. A. (1970): Clin. Exp. Immun. 6:681.
Coombs, R. R. A., et al. (1970): Int. Arch. Allerg. Appl. Immun. 39:658.
Froland, S. S., and Natvig, J. B. (1972): J. Exp. Med. 136:409.
Jondal, M., Holm, G., and Wigzell, W. (1972): J. Exp. Med. 136:207.
Lay, W. H., et al. (1971): Nature (London) 230:531.
Papamichaeil, M., et al. (1972): Lancet 2:64.
Park, B. H., and Good, R. A. (1972): Proc. Nat. Acad. Sci., U.S.A. 69:371.
Silveira, N. P. A., Mendes, N. F., Tolnai, M. E. A. J. (1972): J. Immun. 108:1456.
Wybran, J., Carr, M. C., and Fudenberg, H. H. (1972): J. Clin. Invest. 51:2537.
Wybran, J., Chantler, S., and Fudenberg, H. H. (1973): Lancet 1:126.

B-Cells

Aisenberg, A. C., and Bloch, K. J. (1972): New Eng. J. Med. 287:272.
Basten, A., et al. (1972): J. Exp. Med. 135:160.
Basten, A., Warner, N. L., and Mendel, T. (1972): J. Exp. Med. 135:627.
Cooper, M. D., Lawton, A. R., and Bookman, D. E. (1972): Lancet 2:791.
Dickler, H. B., and Kunkel, H. G. (1972): J. Exp. Med. 136:191.
Nussenzweig, J., et al. (1971): In Progress in Immunology, Amos, B. (ed.). New York, Academic Press, p. 73.
Pernis, B., Forni, L., and Amante, L. (1970): J. Exp. Med. 132:1001.
Rabellino, E., et al. (1971): J. Exp. Med. 133:156.
Unanue, E. R., et al. (1971): J. Exp. Med. 133:1188.
Wilson, J. D., and Nossal, G. J. V. (1971): Lancet 1:788.
Gajl-Peczalska, et al. (1973): Fed. Proc. 32:1027.

Index

Page numbers in *italics* refer to illustrations; page numbers followed by t refer to tables.